Global Bariatric Surgery

Rami Lutfi · Mariano Palermo
Guy-Bernard Cadière
Editors

Global Bariatric Surgery

The Art of Weight Loss Across the Borders

Springer

Editors
Rami Lutfi
University of Illinois at Chicago
Chicago, IL
USA

Mariano Palermo
University of Buenos Aires
Buenos Aires
Argentina

Guy-Bernard Cadière
Saint-Pierre University Hospital
European School of Laparoscopic
Surgery
Brussels
Belgium

ISBN 978-3-030-06681-9 ISBN 978-3-319-93545-4 (eBook)
https://doi.org/10.1007/978-3-319-93545-4

This Springer imprint is published by the registered company Springer Nature Switzerland AG
The registered company address is: Gewerbestrasse 11, 6330 Cham, Switzerland

To Suhayla, Samira, Edward, Maria, and George, for making me who I am

To Aida, for being the strong base for everything that matters

To Lea, Talia, Doreah, and Isabella, for carrying the torch forward

And to every person struggling with severe obesity, for making my job worthy

— Rami Lutfi

The Editors would like to dedicate this book to the memory of Dr. Eduardo Jacob who passed before seeing his work and contribution.

Dr. Jacob was a great surgeon and teacher. It is on shoulders like his that the mission of advancing surgical science and technology is carried on.

On behalf of our patients and readers, we thank you Edu for your contribution in this book and in the world of surgery.

— The Editors

Foreword

For "Global Bariatric Surgery: The Art of Weight Loss Across the Borders"

As I write these lines, prevalence of obesity in the world is even higher, complex, and uncontrollable, as if a virus had infected the planet, like a communicable process displayed on color maps from the CDC (Centers for Disease Control and Prevention). The life expectancy of many countries, with a few demonstrating a decline, is now threatening and is probably associated, like tobacco, with an upsurge in cancer incidence. Yet, prevention would be the least expensive urgent proposition to counteract this wave, but the aftereffects of such community health changes would be reflected 25 years later, and for those who are affected now, only surgery urgently has the answers, and it is offered to 0.5–1% of patients in Western countries, even lower in others!

It has been 25 years since the first laparoscopic bariatric surgery by Guy-Bernard Cadière, and it is very "a propos" that my friends and editors Rami Lutfi, Mariano Palermo, and Guy-Bernard Cadière have congregated a marvelous book and masterpiece on this subject. In "Global Bariatric Surgery: The Art of Weight Loss Across the Borders," international experts' experience have been assembled and gathered to write the most up-to-date information on bariatric and metabolic surgery with all its known facets. This surgical topic has provided growth to the fastest surgical societies in severe countries and worldwide and has pushed the boundaries on hormonal research in the causation of type-2 diabetes and GI incretins. The comprehensive varying opinions on the management of sleeve gastrectomy, weight regain, gastric bypass, and complex revisions are unique to this time. Not only are differing surgical perspectives presented, but physicians, endoscopists, and researchers also describe alternative methods of management, in complications, future treatments, and understanding of the disease.

Aspiring to be wide-ranging, the content includes developments as well as basic standardized techniques, likely occurring complications, described to help practicians avoid dangerous pitfalls. The editors have, for example, included such topics as the relationship between obesity and cancer, the use of surgery in adolescents, preparation and follow-up care, as well as the use of interventional radiology. The latest scientific evidence concerning endoscopy, radiology, robotics, and pharmaceuticals is presented in detail.

Thus, this reference work methodically covers the technique and results of laparoscopic bariatric and metabolic surgery, with an international participation, as obesity and type-2 diabetes are affecting various parts of the world differently, and one with great interest, watches the various approaches taken, and compares them. In letters written by Seneca (64 AC), it is said that reading in the sustenance of a good mind, and will-fortified opinions, and this detailed, authoritative work should do the same to the novice and advanced Bariatric surgeon.

Montreal, Quebec, Canada
April 2018

Michel Gagner

Acknowledgments

I would like to dedicate this book to my wife Gabriela, my two children Agustina and Lucas, my parents Mario and Loly, and also my dear grandmother Lucila, for supporting me to go on progressing in my personal life and also in the field of laparoscopic and bariatric surgery.

Also I am very thankful to all my professors especially those that inspired me to be a better surgeon day by day in the clinical field, teaching, and research and for teaching me the lovely art of surgery.

Mariano Palermo

"When I was a young surgeon, the number one surgical principle was 'big surgeon, big incision.' Now the minimal invasive surgery has become the gold standard. However, this surgery is difficult and needs a good knowledge of anatomy and operative strategy. I hope this book allows the surgeon to have a better understanding of the principles of laparoscopic surgery. Thank you to Dr. Mariano Palermo and Dr. Rami Lutfi for working so hard on this book."

Best regards
Guy-Bernard Cadière

Contents

Contributors

Marianela Aguirre Ackermann, MD Obesity and Diabetes Department, Centro CIEN - Endocrinology, Obesity and Nutrition Center, Corrientes, Buenos Aires, Misiones, Formosa, Argentina

Pablo Acquafresca, MD Department of Surgery, DAICIM Foundation, Buenos Aires, Argentina

Ahmed R. Ahmed, MD, FRCS Department of Bariatric Surgery, St Mary's Hospital, Imperial College London, London, UK

Talat Sh. Al Shaban, MBBS, FRCSI Department of General Surgery, Sheikh Khalifa Medical City, Abu Dhabi, UAE

Ramzi S. Alami, MD, FACS, FASMBS Department of Surgery, American University of Beirut Medical Center, Beirut, Lebanon

Luciano Antozzi, MD Department of Bariatric and Esophago-Gastric Surgery, Hospital Italiano Regional del Sur, Buenos Aires, Argentina

Mario Norberto Antozzi, MD Department of General and Bariatric Surgery, Centro de Cirugías Especiales, Buenos Aires, Argentina

Priscilla Antozzi, MD Department of General and Bariatric Surgery, Centro de Cirugías Especiales, Buenos Aires, Argentina

Kelly Aspinwall EnteroMedics, Roseville, MN, USA

Dan E. Azagury, MD Department of Surgery, Stamford Hospital, Stanford, CA, USA

Ramsen Azizi, MD R.A.M. Plastic Surgery, Chicago, IL, USA

Omar Ezequiel Bellorin-Marin, MD Department of Surgery, New York Presbyterian Hospital, New York, NY, USA

Andrew C. Berry, DO Department of Medicine, University of South Alabama Medical Center, Mobile, AL, USA

Aparna Govil Bhasker, MBBS, MS Bariatric Surgeon, Global and Apollo Hospitals, Mumbai, Maharashtra, India

Laurent Biertho, MD Department of Bariatric and General Surgery, Institut Universitaire de Cardiologie et Pneumologie de Québec – Université Laval, Quebec, QC, Canada

Sébastien Blaye-Felice, MD Department of Bariatric and General Surgery, Institut Universitaire de Cardiologie et Pneumologie de Québec – Université Laval, Quebec, QC, Canada

Katherine S. Blevins, MD, PhD Department of Surgery, Stanford University School of Medicine, Stanford, CA, USA

Camilo Boza, MD Department of Digestive Surgery, Clinica Las Condes, Santiago, Chile

Josemberg Campos, MD, PhD Department of Surgery, Federal University of Pernambuco (UFPE), Recife, PE, Brazil

Anthony Choi, MD Division of Gastroenterology and Hepatology, New York Presbyterian-Weill Cornell Medical Center, New York, NY, USA

Jaclyn Clark, MD Department of Surgery, New York University Langone Medical Center, New York, NY, USA

Austin Cottam, MD Bariatric Research, Bariatric Medicine Institute, Salt Lake City, UT, USA

Daniel Cottam, MD Bariatric Research, Bariatric Medicine Institute, Salt Lake City, UT, USA

John Cole Cowling, MD Department of Surgery, UT Health McGovern Medical School, Houston, TX, USA

Giuseppe D'Amico, MD Department of Surgery, University of Illinois at Chicago, Chicago, IL, USA

Federico Davrieux, MD Minimally Invasive Surgery, Fundacion DAICIM, Rosario, Argentina

Cinthia Barbosa de Andrade Department of Surgery, Federal University of Pernambuco (UFPE), Recife, PE, Brazil

Luiz Gustavo de Quadros, MD Department of Surgery, ABC Medical School, Sao Jose Do Rio Preto, SP, Brazil

Maíra Danielle Gomes de Souza, MD Department of Surgery, University Federal of Pernambuco, Recife, PE, Brazil

Joseph Mark Drosdeck, MD, MS General Surgery, The Everett Clinic, Everett, WA, USA

Wayne J. English, MD, FACS Department of Surgical Sciences, Vanderbilt University Medical Center, Nashville, TN, USA

Yaniv Fenig, MD Monmouth Medical Center, Long Branch, NJ, USA

Flávio Coelho Ferreira, MSc Department of Surgery, Federal University of Pernambuco (UFPE), Recife, PE, Brazil

Christine Ren Fielding, MD Department of Surgery, NYU School of Medicine, New York, NY, USA

George Fielding, MD Department of Surgery, NYU School of Medicine, New York, NY, USA

Ricardo Flores, MD Department of Digestive Surgery, Clinica Las Condes, Santiago, Chile

Teresa R. Fraker, MS, RN Metabolic and Bariatric Surgery Accreditation and Quality Improvement Program (MBSAQIP), American College of Surgeons, Chicago, IL, USA

Ricardo Funke, MD Department of Digestive Surgery, Clinica Las Condes, Santiago, Chile

Mariano Gimenez, MD, PhD Department of Surgery, DAICIM Foundation, Buenos Aires, Argentina

Andres Giovannetti, MD Department of Surgery, Mercy Hospital Medical Center, Chicago, IL, USA

Alexandra H. Leon Guerrero, MD Department of Surgery, New York University Langone Medical Center, New York, NY, USA

Kelvin D. Higa, MD Minimally Invasive and Bariatric Surgery, Fresno Heart and Surgical Hospital, Fresno, CA, USA

Carlos Eduardo Jacob, MD, PhD, FACS Division of Gastrointestinal Surgery and Coloproctology – Hospital das Clínicas, University of Sao Paulo School of Medicine, Sao Paulo, Brazil

Mandi Joshi, MD Department of Surgery, DaVita Medical Group, Albuquerque, NM, USA

François Julien, MD Department of Bariatric and General Surgery, Institut Universitaire de Cardiologie et Pneumologie de Québec – Université Laval, Quebec, QC, Canada

Kara J. Kallies, MS Department of Medical Research, Gundersen Medical Foundation, La Crosse, WI, USA

Aarthy Kannappan, MD Department of Surgery, Loma Linda University, Loma Linda, CA, USA

Paul R. Kemmeter, MD, FACS Department of Surgery, Grand Health Partners, Mercy Health Saint Mary's, Grand Rapids, MI, USA

Keith C. Kim, MD Center for Metabolic and Obesity Surgery, Florida Hospital Celebration Health, Celebration, FL, USA

Mark Knudson, PhD EnteroMedics, Roseville, MN, USA

Shanu N. Kothari, MD Department of General Surgery, Gundersen Health System, La Crosse, WI, USA

Eric J. Krebill, MD Department of Surgery, Grand Health Partners; North Ottawa Community Health System, Grand Rapids, MI, USA

David M. Krpata, MD Digestive Disease and Surgery Institute, Cleveland Clinic Foundation, Cleveland, OH, USA

Sachin Kukreja, MD, FACS, FASMBS Minimally Invasive Surgical Associates, Dallas, TX, USA

Marina S. Kurian, MD, FACS, FASMBS Department of Surgery, New York Minimally Invasive Surgery, PLLC, New York, NY, USA

Muffazal Lakdawala, MBBS, MS Department of Bariatric Surgery and Lap Oncosurgery, Saifee Hospital, Mumbai, Maharashtra, India

Stéfane Lebel, MD Department of Bariatric and General Surgery, Institut Universitaire de Cardiologie et Pneumologie de Québec – Université Laval, Quebec, QC, Canada

Aaron Lee, DO Department of General Surgery, Cleveland Clinic Florida – Weston, Weston, FL, USA

Rami Lutfi University of Illinois at Chicago, Chicago, IL, USA

Simon Marceau, MD Department of Bariatric and General Surgery, Institut Universitaire de Cardiologie et Pneumologie de Québec – Université Laval, Quebec, QC, Canada

Samer G. Mattar, MD, FACS, FRCS, FASMBS Swedish Weight Loss Services, Swedish Medical Center, Seattle, WA, USA

Ronald Matteotti, MD The HOPE Tower at Jersey Shore University Medical Center, Neptune, NJ, USA

Epatobiliary and Pancreatic Program Meridian Cancer Care, Neptune, NJ, USA

Hepatobiliary and Pancreatic Surgery JSUMC, Neptune, NJ, USA

Emma Rose McGlone, MBBS, MA(Cantab), MRCS, PGCertEd Department of Endocrinology and Investigative Medicine, Imperial College London, London, UK

Emanuele Lo Menzo, MD, PhD, FACS, FASMBS The Bariatric and Metabolic Institute, Cleveland Clinic Florida – Weston, Weston, FL, USA

Marc Michalsky, MD Department of Pediatric Surgery, Nationwide Children's Hospital, Columbus, OH, USA

Tripurari Mishra, MD Department of Surgery, Advocate Illinois Masonic Medical Center, Chicago, IL, USA

John Magaña Morton, MD, MPH Department of Surgery, Stamford Hospital, Stanford, CA, USA

Blake R. Movitz, MD General Surgery, University of Illinois at Chicago – Metropolitan Group Hospitals, Chicago, IL, USA

Fernando Muñoz, MD Department of Digestive Surgery, Clinica Las Condes, Santiago, Chile

Samer A. Naffouje, MD Department of General Surgery, University of Illinois Hospital and Health Sciences System, Chicago, IL, USA

Marius Nedelcu, MD Centre Chirurgical de l'Obesite, Clinique Saint Michel, Toulon, VAR, France

Manoel Galvao Neto, MD Department of Surgery, Herbert Wertheim College of Medicine - Florida International University, Doral, FL, USA

Abdelrahman Ali Nimeri, MBBCh, FACS, FASMBS Department of Surgery, IFSO Middle East North African, Pan Arab Society for Metabolic and Bariatric Surgery, Sheik Khalifa Medical City, Abu Dhabi, UAE

Patrick Noel, MD, FACS, IFASMBS Bariatric Department, Emirates Specialty Hospital, Dubai, UAE

Samuel Ordoñez Ortega, MD Division of Endocrine and Laparoscopic Surgery, Instituto Nacional de Ciencias Médicas y Nutrición, Mexico City, Mexico

Mariano Palermo, MD, PhD, FACS Department of Bariatric Surgery, Centro Cien-Diagnomed, Buenos Aires, Argentina

Department of Surgery, DAICIM Foundation, Buenos Aires, Argentina

Juan Pablo Pantoja, MD, FACS Division of Endocrine and Laparoscopic Surgery, Instituto Nacional de Ciencias Médicas y Nutrición, Mexico City, Mexico

Isaac C. Payne, DO Department of Surgery, University of South Alabama Medical Center, Mobile, AL, USA

Alfons Pomp, MD FRCSC, FACS, FASMBS Department of Surgery, New York Presbyterian Hospital, New York, NY, USA

Weill Cornell Medicine, New York, NY, USA

Jaime Ponce, MD, FACS, FASMBS CHI Memorial Hospital, Chattanooga, TN, USA

William O. Richards, MD, FACS Department of Surgery, University of South Alabama Medical Center, Mobile, AL, USA

Amy Robinson-Gerace American College of Surgeons, Division of Research and Optimal Patient Care, Chicago, IL, USA

Michael J. Rosen, MD, FACS Digestive Disease and Surgery Institute, Cleveland Clinic Foundation, Cleveland, OH, USA

Raul J. Rosenthal, MD, FACS, FASMBS Department of Surgery, Cleveland Clinic Florida, Weston, FL, USA

Adriana Ruano, MD Department of Surgery, Clinico San Carlos, Madrid, Spain

Eduardo Valdivieso Rueda, MD, PhD Gastrointestinal and Endoscopic Surgery, International Digestive Diseases Center/FOSCAL, Universidad Autónoma de Bucaramanga, La Sabana University, Bogotá, Colombia

Arsalan Salamat, MD General Surgery, Presence Health St. Joseph Hospital, Chicago, IL, USA

George I. Salti, MD Department of Surgery, Division of Surgical Oncology, University Of Illinois at Chicago, Chicago, IL, USA

Cristina Sánchez-del-Pueblo, MD Department of Surgery, Clinico San Carlos, Madrid, Spain

Andrés Sánchez-Pernaute, MD, PhD Department of Surgery, Clinico San Carlos, Madrid, Spain

Bradley F. Schwack, MD, FACS Department of Surgery, New York University School of Medicine – NYU Langone Medical Center, New York, NY, USA

Edgardo Serra, MD Bariatric Surgery, Centro CIEN, Corrientes, Argentina

Shinil K. Shah, DO Department of Surgery, UT Health McGovern Medical School, Houston, TX, USA

Reem Sharaiha, MD Division of Gastroenterology and Hepatology, New York Presbyterian-Weill Cornell Medical Center, New York, NY, USA

Scott A. Shikora, MD Department of Surgery, Brigham and Women's Hospital, Boston, MA, USA

Mauricio Sierra, MD, FACS Division of Endocrine and Laparoscopic Surgery, Instituto Nacional de Ciencias Médicas y Nutrición, Mexico City, Mexico

Lyz Bezerra Silva, MD, MS Department of Surgery, Federal University of Pernambuco, Recife, PE, Brazil

Amit Surve, MD Bariatric Research, Bariatric Medicine Institute, Salt Lake City, UT, USA

Samuel Szomstein, MD The Bariatric and Metabolic Institute, Cleveland Clinic Florida – Weston, Weston, FL, USA

Luciano G. Tastaldi, MD Digestive Disease and Surgery Institute, Cleveland Clinic Foundation, Cleveland, OH, USA

Alfonso Torquati, MD, MSCI, FACS Department of Surgery, Rush University Medical Center, Chicago, IL, USA

Weill Cornell Medicine, New York, NY, USA

Antonio Torres, MD, PhD Department of Surgery, Clinico San Carlos, Madrid, Spain

Milton Ignacio Carvalho Tube, MD Department of Surgery, University Federal of Pernambuco, Recife, PE, Brazil

Kiara Tulla, MD Department of Surgery, University of Illinois at Chicago, Chicago, IL, USA

Katherine Tweden, PhD EnteroMedics, Roseville, MN, USA

Ivo Tzvetanov, MD Department of Surgery, University of Illinois at Chicago, Chicago, IL, USA

Aaron Lee Wiegmann, MD Department of Surgery, Rush University Medical Center, Chicago, IL, USA

Erik B. Wilson, MD Department of Surgery, UT Health McGovern Medical School, Houston, TX, USA

Alan C. Wittgrove, MD Wittgrove Bariatric Center, Del Mar, CA, USA

Kai Tai Derek Yeung, MRCS, BMBS, BMedSci Department of Bariatric Surgery, St Mary's Hospital, London, UK

Hinali Zaveri, MD Bariatric Research, Bariatric Medicine Institute, Salt Lake City, UT, USA

Natan Zundel, MD, FACS, FASMBS General Surgery, FIU Herbert Wertheim College of Medicine, North Miami Beach, FL, USA

Part I

History and Present

History of Bariatric Surgery

1

Mariano Palermo, Tripurari Mishra, and Rami Lutfi

From a symbol of beauty and wealth to a burden of negative stigma, the perception of overweight and obesity has transformed over the years up to our current times, when it is recognized as a chronic disease.

But despite all evidence, obesity continues to be considered by many, even in health care, a choice rather than a disease.

Its complex nature, the lack of understanding, and the significant role of behavioral factors justified, for many, discrimination and negative opinion about obesity and its treatment modalities.

While many believe it to be a product of civilization, obesity dates back as early as our genesis. It was, however, the exception due to its rarity, as opposed to the growing epidemic we see at our recent times where at least one in three Americans is overweight.

Due to its rarity, obesity was once perceived as a sign of beauty, well-being, or wealth. Venus of Hohle Fels, found in Germany, is an obese female figurine [1] that dates back to 35,000 BC (Fig. 1.1), and according to the *New York Times*, Hatshepsut's mummy is that of an obese, diabetic 50-year-old woman [2].

The prevalence of obesity remained constantly low until last century when science and technology allowed us to have machines and tools to help alleviate most physical work and shifting most jobs from a physical to intellectual ones.

That technology came also into our homes where we stopped getting up to change the TV channel and our kids mastered sports digitally without going in the field and running. As a result, obesity has rapidly uptrended even in our kids, who, in the USA, are expected to be the first generation that would not outlive their parents.

With the alarming growth of the complex problem came the need for better understanding and search for potential solutions. The concept of body mass index was created, and soon this was tied to morbidity and earlier mortality. Because of the alarming data, an official call was made in 2001 by the US Surgeon General for action to prevent and treat obesity [3]. Surgeons were always at the front line of that battle starting in the midst of last century, designing different operations to make weight loss meaningful and long lasting.

Between restricting food intake for earlier satiety and redirecting ingested food to decrease absorption, the operations have shifted back and forth with many combining both mechanisms. Interestingly, the concept for bariatric surgery (in restriction and malabsorption) was initially

M. Palermo
Department of Bariatric Surgery, Centro Cien-Diagnomed, Buenos Aires, Argentina

Department of Surgery, DAICIM Foundation, Buenos Aires, Argentina

T. Mishra
Department of Surgery, Advocate Illinois Masonic Medical Center, Chicago, IL, USA
e-mail: Tripurari.mishra@advocatehealth.com

R. Lutfi (✉)
University of Illinois at Chicago, Chicago, IL, USA

R. Lutfi et al. (eds.), *Global Bariatric Surgery*, https://doi.org/10.1007/978-3-319-93545-4_1

Fig. 1.1 Venus of Hohle Fels, found in Germany, is an obese female figurine that dates back to 35,000 BC. Conard [1]. doi:https://doi.org/10.1038/nature07995

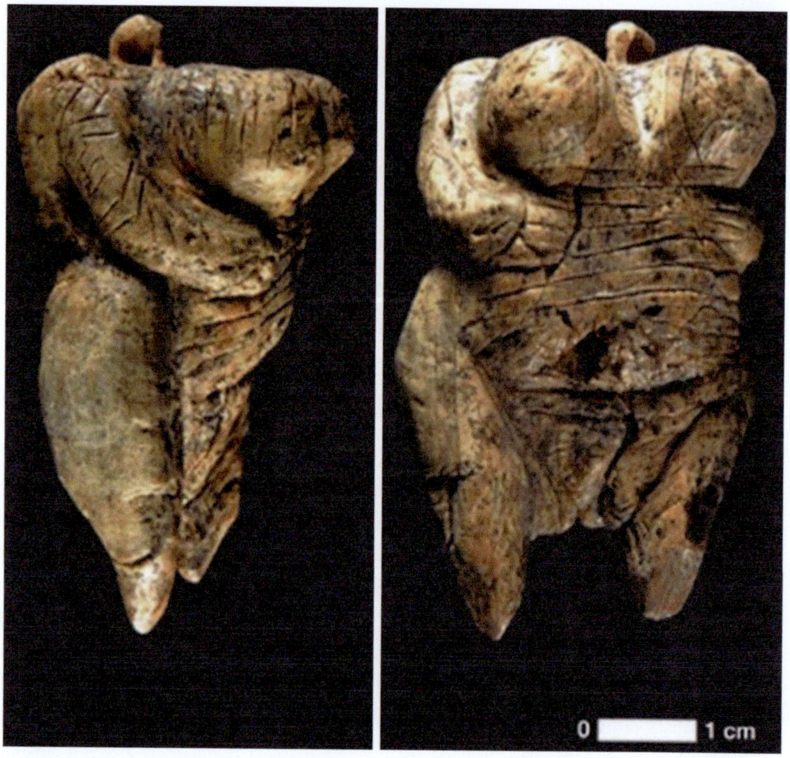

developed from the unintended consequence of weight loss after gastrointestinal surgery for ulcer and cancer. Removing large parts of stomachs or intestine caused severe postoperative weight loss, which some surgeons recognized to be advantageous in the morbidly obese patients.

It all started in the 1950s, when Linnear performed the earliest purely malabsorptive procedure for weight loss by creating a jejunoileal bypass and functionally removing varying lengths of small bowel. This procedure evolved into two variants based on the choice of the enteroenterostomy, while the common channel remained always the same length at 35 cm.

The classic jejunoileal bypass was described by Payne and Dewind in 1969 [5] with end-to-side jejunoileostomy (Fig. 1.2). This was designed as a less malabsorptive operation than their original 1963 jejuno-transverse colostomy bypass (Fig. 1.3). In that operation, they bypassed a much longer segment of intestine hoping for better weight loss. They reported on ten patients [6] but soon realized the severe electrolyte abnormalities and dehydration from uncontrolled diarrhea necessitating revision to their classic jejunoileal bypass.

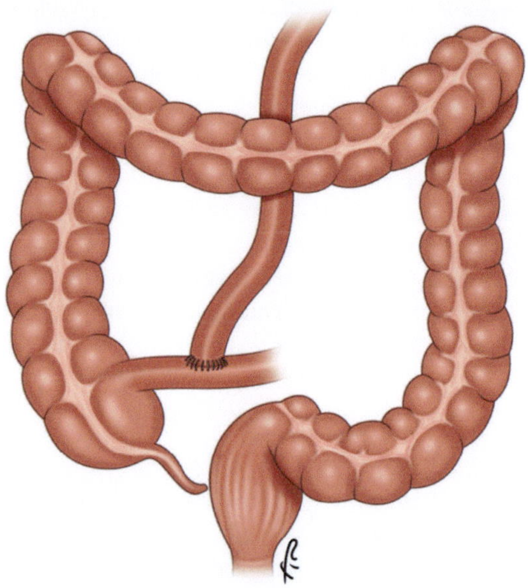

Fig. 1.2 Classic JIB by Payne and Dewind (end-to-side anastomosis)

In 1973 JIB was modified by Scott and Dean [7] to an end-to-end anastomosis reconstruction with drainage ileosigmoidostomy (Fig. 1.4).

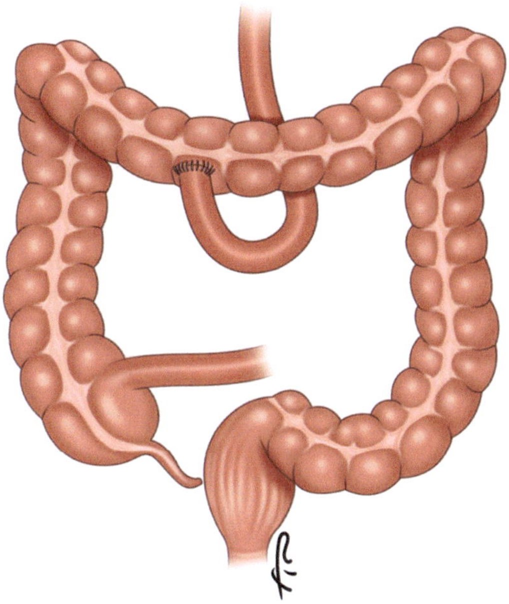

Fig. 1.3 Jejuno-transverse colostomy bypass by Payne and DeWind

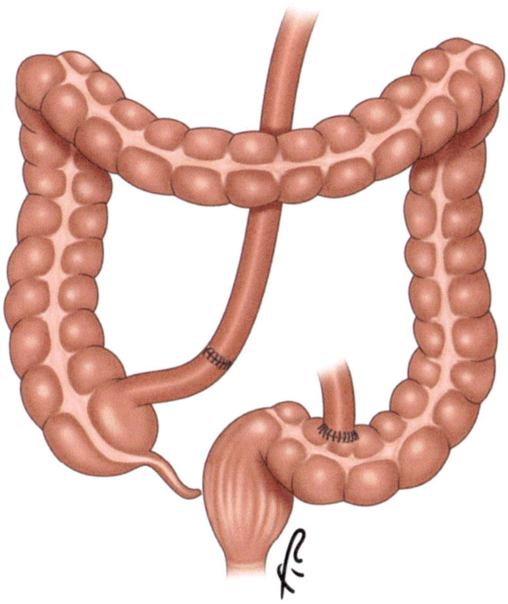

Fig. 1.4 Modified JIB by Scott and Dean with end-to-end anastomosis

Soon after adopting these malabsorptive operations, it became apparent that there is a high price for the significant postoperative weight loss. Many, previously rare, short- and long-term complications were starting to be well described as these operations became more common. Most technical ones were related to the long defunctionalized limb of intestine (in end-to-side technique), where the lack of flow led to bacterial overgrowth which, in many instances, was toxic and life threatening. In addition, liquid contents refluxed in antiperistaltic direction and got gradually absorbed causing in many patients weight regain and long-term failures [8]. Aggressive, significant malabsorption, while thought to be critical for durable significant weight loss, proved to be often morbid and potentially lethal, leading surgeons to eventually abandon these operations.

Bypassing the segment for bile acid resorption reduced the absorption of fat and fat soluble vitamins (A, D, E, and K) leading to deficiencies that were not described before that era. Uncommon condition became common such as osteoporosis-associated pathological fractures due to vitamin D deficiency and night blindness due to vitamin A deficiency. Furthermore, gallstones were very common due to the loss of bile salts. Lastly, the increased exposure of colonic mucosa to these bile salts caused voluminous secretions of water and electrolytes causing severe cramping and diarrhea resulting in wide array of adverse outcome ranging from poor quality of life to life-threatening dehydration.

Alongside the work on malabsorption, the concept of restriction and portion control carried much enthusiasm as complications from the malabsorptive operations were increasingly reported. Horizontal gastroplasty was the first restrictive procedure to be described (Fig. 1.4), in which around 30 cc of fundus is partitioned from the remaining stomach below using a single row of staples. Continuity is reestablished by creating a narrow outlet removing three or less staples and reconnecting the two compartments (Fig. 1.5). Food passes slowly causing prolonged premature stretching of the fundus and therefore early prolonged satiety [9].

Avoiding small bowel bypass with its negative consequences of severe malabsorption, along with the technical simplicity and safety of this operation, made restriction a very appealing

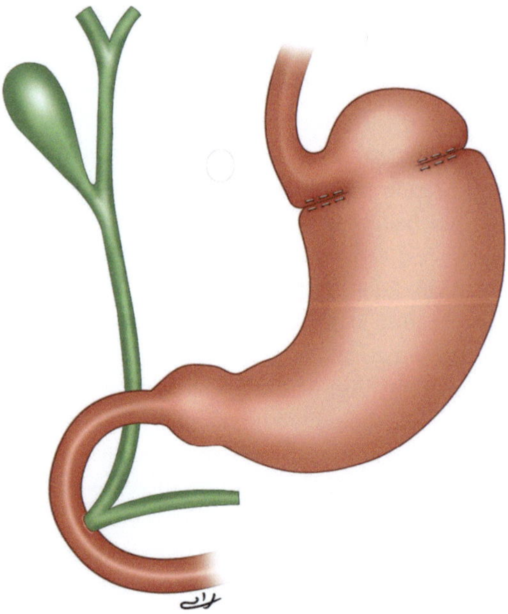

Fig. 1.5 Horizontal gastroplasty

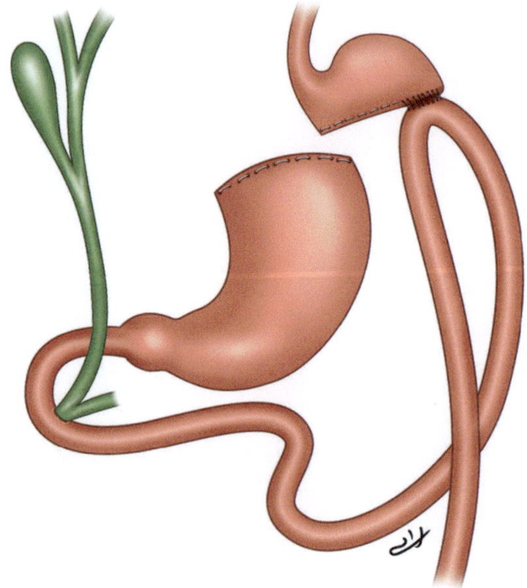

Fig. 1.6 Gastric bypass as described by Dr. Mason

concept. Unfortunately, like any novel weight loss procedure, the hopes were short lived, and weight regain occurred as early as 6–9 months postoperatively. The staple line dehisced and the normal volume of the stomach was restored allowing consumption of normal larger meals causing weight regain [4].

Despite the many technical modifications in stapling, and changing the size of the fundus to cause durability, it was realized that the horizontal design of the staple line cannot hold against the forward peristalsis of the gastric wall. This understanding led Dr. Mason from the University of Iowa to separate the two gastric components, applying the principle of partial gastrectomy to weight loss while leaving the distal stomach in situ. Continuity was restored with gastrojejunostomy, bypassing the duodenum and part of the jejunum. This was the first concept of combined restriction and malabsorption and the birth of modern bariatric surgery as we know it today.

Dr. Mason's operation, described in 1967, was called gastric bypass and remains the cornerstone of bariatric surgery up to this time [10]. It consisted of a completely divided 30 ml gastric pouch using surgical stapler and reconstruction using loop gastrojejunostomy with 0.8–1 cm anastomosis (Fig. 1.6) bypassing the duodenum and the first few inches of the small intestine.

There was significant excitement about this "combination" surgery, but it was far from being ready for widespread use. Many problems occurred with the surgery that required modifications and caused significant variation in outcome. Surgeons soon realized the need to standardize this operation in order to optimize results.

The pouch size was agreed upon to be less than 50 cc and the outlet need to be less than 1 cm in diameter. The most significant modification was switching reconstruction from loop configuration to Roux-en-Y, in order to prevent the bile from refluxing through the afferent jejunal limb into the gastric pouch.

It is worth noting that the anatomical configuration of the gastric bypass as an operation was described almost a century prior to that intended for weight loss. In 1892, Dr. Cesar Roux, from Switzerland, designed the "roux" configuration to bypass gastric obstruction. However, he later abandoned the procedure in 1910 due to high rates of marginal ulcer and nutritional deficiency.

As for weight loss, Dr. Griffin, in 1977, is credited for changing the "loop" to the "Y" configuration in order to prevent reflux (Fig. 1.7).

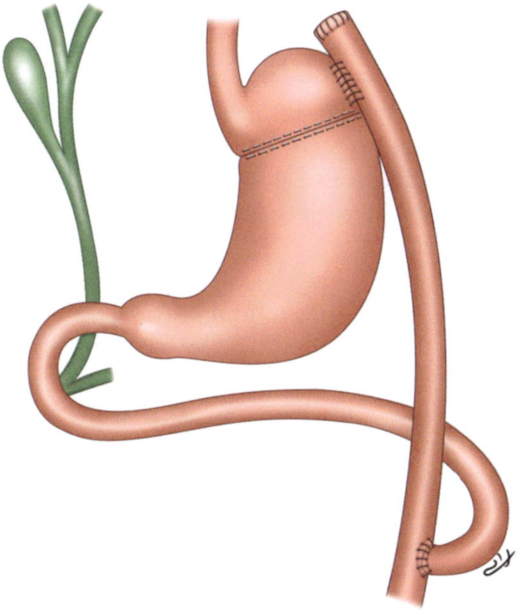

Fig. 1.7 Horizontal gastric bypass with Roux reconstruction as per Griffin

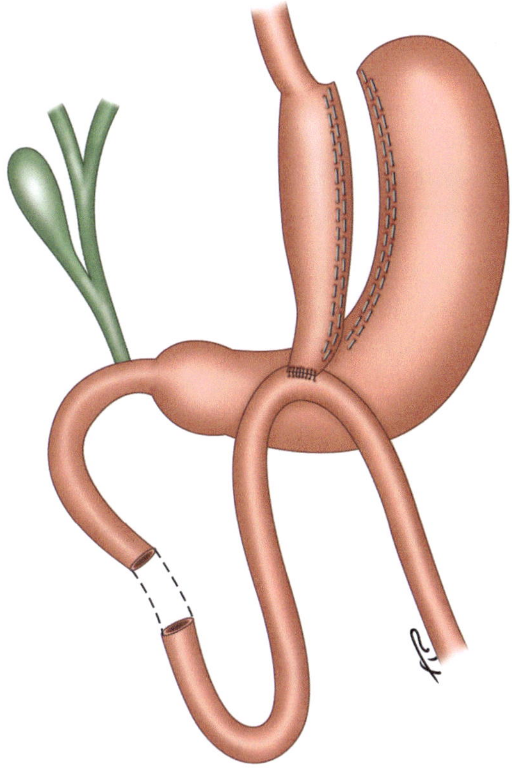

Fig. 1.8 Mini-gastric bypass

He is also credited for changing the design of the gastric pouch to be based on the lesser, rather than greater, curvature by changing the direction of the staple line from horizontal to vertical [4, 11]. However, he did go back to the undivided pouch, which again, failed overtime due to dehiscence of the staple line. This was later modified again to the complete separation with oversewing of the cut edges [4].

As for the intestinal bypass, the small bowel was divided approximately 45 cm from ligament of Treitz, and the Roux limb was found to be optimal at about 100–150 cm length to optimize the malabsorption while limiting its unintended consequences. Furthermore, retrocolic, retrogastric route was thought to be a safer alternative that provides a tension-free, well-perfused gastrojejunostomy.

Many modifications occurred over the years; but the one that stood out came from Chapel Hill, North Carolina, in 1997 after an emergency surgery performed by Dr. Robert Rutledge for penetrating trauma where he used Billroth II antecolic gastrojejunostomy for reconstruction. In the morning, he had an elective gastric bypass and thought of using the same type of reconstruction again to make the operation easier to perform laparoscopically. Rutledge thought that using a long narrow pouch with loop gastrojejunostomy reconstruction without the need for a second anastomosis (jejuno-jejunostomy) would make this operation shorter, simpler, and easier to standardize and teach (Fig. 1.8). This came at a time when laparoscopy was challenging for these complex surgeries and gastric bypass still had high rate of morbidity.

He reported his first series on over 1200 patients with significantly short operating time averaging 37 min. Excess weight loss was 77% at 2 years with a leak rate of 1.6% and only one death in his large series [12]. This single anastomosis gastric bypass (that he named *mini-gastric bypass*) was and remains to this date controversial in the USA, while it has been widely accepted in the rest of the world. Concerns over significant malabsorption, bile reflux, ulceration, and eventual cancer led many American surgeons to oppose it. This opposition was also based on the failure of the loop reconstruction described by Dr. Mason (described earlier in chapter, Fig. 1.6). Rutledge argued that in his version, the anastomosis is further down from the esophagus due to the long pouch, eliminating the increased risk of malignancy, and he also argued that his data shows an acceptable rate of marginal ulcers despite, what he called, *theoretical* increase in risk due to loop configuration.

Today, Roux-en-Y gastric bypass is the cornerstone operation for bariatric surgery worldwide. Bypass, however, is a complex operation that carried early on significant risk of morbidity [13]. These risks were even higher in the days of open surgery where wound complications such as hernias and infections were unacceptably high in this population. Due to the prejudiced views against obesity, technical complications, universal to any surgery such as leak and obstruction, were always used to question the value of this operation and to some extent, bariatric surgery as a whole!

Bariatric surgeons realized the need of large studies to prove the long-term safety of bariatric surgery. Pories was the first to publish such long-term data reporting on 600 patients who underwent a standardized operation with up to 14-year follow-up [14]. He showed mortality of 1.5% and morbidity of 8.5% in the 1980s at a time gastric bypass was under heavy scrutiny. His patients maintained average weight of about 200 lb at 14 years from a starting weight over 300 lb. He was first to clearly demonstrate improvements in diabetes, hypertension, sleep apnea, heart failure, arthritis, and infertility. Furthermore, survival benefit was reported for patients who undergo bariatric surgery as shown by the Utah group. They looked at almost 10,000 patients over 7-year span and were able to show a marked decrease in adjusted long-term all-cause mortality in the surgery group by 40%, as compared with the control group [15].

Dr. Mason was an incredible thinker and innovator who never stopped his pursuit of the optimal weight loss operation. He was not satisfied with the overall results of his bypass operation from a safety standpoint and continued his search for the ideal risk/benefit balance. In his mind, restriction was eventually the way forward. To achieve that safely, he aimed to eliminate the risk of leak by avoiding dividing the stomach. For long-term success, his pouch was based on the less distensible lesser curvature of the stomach, and the outlet was made tight and reinforced with pliable ring to prevent stretching and have long-lasting effect.

With these principles, he created the vertical banded gastroplasty (VBG) in the early 1980s (Fig. 1.9) placing a vertical staple line parallel to the lesser curvature to create the pouch and fixed its outlet using a 5 cm long polypropylene band around the stoma [16].The ease of construction and the high safety profile of this operation without leaks or vitamin deficiencies made it very popular operation for many years to follow.

High hopes, once again, fell short. Staple line dehiscence was common and made weight loss short lived, while mesh complications piled up causing severe reflux, obstruction, and erosion. These adverse events caused the rapid enthusiasm to fade away gradually until VBG became of

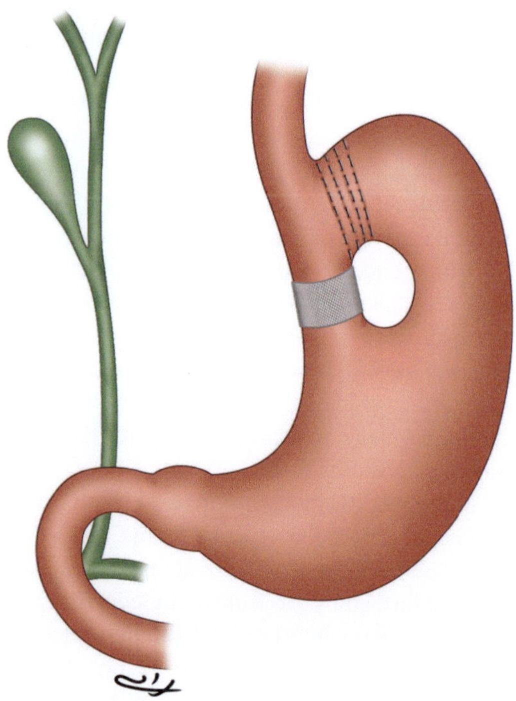

Fig. 1.9 Vertical banded gastroplasty (VBG)

only a historical value. Gastric bypass remained the "best" available operation and the operation of choice to revise complicated VBGs up to our current days.

While Dr. Mason was working out of University of Iowa on the bypass and VBG, a young man in Rome named Dr. Nicola Scopinaro was working on improving the results of the jejunoileal bypass. He saw the problem with this operation to be mainly related to the long defunctionalized small bowel left when the bypass is constructed. His plan to eliminate stasis was achieved by having each limb connected to a source of constant flow. To do that, he performed a limited distal gastrectomy by dividing the duodenum (the pylorus was excised with the specimen causing dumping in many patients). The *alimentary limb* had constant flow from the proximal stomach (gastrojejunostomy), while the remaining long *biliary limb* (that would be defunctionalized in JIB) now had constant natural flow of bile from the duodenum. The two limbs connected distally with an end-to-side anastomosis taking the Roux-en-Y configuration. His procedure, described in 1979, became known as the biliopancreatic diversion (BPD) (Fig. 1.10).

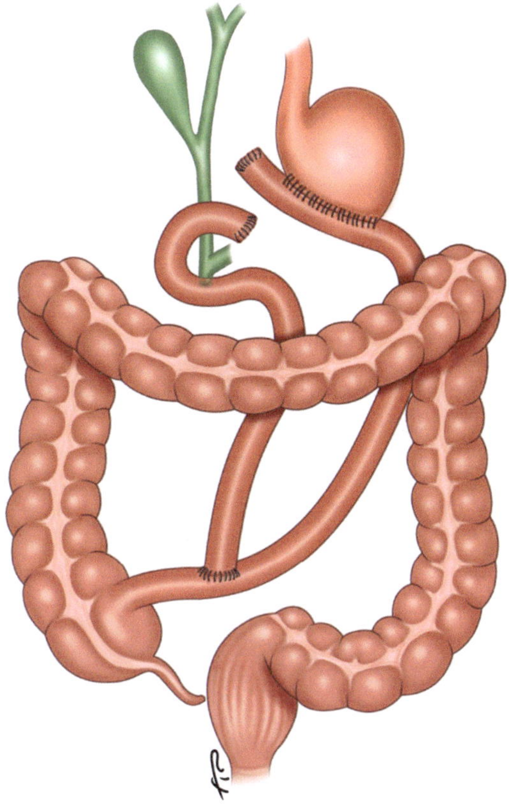

Fig. 1.10 Biliopancreatic diversion as described by Dr. Scopinaro

This was mainly a malabsorptive operation as the common channel measured only 50 cm, while restriction was only minimal due to limited gastrectomy leaving a generous 250–400 cc pouch [17].

While very successful in weight loss and much improved from prior purely restrictive historical operations, the disadvantage of loose, foul-smelling stool and stomal ulcers was significant. Malnutrition caused severe hypoalbuminemia, anemia, edema, and many other severe complications that necessitated lifelong strict follow-up, significant dietary supplementation, and in many cases revisions and reversals [4].

The high incidence of complications resulting from the distal gastrectomy in the Scopinaro operation (dumping, marginal ulcers, biliary reflux) led Dr. Douglas Hess in 1986 to incorporate the duodenal switch, described by Tom R. DeMeester in the 1980s for biliary reflux, to the Scopinaro operation in order to prevent the aforementioned complications [17]. This hybrid operation was appropriately referred to as the biliopancreatic diversion with duodenal switch (BPD-DS) or, less commonly, GR-DS (gastric reduction-duodenal switch) (Fig. 1.11).

It consisted of dividing the duodenum just distal to the pylorus with a duodeno-ileostomy to proximal duodenum (the distal duodenal side stays as a stapled stump). Gastric volume was also reduced, but as opposed to the Scopinaro operation, the gastric continuity was preserved and the resection was of the lateral greater curvature part of the stomach, leaving a sleeve-like conduit for food passage. While the incidence of malabsorptive complications did not change (length of the common channel remains constant), biliary reflux, ulcerations, and dumping syndrome were all eliminated by preserving the pylorus. The significant malabsorption necessitated supplementation and surveillance. Still, even in compliant patients, deficiencies and complications occurred and were

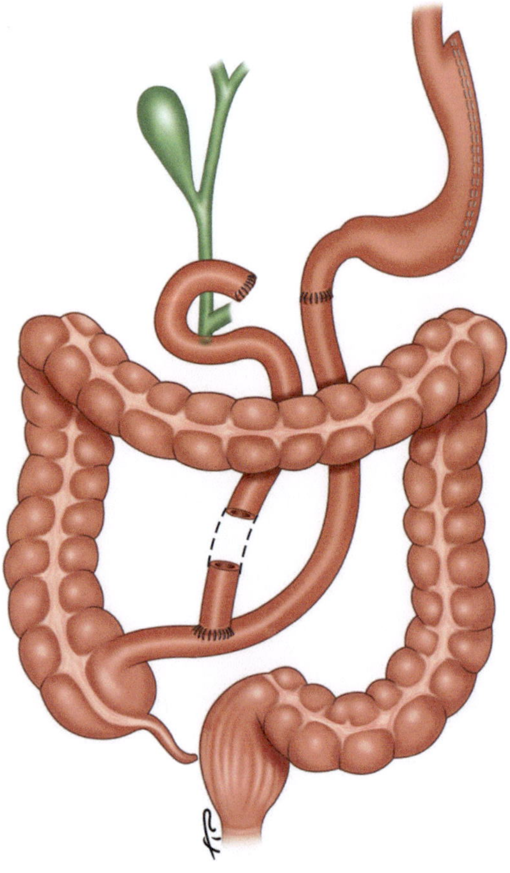

Fig. 1.11 Biliopancreatic diversion with duodenal switch

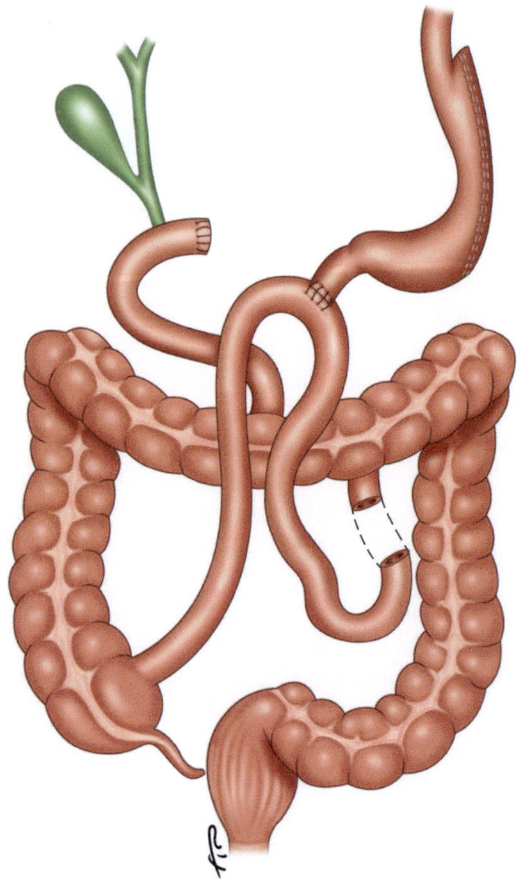

Fig. 1.12 Single anastomosis duodenal switch

in many instances dangerous and life threatening [4]. These complications, along with technical complexity, prevented this operation from ever becoming a popular one, with steady low prevalence around 1%.

The only major modification to the BPD-DS came many years later from Spain where Dr. Antonio Torres [18] tried to make this complex operation easier to perform.

He described a simpler alternative, eliminating the need for the distal small bowel anastomosis. Instead, he reconstructed (after dividing the duodenum) with a single, end-to-side duodeno-ileostomy at 200 cm proximal to the ileocecal valve (Fig. 1.12). Results were encouraging and the operation was indeed much easier to perform, teach, and reproduce than that described by Hess. This alteration finally sparked interest in duodenal switches and caused increased adoption worldwide, both as a stand-alone and revisional surgery after failed sleeve gastrectomy. Of note, as of the day we write this chapter, single anastomosis duodenal switch remains "investigational" in the USA until more data is collected.

From a totally different mind-set emerged the concept of gastric banding based on safety and simplicity and accepting perhaps inferior weight loss in exchange for (perceived) safety and preservation of the anatomy (Fig. 1.13).

The work of many innovators over the span of half a decade led to the idea of a gastric band placement around the upper part of the stomach. This was described by Wilkinson and Peloso in 1978 [19], Kolle in 1982 [20], and Molina and Oria in 1983 [21]. The idea was to cause restriction without any suturing or division of the stomach. This is rather achieved by

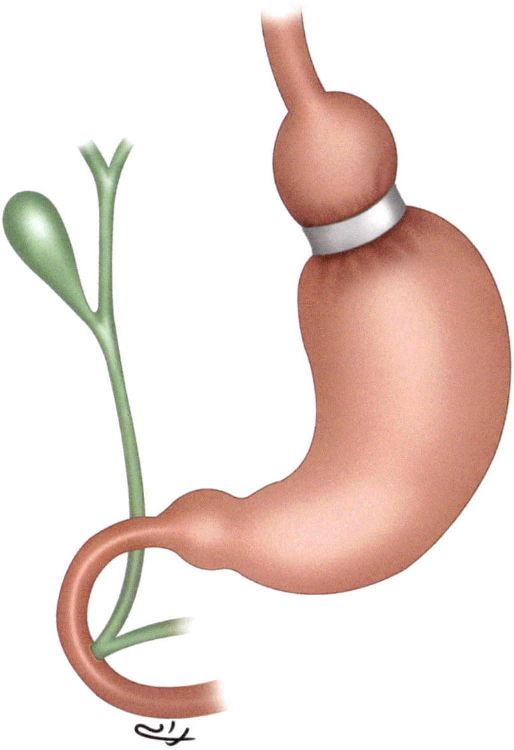

Fig. 1.13 Gastric band

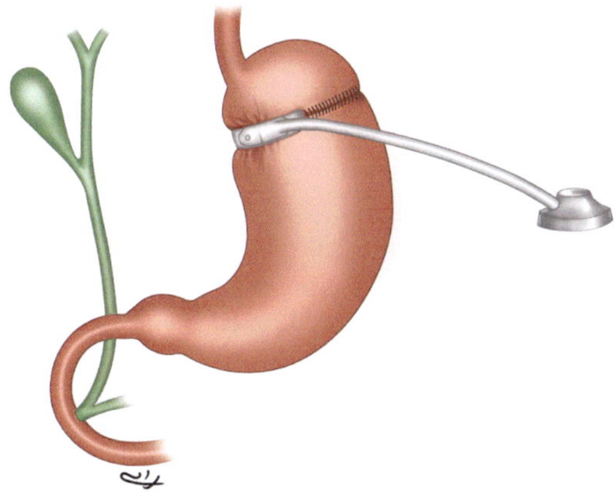

Fig. 1.14 Kuzmak adjustable silicone gastric band

simply placing a band around the top of the stomach creating a narrow outlet with a small stoma that measures 15–30 cc [4]. The operation was indeed simple and safe at a time when safety was a major concern to patients, and complexity was a major limiting factor stopping many surgeons from adopting bariatric surgery. Soon, however, a whole new armamentarium of complications was described, such as slippage and erosion of the band. While these complications were not life threatening, they were very common. The unpredictable response of patients to hunger and weight loss after surgery caused wide variation of results and questioned if "one size band fits all." To address that, Kuzmak in 1986 [22] made the band *adjustable* aiming to customize the restriction to individual needs, compliance, and weight loss. The device consisted of a silicone band with an inflatable balloon connected via a tube to a reservoir placed under the skin and used for adjustments (Fig. 1.14).

The first successful laparoscopic banding procedure was published in 1993 by Broadbent [23]. During the same time, Belachew [24] designed an adjustable gastric band (similar to that designed by Kuzmak) that could be placed using laparoscopic techniques. He described this procedure in a porcine model a decade after the original report by Kuzmak [22].

While unlimited adjustability was conceptually a way for long-term success, the results never reached the desired long-term success. We know now that the inferior results were, in part, due to the lack of the metabolic effect which are achieved in stapling procedures that excise or bypass the fundus of the stomach. While the excitement of banding was significant due to the perceived safety and reversibility, it quickly faded away with inferior long-term results, increased number of revisions, and improved safety profile of other stapling procedures that were once deemed "too risky." Today, banding is not even an option in many countries around the world and continues to be on the decline in the rest.

Last but not least is the sleeve gastrectomy which has quickly become the fastest-growing bariatric surgery worldwide, constituting more than 50% of all bariatric surgeries performed in the USA in 2015 [25].

The early concept dates back to Johnston in 1987, who performed the first Magenstrasse and Mill procedure [26]. The Magenstrasse referred to a thin tube created based on the lesser curvature of the stomach, and the Mill referred to the antrum. The operation would start by creating a defect in the antrum using circular stapler and then stapling cephalad along 40 fr bougie creating a narrow tube along the lesser curvature (Fig. 1.15).

Natural evolution led to resecting the lateral remaining part of the stomach instead of keeping the antral connection. This resulted in a sleeve-like stomach similar to what was previously described by Hess as part of the restrictive component of the duodenal switch [27]. Sleeve gastrectomy (Fig. 1.16) as a bariatric procedure was initially performed as first of a two-step procedure in high-risk patients that may not tolerate the long and complex laparoscopic gastric bypass or duodenal switch. Splitting the operation proved valuable in decreasing the morbidity and mortality in this high-risk group [28–30].

The sleeve gastrectomy when performed as a first step had significant success as far as safety and early weight loss. This led increasing numbers of patients to decline proceeding with the second intestinal part (completion gastric bypass or duodenal switch). The encouraging early results of the sleeve gastrectomy (without the completion intestinal bypass) led some surgeons like Dr. Michel Gagner to look at the value of the sleeve as a stand-alone operation [31]. This quickly changed the demographics of bariatric surgery in the USA and worldwide introducing what became quickly the most popular and fastest-growing operation of our times [25].

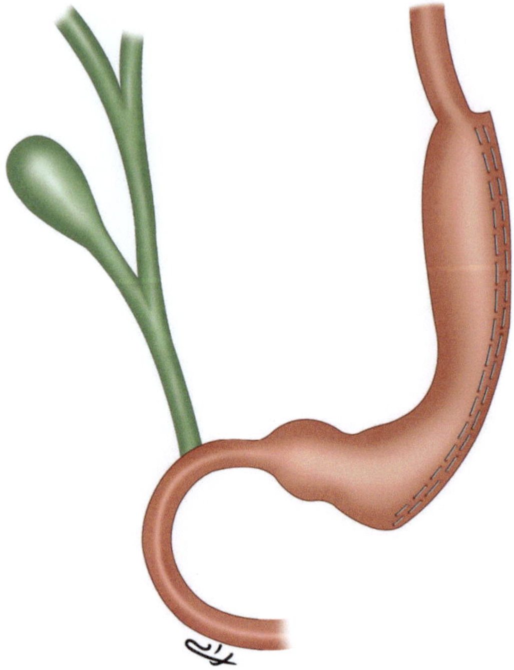

Fig. 1.16 Sleeve gastrectomy

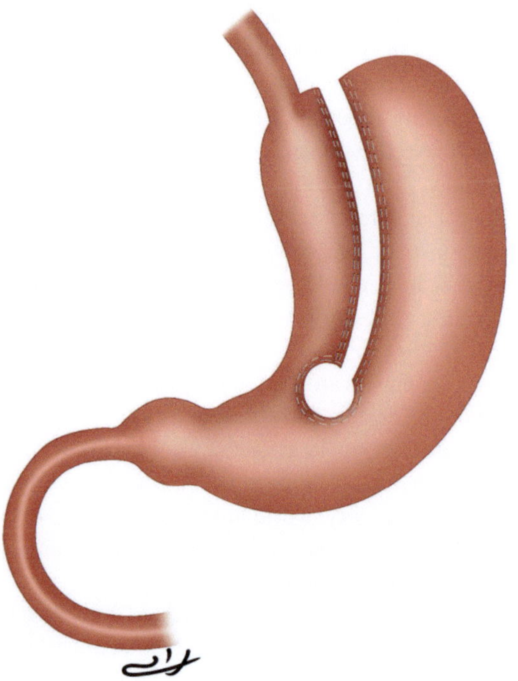

Fig. 1.15 Magenstrasse and mill operation

Lastly, and aside from the actual design of the operation, perhaps the single most significant technical innovation to surgery as a whole has been the evolution of laparoscopic surgery. This was particularly significant in the field of bariatric surgery as our patients would benefit most from avoiding large abdominal incisions given their large pannus and the resulting high prevalence of wound infection, breakdown, and hernias.

Dr. Alan Wittgrove from California was the first to successfully perform laparoscopic Roux-en-Y gastric bypass in 1994 [31]. Of course, in the early days of laparoscopy, completing such a complex operation laparoscopically was a major technical challenge especially in morbidly obese patients with large fatty livers. Performing the gastrojejunal anastomosis was and still remains the most challenging part of this operation. Therefore, there was an agreement that using the circular stapler provides the only way for a reliable anastomosis, although the route to delivering the anvil remained an area of debate [32].

As complications from the anvil and circular stapler started to appear (esophageal injuries, strictures, and wound infections), alternative techniques were sought. Kelvin Higa, also from California, was first to be able to perform a completely hand-sewn anastomosis laparoscopically [33]. Mastering laparoscopic suturing and knot tying opened the door for wider application for laparoscopy to be attempted on the most complex open surgeries. In the year 2000, Ren et al. reported on successful completion of 40 duodenal switch surgeries laparoscopically without conversion [34]; these were high-risk patients with median BMI of 65. There was one mortality, one leak, and four staple line bleeds. The authors concluded that laparoscopy, while technically challenging, is feasible in this complex operation.

Introduction of laparoscopy to bariatric surgery may be the single most important milestone in its evolution and acceptance by an apprehensive public opinion. Shorter hospitalization, early mobility, faster recovery with less pain convinced many who were reluctant to consider the operation. Despite this great advancement in technology and proven safety and efficacy [35], we continue to operate on only 1% of the morbidly obese patients who qualify for surgery.

Unrealistic fear, concerns regarding general anesthesia, or having an actual operation still hold most morbidly obese patients from coming to see a surgeon. Therefore, there was a need for less aggressive treatment to fill the gap between medical behavioral therapy and surgery, similar to stenting for coronary artery disease instead of open heart surgery when medical therapy fails. This gap in obesity treatment was filled with *Bariatric Endoscopy.*

At this date, intragastric balloons are the most prevalent well-studied endoscopic procedures performed for weight loss. While relatively new, the idea of occupying the intragastric space for restriction and weight loss goes back about a century, where Dr. DeBakey, in 1938, observed and described weight loss as a long-term complication of bezoar [36]. It was not until 1979 when Dr. Miller from the University of Mississippi took that observation to the lab and placed 250 cc polyethylene bottles in nine dogs via laparotomy to test for decreased oral intake. His experiment however, failed to show a difference in weight loss between the surgical and sham group [37]. In Santa Ana, California, Drs. Lloyd and Mary Garren (gastroenterologists from Delaware) had a different opinion. They designed a cylinder shape "bubble" made of elastomer plastic and filled with 200 cc of air to stay in the stomach for 3 months. This was manufactured by American Edwards Labs and carried the name "Edward Garren-Edwards Bubble." Their data got them FDA approval in the USA in 1985. Concerns about the safety of weight loss surgery at that time led to high demand for these bubbles with more than 20,000 devices sold in the 1st year alone. It was soon discovered, however, that the procedure is not as benign as was thought, mainly due to the device itself causing tears, erosions, ulcers, and even bowel obstruction from migration [38]. These complications led the company to stop manufacturing the balloon in 1988 and recall the product in 1992.

Despite repeated failures, interest remained high in this concept leading many international experts to organize a multidisciplinary meeting looking at what would constitute the ideal device to achieve restriction without compromising safety. They met in Tarpon Spring in Florida in 1987 and came up with what they called the *Tarpon Spring criteria for the ideal balloon.* They envisioned that to be large (to prevent distal migration), smooth, round, filled with saline instead of air, and made of durable long-lasting material that can withstand the acidity of the stomach. Based on these criteria, many types of balloons were later invented in different countries with varying degree of success and risks. It took close to three decades to have a commercial type be approved by the FDA for use in the USA.

In addition to placing balloons, the field of endoscopy grew widely, and advanced technology allowed complex tasks to be performed endoscopically, potentially eliminating completely the need for surgery. Endoscopic suturing allowed for revising a dilated pouch or anastomosis for weight regain and also was applied to perform a full weight loss procedure such as the gastric sleeve. Innovators did not stop at restriction but also replicated malabsorption by using endoscopy to place a barrier in the proximal jejunum mimicking the effects of gastric bypass by preventing absorption in the covered areas. To take this further, upper and lower endoscopy are now used together to place magnets in the jejunum and ileum that would "mate" causing local necrosis of the tissues in between, creating an actual anastomosis and bypassing the entire segment of bowel in between.

Last but not least, in addition to restriction and malabsorption, much work is now done on vagal stimulation to affect hunger and satiety signals. Different types of electrodes and devices are now in market with one at this time available in the USA after obtaining FDA approval. These must be placed laparoscopically at this time, but by the time many read this chapter, endoscopically placed electrodes to stimulate satiety may be available.

In summary, after almost a century of battling severe obesity with the search of the optimal operation, we learned that obesity is a very complex chronic progressive disease, and hence, its therapy cannot be simply achieved by an hour or so operation or intervention.

Between laparoscopy and endoscopy and restriction, malabsorption, or electrical stimulation, the optimal surgery or intervention can only be reached when a mutual decision is made by a well-informed patient who has the same success criteria as the surgeon. A well-informed patient and a competent surgeon along with a comprehensive team in a specialized center is the backbone for any successful bariatric surgery or intervention.

References

1. Conard NJ. A female figurine from the basal Aurignacian of Hohle Fels Cave in southwestern Germany. Nature. 2009;459:248–52.
2. Wilford JN. Tooth may have solved mummy mystery. Tooth may have solved mummy mystery. 2007. Retrieved 2 Feb 2017, from http://www.nytimes.com/2007/06/27/world/middleeast/27mummy.html.
3. Calle EE, Thun MJ, Petrelli JM, Rodriguez C, Heath CW. Body-mass index and mortality in a prospective cohort of U.S. adults. Engl J Med. 1999;341(15):1097–105.
4. Bariatric surgery—history. 2003. Available: http://bariatrics.ucsf.edu/patient/history.html.
5. Payne JH, DeWind LT. Surgical treatment of obesity. Am J Surg. 1969;118:141.
6. Payne JH, DeWind LT, Commons RR. Metabolic observations in patients with jejunocolic shunts. Am J Surg. 1963;106:273–89.
7. Scott HW, Dean R, Shull HJ, et al. Considerations in the use of jejuno-ileal bypass in patients with morbid obesity. Ann Surg. 1973;177:323–35.
8. MacGregor A. The story of surgery for obesity. Am Soc Bariatric Surg. 2002. http://www.asbs.org/html/story/chapter1.html.
9. Balsiger BM, Murr MM, Poggio JL, Sarr MG. Bariatric surgery: surgery for weight control in patients with morbid obesity. Med Clin N Am. 2000;84:477–89.
10. Mason EE, Ito C. Gastric bypass in obesity. Surg Clin N Am. 1967;47:1345–51.
11. Griffen WO, Young VL, Stevenson VV. A prospective comparison of gastric and jejunoileal bypass procedures for morbid obesity. Ann Surg. 1977;186:500–9.
12. Rutledge R. The mini-gastric bypass: experience with the first 1,274 cases. Obes Surg. 2001;11:276–80.
13. Flickinger EG, Pories WJ, Meelheim HD, Sinar DR, Blose IL, Thomas FT. The Greenville gastric bypass. Progress report at 3 years. Ann Surg. 1984;199:555–62.
14. Pories WJ, Swanson MS, MacDonald KG, et al. Who would have thought it? An operation proves to be the most effective therapy for adult-onset diabetes mellitus. Ann Surg. 1995;222:339–52.
15. Adams TD, Gress RE, Smith SC, Halverson RC, Simper SC, Rosamond WD, LaMonte MJ, Stroup AM, Hunt SC. Long term mortality of gastric bypass surgery. N Engl J Med. 2007;357(8):753–61.
16. Mason EE. Vertical banded gastroplasty for obesity. Arch Surg. 1984;117:701–6.
17. Hess DS, Hess DW. Biliopancreatic diversion with a duodenal switch. Obes Surg. 1998;8:267–82.
18. Sanchez-Pernaute A, Herrera MAR, Perez-Aguirre E, Perez JCG, Cabrerizo L, Valladares LD, Fernandez C, Talavera P, Torres A. Proximal duodenal-ileal end-to-side bypass with sleeve gastrectomy: proposed technique. Obes Surg. 2007;17(12):1614–8.
19. Wilkinson LH, Peloso OA. Gastric (reservoir) reduction for morbid obesity. Arch Surg. 1981;116:602–5.
20. Kolle K. Gastric banding. OMGI 7th Congress, Stockholm, Sweden. 1982. Abst No 145).
21. Molina M, Oria HE. Gastric segmentation: a new, safe, effective, simple, readily revised and fully reversible surgical procedure for the correction of morbid obesity. Iowa City: 6th Bariatric Surgery Colloquium. June 2–3, 1983. p. 15.

22. Kuzman LI. Silicone gastric banding; a simple and effective operation for morbid obesity. Contemp Surg. 1986;28:13–8.
23. Broadbent R, Tracey M, Harrington P. Laparoscopic gastric banding: a preliminary report. Obes Surg. 1993;3:63.
24. Belachew M, Legrand MJ, Defecherux TH, Burtheret MP, Jacquet N. Laparoscopic adjustable silicone gastric banding in the treatment of morbid obesity. A preliminary report. Surg Endosc. 1994;8:1354–6.
25. Ponce J, DeMaria EJ, Nguyen NT, Hutter M, Sudan R, Morton JM. American Society for Metabolic and Bariatric Surgery estimation of bariatric surgery procedures in 2015 and surgeon workforce in the United States. Surg Obes Relat Dis. 2016;12(9):1637–9.
26. Johnston D, Dachtler J, Sue-Ling HM, King RF, Martin LG. The magenstrasse and mill operation for morbid obesity. Obes Surg. 2003;13(1):10–6.
27. Marceau P, Biron S, Bourque RA, Potvin M, Hould FS, Simard S. Biliopancreatic diversion with a new type of gastrectomy. Obes Surg. 1993;3(1):29–35.
28. Chu CA, Gagner M, Quinn T, et al. Two-stage laparoscopic bilio-pancreatic diversion with duodenal switch: an alternative approach to super-super morbid obesity (abstr). Surg Endosc. 2002;16:S069.
29. Regan JP, Inabnet WB, Gagner M, et al. Early experience with two stage laparoscopic Roux-en-Y gastric bypass as an alternative in the super-super obese patient. Obes Surg. 2003;13:861–4.
30. Moy J, Pomp A, Dakin G, Parikh M, Gagner M. Laparoscopic sleeve gastrectomy for morbid obesity. Am J Surg. 2008;196(5):e56–9.
31. Wittgrove AC, Clark GW, Tremblay LJ. Laparoscopic gastric bypass, Roux-en-Y preliminary report of five cases. Obes Surg. 1994;4:353–7.
32. De la Torre RA, Scott JS. Laparoscopic Roux-en-Y gastric bypass totally intra-abdominal approach—technique and preliminary report. Obes Surg. 1999;9:492–8.
33. Higa KD, Boone KB, Ho T. Laparoscopic Roux-en-Y gastric bypass for morbid obesity in 850 patients, technique and follow-up. Poster at the American Society of Bariatric Surgery, American Society of Bariatric Surgery; 1999.
34. Ren CJ, Patterson E, Gagner M. Early results of laparoscopic bilio-pancreatic diversion with duodenal switch: a case series of 40 consecutive patients. Obes Surg. 2000;10:514–23.
35. Chang SH, Stoll CR, Song J, et al. The effectiveness and risks of bariatric surgery: an updated systematic review and meta-analysis, 2003–2012. JAMA Surg. 2014;149:275–87.
36. DeBakey M, Ochsner A. Bezoars and concretions: a comprehensive review of the literature with an analysis of 303 collected cases and a presentation of 8 additional cases. Surgery. 1938;4(934–9630):132–60.
37. Miller JD. Intragastric prosthesis for management of obesity. World J Surg. 1982;6:492.
38. Benjamin SB, Maher KA, EL C Jr, et al. Double-blind controlled trial of the Garren-Edwards gastric bubble: an adjunctive treatment of exogenous obesity. Gastroenterology. 1988;48(3):592–4.

Bariatric Surgery: Current State of Affairs

2

Katherine S. Blevins, Dan E. Azagury, and John Magaña Morton

Introduction

Obesity and bariatric surgery are of increasing importance in the USA and globally. In 2014, it was estimated that 39% of adults were overweight and 13% of adults were obese worldwide. Additionally, 41 million children under age 5 were overweight or obese [1]. Obesity has more than doubled since 1980, with now over 600 million obese adults across the globe [1]. The implications of obesity on health, including the association with increased risk of cardiovascular disease, dyslipidemia, diabetes mellitus, sleep apnea, osteoarthritis, and certain cancers, were officially recognized by the National Institutes of Health (NIH) in 1985 [2]. Additionally, it has been shown that class II and III obesities are associated with a significantly higher all-cause mortality [3]. The increasing prevalence and health implications make obesity one of the most important epidemics today [4].

Electronic Supplementary Material The online version of this chapter (doi:10.1007/978-3-319-93545-4_2) contains supplementary material, which is available to authorized users.

K. S. Blevins
Department of Surgery, Stanford University School of Medicine, Stanford, CA, USA
e-mail: blevinsk@stanford.edu

D. E. Azagury · J. M. Morton (✉)
Department of Surgery, Stamford Hospital, Stanford, CA, USA
e-mail: dazagury@stanford.edu; morton@stanford.edu

Bariatric surgery has been shown to be an effective treatment for clinically severe obesity in multiple measures including improvement or remission of obesity-related comorbidities, sustained weight loss, improvement of quality of life, and survival benefit [5–8]. Since first described over 50 years ago, bariatric surgery has evolved dramatically. In the mid-1960s, Edward Mason described a method for surgical weight loss achieved by a restrictive and malabsorptive gastrointestinal procedure, the gastric bypass [9]. Initially described as gastric bypass with a single-loop anastomosis, the operation was later modified to a Roux-en-Y configuration to minimize alkaline reflux gastritis [10]. Since then, the evolution of bariatric surgery has been shaped by development of laparoscopic approach, technical refinements, and the invention of various surgical devices [11].

There are currently four bariatric operations commonly performed: Roux-en-Y gastric bypass (RYGB), sleeve gastrectomy, adjustable gastric banding, and biliopancreatic diversion with (or without) duodenal switch (BPD-DS). RYGB has been performed the greatest number of times and remains the most commonly performed procedure worldwide [10]. However, sleeve gastrectomy has recently become the most frequently performed bariatric procedure in the USA [12]. Adjustable gastric banding use has steadily declined since the adoption of the sleeve gastrectomy.

R. Lutfi et al. (eds.), *Global Bariatric Surgery*, https://doi.org/10.1007/978-3-319-93545-4_2

Adoption Across the Globe

The adoption of bariatric surgery as a safe, effective treatment for obesity has been a process over the last four decades that continues today. The 1991 NIH consensus statement on obesity surgery recommended surgical management for patients with severe obesity with a BMI of ≥35 kg/m^2 with at least one comorbid condition (type 2 diabetes mellitus, hypertension, obstructive sleep apnea) or a BMI of ≥40 kg/m^2 [13]. The safety of bariatric surgery has improved since the late 1990s with mortality dropping from 0.5% to 1% to current mortality rates around 0.1–0.3% [14, 15]. In the USA, the adoption of bariatric surgery continues to spread. It is estimated that there were 196,000 bariatric operations performed in the USA in 2015, up from 158,000 in 2011 [16]. Of the operations in 2015, approximately 53.8% were sleeve gastrectomy, 23.1% RYGB, 5.7% laparoscopic adjustable gastric banding, and 0.6% BPD-DS. Although the number of operations is increasing, in the USA, it is estimated that only 1.24% of estimating those eligible for surgical intervention underwent bariatric surgery [16]. Worldwide, in 2013 there were 468,609 bariatric procedures, 95.7% performed laparoscopically [17].

A major factor in the spread of bariatric surgery in the USA is insurance coverage. The economic impact of obesity in the USA has been estimated at $147 billion in direct medical costs [18]. Studies have shown that metabolic and bariatric surgeries are cost-effective and provide a return on investment in as little as 25 months to 5 years [19–22]. Despite evidence of the safety and benefits, universal insurance coverage has not been established. In 2004 the Centers for Medicare and Medicaid Services (CMS) convened a Medicare Coverage Advisory Committee to determine whether CMS should cover bariatric surgery. In 2006, CMS published a favorable national coverage decision supporting coverage for Roux-en-Y gastric bypass, open and laparoscopic biliopancreatic diversion with duodenal switch (BPD/DS), and laparoscopic adjustable gastric banding for patients with BMI >35 with at least one comorbidity related to obesity and has been unsuccessful with medical treatment for obesity, limiting to operations performed at facilities that were certified by the American College of Surgeons as a Level 1 Bariatric Surgery Center or certified by the American Society for Bariatric Surgery as a Bariatric Surgery Center of Excellence. In 2009, the decision was updated to include type 2 diabetes mellitus as a comorbidity for coverage. In 2012, laparoscopic sleeve gastrectomy was added to the list of covered operations. In 2013, the requirement that facilities be certified was removed by CMS; however, all major private insurers still require accreditation by the combined Metabolic and Bariatric Surgery Accreditation Quality Improvement Program from the American Society for Metabolic and Bariatric Surgery and American College of Surgeons [23]. Although there is a favorable national coverage decision for Medicare beneficiaries, there is no universal insurance coverage, and often coverage can be dependent on insurance-mandated preoperative weight loss requirements. The American Society of Metabolic and Bariatric Surgery recently updated their position on these requirements, recommending the abandonment of insurance-mandated preoperative weight loss [24].

In the UK, examining the National Health Service (NHS) reveals similarities in coverage and use of bariatric surgery. The National Institute for Health and Care Excellence (NICE) recommends that after all nonsurgical measures have been tried without achieving or maintaining weight loss, bariatric surgery is considered for people with BMI >40, BMI ≥35 with onset of type 2 diabetes in the past 10 years with consideration for surgery with BMI 30–34.9, and is recommended as the option of choice for adults with a BMI >50 when other interventions have not been effective [25]. This means 2.6 million people in the UK meet criteria for surgery. Despite this, NHS bariatric procedures have been dropping. From 2011–2012 to 2014–2015, the number of operations dropped from 8794 to 6032, much less than 1% of those eligible for surgery [26]. Although coverage is described within the NHS according to NICE guidelines, restructuring in 2012 resulted in a four-tier model of care [27]. This pathway requires patients to go through several steps before referral for surgery, including evaluation by a general practitioner (tier 2) and referral and treatment by a multidisciplinary team approach for 12–24 months (tier 3) before referral for evaluation for surgical treatment (tier 4) [28]. There is continued discussion about the access barrier this presents [28].

Obesity Is a Disease

Discrimination against the obese is also an important factor in the spread of bariatric surgery. Experiences of weight discrimination have been reported in various settings, including employment, healthcare, educational institutions, public health, and interpersonal relationships [10, 29]. As obesity is generally perceived as being under volitional control, it is stigmatized. Studies have documented that overweight and obese individuals are perceived as lazy, weak-willed, unintelligent, and lack self-discipline and are non-compliant with weight loss care plans [30, 31]. Although stigma about obesity is prevalent, there is considerable scientific evidence that shows many significant factors that contribute to obesity are beyond the control of individuals. Genetic and biological factors contribute to the regulation of body weight, and social and economic factors influence a complex environment that promotes and reinforces obesity.

The WHO has additionally developed the "Global Action Plan for the Prevention and Control of Noncommunicable Diseases 2013–2020" with a specific goal of a 25% relative reduction in premature mortality from noncommunicable diseases by 2025 and a halt in the rise of global obesity to match the rates in 2010 [1]. The worsening of the obesity epidemic despite increased awareness highlights the need for increased awareness and education about the complexity of obesity. Obesity is a chronic disease with complex etiology, and bariatric surgery is and will continue to be an important part of multidisciplinary care for this disease.

Future Directions

The future of bariatric surgery will be an evolving landscape. With only 1% of those who qualify for surgical treatment of obesity actually having an operation, there is opportunity in the gap. Although the number of operations is increasing in the USA, there is still an unmet need in the treatment of obesity. This gap may be partially addressed by the emergence of new technology around novel and less invasive procedures. Since the approval of the Realize Band in 2007, there was a drought of new devices approved by the FDA for the treatment of obesity. In the last 2 years, there has been a surge of new technologies. Specifically, five novel technologies have been approved by the FDA since 2015 for usage in the USA: VBLOC (vagal blocking therapy for obesity), the AspireAssist device for percutaneous mechanical gastric emptying, and three endoscopically placed intragastric balloon systems (ReShape™ Dual Balloon, Orbera™ Intragastric Balloon System, and Obalon ® Balloon System) [32]. Each technology has specific indications as well as outcomes [33]. These and other new technologies may help bridge the gap in treating obesity, although long-term efficacy remains to be seen.

References

1. WHO | Obesity and overweight. WHO. Available at: http://www.who.int/mediacentre/factsheets/fs311/en/. Accessed: 8 Jan 2017.
2. Health implications of obesity. National Institutes of Health consensus development conference statement. Ann Intern Med. 1985;103:147–51.
3. Flegal KM, Kit BK, Orpana H, Graubard BI. Association of all-cause mortality with overweight and obesity using standard body mass index categories: a systematic review and meta-analysis. JAMA. 2013;309:71–82.
4. Nguyen NT, Varela JE. Bariatric surgery for obesity and metabolic disorders: state of the art. Nat Rev Gastroenterol Hepatol. 2016. https://doi.org/10.1038/nrgastro.2016.170.
5. Mingrone G, et al. Bariatric-metabolic surgery versus conventional medical treatment in obese patients with type 2 diabetes: 5 year follow-up of an open-label, single-centre, randomised controlled trial. Lancet Lond Eng. 2015;386:964–73.

6. Adams TD, et al. Health benefits of gastric bypass surgery after 6 years. JAMA. 2012;308:1122–31.
7. Colquitt JL, Pickett K, Loveman E, Frampton GK. Surgery for weight loss in adults. Cochrane Database Syst Rev. 2014;CD003641. https://doi.org/10.1002/14651858.CD003641.pub4.
8. Sjöström L, et al. Effects of bariatric surgery on mortality in Swedish obese subjects. N Engl J Med. 2007;357:741–52.
9. Mason EE, Ito C. Gastric bypass in obesity. Surg Clin N Am. 1967;47:1345–51.
10. Nguyen NT. The ASMBS textbook of bariatric surgery – volume 1: bariatric. Springer 2017.
11. Ng M, et al. Global, regional, and national prevalence of overweight and obesity in children and adults during 1980–2013: a systematic analysis for the Global Burden of Disease Study 2013. Lancet. 2014;384:766–81.
12. Esteban Varela J, Nguyen NT. Laparoscopic sleeve gastrectomy leads the U.S. utilization of bariatric surgery at academic medical centers. Surg Obes Relat Dis Off J Am Soc Bariatr Surg. 2015;11:987–90.
13. NIH conference. Gastrointestinal surgery for severe obesity. Consensus Development Conference Panel. Ann Intern Med. 1991;115:956–61.
14. Nguyen NT, Vu S, Kim E, Bodunova N, Phelan MJ. Trends in utilization of bariatric surgery, 2009–2012. Surg Endosc. 2016;30:2723–7.
15. Chang S-H, et al. The effectiveness and risks of bariatric surgery: an updated systematic review and meta-analysis, 2003–2012. JAMA Surg. 2014;149:275–87.
16. Ponce J, et al. American Society for Metabolic and Bariatric Surgery estimation of bariatric surgery procedures in 2015 and surgeon workforce in the United States. Surg Obes Relat Dis Off J Am Soc Bariatr Surg. 2016;12:1637–9.
17. Angrisani L, et al. Bariatric surgery worldwide 2013. Obes Surg. 2015;25:1822–32.
18. Finkelstein EA. How big of a problem is obesity? Surg Obes Relat Dis Off J Am Soc Bariatr Surg. 2014;10:569–70.
19. Gallagher SF, et al. The impact of bariatric surgery on the Veterans Administration healthcare system: a cost analysis. Obes Surg. 2003;13:245–8.
20. Sampalis JS, Liberman M, Auger S, Christou NV. The impact of weight reduction surgery on health-care costs in morbidly obese patients. Obes Surg. 2004;14:939–47.
21. Cremieux P-Y, et al. A study on the economic impact of bariatric surgery. Am J Manag Care. 2008;14:589–96.
22. Klein S, Ghosh A, Cremieux PY, Eapen S, McGavock TJ. Economic impact of the clinical benefits of bariatric surgery in diabetes patients with BMI ≥35 kg/m. Obes Silver Spring Md. 2011;19:581–7.
23. National Coverage Determination (NCD) for Bariatric Surgery for Treatment of Morbid Obesity. Available at: https://www.cms.gov/medicare-coverage-database/details/ncd-details.aspx?NCDId=57&ncdver=5&NCAId=160&NcaName=Bariatric+Surgery+for+the+Treatment+of+Morbid+Obesity&ExpandComments=y&CommentPeriod=0&TAId=47&bc=ACAAAAAAAQAAAA%3d%3d&.
24. Kim JJ, Rogers AM, Ballem N, Schirmer B, American Society for Metabolic and Bariatric Surgery Clinical Issues Committee. ASMBS updated position statement on insurance mandated preoperative weight loss requirements. Surg Obes Relat Dis Off J Am Soc Bariatr Surg. 2016;12:955–9.
25. Stegenga H, Haines A, Jones K, Wilding J. Identification, assessment, and management of overweight and obesity: summary of updated NICE guidance. BMJ. 2014;349:g6608.
26. Welbourn R, le Roux CW, Owen-Smith A, Wordsworth S, Blazeby JM. Why the NHS should do more bariatric surgery; how much should we do? BMJ. 2016;353:i1472.
27. Capehorn MS, Haslam DW, Welbourn R. Obesity treatment in the UK health system. Curr Obes Rep. 2016;5:320–6.
28. Welbourn R, et al. NICE-accredited commissioning guidance for weight assessment and management clinics: a model for a specialist multidisciplinary team approach for people with severe obesity. Obes Surg. 2016;26:649–59.
29. Andreyeva T, Puhl RM, Brownell KD. Changes in perceived weight discrimination among Americans, 1995–1996 through 2004–2006. Obes Silver Spring Md. 2008;16:1129–34.
30. Budd GM, Mariotti M, Graff D, Falkenstein K. Health care professionals' attitudes about obesity: an integrative review. Appl Nurs Res ANR. 2011;24:127–37.
31. Teachman BA, Brownell KD. Implicit anti-fat bias among health professionals: is anyone immune? Int J Obes Relat Metab Disord J Int Assoc Study Obes. 2001;25:1525–31.
32. Obesity Treatment Devices – FDA Approved Obesity Treatment Devices. Available at: http://www.fda.gov/MedicalDevices/ProductsandMedicalProcedures/ObesityDevices/ucm350134.htm.
33. Rafid R, Azagury D. Novel technologies and techniques in bariatric surgery. Minerva Chir. 2016;16:1683–4. [Epub ahead of print].

Accreditation, Quality, and Centers of Excellence

3

Wayne J. English, Teresa R. Fraker, and Amy Robinson-Gerace

Introduction

This chapter reviews the history of quality measurement and improvement and discusses its development with the current efforts surrounding accreditation and quality improvement programs being utilized by metabolic and bariatric surgeons today.

History and Timeline of Quality Improvement

Standardization of care can be traced back to 1847, when Ignaz Semmelweis in Vienna, Austria, established hand hygiene protocols in an effort to reduce maternal mortality rates attributable to puerperal fever after realizing hospital-acquired diseases were transmitted via the hands of healthcare workers [1].

W. J. English (✉)
Department of Surgical Sciences, Vanderbilt University Medical Center, Nashville, TN, USA
e-mail: wayne.english@vanderbilt.edu

T. R. Fraker
Metabolic and Bariatric Surgery Accreditation and Quality Improvement Program (MBSAQIP), American College of Surgeons, Chicago, IL, USA
e-mail: tfraker@facs.org

A. Robinson-Gerace
American College of Surgeons, Division of Research and Optimal Patient Care, Chicago, IL, USA
e-mail: agerace@facs.org

Florence Nightingale, during the Crimean War in 1850, recognized correcting sanitation issues and improving hand hygiene could significantly improve the mortality rate among soldiers treated at army hospitals with poor ventilation, sanitation, and hygiene standards [2].

Ernest Amory Codman, considered the pioneer of outcome-based quality improvement, developed a system in which he would follow up with his patients for years after treatment and record the end result to determine the effectiveness of care. His concept influenced the founding of the American College of Surgeons (ACS) in 1917 and would eventually transform into the hospital standardization movement, a forerunner to what we readily recognize today as The Joint Commission [3].

Federal supervision of healthcare would eventually follow as Congress passed the Social Security Amendments Act of 1965 mandating that hospitals participating in Medicare must be accredited by JCAH (conferred "deemed status") and be in compliance with the Medicare "Conditions of Participation." This would be revised in 1986 [4].

Avedis Donabedian, in 1966, described a conceptual framework for defining and assessing quality of healthcare services. He identified three basic components essential to quality of care (*structure, process, and outcome*), emphasizing that properly integrating these components is critical in improving the quality of care [5].

R. Lutfi et al. (eds.), *Global Bariatric Surgery*, https://doi.org/10.1007/978-3-319-93545-4_3

In 1970, the National Academy of Science established the Institute of Medicine (IOM), a nonprofit independent scientific advisor, to improve healthcare in America. The IOM changed its name to the National Academy of Medicine in 2015 [6].

In 1989, the Agency for Healthcare Policy and Research was established, currently known as the Agency for Healthcare Research and Quality (AHRQ), a public health service agency within the Department of Health and Human Services, since 2011 [7].

The National Committee for Quality Assurance (NCQA) was established in 1990 to oversee the accreditation program for managed care organizations. Performance was measured through the Health Plan Employer Data and Information Set (HEDIS), looking at six categories: access and availability, effectiveness of care, utilization of services, member satisfaction, cost of care, and health plan stability. Another instrument used to measure performance was the Consumer Assessment of Healthcare Providers and Systems (CAHPS) survey [8].

In 1992, the Health Care Financing Administration (HCFA) proposed a quality improvement initiative in an effort to achieve evidence-based continuous quality improvement based on claims data [9].

The National Patient Safety Foundation (NPSF) was established in 1996 to provide a unified voice for the patient consumer [10].

The IOM initiated several healthcare quality campaigns evaluating, informing, and improving healthcare quality in America. In 1998, the Quality of Healthcare in America initiative aimed to improve outcomes over a period of 10 years. The initial focus was on medical errors and eventually led to a report "To Err is Human: Building Safer Health Systems" [11]. It was stunning to learn that up to 98,000 deaths annually were caused by medical errors. This report prompted a number of regulatory and legislative initiatives aimed at documenting errors and seeking solutions.

In 1999, the National Quality Forum (NQF) was established with a mission to lead national collaboration to improve health and healthcare quality through measurement. NQF efforts focused on developing a national consensus with implementing standardized performance and quality metrics. NQF has a diverse membership, which includes hospitals, healthcare providers, consumer groups, purchasers, accrediting bodies, and research and healthcare quality improvement organizations [12].

In 2002, JCAHO announced a new program to sharpen the focus of the accreditation process on care systems critical to safety and quality of care. In 2003, they announced the first set of National Patient Safety Goals, which include improving the following aspects of patient care: accuracy of patient identification, effectiveness of communication among caregivers, safety of using high-alert medications, safety of using infusion pumps, and effectiveness of clinical alarm systems. An additional measure focuses on eliminating wrong site, wrong patient, and wrong procedure surgery [13].

The History of Metabolic and Bariatric Surgery and the Growing Need for Quality Improvement

The dawn of metabolic and bariatric surgery began in the 1950s with the introduction of the jejunoileal bypass. However in the 1970s, patients were advised to undergo reversal or conversion to another metabolic and bariatric procedure in order to prevent development or progression of the subsequent development of severe nutritional deficiencies, hepatic cirrhosis, and even death [14].

In 1966, Edward Mason performed the first gastric bypass connecting a loop of jejunum to the gastric pouch [15]. This technique would later be modified in 1977, introducing the Roux-en-Y configuration to replace the loop gastrojejunostomy [16].

In 1971, Dr. Mason introduced the vertical-banded gastroplasty (VBG) in an attempt to avoid the complications associated with JIB [17]. Unfortunately, less than half of the patients would maintain satisfactory weight loss after 5 years, and many patients went on to require reoperations due to staple line dehiscence, pouch dilation, band erosions, and weight loss failure [18].

In 1985, the inflatable gastric band was introduced, and, in the 1990s, the sleeve gastrectomy would be described as a component of the biliopancreatic diversion with duodenal switch procedure [19, 20].

Dr. Mason would eventually become a significant contributor in the development of the National Bariatric Surgery Registry in 1986, which produced data revealing that metabolic and bariatric surgery could be performed safely with a low mortality rate [21].

Metabolic and bariatric surgery became more widely accepted in the 1990s as Dr. Mason's and additional mounting evidence demonstrated low mortality rates, durable weight loss, and comorbidity remission. Laparoscopic techniques were described, thus initiating an expansion of the field of metabolic and bariatric surgery. However in 2005, Flum et al. revealed data indicating the risk of early death after metabolic and bariatric surgery is considerably higher than previously suggested [22].

Since the introduction of laparoscopic metabolic and bariatric surgery, there has been a steady increase in the number of surgeons performing laparoscopic metabolic and bariatric surgery. The metabolic and bariatric surgery rate per 100,000 adults increased from 6.3 in 1998 to 67.95 in 2012 [23].

In 1998, the number of metabolic and bariatric operations performed annually in the United States was 12,775, which increased to 70,256 in 2002, 135,985 in 2004, and over 196,000 in 2015. The number of metabolic and bariatric surgeons with active membership in the ASMBS increased from 131 in 1998 to 1810 in 2015. Only 2.1% of all metabolic and bariatric surgery procedures were completed laparoscopically in 1998. This proportion increased to 17.9% in 2002, greater than 90% in 2008, and greater than 98.5% in 2015 [24–27].

The expansion in the field of metabolic and bariatric surgery was not confined to the United States as an increase in procedure volume was realized in many countries worldwide. In 2013, the number of metabolic and bariatric procedures performed worldwide was 468,609 with over 95.7% of the procedures being completed laparoscopically [28].

During the growth period, many surgeons would become inadequately trained after attending an introductory course and start performing metabolic and bariatric surgery without the appropriate infrastructure necessary to provide safe care for the patient. Subsequently, significant complications occurred, high mortality rates were realized, and adverse news was regularly broadcasted on prominent national news programs. Consequently, the public and payors were seriously questioning the importance and role of metabolic and bariatric surgery as a means of treating morbid obesity. Many payors simply stopped providing insurance coverage, branding the procedures as cost-prohibitive.

The Commitment to Metabolic and Bariatric Surgery Accreditation

As the future of metabolic and bariatric surgery was at a despairing crossroad, critical measures were necessary to preserve the integrity and reputation of the profession. Intensive scrutiny and quality improvement of the services being provided by surgeons were crucial if metabolic and bariatric surgery were to become more widely accepted as a viable treatment option for morbid obesity.

In an effort to resolve these issues, the American Society for Metabolic and Bariatric Surgery (ASMBS) and the American College of Surgeons (ACS) decided to establish separate, but similar, accreditation programs to improve the quality of metabolic and bariatric surgery care.

The ASMBS Bariatric Surgery Center of Excellence (BSCOE) program was developed in 2004 to provide a mechanism that would identify programs providing high quality of metabolic and bariatric surgery care. These measures included comprehensive standardized surgical care, long-term follow-up, and management of the morbidly obese patient. The ASMBS BSCOE Program was administered by the Surgical Review Corporation.

In a parallel effort, the ACS, in 2005, gave highest priority for developing the Bariatric

Surgery Center Networks (BSCN) to improve quality and facilitate access to care for morbidly obese patients.

Both programs consisted of standards that provided an opportunity for metabolic and bariatric surgery centers to develop the infrastructure, process and outcomes to improve their standards, and education and training necessary to meet specific guidelines. Uniform data elements would be collected and outcomes compiled to provide programs with an opportunity to assess and verify risks and benefits of metabolic and bariatric surgery. The data registries for both programs in 2011 had greater than 100,000 patients per year being entered into one of the two registries.

Surgical Quality Improvement

Veterans Administration and National Surgical Quality Improvement Program (NSQIP)

The ACS NSQIP was established as a result of a government mandate to improve the quality of surgical care within the 133 Veterans Administration (VA) hospitals. In 1985, a report cited unacceptably high mortality and complication rates within the VA hospital system. A mandate in 1986 led to annual outcomes reporting in all VA hospitals and ultimately improvement in the overall quality of surgical care at VA hospitals. Risk-adjustment models were developed that would take into account the patient's severity of illness in order to level the playing field for comparison. In 1994, the VA NSQIP was created so that all VA hospitals could work in a collaborative manner to comply with the legislative mandate. As a result, mortality and morbidity rates were reduced by 27% and 45%, respectively [29]. In 1999, the ACS initiated a pilot program involving 14 academic centers and 7 private community hospitals due to the great success of the VA NSQIP. The study validated the VA NSQIP results, and thus the ACS NSQIP was officially established in 2004 [30].

Michigan Bariatric Surgery Collaborative

Additional collaborative quality improvement programs were developing across the United States in an effort to achieve the best possible patient care outcomes at the lowest reasonable cost. In 2006, the Michigan Bariatric Surgery Collaborative (MBSC) was developed and quickly gained traction with quality improvement efforts in metabolic and bariatric surgery. Collecting standardized data, there was significant variation in resource utilization and outcomes noted among participating hospitals. This ultimately resulted in the development of numerous protocols for quality and process improvement.

When data was initially collected, it was noted that approximately 10% of patients had preoperative inferior vena cava (IVC) filters inserted to prevent venous thromboembolism (VTE). There was wide variation in the use of IVC per hospital, ranging from 0% to 35%, but most IVC filter insertions were concentrated within only 5 of the 20 participating centers. The data revealed that over 50% of the mortality and permanent disability were associated with the IVC filter [31].

As a result, the members of the MBSC agreed to develop and implement statewide guidelines for a standardized approach to administering VTE prophylaxis to minimize the risks of postoperative VTE as well as reducing complications associated with IVC filters and bleeding. A risk prediction model was developed, and anticoagulation pathways were developed depending on the VTE risk assigned [32]. This effort significantly reduced the number of IVC filters being placed for metabolic and bariatric surgery patients throughout Michigan and resulted in an overall cost savings of over $4 million.

The Pitfalls of the Original Metabolic and Bariatric Surgery Accreditation Programs

There were several drawbacks with the accreditation process at the time as programs were accredited based on structural and process elements only. Accreditation was based on volume, but not on outcomes. Therefore, the accreditation process could not truly differentiate between those programs that were “excellent” and those that were not. Additionally, the existence of two accreditation programs created confusion due to slight dissimilarities within the standards, and some centers duplicated effort in data collection. Finally, access to care would be restricted as the Centers for Medicare and Medicaid Services (CMS) and some insurance payors would require one of these designations in order for metabolic and bariatric surgery centers to provide care to beneficiaries within their network. Many facilities offering high-quality service for metabolic and bariatric surgery patients could not become accredited due to difficulty meeting annual volume requirements. In 2012, it was discouraging to learn that at least one third of the ACS-accredited programs would be unable to meet the volume requirements to maintain accreditation status if the existing accreditation process were to continue.

The center of excellence (COE) program appeared to have directly contributed to improve patient outcomes as data from the Nationwide Inpatient Sample revealed in-patient mortality associated with metabolic and bariatric surgery dramatically improved from 0.8% in 1998 to 0.21% in 2003 and would decrease even further to 0.1% in 2008 [24, 25].

However, studies looking at CMS’s policy limiting metabolic and bariatric surgery coverage only to hospitals designated as “centers of excellence” found no difference in adjusted rates of complications and reoperations, as well costs savings, in the time before and after the national coverage decision [33, 34]. This would eventually lead to a policy change in which patients are no longer required to undergo surgery only at programs participating in the ASMBS BSCOE or ACS BSCN [35]. This generated a debate regarding the importance of COE programs, as there was also data strongly suggesting that COE centers were indeed the foundation of improving quality in metabolic and bariatric surgery [36, 37].

Maturation of the metabolic and bariatric surgery accreditation process allowed new evidence to emerge in order to alleviate the notorious volume requirement embedded within the previous accreditation program standards. Growing evidence supported reducing the annual volume criteria from 125 total procedures to 50 stapling cases, thus improving access to care for morbidly obese patients to undergo metabolic and bariatric surgery, while keeping a balance of maintaining high quality and safe care [38].

The New Era in Metabolic and Bariatric Surgery Quality Improvement: Metabolic and Bariatric Surgery Accreditation and Quality Improvement Program (MBSAQIP)

Lessons were learned from the previous metabolic and bariatric surgery accreditation programs, but it was NSQIP and the Michigan model that helped provide further insight allowing collaborative quality improvement to emerge as an important concept for the future development of the new accreditation program.

In 2012, the ACS and ASMBS announced that it combined their respective national metabolic and bariatric surgery accreditation programs into a single unified national accreditation program for metabolic and bariatric surgery centers, the Metabolic and Bariatric Surgery Accreditation and Quality Improvement Program (MBSAQIP). A metabolic and bariatric surgery center would achieve accreditation after following a rigorous review process to prove it can meet and maintain specific requirements. MBSAQIP provides a platform for continuous monitoring of outcomes and resource utilization, emphasizing continuous quality improvement. Currently, there are approximately 750 MBSAQIP-accredited programs in the United States [39].

Within a short period of time since the inception of MBSAQIP, a collaborative effort was undertaken to improve the value of care metabolic and bariatric surgeons provide to their patients by decreasing readmissions. The “Decreasing

Readmissions with Opportunities Provided" (DROP) project was a nationwide effort to standardize patient care pathways and identify patients at risk for readmission. Of the over 120 programs participating in the study, those with baseline readmission rates within the highest quartile realized a 32% reduction in their readmission rates. The readmission rate for all participating hospitals was decreased by 10% [40].

Several studies have demonstrated a 30-day readmission rate of between 5.1% and 7.3% for laparoscopic gastric bypass (LGBP) and approximately 5.5% for laparoscopic sleeve gastrectomy (LSG) [41–43]. More recently, MBSAQIP data revealed that the average procedure-related readmission rate for LGBP and LSG is 7.0% and 3.9%, respectively [27].

A study of insurance claims from metabolic and bariatric procedures during 2001–2002 found that the most costly aspect of metabolic and bariatric surgery was readmission. The study suggested that savings of approximately $38,000 could be realized per avoided readmission. The total risk-adjusted healthcare payments were $65,031 for readmitted patients with complications within 6-month after surgery, compared to $27,125 for non-admitted patients with complications [44]. In another study looking at costs in patients undergoing major noncardiac surgery, the average difference between patients with and without complications was $29,876 [45]. With approximately 190,000 new metabolic and bariatric surgery procedures being performed annually in the United States, approximately 9500 patients are readmitted within 30 days of their index procedure. A 10% reduction in the 30-day readmission rate, as reported in the DROP study, could possibly result in costs savings of approximately 28–36 million dollars annually.

Developing an Accredited Center and Maintaining Quality Improvement Standards

Embracing a culture of quality is critical in developing an accredited center. Formal structure and process allow objective assessment to monitor the quality and value of services provided. The following key elements must be taken into consideration when developing a high-quality metabolic and bariatric surgery program and in concordance with the current MBSAQIP standards for accreditation [46].

1. Commitment to quality care
   (a) Leadership and governance (physician and executive)
   (b) Credentialing
   (c) Designated personnel
2. Infrastructure
   (a) Equipment
   (b) Critical care support
3. Annual procedure volume and patient selection
4. Clinical pathways outlining the continuum of care
5. Data collection and analyzing evidence
6. Developing and maintaining continuous quality improvement

Safety, timeliness, effectiveness, efficiency, equitability, and patient centeredness are six key elements recommended by the IOM to accomplish fundamental changes within the healthcare system [47]. A systematic approach to quality improvement involves dedicated leaders, properly trained staff, and precise data collection. After truthful and accurate data is collected, regular data review must be performed to identify strengths and weaknesses within the center. Plans must then be implemented to correct any gaps in patient care.

Commitment to Quality Care

Leadership: Surgeon Director and Hospital Administrative Champions

One of the key components of developing a successful metabolic and bariatric surgery program is to have strong surgeon and hospital administration leadership. The surgeon director would not be expected to fully understand the business aspect of running a practice or organizing staff nor should an administrator be expected to fully understand the clinical and technical aspects of metabolic and bariatric surgery.

Once dedicated parties are involved, the center should reference the MBSAQIP standards as a guide to achieve their goals of developing and maintaining a high-quality metabolic and bariatric surgery center.

Metabolic and Bariatric Surgery (MBS) Committee

The control of the program resides in the MBS Committee and should involve, at a minimum, a surgeon director, all surgeons performing metabolic and bariatric surgery at the center, coordinator, clinical reviewer, and institutional administration representatives involved in the care of metabolic and bariatric surgical patients. While it is necessary to have a surgeon champion and administrator lead the charge in the metabolic and bariatric surgery quality movement, it is just as critical to have all surgeons practicing metabolic and bariatric surgery at the center participate on the committee. All participants of the committee should provide input toward the final decisions in developing the structure, process, and improvement plans for the metabolic and bariatric surgery program.

Other members of the MBS Committee can include, but are not limited to, charge nurses for dedicated patient areas and personnel that can provide information on services provided with patient transportation, central supply, radiology, and equipment purchasing.

The center's mission, vision, goals, and objectives of the program are discussed and agreed upon, within the MBS Committee. It provides a setting for sharing best practices, reducing practice variation, and responding to adverse events. After identifying opportunities for improvement, committee team members must be willing to enact changes in an effort to decrease complication rates, as well as improve the patient's overall experience at the center.

Surgeon Credentialing

Well-trained surgeons are essential in delivering high-quality care to metabolic and bariatric surgery patients in a consistent manner. Uniform credentialing guidelines assist centers in preparing their local credentialing criteria for metabolic and bariatric surgeons and should also include recommendations for surgeons with little or no experience. Credentialing criteria for metabolic and bariatric surgeons should be thoroughly discussed among the MBS committee members and approved before being submitted to the hospital's credentialing committee for official use by the hospital.

Metabolic and Bariatric Surgery Coordinator (MBS Coordinator)

A designated coordinator assists in center development, managing the accreditation process and ensuring continuous compliance with accreditation bodies. Other essential duties include maintaining relevant policies and procedures, patient education, outcome data collection, quality improvement efforts, and education of relevant institution staff. The coordinator supports the development of written patient care pathways and education of nurses detailing the rapid communication and basic response to critical vital signs to minimize delays in the diagnosis and treatment of serious adverse events. The coordinator also serves as the liaison between the hospital and all surgeons performing metabolic and bariatric surgery at the center.

Data Collection and the Metabolic and Bariatric Surgery Clinical Reviewer (MBSCR)

Managing data is a critical component of optimizing performance. The center must designate a person or department that is accountable for gathering the data and making it available when deemed necessary. In an effort to maintain integrity of the data and eliminate bias, the designated MBSCR should not be contributing to patient care and should work closely with the institution and clinicians to ensure that appropriate short-term and long-term data points are properly entered and available in the medical records and the database.

Annual Procedure Volume, Patient Selection, and Procedure Choice

Deciding what operation to perform or on which patient we should strongly consider not offering a surgical alternative for treatment can often be difficult. Simply put, complex cases should not be performed at a center that only performs a few metabolic and bariatric procedures per month. The MBSAQIP standards outline that more complex procedures should only be performed at centers performing at least 50 stapling procedures annually. If a center is performing fewer cases, then patient selection must be restricted to lower-risk patients.

Centers should take the necessary precautions and additional supportive measures to further assess known and undiagnosed conditions with the ultimate goal of optimizing surgical outcomes. Risk assessment should be performed on every patient and should not only apply to patient factors (BMI, comorbidities, etc.) as surgeons are deciding which procedure to perform. Additionally, resource availability, infrastructure, and surgeon and staff expertise needs to be taken into strong consideration when selecting patients for surgery. Surgeons must consider the learning curves of the personnel within the institution and should only consider operating on lower-risk patients until the center is mature enough to handle higher-risk patients appropriately.

Risk prediction models can be used to assess the patient's overall risk associated with metabolic and bariatric surgery [48–53].

Appropriate Equipment

Patient safety is the ultimate priority when maintaining a metabolic and bariatric surgery center. The center must maintain appropriate equipment and instruments for the care of metabolic and bariatric surgical patients. Personnel caring for the metabolic and bariatric surgery patient must be trained to maintain patient and staff safety while the patient is on the hospital unit and being transported to other areas of the hospital.

Critical Care Support and Training for Patient Safety

All relevant staff must be educated on the care pathway, patient safety, and complication recognition to prevent "failure to rescue" situations, in which differences in mortality are proposed to result from the failure to timely recognize, and effectively manage, a postoperative complication. Additional training for the surgical teams and the integrated health personnel in postoperative complication recognition and management may improve outcomes.

Data Review and Identifying Deficiencies and Implementing Quality Improvement

Accurate data collection, feedback, and data review are necessary in developing a high-quality metabolic and bariatric surgery program. Critical analysis and interpretation of data will help identify opportunities for improvement. Once deficiencies are recognized, the center can apply interventions for quality improvement.

Participating MBSAQIP centers have the capability of comparing their individual center data to all centers entering data into the MBSAQIP database; thus they can determine where they rank among their cohorts. This data can be critically analyzed between all surgeons at the center, which would be known as the institutional collaborative, and can take place during the MBS Committee meetings. Collectively, decisions can be made based on the data to assist in developing and implementing quality improvement measures. The camaraderie that develops from these discussions can be extremely helpful in reducing practice variation and ultimately resource utilization due to complications.

A cornerstone of the data collection and review process is the MBSAQIP Semiannual Report (SAR). The SAR is provided to participating MBSAQIP centers twice yearly in order for the center to measure their outcomes against an aggregate data set of approximately 150,000 principal operative procedures of gastric bypass, adjustable gastric band, and sleeve gastrectomy procedures. Each SAR is prepared using sophisticated modeling by expertly trained biostatisticians. While risk adjustment involves complicated statistical methods, its goal for MBSAQIP is clear: to correct for differences in patient and procedure mix so that centers can be more fairly compared. An effective risk-adjustment process based on logistic or hierarchical modeling allows centers to be compared even if there are differences in patient comorbidities or differences in the complexity of (or risks associated with) procedures performed. MBSAQIP adjusts for procedure mix by splitting procedure types into separate models. It should be kept in mind that statistical models are only approximations to reality and that no risk-adjustment process is perfect. Nevertheless, because MBSAQIP employs a large number of clinically relevant and accurately recorded risk-adjustment variables using accepted statistical methods, it seems evident that risk-adjustment is effective and useful.

In addition, institutions can elect to develop a local, statewide, or regional (involving multiple states) collaborative to establish a forum in which they can share data with one or more institutions in order to share best practices. Metabolic and bariatric surgeons can choose to meet face-to-face or arrange conference calls on a regularly scheduled basis to discuss clinical outcomes and complications based on data being entered into the MBSAQIP database.

International Participation in Data Registries and Quality Improvement

International data registries used to improve patient care in the field of metabolic and bariatric surgery include the following:

1. *Scandinavian Obesity Surgery Registry (SOReg)*: In 2004, the Scandinavian Obesity Surgery Registry (SOReg) was started, and government financing was secured to develop a national database covering all public and private hospitals. Currently, the database exceeds over 40,000 patients with participation of over 99% of the metabolic and bariatric surgery centers in Sweden [54].
2. *Bariatric Registry – Ontario Bariatric Network (OBN)*: The network was developed in an effort to examine provincial outcomes and current practices in Ontario. The registry is managed by the Centre for Surgical Intervention and Innovation in collaboration from the OBN, the Population Health Research Institute, and the Ministry of Health and Long-Term Care [55].
3. *Italian National Registry*: The Italian Society of Obesity Surgery entered data into a registry from 1996 to 2006 that included 13,871 patients, reporting that metabolic and bariatric surgery can be safely performed with low mortality [56].
4. *National Bariatric Surgery Registry-United Kingdom (NBSR-UK)*: The registry was developed in 2009 in collaboration with the Association of Laparoscopic Surgeons of Great Britain and Ireland, Association of Upper gastrointestinal Surgery, British Obesity and Metabolic Surgery Society, and Dendrite Clinical Systems, Ltd. Currently, the NBSR is the major source of data on the effectiveness of weight loss surgery in the United Kingdom. The latest published report in 2014 includes data on 18,283 procedures performed from 2010 to 2013 and contained data compiled from 161 surgeons from 137 hospitals [57].
5. *International Federation for Surgical Obesity Center of Excellence Program (IFSO-COE)*: IFSO-COE officially started in 2009 and is overseen by the European Accreditation Council for Bariatric Surgery (EAC-BS). Participating surgeons are required to submit data prospectively in the International Bariatric Surgery registry (IBAR™). At present, there are 81 centers that are certified, or under evaluation for certification, in

countries within Europe, the Middle East, and Africa [58].

6. *Bariatric Outcomes Longitudinal Database (BOLD)*: The Surgical Review Corporation (SRC) administrates the Center of Excellence (COE) and Surgeon of Excellence programs, in which there are many participating international metabolic and bariatric surgery centers, with 51 participating COE programs worldwide. Countries represented in the program include centers from Australia (1), Bahrain (2), Brazil (13), Canada (1), India (2), Mexico (2), Qatar (1), Romania (1), Saudi Arabia (2), Taiwan (1), Turkey (2), the United Arab Emirates (3), the United States (20), and the United Kingdom (1). BOLD data is used to collect long-term data to evaluate the safety and efficacy of metabolic and bariatric surgery and to establish best practices for treating obesity [59].

International Centers Participating in MBSAQIP

International Data Collection Centers is an option offered by MBSAQIP as of the first quarter of 2017. This option enables those international centers, who desire participation in the data registry, access to the reporting and benchmarking capabilities offered by MBSAQIP as is the case with domestic (the United States and Canada) centers. While International Data Collection Centers are not formally accredited by MBSAQIP, the benefits of receiving feedback on the centers' outcomes versus the aggregate data set (inclusive of the United States and Canada) are of extreme value, considering the likely different approaches to metabolic and bariatric surgical care across the globe.

One requirement to participation in the MBSAQIP data registry internationally is that the center must document in the local medical record using the English language. This is necessary in order for MBSAQIP to conduct a valid data integrity audit to measure the center against the variables and definitions used in the registry and to ensure that all MBSCRs are using and applying the definitions in a standardized fashion. Second, the center must use Current Procedural Terminology (CPT) medical coding of assigning the types of metabolic and bariatric surgical procedures that the center performs. Again, this is necessary to ensure that all centers are following the same logic as is applies to nomenclature of the most common surgical procedures such as sleeve gastrectomy and gastric bypass.

While at the present time, there are no immediate plans for MBSAQIP to evolve into the international accreditation business, this will be an area of exploration as the program continues to grow and evolve. Privacy laws and local legislative laws of each country would need to be fully investigated with adequate resources assigned to achieve such an endeavor. As the international data collection option evolves, there may be an interest by the centers to participate as a collaborative (i.e., a Middle Eastern, European, or South America collaborative), but this is yet to be determined at the present time.

Conclusion

A highly successful metabolic and bariatric surgery program requires embracing a change in safety culture, effective leadership, and a rich data registry but, mostly, a commitment to provide standardized high-quality care for metabolic and bariatric surgery patients.

Standardization of care is the basis of quality improvement and participating in an accreditation or data collection program provides the foundation necessary to ensure all metabolic and bariatric surgery centers achieve the best possible outcomes for their patients. All MBSAQIP centers are measured equitably, with the same set of standards and uniform definitions that describe patient demographics, comorbidities, and postoperative events. This robust database is an excellent resource for centers to maximize opportunity to correct deficiencies identified during regularly scheduled data review.

By participating in a program with standardized data collection, one cannot overemphasize the immeasurable value for patients as they receive care with greater efficiency, higher quality, and lower complication rates.

References

1. Best M, Neuhauser D. Heroes and martyrs of quality and safety: Ignaz Semmelweis and the birth of infection control. Qual Saf Health Care. 2004;13:233–4.
2. Marjoua Y, Bozic KJ. Brief history of quality improvement in US healthcare. Curr Rev Musculoskelet Med. 2012;5:265–73.
3. Chun J, Bafford AC. History and background of quality measurement. Clin Colon Rectal Surg. 2014;27:5–9.
4. Center for Medicare and Medicaid Services. Title XVIII of the social security act, in title 42. Center for Medicare and Medicaid Services, Editor; 1965.
5. Donabedian A. Evaluating the quality of medical care. Milbank Mem Fund Q. 1966;3(pt 2):166-2-3.
6. About the National Academy of Medicine. https://nam.edu/about-the-nam/. Accessed 4 Jan 2017.
7. Working for quality: About the National Quality Strategy (NQS) https://www.ahrq.gov/workingforquality/about.htm. Accessed 4 Jan 2017.
8. Sennett C. An introduction to the National Committee for quality assurance. Pediatr Ann. 1998;27:210–4.
9. Gagel BJ. Health care quality improvement program: a new approach. Health Care Financ Rev. 1995;16:15–23.
10. United for Patient Safety. National patient safety foundation progress report 2014–2015.
11. To Err is Human. Building a safer health system. In: Kohn LT, Corrigan JM, Donaldson MS, editors. Institute of Medicine (US) committee on quality in healthcare. Washington, DC: National Academies Press (US); 2000.
12. National Quality Forum: NQFs History. http://www.qualityforum.org/about_nqf/history/. Accessed 4 Jan 2017.
13. The Joint Commission: National Patient Safety Goals 2017. https://www.jointcommission.org/hap_2017_npsgs/. Accessed 5 Jan 2017.
14. Griffen WO Jr, Bivins BA, Bell RM. The decline and fall of the jejunoileal bypass. Surg Gynecol Obstet. 1983;157:301–8.
15. Mason EE, Ito C. Gastric bypass in obesity. Surg Clin North Am. 1967;47:1345–51.
16. Griffen WO, Young VL, Stevenson CC. A prospective comparison of gastric and jejunoileal bypass procedures for morbid obesity. Ann Surg. 1977;186(4):500–9.
17. Mason EE. Vertical banded gastroplasty for obesity. Arch Surg. 1982;117:701–6.
18. Eckhout GV, Willbanks OL, Moore JT. Vertical ring gastroplasty for morbid obesity. Five year experience with 1,463 patients. Am J Surg. 1986;152:713–6.
19. Kuzmak LI, Yap IS, McGuire L, et al. Surgery for morbid obesity. Using an inflatable gastric band. AORN J. 1990;51:1307–24.
20. Hess DS, Hess DW. Biliopancreatic diversion with a duodenal switch. Obes Surg. 1998;8:267–82.
21. Mason EE, Tang S, Renquist KE, Barnes DT, Cullen JJ, Doherty C, et al. A decade of change in obesity surgery. National Bariatric Surgery Registry (NBSR) contributors. Obes Surg. 1997;7(3):189–97.
22. Flum DR, Salem L, Elrod JA, Dellinger EP, Cheadle A, Chan L. Early mortality among Medicare beneficiaries undergoing bariatric surgical procedures. JAMA. 2005;294(15):1903–8.
23. Johnson E, Simpson A, Harvey J, Simpson K. Bariatric surgery implementation trends in the USA from 2002 to 2012. Implement Sci. 2016;11:21 Open Access. https://doi.org/10.1186/s13012-016-0382-x.
24. Nguyen NT, Root J, Zainabadi K, Sabio A, Chalfoux S, Stevens CM, Mavandadi S, Longoria M, Wilson SE. Accelerated growth of bariatric surgery with the introduction of minimally invasive surgery. Arch Surg. 2005;140(12):1198–202.
25. Nguyen NT, Masoomi H, Magno CP, Nguyen XM, Laugenour K, Lane J. Trends in use of bariatric surgery, 2003–2008. J Am Coll Surg. 2011;2013(2):621–6.
26. Ponce J, DeMaria EJ, Nguyen NT, Hutter M, Sudan R, Morton JM. American Society for Metabolic and Bariatric Surgery estimation of bariatric surgery procedures in 2015 and surgeon workforce in the United States. Surg Obes Relat Dis. 2016;12(9):1637–9.
27. MBSAQIP Public Use File. Data from January 1, 2015 to December 31, 2015.
28. Angrisani L, Santanacola A, Iovino P, Formisano G, Buchwald H, Scopinaro N. Bariatric surgery worldwide 2013. Obes Surg. 2015;25:1822–32.
29. Khuri SF, Dalet J, Henderson WG. The comparative assessment and improvement of quality of surgical care in the Department of Veterans Affairs. Arch Surg. 2002;1367(1):20–7.
30. Fink AS, Campbell DA, Mentzer RM, et al. The national surgical quality improvement program in non-veterans administration hospitals: initial demonstration of feasibility. Ann Surg. 2002;236:344–54.
31. Birkmeyer NJ, Share DA, Baser O, Carlin AM, Finks JF, Pesta CM, et al. Preoperative placement of inferior vena cava filters and outcomes after gastric bypass surgery. Ann Surg. 2010;252(6):1000–103.
32. Finks JF, English WJ, Carlin AM, Krause KR, Share DA, Banerjee M, Birkmeyer JD, Birkmeyer NJ. Predicting risk for venous thromboembolism with bariatric surgery: results from the Michigan bariatric surgery collaborative. Ann Surg. 2012;255(6):1100–4.
33. Dimick J, Nicholas LH, Ryan AM, Thumma JR, Birkmeyer JD. Bariatric surgery complications before vs. after implementation of a national policy restricting coverage to centers of excellence. JAMA. 2013;309(8):792–9.
34. Scally CP, Shih T, Thumma JR, Dimick JB. Impact of national bariatric surgery center of excellence program on medicare expenditures. J Gastrointest Surg. 2016;20(4):708–14.
35. Decision Memo for Bariatric Surgery for the Treatment of Morbid Obesity – Facility Certification Requirement (CAG-00250R3). https://www.cms.gov/medicare-coverage-database/details/nca-decision-

memo.aspx?NCAId=266&NCDId=57&ncdver=5&IsPopup=y&bc=AAAAAAAAAgAAAA%3d%3d&. Accessed 26 Jan 2017.
36. Young MT, Jafari MD, Gebhart A, Phelan MJ, Nguyen NT. A decade analysis of trends and outcomes of bariatric surgery in Medicare beneficiaries. J Am Coll Surg. 2014;219(3):480–8.
37. Azugary D, Morton JM. Bariatric surgery outcomes in US accredited vs. non-accredited centers: a systematic review. L Am Coll Surg. 2016;223(3):469–77.
38. Zevin B, Aggarwal R, Grantcharov TP. Volume-outcome association in bariatric surgery: a systematic review. Ann Surg. 2012;256(1):60–71.
39. American College of Surgeons. https://www.facs.org/search/bariatric-surgery-centers?allresults=. Accessed 26 Feb 2017.
40. Morton J, Brethauer S, Fraker T, Bradford J, Huffman K, Berger K, Petrick A, Ko C. Decreasing readmissions through opportunities provided (DROP): the first national quality improvement collaborative from the metabolic and bariatric surgery accreditation and quality improvement program (MBSAQIP). Surg Obes Relat Dis. 2016;12:S1–2.
41. Birkmeyer NJ, Dimick JB, Share D, Hawasli A, English WJ, Genaw J, et al. Hospital complication rates with bariatric surgery in Michigan. JAMA. 2010;304:435–42.
42. Saunders JK, Ballantyne GH, Belsley S, et al. 30-day readmission rates at a high volume bariatric surgery center: laparoscopic adjustable gastric banding, laparoscopic gastric bypass, and vertical banded gastroplasty-Roux-en-Y gastric bypass. Obes Surg. 2007;17(9):1171–7.
43. Hutter MM, Schirmer BD, Jones DB, et al. First report from the American College of Surgeons Bariatric Surgery Center Network: laparoscopic sleeve gastrectomy has morbidity and effectiveness positioned between the band and the bypass. Ann Surg. 2011;254(3):410–20.
44. Encinosa WE, Bernard DM, Chen C, et al. Healthcare utilization and outcomes after bariatric surgery. Med Care. 2006;44(8):706–12.
45. MBSAQIP Standards Manual v2.0. Resources for optimal care of the metabolic and bariatric surgery patient 2016.
46. Institute of Medicine (IOM). Crossing the quality chasm: a new health system for the 21st century. Washington, DC: National Academy Press; 2001.
47. DeMaria EJ, Portenier D, Wolfe L. Obesity surgery mortality risk score: proposal for a clinically useful score to predict mortality risk in patients undergoing gastric bypass. Surg Obes Relat Dis. 2007;3(2):134–40.
48. Finks JF, Kole KL, Yenumula PR, English WJ, Krause KR, Carlin AM, Genaw JA, Banerjee M, Birkmeyer JD, Birkmeyer NJ. Predicting risk for serious complications with bariatric surgery: results from the Michigan bariatric surgery collaborative. Ann Surg. 2011;254(4):633–40.
49. Ramanan B, Gupta PK, Gupta H, Fang X, Forse RA. Development and validation of a bariatric surgery mortality risk calculator. J Am Coll Surg. 2012;214(6):892–900.
50. Gupta PK, Franck C, Miller WJ, Gupta H, Forse RA. Development and validation of a bariatric surgery morbidity risk calculator using the prospective, multicenter NSQIP dataset. J Am Coll Surg. 2011;212(3):301–9.
51. Benotti P, Wood GC, Winegar DA, Petrick AT, Still CD, Argyropoulos G, Gerhard GS. Risk factors associated with mortality after Roux-en-Y gastric bypass surgery. Ann Surg. 2014;259(1):123–30.
52. Aminian A, Brethauer SA, Sharafkhah, Schauer PR. Development of a sleeve gastrectomy risk calculator. Surg Obes Relat Dis. 2015;11(4):758–64.
53. Hedenbro JL, Naslund E, Boman L, Lundeggard G, Bylund A, Ekelund M, Laurenius A, Moller P, Olbers T, Sundborn M, Ottosson J, Naslund I. Formation of the Scandinavian obesity surgery registry, SOReg. Obes Surg. 2015;25(10):1893–900.
54. Ontario Bariatric Network. http://www.ontariobariatricnetwork.ca/our-programs/surgical-program. Accessed 26 Jan 2017.
55. Morino M, Toppino M, Forestieri P, Angrisani L, Allaix ME, Scopinaro N. Mortality after bariatric surgery: analysis of 13,871 morbidly obese patients from a national registry. Ann Surg. 2007;246(6):1002–7.
56. Welbourn R, Small P, Finlay I, Sareela A, Somers S, Mahawar K on behalf of the NBSR Data Committee. The NBSR Second Registry Report 2014.
57. IFSO-endorsed COE. http://www.eac-bs.com/site/. Accessed 26 Jan 2017.
58. Surgical Review Corporation. http://www.surgicalreview.org/find-a-provider/specialties/. Accessed 27 Jan 2017.

Part II

Global Bariatric Surgery

4 Global Certifications for Surgeons and Centers

Joseph Mark Drosdeck and Samer G. Mattar

Abbreviations

ASMBS	American Society for Metabolic and Bariatric Surgery
IFSO	International Federation for the Surgery of Obesity and Metabolic Disorders
LRYGB	Laparoscopic Roux-en-Y gastric bypass
LSG	Laparoscopic sleeve gastrectomy

Introduction

The increasing prevalence of morbid obesity throughout the world presents an opportunity for bariatric surgeons to improve the longevity and quality of life for patients afflicted with this disease and its associated comorbidities [1]. However, this opportunity also challenges the international bariatric community to ensure that bariatric providers have adequate training and resources to provide the best outcomes. Surgeons, for example, must acquire the requisite skill set and experience to perform technically demanding procedures, such as the laparoscopic Roux-en-Y gastric bypass (LRYGB) and laparoscopic sleeve gastrectomy (LSG). Mastery of this procedure requires a significant learning curve, estimated at 75–100 procedures [2–4]. During this learning curve, complication rates may be significantly higher [2, 3]. Additionally, patient selection, preoperative optimization, and long-term follow-up are crucial for excellent outcomes. In order to maximize safety and establish an effective, standardized training curriculum in the USA, the American Society for Metabolic and Bariatric Surgery (ASMBS) published guidelines for bariatric privileges in 2006 [5]. With similar intentions, the International Federation for the Surgery of Obesity and Metabolic Disorders (IFSO) published guidelines in 2007 [5]. Unlike the USA, however, many countries do not have well-established fellowship programs that allow junior surgeons to perform bariatric procedures under the supervision of experienced mentors [5]. Heterogeneity, variability, and inconsistency in bariatric training are therefore among the challenges that must be addressed in order to meet the worldwide demand for skilled bariatric surgeons.

Bariatric Surgery in the USA

The USA experienced exponential growth in the volume of bariatric operations performed between 1997 and 2004, a period also characterized by a

J. M. Drosdeck
General Surgery, The Everett Clinic, Everett, WA, USA
e-mail: Jdrosdeck@everettclinic.com

S. G. Mattar (✉)
Swedish Weight Loss Services, Swedish Medical Center, Seattle, WA, USA
e-mail: mattar@ohsu.edu

R. Lutfi et al. (eds.), *Global Bariatric Surgery*, https://doi.org/10.1007/978-3-319-93545-4_4

paradigm shift from open to laparoscopic procedures. According to insurance company data, albeit unpublished, this was associated with an increase in operative morbidity and mortality [3]. However, this finding may be a manifestation of the learning curve for the adoption of the laparoscopic approach to bariatric surgery, well recognized to add a technically challenging dimension to already complex procedures. Since that time, there has been a focus on the role of both surgeon and institutional volume in relation to patient outcomes. High-volume surgeons and institutions have both been associated with significant improvements in morbidity and mortality [6–8]. With regard to surgeons, the goal is to identify the best method of guiding trainees through the learning curve of laparoscopic bariatric surgery safely and efficiently.

The first opportunity to initiate this process is during general surgery residency, as it is clear that general surgery residents currently lack the necessary skill set to perform bariatric procedures and achieve the same outcomes as experienced bariatric surgeons. Untrained resident participation in these complex cases may have a negative impact on patient outcomes. For example, Krell et al. reported that resident participation in laparoscopic gastric bypass was an independent risk factor for two postoperative complications likely mediated by longer operative times: wound infections and venous thromboembolism [9]. These findings highlight the need to identify strategies to improve technique and proficiency prior to assisting in the operating room. Furthermore, general surgery residency often provides inadequate training for advanced subspecialty fellowships. A global assessment survey designed by the Fellowship Council research committee was sent to fellowship program directors in minimally invasive, bariatric, colorectal, hepatobiliary, and thoracic surgery specialties. The disappointing results revealed significant deficiencies across multiple domains, including independent practice ability, patient responsibility, motor skills, and academic interest. Respondents stated that 21% of incoming fellows arrived unprepared for the operating room, 30% could not independently perform a laparoscopic cholecystectomy, and 66% were unable to operate for 30 unsupervised minutes during a major procedure. With regard to laparoscopy, 30% could not manipulate tissues atraumatically, 26% could not recognize tissue planes, and 56% could not suture [10]. Clearly, this highlights a significant challenge faced by residency and fellowship program directors with implications beyond bariatric surgery training. However, it emphasizes the need for accreditation bodies to adapt general surgery training to keep pace with the technological advancements and changing skill sets that have reshaped the modern-day practice of bariatrics and general surgery.

For those who have completed general surgery residency and seek additional bariatric training, there are currently several options. The most comprehensive training regimen is a year-long minimally invasive/bariatric surgery fellowship. Offered at numerous academic and private bariatric centers throughout the USA, these fellowships provide comprehensive experience in the surgical and perioperative care of bariatric patients under the mentorship of experienced bariatric surgeons. There is evidence supporting the efficacy of this training model. Hsu et al. suggest that the training background of practicing bariatric surgeons influences patient outcomes. Using a retrospective analysis, they identified significant differences in intraoperative blood loss and complications, hospital length of stay, admission to intensive care unit, and late complications. They suggested that participation in a dedicated laparoscopic fellowship may improve outcomes during the learning curve [11]. This assertion has also been echoed by others. In a pilot study by Oliak et al., the outcomes of two practicing bariatric surgeons, one with and one without fellowship training, were compared. The fellowship trained surgeon had significantly less major complications and operative times [2]. Stronger evidence comes from Ali et al., who evaluated complication rates among newly graduated minimally invasive/bariatric fellows during their first 100 consecutive LRYGBs and found them to be comparable to that of the fellows' experienced mentors. They concluded that fellowship graduates can immediately achieve excellent outcomes, and year-long fellowships can eliminate the learning curve for laparoscopic bariatric surgeons who newly embark on this career without prior fellowship training [12].

With the growing obesity epidemic, however, there is concern that the limited number of bariatric fellowships is unlikely to produce enough bariatric surgeons to meet the demand. Therefore, alternate training methods have been established. For experienced community surgeons desiring to incorporate bariatrics into their practice, a year-long fellowship may be impractical and unnecessary. For these individuals, the mini-fellowship concept provides a focused 6-week training program in laparoscopic bariatric surgery. This program supplements existing knowledge and skill, allowing fully trained surgeons to safely and successfully incorporate bariatrics into their current practice [13]. There is evidence to suggest that with the appropriate skill set and mentorship, the learning curve for LRYGB can be mitigated, and bariatric procedures can be safely incorporated into the repertoire of the experienced community laparoscopic surgeon [14].

Current recommendations to obtain privileges in bariatric surgery come from two major surgical societies: the American Society for Metabolic and Bariatric Surgery (ASMBS) and the Society of American Gastrointestinal and Endoscopic Surgeons (SAGES). They determine the minimum amount of experience, expertise, and support necessary for general surgeons who wish to acquire hospital privileges in bariatric surgery. SAGES published their guidelines in 2003 and 2011 with the following recommendations: completion of a general surgery residency program and formal training in both open and laparoscopic bariatric surgery. They further recommended a structured curriculum for those without formal residency or fellowship training in bariatric surgery with documented practical experience. Additionally, practical experience must be documented [15, 16]. However, these recommendations do not specify a specific number of cases to be performed.

The American Society for Metabolic and Bariatric Surgery, formerly the American Society for Bariatric Surgery (ASBS), also published guidelines in 2003 with updates in 2006. For global credentialing requirements, applicants should achieve four main criteria: (1) have credentials at an accredited facility; (2) work with an integrated, multidisciplinary team providing comprehensive care to bariatric patients (nurses, dietitians, psychologists); (3) establish a program to prevent, monitor, and manage all postoperative complications; and (4) establish a system that provides adequate follow-up for patients. For procedures, they distinguish between procedures that require stapling/division of the gastrointestinal tract and those that do not. They also recommend that a certain number of procedures be performed under the supervision of an experienced bariatric surgeon in residency or post-residency training. Fifteen open cases are required for open bariatric privileges, whereas 50 laparoscopic stapling procedures are required for laparoscopic privileges. Furthermore, they emphasize comprehensive pre- and postoperative care of bariatric patients, as well as long-term follow-up [17].

While there is general agreement that skill level correlates positively with experience, the minimum number of procedures to achieve competence in bariatric surgery is unclear. Current case volume requirements for bariatric surgery fellows were developed by the Fellowship Council and the ASMBS. To receive certification, fellows are required to act as the primary surgeon during 51 procedures requiring stapling of anastomosis of the gastrointestinal tract and 10 gastric restrictive procedures. Overall, they must complete 100 weight loss operations [18].

Although case volume provides an easy method for gaging trainee experience, it does not necessarily ensure competence. Thus, a competency-based platform has emerged in the USA for bariatric surgery trainees and is currently being piloted at select centers across the country. Participants in this new program are fellows in minimally invasive/bariatric surgery who have successfully completed general surgery residency. In addition to recording case volume, competence in bariatric procedures will be assessed by instructors via a modular program utilizing entrustable professional activities

(EPAs). Among the major benefits of entrustment-based assessments are that they compare current performance against what will be required in future independent practice. This provides the basis for assessing a trainee's progression to competence and their readiness for independent practice [19]. With the increasing prevalence of competency-based medical education, it seems plausible that training programs utilizing EPAs may someday become the standard in bariatrics and other sub-specialties.

Bariatric Surgery in Europe

Like most of the world, European nations have also experienced a drastic rise in obesity in the twenty-first century [1] which have coincided with an increase in bariatric procedures [20]. Gastric bypass is the most common bariatric procedure performed (38% of all bariatric procedures) but is closely followed by sleeve gastrectomy (37%), which has rapidly increased. Although there is variability among nations, throughout the continent as a whole, 97% of bariatric procedures are performed laparoscopically [20]. The struggle for European surgeons to meet the demand for bariatric procedures mirrors that of the USA. Factors contributing to this challenge include the technically challenging nature of the procedures, need for multidisciplinary resources for comprehensive care with long-term follow-up, and lack of well-established fellowship training programs [5].

To fill this void, several medical societies have published guidelines for training and obtaining practice privileges. The International Federation for the Surgery of Obesity and Metabolic Disorders (IFSO) recommends formal bariatric training in the form of 2-day courses, mini-fellowships, or mentoring programs [5]. Similarly, the Spanish Society of Surgery Obesity and Metabolic Diseases (SECO) developed a training program which includes practical courses, a 2-month fellowship, and a mentoring program during the first 40 cases for new bariatric surgeons. This mentor-initiated approach was offered to address the marked diversity in bariatric training previously being offered [5]. A systematic review published by Sanchez-Santos et al. suggests that this mentorship approach lead by an experienced bariatric surgeon significantly reduces complications during early cases performed by a new bariatric surgeon to acceptable levels equivalent with experienced groups [5]. This training paradigm may prove to be an effective strategy to meet the demand for bariatric surgeons in Europe.

Bariatric Surgery in Asia

Obesity is increasing in Asia with the adoption of a Western diet and lifestyle [1, 21]. This has led to a marked increase in the number of bariatric procedures being performed. In an investigation of a 5-year trend in bariatric procedures from 2005 to 2009, Lomanto et al. report a 449% absolute growth rate of bariatric surgery in Asia with laparoscopic adjustable gastric banding (LAGB) and LRYGB being the most common procedures performed at 35.9% and 24.3%, respectively [22]. However, bariatric surgery is still a relatively uncommon procedure outside of Taiwan and South Korea [21, 22]. In fact, Lomanto et al. reported a mere 155 bariatric surgeons throughout Asia during their 5-year span of their investigation [22]. Although there are notable limitations of their dataset (incomplete date, omission of China), the numbers are surprising and indicate a dire need to provide these countries with qualified bariatric surgeons. This is especially true when considering the decreased utilization of LAGB by many bariatric surgeons in other parts of the world, which has been supplanted by LRYGB and LSG, procedures with better long-term results but are more technically challenging. Additionally, the propensity for individuals of Asian descent to develop comorbid diseases at a lower BMI has led to a reduction in the BMI threshold to define one as overweight and obese to 23 and 27.5, respectively [22]. These represent some of the unique challenges that must be addressed in order to adequately address the obesity epidemic in Asia.

The Asian-Pacific Bariatric Surgery Group (APBSG) was established in Seoul in 2004 and publishes professional guidelines for providers in the region. Current qualifications for bariatric surgery in Asian populations include BMI > 37 or BMI > 32 with concurrent diabetes or two other significant obesity-related comorbidities, failure of medical weight loss, and age 18–65 [21, 23]. Additionally, the APBSG acknowledges the need for additional bariatric surgeons to meet the growing demand. However, the increase in bariatric procedures being performed in Asia has been associated with escalating complications. The APBSG is therefore developing training centers and recruiting experienced surgeons to help new surgeons safely navigate the learning curve. Interestingly, the APBSG recommended that LAGB be considered as the primary bariatric procedure for Asian countries at the beginning of surgical treatment of obesity due to its lower short-term complications [23]. It seems likely, however, that this recommendation will change, with practice patterns favoring LRYGB and LSG, in suit with trends in the rest of the world.

As the world's most populous country affected by the global obesity epidemic, China may be facing the greatest demand for bariatric surgeons. However, there is a surprising lack of data about the practice of bariatric surgery in China. Central to this problem is a lack of a national registry which would provide useful demographic information about patients and the practice patterns of bariatric surgeons. However, Du et al. published the first investigation of trends in bariatric surgery in China between 2001 and 2015. They concluded that although bariatric surgery is at an early stage, it is experiencing tremendous growth – the number of bariatric procedures increased 148.7 times in the last 5 years compared to 2001–2005. Of all procedures performed, 89.4% were performed laparoscopically, and the most common procedure was LRYGB (55.5%) followed by LAGB (19%) and LSG (11.5%) [24]. In order to advance bariatric practices in China, the Chinese Society for Metabolic and Bariatric Surgery aims to develop a national registry and establishes indications for surgery and treatment standards specific to the Chinese population [24]. This will be a crucial first step toward meeting the extraordinary demand for bariatric surgery in China.

Bariatric Surgery in Latin America

Latin America is a region with great potential for growth and development of laparoscopic bariatric surgery, and perhaps the country with the highest demand for bariatric surgeons is Brazil. With 52% of its population overweight or obese, millions of people are affected [25]. Currently, Brazil is second only to the USA with regard to the annual number of bariatric operations performed and experienced a 300% growth in the number of bariatric operations performed in the last 10 years [26]. However, there remains a significant need for bariatric surgeons in this country and throughout Latin America. With the goal of addressing this need, the Brazilian Society for Bariatric Surgery (now the Brazilian Society for Bariatric and Metabolic Surgery – SBCBM) was founded in 1996 and is 1 of 17 National Societies of the Latin American Chapter of the IFSO [26]. Their achievements provide an excellent example of the positive impact that can be accomplished by a professional medical society tasked with the goal of improving access to quality care. For instance, the SBCBM worked with the Brazilian government to increase the percentage of operations covered by the Unified Brazilian Health System, collaborated with other Brazilian surgical societies to create guidelines aimed at improving safety and outcomes after bariatric surgery, and advocated for the use of laparoscopy in public hospitals [25, 26]. The important and ongoing work of the SBCBM highlights the success that can be achieved by a dedicated medical society, one that may be useful model for other countries in Latin America, and worldwide, seeking to develop the medical infrastructure to provide quality bariatric services.

Role of Simulation in Bariatric Training

Due to the steep learning curve of laparoscopic bariatric procedures and the increased rates of complications associated with early experience, much focus has been placed on the ideal training method for bariatric procedures. Simulation represents an attractive modality by offering the ability to develop technical skills in a low-stakes setting. Published studies have demonstrated that simulation reduces the learning curve for basic laparoscopic procedures and may improve technical performance in the operating room [27]. This can serve as a useful compliment to real-world operative experience, which is particularly important for laparoscopic bariatric procedures that have a steep learning curve. Current modalities for laparoscopic simulation include anesthetized animals, human cadavers, virtual reality simulators, and laparoscopic box trainers. Although anesthetized animals and human cadavers offer a more realistic experience, these resources are more difficult to acquire and more expensive. However, teaching LRYGB in the operating room also carries a significant expense. It has been estimated that the cost of teaching a two-layer enteroenterostomy to a surgical trainee in the operating room is € 1082 ($1215) [27]. Moreover, the increasing global attention to improving patient quality and safety outcomes is compelling mentors and trainees to identify training techniques outside the operating room. Zevin et al. present a framework for a comprehensive ex vivo training curriculum in laparoscopic bariatric surgery defined by the following steps: knowledge-based learning, deconstruction of procedures into tasks, training in the laboratory environment, transfer of skills to the real environment, and lastly, granting privileges for operating room practice [27]. This conceptual training platform represents a proficiency-based framework of graduated responsibility that balances trainee education with patient safety.

Endoscopy in Bariatric Patients

Ensuring good outcomes for bariatric patients extends beyond the operative skills, and bariatric surgeons should be capable of providing comprehensive care for their patients before and after surgery. Upper endoscopy (UE) plays a significant role in perioperative care and should be in the armamentarium of all bariatric surgeons. An important area of controversy, however, is the role of preoperative screening endoscopy. This provides the theoretical advantage of diagnosing pathologies that could change clinical management, such as peptic ulcer disease, hiatal hernia, gastroesophageal reflux disease, and *Helicobacter pylori* infection. However, UE is an invasive procedure associated with significant cost and some risk. Additionally, there is controversy regarding the actual actionable yield of UEs that lead to changes in surgical management. Although professional societies provide their own recommendations, there is no global consensus. This will be an important topic as countries throughout the world combat the obesity epidemic and bariatric procedures become more common.

The European Association for Endoscopic Surgery (EAES) guidelines state that UE is advisable prior to all bariatric procedures (grade C recommendation) and is strongly recommended prior to gastric bypass (grade B recommendation) [28]. However, this practice does not seem to be universally adopted throughout Europe. A survey of British Obesity and Metabolic Surgery Society members at National Health Service bariatric units throughout the United Kingdom indicates that 44 of 49 responding units (90%) use preoperative UE either routinely (15 units; 31%) or selectively (29 units; 59%). Five units (10%), however, deemed preoperative UE unnecessary or too risky [29]. In contrast, SAGES recommends preoperative UE "if suspicion for gastric pathology exists" [30]. Similarly, ASMBS guidelines recommend evaluation of "clinically significant gastrointestinal symptoms" with UE or upper gastrointestinal series (grade D recommendation) [31]. A systematic review and meta-analysis by Bennett et al. reveal that endoscopic findings result in alteration of surgical management in 0.4–7.8% of patients, depending on the interpretation by the surgeon. They conclude that routine preoperative UE is therefore unnecessary in the absence of clear clinical indications [32].

Currently, there are no recommendations from IFSO or any Asian medical society on this topic. As such, Lee et al. set out to define the prevalence of clinically significant lesions in the Chinese bariatric population. In a retrospective analysis, they report that 27% had abnormalities on UE that may delay or change surgical approach and therefore recommend routine preoperative UE for all bariatric patients [33]. It is possible that regional, environmental, and ethnic differences may play a role in determining the utility of UE before bariatric surgery, but further data is needed before firm recommendations can be made.

There is, however, a more significant need for the acquisition of endoscopic skills, such as the therapeutic aspect of this modality. Many bariatric patients will need postoperative evaluation of their foregut for a variety of symptoms related to bleeding marginal ulcers, strictures, gastrogastric fistulas, staple line leaks, etc. For example, stent placement and endoluminal suturing are two examples of therapeutic endoscopy that are now commonly being performed by bariatric surgeons. Additionally, there is a growing interest among providers and patients in endoscopic weight loss devices, such as intragastric balloons, intestinal liners, and modified gastrostomy tube-type devices (Aspire).

Future Directions

The current obesity epidemic represents an opportunity for general surgeons to improve the duration and quality of life for many people throughout the world. However, numerous countries affected by the obesity epidemic lack an established training infrastructure capable of producing qualified bariatric surgeons to meet the demands of the population. This represents an equally significant challenge and opportunity. Established leaders in bariatric surgery and surgical societies can provide mentorship to developing centers and help institute established, effective training protocols. Certainly, adaptation of a universal training standard faces many barriers. Differences in existing training techniques, institutional resources, and financial constraints vary by region and represent some of the challenges to be overcome. However, there is a growing body of evidence that the year-long fellowship model established in the USA mitigates the learning curve for bariatric procedures and correlates with improved outcomes [2, 12, 34]. This may serve as a valuable template for developing bariatric centers who seek credentialing and desire to institute and customize a training curriculum that fits with the needs and resources of their community. It would also serve to protect patients from unsafe practices and ensure oversight of new technologies as they become available. International collaboration with a focus on proficiency standards, accreditation, and effective use of simulation represents some of the cornerstones required for the global bariatric community to ensure effective training for surgeons and quality care for patients.

References

1. Ahima RS. Digging deeper into obesity. J Clin Invest. 2011;121:2076–9.
2. Oliak D, Owens M, Schmidt HJ. Impact of fellowship training on the learning curve for laparoscopic gastric bypass. Obes Surg. 2004;14:197–200.
3. Schirmer BD, Schauer PR, Flum DR, Ellsmere J, Jones DB. Bariatric surgery training: getting your ticket punched. J Gastrointest Surg. 2007;11:807–12.
4. Schauer P, Ikramuddin S, Hamad G, Gourash W. The learning curve for laparoscopic Roux-en-Y gastric bypass is 100 cases. Surg Endosc. 2003;17:212–5.
5. Sanchez-Santos R, Estevez S, Tome C, et al. Training programs influence in the learning curve of laparoscopic gastric bypass for morbid obesity: a systematic review. Obes Surg. 2012;22:34–41.
6. Courcoulas A, Schuchert M, Gatti G, Luketich J. The relationship of surgeon and hospital volume to outcome after gastric bypass surgery in Pennsylvania: a 3-year summary. Surgery. 2003;134:613–21; discussion 21–3.
7. Flum DR, Dellinger EP. Impact of gastric bypass operation on survival: a population-based analysis. J Am Coll Surg. 2004;199:543–51.
8. Nguyen NT, Paya M, Stevens CM, Mavandadi S, Zainabadi K, Wilson SE. The relationship between hospital volume and outcome in bariatric surgery at academic medical centers. Ann Surg. 2004;240:586–93; discussion 93–4.
9. Krell RW, Birkmeyer NJ, Reames BN, et al. Effects of resident involvement on complication rates after laparoscopic gastric bypass. J Am Coll Surg. 2014;218:253–60.
10. Mattar SG, Alseidi AA, Jones DB, et al. General surgery residency inadequately prepares trainees for fellowship: results of a survey of fellowship program directors. Ann Surg. 2013;258:440–9.

11. Hsu GP, Morton JM, Jin L, Safadi BY, Satterwhite TS, Curet MJ. Laparoscopic Roux-en-Y gastric bypass: differences in outcome between attendings and assistants of different training backgrounds. Obes Surg. 2005;15:1104–10.
12. Ali MR, Tichansky DS, Kothari SN, et al. Validation that a 1-year fellowship in minimally invasive and bariatric surgery can eliminate the learning curve for laparoscopic gastric bypass. Surg Endosc. 2010;24:138–44.
13. Cottam D, Holover S, Mattar SG, et al. The mini-fellowship concept: a six-week focused training program for minimally invasive bariatric surgery. Surg Endosc. 2007;21:2237–9.
14. Shin RB. Evaluation of the learning curve for laparoscopic Roux-en-Y gastric bypass surgery. Surg Obes Relat Dis. 2005;1:91–4.
15. Clements R, Saber A, Teixeira J, et al. Guidelines for institutions granting bariatric privileges utilizing laparoscopic techniques. Society of American Gastrointestinal and Endoscopic Surgeons Guidelines Committee. Surg Endosc. 2011;25:671–6.
16. Society of American Gastrointestinal Endoscopic S. Guidelines for institutions granting bariatric privileges utilizing laparoscopic techniques. Society of American Gastrointestinal Endoscopic Surgeons (SAGES) and the SAGES Bariatric Task Force. Surg Endosc. 2003;17:2037–40.
17. Committee ABT. American Society for Bariatric Surgery's guidelines for granting privileges in bariatric surgery. Surg Obes Relat Dis. 2006;2:65–7.
18. The Fellowship Council and The American Society for Metabolic and Bariatric Surgery Advanced GI Surgery Curriculum for Bariatric Surgery Fellowship. 2007. At https://fellowshipcouncil.org/wp-content/uploads/2012/02/Bariatric-Surgery1.pdf.
19. Rekman J, Gofton W, Dudek N, Gofton T, Hamstra SJ. Entrustability scales: outlining their usefulness for competency-based clinical assessment. Acad Med. 2016;91:186–90.
20. Angrisani L, Santonicola A, Iovino P, Formisano G, Buchwald H, Scopinaro N. Bariatric surgery worldwide 2013. Obes Surg. 2015;25:1822–32.
21. Kasama K, Tagaya N, Kanahira E, et al. Has laparoscopic bariatric surgery been accepted in Japan? The experience of a single surgeon. Obes Surg. 2008;18:1473–8.
22. Lomanto D, Lee WJ, Goel R, et al. Bariatric surgery in Asia in the last 5 years (2005–2009). Obes Surg. 2012;22:502–6.
23. Lee WJ, Wang W. Bariatric surgery: Asia-Pacific perspective. Obes Surg. 2005;15:751–7.
24. Du X, Dai R, Zhou HX, et al. Bariatric surgery in China: how is this new concept going? Obes Surg. 2016;26(12):2906–12. Review.
25. Campos JM. The Brazilian Society of Bariatric and Metabolic Surgery – Sbcbm – prioritizes encouraging of scientific production. Arq Bras Cir Dig. 2015;28(Suppl 1):1.
26. Campos JM, Ramos AC, Cohen R. The importance of Brazilian Society of Metabolic and Bariatric Surgery and its interaction with the Xxi world congress of Ifso in Brazil. Arq Bras Cir Dig. 2016;29(Suppl 1):1–2.
27. Zevin B, Aggarwal R, Grantcharov TP. Simulation-based training and learning curves in laparoscopic Roux-en-Y gastric bypass. Br J Surg. 2012;99:887–95.
28. Sauerland S, Angrisani L, Belachew M, et al. Obesity surgery: evidence-based guidelines of the European Association for Endoscopic Surgery (EAES). Surg Endosc. 2005;19:200–21.
29. Zanotti D, Elkalaawy M, Hashemi M, Jenkinson A, Adamo M. Current status of preoperative oesophago-gastro-duodenoscopy (OGD) in bariatric NHS units-a BOMSS survey. Obes Surg. 2016;26:2257–62.
30. Committee SG. SAGES guideline for clinical application of laparoscopic bariatric surgery. Surg Endosc. 2008;22:2281–300.
31. Mechanick JI, Youdim A, Jones DB, et al. Clinical practice guidelines for the perioperative nutritional, metabolic, and nonsurgical support of the bariatric surgery patient – 2013 update: cosponsored by American Association of Clinical Endocrinologists, the Obesity Society, and American Society for Metabolic & Bariatric Surgery. Surg Obes Relat Dis. 2013;9:159–91.
32. Bennett S, Gostimir M, Shorr R, Mallick R, Mamazza J, Neville A. The role of routine preoperative upper endoscopy in bariatric surgery: a systematic review and meta-analysis. Surg Obes Relat Dis. 2016;12:1116–25.
33. Lee J, Wong SK, Liu SY, Ng EK. Is preoperative upper gastrointestinal endoscopy in obese patients undergoing bariatric surgery mandatory? An Asian perspective. Obes Surg. 2017;27(1):44–50. https://doi.org/10.1007/s11695-016-2243-8.
34. Kim PS, Telem DA, Altieri MS, et al. Bariatric outcomes are significantly improved in hospitals with fellowship council-accredited bariatric fellowships. J Gastrointest Surg. 2015;19:594–7.

5 Bariatric and Metabolic Surgery in Latin America

Camilo Boza, Ricardo Funke, Ricardo Flores, and Fernando Muñoz

Introduction

Obesity could be defined as an excess of body fat, accompanied by an increase of the relation between weight and height. Operationally, obesity can be considered as the condition in which body mass index (BMI) is greater than 30.1 kg/m^2.

The etiology is multifactorial. It is result of the conjunction of biological, genetic, and ambient factors. The greater association is with lifestyle [1, 2].

The concern about obesity lies not only in its effects on health and quality of life of people who suffer from it but also in its association with the most prevalent non-transmissible diseases of actuality such as cardiovascular diseases, diabetes, high blood pressure, osteomuscular diseases, and some kinds of cancer. Obesity could reduce life expectations and represent a high economic cost for patients and society [3].

Obesity is a public health problem. It affects mostly First World countries and developing countries [2]. A question to resolve is to determine if the observed prevalence constitutes a public health problem or is a speculation derived from the situation in the most developed countries [4]. This assertion would be based on an almost linear projection of the epidemiological transition, without regard to the dynamics of corrections [4].

Another factor that should be addressed is whether the situation is homogeneous in the different countries of Latin America or varies according to the stages of the epidemiological transition or the level of economic development achieved. This would determine if in some geographical areas, we would be facing an epidemic of obesity, or it would be more appropriate to point out that it is a localized endemic or a simple temporary trend change [5].

Trends and Extent of the Problem

The evolution of obesity has been observed in countries such as Chile, Mexico, Brazil, Argentina, Peru, Colombia, Guatemala, and Bolivia among others [6].

In Brazil, for example, national studies show an increase in the prevalence of obesity from 1974 to the present from 2% to 5% and from 7% to 12% in men and women, respectively.

In Mexico, national studies showed an increase in the prevalence of obesity in the female population, increasing from 9.4% to 24.44%.

Studies in Chile also showed an alarming increase in obesity numbers from 6% in 1987 to 18% in 2000 [8].

The population in Latin America and the Caribbean has increased systematically.

C. Boza (✉) · R. Funke · R. Flores · F. Muñoz
Department of Digestive Surgery, Clinica Las Condes, Santiago, Chile
e-mail: CBOZA@CLC.CL; RFUNKE@CLC.CL

R. Lutfi et al. (eds.), *Global Bariatric Surgery*, https://doi.org/10.1007/978-3-319-93545-4_5

According to the records of the United Nations, an estimated total of 632,381,000 inhabitants is estimated by 2015. Of these total, according to the IFSO 2016 register of member countries, a total population of 536,664,563 inhabitants (84.8%) is registered. Of these, Brazil and Mexico represent the most populated, representing about 56% of the population of Latin America. This has a direct economic implication, since Mexico presents a 30% of obesity in their total population and Brazil a 13.9% of obesity in their total population. Between the two countries, it's estimated 60 million obese people (Table 5.1).

Venezuela is the country with the highest percentage of obese population (30.3%), followed by Mexico with 30% and Argentina with 29.7% (Table 5.1). In Latin America, according to countries that have adequate records of their population, the percentage of obese people is near 27% with a total close to 61 million.

In the United States, it is estimated that there live an about 47 million Hispanics which represent 15% of the total population. In 2010, the National Hispanic Caucus of State Legislators in a policy summary report the growth of obesity in this population compared to non-Hispanic whites. By comparing rates of overweight and obesity, Latinos outnumber the general population by ten percentage points. Compared to the general female population, Mexican-American women have the highest percentage of overweight and obesity (73%) (Table 5.2) [7].

Bariatric Surgery in Latin America

Since Friedman et al. published in 1955 their observations in three diabetic patients undergoing partial gastrectomy with gastrojejunal reconstruction who improved from the viewpoint of hyperglycemia, a breakthrough was initiated with multiple studies. In Latin America, Álvarez Cordero (Mexico) was a pioneer in introducing bariatric surgery and observing their metabolic effects [8].

Table 5.2 Overweight and obesity in Hispanic American population

	Overweight (obesity included)		Obesity	
	20–74 years, adjusted age			
	1976–1980	2003–2006	1976–1980	2003–2006
	Population percentage			
General population (both genders)	47.4	66.9	15.1	34.1
Males	52.9	72.6	12.8	33.1
Females	42	61.2	17.1	35.2
Mexican males	61.6	77.3	15.7	30.4
Mexican females	61.7	74.4	26.6	42.6

Table 5.1 Percentage of obese people according to the IFSO 2016 records

Ranking	Country	Total population	% of obese population	Total obese population
1	Venezuela	33,221,865	30.3%	10,066,225
2	Mexico	109,219,200	30.0%	32,765,760
3	Argentina	41,446,246	29.7%	12,309,535
4	Panama	3,608,431	25.4%	916,506
5	Chile	17,248,000	25.1%	4,329,248
6	Costa Rica	4,586,353	23.7%	1,086,965
7	Ecuador	15,223,680	21.4%	3,257,867
8	Dominican Republic	9,445,281	21.2%	2,002,399
9	Guatemala	14,388,929	19.2%	2,762,674
10	Bolivia	9,786,000	17.9%	1,751,694
11	Paraguay	6,802,295	17.9%	1,217,610
12	Peru	30,911,183	17.5%	5,409,457
13	Colombia	46,044,600	17.3%	7,965,715
14	Brazil	194,732,500	13.9%	27,067,817
	Total	209,330,095	27.4%	61,474,239

Due to the magnitude of the problem, as a worldwide epidemic associated with high morbidity and mortality, the International Federation for the Surgery of Obesity (IFSO) was created in 1995 with 8 member countries progressively increasing to 31 nations in 2003 [9, 10].

Due to the lack of international data in bariatric surgery, the data collection begins with four general questions to the members:

1. How many bariatric surgeries are being performed annually in your country?
2. How many surgeons practice bariatric surgery in your country?
3. When did bariatric surgery begin in your country?
4. When did your country join IFSO?

From Latin America only Argentina, Brazil, Panama, and Mexico participated in this study. The results are shown in Table 5.3.

According to the 2002–2003 data, a total number of 146.301 surgeries were estimated. In that ranking, Brazil was in the fourth place worldwide with 4000 surgical procedures [11].

The number of surgeries performed in Latin America increases exponentially until 2013 with a total of 468,609 reported, an increase of 39% between the years 2011 and 2013. This number represents 30.5% of the total worldwide bariatric surgeries (Table 5.4 – Fig. 5.1).

Respecting the types of bariatric surgery performed in Latin America, the trend shows that from 2003 to 2008, gastric bypass (RYGB) has increased sharply, with a plateau of 57.9% in 2011 and 65% in 2013; however, RYGB still represents the most accomplished bariatric/metabolic procedure in Latin America, which is heavily influenced by Brazil, with a total of 66,000 RYGB (67.7%) out of a total of 97,480 bariatric surgeries [12].

Vertical gastrectomy (SG) increased from 0.0% in 2003 to 9.2% in 2008 to 30.1% in 2011 but decreased in 2013 (−5.1%). The AGB fell from 61.5% in 2003 to 20.4% (−41.1%) in 2008 and continued to decline in 2011 (−15.1%) and 2013 (−1.3%) (Tables 5.5 and 5.6; Figs. 5.2 and 5.3).

Obesity as a global epidemic has forced the development of government policies to stop the socioeconomic impact of this pathology and its associated comorbidities. The development of dietary guidelines for different age groups, especially the infant as a more susceptible group, will enable to tackle obesity early.

In the future, it is likely that the number of bariatric surgeries in Latin America will continue to increase, observing that the vertical gastrectomy and laparoscopic gastric bypass are the two most frequent surgeries; however, there are other surgical and endoscopic techniques that will be developed and consolidating that will be a complement in the therapeutic arsenal against this global disease.

Table 5.4 Number of bariatric surgeries worldwide and in Latin America between 2003 and 2013

	Worldwide	Latin America	%
1997	40,000		
2003	146,301	2700	1.8
2008	344,221	44,242	12.9
2011	340,768	102,984	30.2
2013	468,609	143,038	30.5

Table 5.3 IFSO global survey 2003

	Question 1	Question 2	Question 3	Question 4
Argentina	200	30	1988	2000
Brazil	4000	510	1973	1996
Panamá	60	5	1971	2002
México	2500	200	1989	1995

Fig. 5.1 Number of bariatric surgeries worldwide and in Latin America between 2003 and 2013

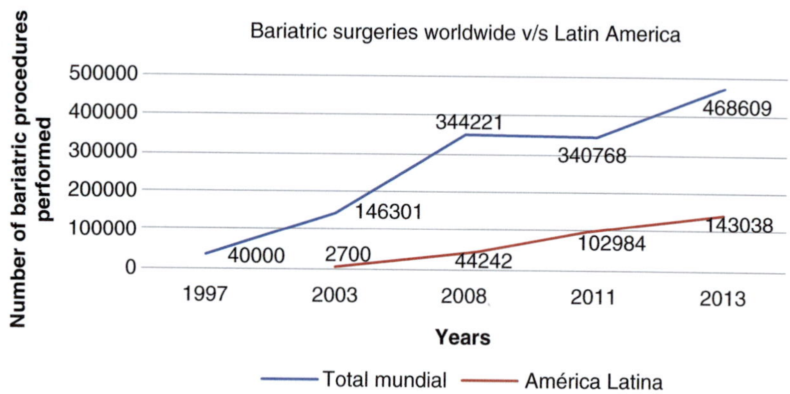

Table 5.5 Numbers of bariatric surgeries from 2003 to 2008 to 2011 to 2013 in Latin America

	2003	2008	2011	2013
RYGB	545	29,176	59,659	85,371
SG	0	4076	30,949	35,349
AGB	1660	9028	5418	5513
BPD/DS	58	1370	4376	3487

Table 5.6 Percentage of bariatric surgeries from 2003 to 2008 to 2011 to 2013 in Latin America

	2003	2008	2011	2013
RYGB	20,2	65,9	57,9	59,7
SG	0	9,2	30,1	24,7
AGB	61,5	20,4	5,3	3,8
BPD/S	2,2	3,1	4,3	2,4

Fig. 5.2 Numbers of bariatric surgeries from 2003 to 2008 to 2011 to 2013 in Latin America

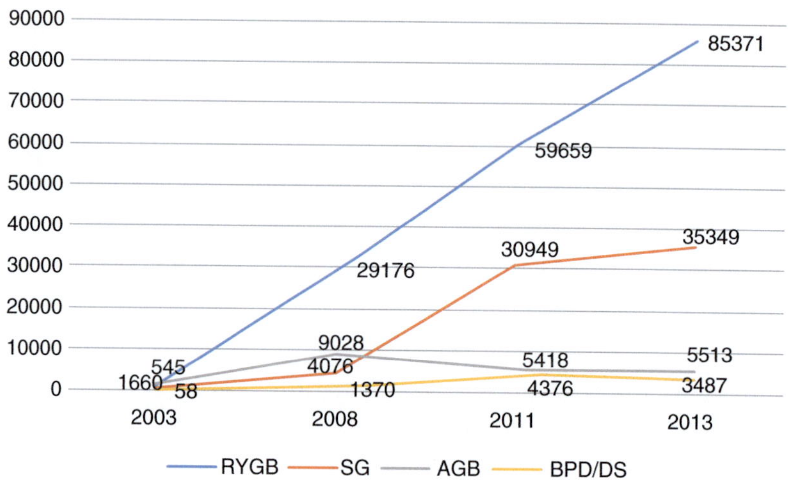

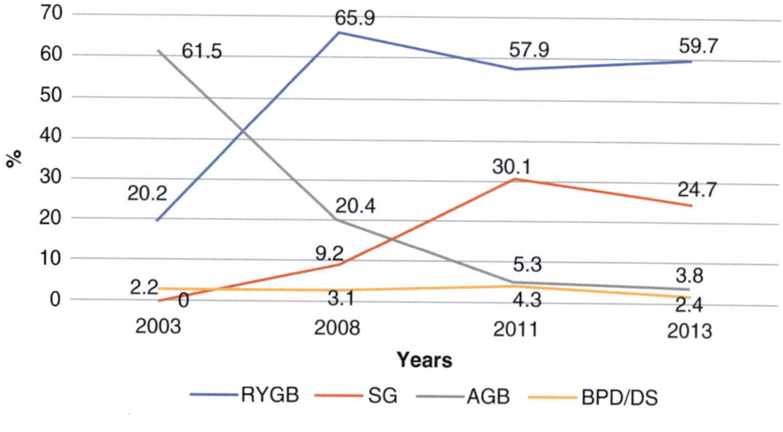

Fig. 5.3 Percentage of bariatric surgeries from 2003 to 2008 to 2011 to 2013 in Latin America

References

1. Begué C, Galante M, Gaudio M. Boletín de Vigilancia. Enfermedades No Transmisibles y Factores de Riesgo. Obesidad: Determinantes, epidemiología y su abordaje desde la salud pública. Ministerio de Salud Argentino. 2016.
2. Braguinsky J. Prevalencia de obesidad en america latina. Obesity prevalence in latin America. An Sis San Navarra. 2002;25(Supl. 1):109–15.
3. Welbourn R, Dixon J, Higa K. International Federation for the surgery of obesity and metabolic disorders. The IFSO Global Registry. 2016.
4. Romero C. Cirugia metabolica en America Latina. Metabolic surgery in Latin America. Cirujano Gen. 2010;32(2):121–4.
5. Lanas F, Bazzano L, Rubinstein A. Prevalence, distributions and determinants of obesity and central obesity in the Southern Cone of America. PLoS One. 2016;11(10):e0163727.
6. Ibañez L. El Problema de la Obesidad en América. Rev Chil Cir. 2007;59(6):399–400.
7. Faña C. Hispanic obesity: an American crisis. National Hispanic Caucus of state Legislators (NHCSL). 2010.
8. Figueroa D. Obesidad y pobreza: marco conceptual para su análisis en latinoamerica. Obesity and poverty: conceptual references for its analysis in Latin America. Saúde Soc Sao Paulo. 2009;18(1):103–17.
9. Amigo H. Obesidad en el niño en America Latina: situación, criterios de diagnostico y desafíos. Obesity in Latin American children: situation, diagnostic criteria and challenges. Cad Saude Publica, Rio de Janeiro. 2003;19(Sup.1):S163–70.
10. Buchwald H, Williams SE. Bariatric surgery worldwide 2003. Obes Surg. 2004;14(9):1157–64.
11. Buchwald H, Oien DM. Metabolic/bariatric surgery worldwide 2011. Obes Surg. 2013;23(4):427–36.
12. United nations desa/population division. World population prospects. 2017. https://esa.un.org/unpd/wpp/DataQuery/. Consulta on line 27/06/17.

Bariatric and Metabolic Surgery in the Middle East

6

Talat Sh. Al Shaban, Ramzi S. Alami, and Abdelrahman Ali Nimeri

The Middle East region is defined by WHO as the Arabic-speaking countries (excluding Algeria) in addition to Turkey, Israel, Iran, and Afghanistan. This region is one of the regions in the world with the highest prevalence of obesity and type II diabetes [1]. In addition, two major studies showed that adult men and women in the Middle East have the highest mean BMI after the USA. Furthermore, women in the Middle East region have the highest waist-to-hip ratio compared to all other regions [2, 3].The prevalence of being overweight among school children and adolescents (6–18 years) in the Middle East ranges from 5.4% to 32%, while the prevalence of obesity ranges from 1.6% to 24.8%. Similarly, the prevalence of being overweight among adult men in the Middle East region ranges from 19.2% to 51.7% and 21.1% to 71% in women. Likewise the prevalence of obesity in the Middle East ranges from 5.7% to 39% in men and 7.1 to 53% in women [4, 5]. In particular, the Gulf region represents the area in the Middle East with the highest burden for obesity and type II DM with Kuwait having the highest prevalence of both overweight and obesity in the different age groups [6]. Additionally, for the last four decades, the Middle East has the greatest rise in diabetes prevalence worldwide and is currently the WHO region with the highest prevalence of diabetes (13.7%) [5, 6, 9] . Furthermore, a report issued by the International Diabetes Federation (IDF) in 2009 showed that five of Middle East countries are among the top ten countries by percentage of adult population living with diabetes worldwide. These five countries are United Arab Emirates (18.7%), Saudi Arabia (16.8%), Bahrain (15.4%), Kuwait (14.6%), and Oman (13.4%).

The burden of obesity and type II diabetes in the Middle East region does not come without a heavy cost. For example, the worldwide rate of death attributed to type II DM is the highest in the Middle East [7]. There is compelling evidence that the high rates of obesity and type II diabetes are mainly due to the urbanization associated with the increased prosperity in the Middle East over the past few decades [8]. This has led to abundance of food with more exposure to fast food and consequently increased consumption of calorie-rich diet [9]. In addition, the improved socioeconomic status and the availability of technology (cars, electric appliances, televisions, computers, electronic gaming, and the Internet) have encouraged a more sedentary lifestyle and physical inactivity [10–13].

A recent review to assess physical activity in the countries of the Gulf Cooperation Council

T. S. Al Shaban
Department of General Surgery, Sheikh Khalifa Medical City, Abu Dhabi, UAE

R. S. Alami
Department of Surgery, American University of Beirut Medical Center, Beirut, Lebanon

A. A. Nimeri (✉)
Department of Surgery, IFSO Middle East North African, Pan Arab Society for Metabolic and Bariatric Surgery, Sheik Khalifa Medical City, Abu Dhabi, UAE

R. Lutfi et al. (eds.), *Global Bariatric Surgery*, https://doi.org/10.1007/978-3-319-93545-4_6

showed that the prevalence of adults being physically active for at least 150 min week is low based on the international standard definition, ranging from 39.0% to 42.1% for men and 26.3% to 28.4% for women [13]. Several other factors are associated with the high prevalence of being overweight or obese in the Middle East region. For example, cultural factors related to traditional standards of beauty and cultural preference of body fatness among women. In addition, historically in the Middle East region, a higher body weight was linked to being healthy among adults and children. Other traditional factors include loose clothing, without a defined waist, unlike pants and skirts, resulting in delayed awareness of weight gain. Furthermore, limited outdoor activity due to hot weather, lack of exercise among women, and the habit of the entire family eating together from a large plate result in unawareness of the amount consumed by each individual. Other factors include the high number of pregnancies with weight gain with each pregnancy that is not lost after each pregnancy. All these factors lead to long-term weight gain and are all believed to be contributing factors to the increasing rates of obesity in women in the Middle East, but further studies are needed to prove these theories [14, 15].

History of Bariatric Surgery in the Middle East Bariatric surgery worldwide has been shown to be an effective and durable treatment for morbid obesity [16]. In addition, when it comes to the treatment of type II diabetes (DM II), bariatric surgery has been shown to be more effective than intensive medical therapy in several randomized controlled trials [17–21]. A worldwide assessment, by Buchwald et al. of the prevalence of different types of bariatric surgeries over time, has shown that some bariatric surgeries have lost their popularity, while others have become more popular [22]. In this worldwide assessment, laparoscopic adjustable gastric banding (LAGB) has fallen out of favor since its introduction at the turn of the last century. Similarly, the gold standard for bariatric surgery for more than 50 years, the laparoscopic Roux-en-Y gastric bypass (LRYGB), has lost significant ground worldwide for the newly introduced laparoscopic sleeve gastrectomy (LSG). In contrast, the prevalence of malabsorptive surgeries like biliopancreatic diversion (BPD) and its duodenal switch version (BPD-DS) has remained very low worldwide.

In contrast to the progress of bariatric surgery worldwide, the progress of bariatric surgery in the Middle East region is lagging behind Europe and North and South America when we consider the magnitude of the problem. Moreover, the bariatric practice in the Middle East is still deficient in several areas when compared to the progress achieved in Europe and North and South America. These areas include, with few exceptions, the lack of a multidisciplinary approach (MDT) to bariatric surgery, lack of prospective registries and outcome databases, very few centers adopting outcomes data reporting programs to assess and maintain quality of care, and paucity of bariatric surgery fellowship programs. On top of that, no clear guidelines are published in the Middle East region, with some countries in the Middle East having regulations that are less strict thereby encouraging the performance of nonstandard and, sometimes, experimental procedures.

The majority of published bariatric surgery outcomes from the Middle East region, with few exceptions (Table 6.2), consist of retrospective or small prospective case series with few large prospective series or randomized controlled trials [23–71] (Tables 6.1, 6.2, and 6.3). Initially, reports published from the Middle East in the 1980s and 1990s showed that the most commonly

Table 6.1 Overall bariatric surgery publications in the Middle East by country

Country	Number of studies
Israel	217
Turkey	140
Lebanon	75
Saudi Arabia	63
Egypt	54
Iran	38
Kuwait	36
Jordan	19
United Arab Emirates	15

performed bariatric surgeries were LAGB, open RYGB (ORYGB), and open VBG. In contrast, reports published in the last two decades show that the commonest procedures performed are LSG, OAGB/MGB, and to a lesser degree LRYGB and laparoscopic greater curvature plication (LGCP) [23–71] (Table 6.4). Similarly, the types of bariatric surgeries performed in Asia based on a survey of all the representatives of the Asia Pacific Metabolic and Bariatric Surgery Society (APMBSS) have changed over time [73]. Initially, this survey showed that the commonest procedures performed in Asia were LAGB (35.9%), LRYGB (24.3%), LSG (19.5%), and MGB (15.4%). APMBSS constitutes all 12 leading Asian countries, except China; in this survey, a total of 6598 bariatric procedures were performed by 155 surgeons. In addition, similar to the Middle East, LSG increased from 1% to 24.8% and LRYGB from 12% to 27.7%, a relative increase of 24.8 and 2.3 times, respectively, among APMBSS surgeons from 2005 to 2009. In contrast to the Middle East during the same period, LAGB and mini gastric bypass decreased from 44.6% to 35.6% and 41.7% to 6.7%, respectively. However, during the same 5 years, the absolute growth rate of bariatric surgery in Asia was 449%. There is no data available regarding the exact growth of bariatric surgery in the Middle East region [72].

Table 6.2 Pediatric and adolescent bariatric surgery publications by country

Country	Number of studies
Saudi Arabia	17
Israel	10
Egypt	3
Iran	2
Lebanon	2
Jordan	1
Kuwait	1
Turkey	1

Revisional Bariatric Surgery Revisional surgery for weight recidivism or correction of complications of bariatric surgery is not uncommon after primary bariatric surgery. Recently, the

Table 6.3 Small bariatric surgery series <100 patients

Procedure	Number	Year	BMI	%EWL (FU)	M&M
1. VBG	39	1988–1992	>40	42% (4 years)	13% failure
					2.5% mortality
2. LAGB	39	1997	44	BMI 35 (6 months)	15.3% morbidity
				72% FU rate	1% PE
3. LAGB	50	1998–1999	50 (36–63)	62% (22–86%) 1 year	Bleeding 2%
4. LAGB	51	2005–2007	49.9	42% 6 months	1 port reposition
			38–63	60% 12 months	FU 16 m [3–34]
5. LAGB	94	1999–2003	BMI 50.8	Mean BMI 35 at 2 years	Wound inf 1
					PE death 2
					SQ heparin TID
6. LRYGBP	90	1999–2001	47	70% (1 year)	Leak 5.5%
7. VBG		1993–1999	52.3 kg/m^2 (41–77.8)	64.1% (21.2–92.3)	Early and late complication rates were 7.9% and 15.8%
8. LSG	61	2007	47.5±9.6	30.5±6.5 (1 year)	Iron did not decrease
					Vitamin B12 and folate did
9. RYGB Egypt	70	2008	48 (7 SD)	32 (SD 4)	PTH did not increase
10. LSG	75	2006–2009	58(33–77)	65% (2 years)	One death from PE, DM 75%, HTN 85%, Dys 87%
11. LSG	70	06–2007	40.7±7.8	63 (1 year)	Leak 1.4%, Stricture 1.4% FU 7.1 +/− 5 months

Table 6.4 Large bariatric surgery series >100 patients

Study	Surgeon Country	Number of patients	Year	BMI kg/m^2	Weight loss %EWL	Morbidity Mortality
12. LAGB 10 years FU	Biagini Lebanon	591	1996–2006	41.95 (+/− 8.7)	66% 12 months 82.7% 8 years	23% morbidity 8.6% removal 9.3% failure 5.3% slippage 4.6% erosion 2.4% infection
13. OAGB/MGB 1000 patients	Noun Lebanon	1000	2012	42.5 (+/− 6)	72.5% 18 months	0.5% leak No mortality
14. LAGB SAGB	Al Momen Saudi Arabia	140	2001 2004	45 ± 6.3	52 kg wt lost 12 months 75 kg and mean BMI 29 at 30 months	Conversion 0 Mortality 0
15. LAGB SAGB	Nowara Egypt	108	1998–2001	48.8	Mean BMI 37.2 12 months 34.3 in 24 months	Conversion 2 Slippage 3 Port complic 6 Gastric perf 1 Mortality 0
16. Lap Vertical Gastric Plication	Taleb Pour Iran	100	1996–2006	47 (36–58)	61% 12 months 57% 3 years (11 patients) FU 18 months	Vomiting Gastric perforation 1% Leak 1%
17. LSG	Nimeri et al. UAE	310	2009–2015	45 (35–65)	–	Leak primary 0% revision 12.5% Stenosis 0%
18. LRYGB	Hadad et al. UAE	342	2009–2014	48 (35–92)	–	Leak primary 0.3% Revision 3% Stenosis 0.88%
19. LRYGBP 55% LSG 44% LAGB 1%	Nimeri et al. UAE	275	2009–2013	45.8 (35–78)	LRYGBP 74.5% LSG 62% LAGB 45% 12 months (82% FU)	Conversion 1% Leak 0.5% Mortality 0

American Society of Metabolic and Bariatric Surgery (ASMBS) has recommended the use of three terms to define revisional bariatric surgery for weight recidivism or correction of complications [73]. The first of these terms is conversion, when a procedure is changed to another procedure (LAGB to LRYGB or LSG). The second of these terms is correction, when a procedure is corrected (gastro-gastric fistula after RYGB). The third term is reversal when the procedure is returned to normal anatomy (LAGB removal). Revisional bariatric surgery carries a higher complication rate when compared to primary bariatric surgery [74]. In addition, some series have shown that the weight loss outcomes might not be as good as primary bariatric surgery [75]. Hence, the decision to offer a patient revisional bariatric surgery has to be taken after considerable consideration for the causes of weight recidivism and the current anatomy of the patient. In addition, potential candidates for revisional bariatric surgery must be managed by a multidisciplinary team, and the revisional procedure should be performed by an experienced bariatric surgeon at a center capable of dealing with various pre- and postoperative complications. Finally, the type of revisional procedure should be determined preoperatively, taking into consideration the presence of reflux, concomitant type II diabetes, patient's weight, as well as the patient's preference, while maintaining some degree of flexibility to switch to another procedure intraoperatively based on the operative findings. Published studies of revisional bariatric surgery from the Middle East are limited, and most of the studies are single center small series for management of weight recidivism or complications with short- to medium-term outcomes at best [36, 41, 45, 50, 54, 55, 61, 65–71]. The main reason for revisional bariatric surgery published in the Middle East region was failed restrictive procedures such as the VBG, silastic ring VBG, LSG, and LAGB. LAGB used to be a very popular procedure in the Middle East in the late 1990s as it was considered safe and effective. However, in the past 10 years, several published studies with long-term outcomes after LAGB have indicated that although LAGB has low complications in the short term, the long-term outcomes show a high rate of revisional surgery for inadequate weight loss, weight regain, or mechanical complications (erosion, slippage, dysphagia, reflux) [75–78] (Table 6.5). Similarly, a study from Iran reported the outcome of 80 patients who had LAGB between 2001 and 2006 after 13 years of follow-up and showed that 84.8% of patients had at least one complication. The most common complications were band erosion (25%) and weight regain (16%), and revisional surgery was required in 78.5% of patients [64].

The LAGB was not the only restrictive procedure revised; studies published from Israel described conversion of a VBG or SRVBG to RYGB or bilio-pancreatic diversion (BPD) with or without duodenal switch. Both conversion

Table 6.5 Small revisional bariatric surgery series <100 patients

Type of surgery	Number	BMI kg/m² preop	Year	Length since primary surgery	BMI kg/m² post-op	Morbidity/mortality
20. VBG or AGB to MiniGB	33	39.5 (28–58)	2005–2006	36 (12–84) m	30.6 (24–50) 6 months FU	6 patients with prep reflux cured
21. VBG to LAGB	23	Referred for dysphagia	2003	19 (9–72) m	7(3–16) months FU	None
22. 4VBG or 37 LAGB to RYGBP	42	45 ± 7	2005–2009	Lap 39 open 3 conversion 2.5%	35 ± 6.7 ESWL% 42%	Reoperation 9.5%
					FU (15.8 ± 13.4 m)	No mortality
23. 15 VBG	17	58.4 ± 16.9	1998–2000	15.6 (1–72) m	5/17 referred	Short FU
1 LAGB				5/17 referred	12/17 (5.9%) reoperation	Dysphagia/ recidivism
1 RYGP						
24. VBG/LAGB 2 RYGB Khoursheed et al.	42	2005–2009	35 ± 6.7	%EWL 42%	–	12. VBG/LAGB 2 RYGB Khoursheed et al.
25. LSG to re-LSG or RYGB	12 LRYGB	52 LRYGB	2009–2014	–	EWL 61%	None
	24 LRSG	50 LRSG			EWL 57%	
26. LAGB to LSG	56	44 (SD 7)	2007–2012	–		5.5% complication
27. LAGB to LRYGB	40	35–62	2009–2015	–	60% EWL (18–111%)	Leak 5%
						Mortality 0%
28. LAGB to LSG or RYGB	42 LSG	38.5 LSG	2005–2012	–	47.4% LSG	RYGB leak 2%
	53 RYGB	43 RYGB			45.6% RYGB	
29. LAGB to LSG	40	44 (SD 7)	2009–2012	6–36 months	56.9%	–

methods were found to be safe and effective. However, BPD was associated with high, sometimes prohibitive, complication rates (28–42%). In contrast, conversion to RYGB was as effective in treating complications of VBG and SRVBG and did carry significant but fewer complications than BPD (14.2–20.8%). Weight loss after conversion to RYGB was comparable to weight loss after conversion to BPD at 1 year but inferior at 3 years [65, 66].

Recently, the most common revisional procedure published in the Middle East is conversion of LAGB to LSG followed by LRYGB [67–70]. The outcomes of conversion of LAGB to LSG in terms of safety (complication rates 5.5–7.1%) and efficacy (%EWL at 12 months 47.4–53% and at 24 months 51–80.1%) were reproducible by at least three bariatric centers in the region (Khoursheed et al., Alqahtani et al., and Goitein et al.). In addition, the series of Khoursheed et al. and Nimeri et al. included conversion to LSG and RYGB. Furthermore, Alqahtani et al. found that the results of revisional LSG were comparable to primary LSG (complications rate 5.5% vs 7% and %EWL at 24 months 80.1% vs 84.6%, respectively).

We predict that similar to the LAGB, a large number of patients with weight recidivism after LSG will need revision in the future. Al Sabah et al. described algorithm to manage patients with weight recidivism after LSG as well as operative management by re-sleeve gastrectomy or conversion to RYGB [72].

Adolescent Bariatric Surgery

Youth is the predominant age group in the Middle East. In 2014, 54% of the population were still under the age of 25 years, and 31% were younger than 15 years of age [79, 80]. Similar to the adult population, the increase in obesity prevalence among children and adolescents (aged 2–18 years) in the Middle East region is alarming. In addition, the incidence of obesity-related conditions, particularly type II diabetes, is increasing [81]. The etiology of adolescent obesity is believed to be similar to that in adults and is related to urbanization, improved socioeconomic status, decreased physical activity, and increased consumption of calorie-rich diet. The cultural factors also play a similar role as among the adult, whereby overweight is perceived as healthy and a beauty criterion.

There are different definitions of overweight and obesity in children adopted by different bodies. These different bodies include the World Health Organization (WHO), US Center for Disease Control and Prevention (CDC), and World Obesity Federation through their International Obesity Task Force (IOTF). The definitions adopted in children are somewhat overlapping, resulting in loss of precise boundaries between normal weight, overweight, and obesity estimates. This lack of consensus on definitions, which was obvious in various publications from different countries in the region, had an impact on prevalence estimation and treatment recommendations [82–84].

A meta-analysis conducted by Mirmiran et al. found that the highest prevalence of overweight and obesity was among adolescents in Bahrain and Kuwait (38.5% and 31.2%, respectively). In contrast, the lowest prevalence was in Islamic Republic of Iran and Lebanon (3% and 3.2%, respectively) [85].

We conducted a PubMed search for articles about Bariatric surgery in children and adolescents from the Middle East by country (Table 6.2). Bariatric surgery in children and adolescents is still considered debatable and controversial in the Middle East. The controversy ranges from one extreme considering adolescent bariatric surgery relatively contraindicated to another extreme performing bariatric surgery on children with Prader-Willi syndrome as well as children as young as 2.5 years of age [58, 86]. However, the majority of publications from the Middle East region consider it to be an acceptable solution in properly selected patients, with more evidence showing it to be safe and effective in treating obesity and its associated comorbidities in this age group [47, 49, 51, 52, 57–59].

The initial experience with adolescent bariatric surgery in the Middle East was LAGB due to its safety and efficacy and lower theoretic chance of developing nutritional deficiencies [39]. Over time, this has changed, and most of the publications from the Middle East region over the past few years have described LSG for adolescents. In addition, LSG is either used as a primary procedure or for conversion of LAGB in children and adolescents [47, 49, 51, 52, 57–59].

We did not find any publication describing the role of RYGB in children and adolescents in the Middle East region. Surprisingly, the same cannot be said about the malabsorptive form of gastric bypass (one anastomosis gastric bypass (OAGB) also known as mini gastric bypass). There is a study by Noun et al. describing mini gastric bypass in various age groups including adolescents as young as 14 years of age with good results [87].

Obesity, and concomitant comorbidities, among children and adolescents in the Middle East remains a major challenge to the health-care systems in the region. Bariatric surgery cannot be the solution, except for a small minority of children and adolescents. Since the prevalence is still increasing in an alarming fashion, there needs to be a call for action plan at governmental levels in order to address the issues and educate the public about causes and complications of obesity while encouraging and facilitating healthy eating habits and regular physical activity. Furthermore, access to treatment of obesity and/or its complications (including screening programs) needs to be facilitated by health-care systems. This is challenging in view of the limited resources and poor economy in many countries of the region.

We believe that surgical treatment of obesity in children and adolescents should be carried out by a multidisciplinary team with extensive experience in adult bariatric surgery, at a specialized center, and offered only to selected patients in these age groups as described by Alqahtani et al. [59]. We also believe that the lack of unified definitions of overweight and obesity and the absence of regional guidelines and the variability in the standard of medical practice among health-care systems in the region adds to the challenge of adolescent bariatric surgery in the Middle East region.

Future Perspectives of Bariatric Surgery in the Middle East

Several national bariatric surgery societies were established in most Middle East countries in the last decade. In addition, several regional societies are coming together such as the Gulf Obesity Surgery Society (GOSS) and the Pan Arab Society for Metabolic and Bariatric Surgery (PASMBS). Currently, the main function of these societies is organization of educational activities and continuous medical education conferences. It is hoped that these societies will address some of the challenges of practicing bariatric surgery in the Middle East such as access to bariatric surgery care, unified bariatric surgery guidelines, establishing a unified outcome registries, and accreditation process for bariatric surgery programs. In addition, two of the largest regional societies (Gulf Obesity Surgery Society) and the Pan Arab Society for Metabolic and Bariatric Surgery have come together to form the International Federation for Surgery of Obesity and Metabolic disorder (IFSO) Middle East and North Africa Chapter (IFSO MENAC).

References

1. Abuyassin B, Laher I. Obesity-linked diabetes in the Arab world: a review. East Mediterr Health J. 2015;21(6):420–39.
2. NCD Risk Factor Collaboration (NCD-RisC). Trends in adult body-mass index in 200 countries from 1975 to 2014: a pooled analysis of 1698 population-based measurement studies with 19·2 million participants. Lancet. 2016;387(10026):1377–96. https://doi.org/10.1016/S0140-6736(16)30054-X.
3. Yusuf S, Hawken S, Ounpuu S, Bautista L, Franzosi MG, Commerford P, Lang CC, Rumboldt Z, Onen CL, Lisheng L, Tanomsup S, Wangai P Jr, Razak F, Sharma AM, Anand SS, INTERHEART Study Investigators. Obesity and the risk of myocardial infarction in 27,000 participants from 52 countries: a case-control study. Lancet. 2005;366(9497):1640–9.
4. Musaiger AO, Al-Hazzaa HM. Prevalence and risk factors associated with nutrition-related noncommunicable diseases in the Eastern Mediterranean region. Int J Gen Med. 2012;5:199–217. https://doi.org/10.2147/IJGM.S29663.
5. Lobstein T, Baur L, Uauy R. Obesity in children and young people: a crisis in public

health. Obes Rev. 2004;5:4–85. https://doi.org/10.1111/j.1467-789X.2004.00133.x.
6. Musaiger AO, Al-Mannai M, Tayyem R, et al. Prevalence of overweight and obesity among adolescents in seven Arab countries: a cross-cultural study. J Obes. 2012;2012:981390. https://doi.org/10.1155/2012/981390.
7. International Diabetes Federation. 4th edn. 2009. https://www.idf.org/e-library/epidemiology-research/diabetes-atlas/21-atlas-4th-edition.html.
8. ALNohair S. Obesity in gulf countries. Int J Health Sci. 2014;8(1):79–83.
9. World Health Organization. Global report on diabetes, Part 1: global burden of diabetes, 1.2 prevalence of diabetes and associated risk factors. 2016; p. 25, 26.
10. Musaiger AO. Overweight and obesity in Eastern Mediterranean Region: prevalence and possible causes. J Obes. 2011;2011:407237., 17 pages. https://doi.org/10.1155/2011/407237.
11. Goryakin Y, Suhrcke M. Economic development, urbanization, technological change and overweight: what do we learn from 244 Demographic and Health Surveys? Econ Hum Biol. 2014;14:109–27. https://doi.org/10.1016/j.ehb.2013.11.003.
12. Adeomi AA, Adeoye OA, Bamidele JO. Childhood obesity in developing countries: an emerging menace. IJHSR. 2014;4(6):170–7.
13. Mabry RM, Reeves MM, Eakin EG, Owen N. Evidence of physical activity participation among men and women in the countries of the Gulf Cooperation Council: a review. Obes Rev. 2010;11:457–64. https://doi.org/10.1111/j.1467-789X.2009.00655.x.
14. Musaiger, et al. Strategy to combat obesity and to promote physical activity in Arab countries. Diabetes Metab Syndr Obes. 2011;4:89–97. Epub 2011 Mar 8
15. Musaiger AO, Shahbeek NE, AL-Mannai M. The role of social factors and weight status in ideal body shape preferences as perceived by Arab Women. J Biosoc Sci. 2004;36(6):699–707. https://doi.org/10.1017/S0021932003006412.
16. Weiner RA, et al. Indications and principles of metabolic surgery. US Natl Libr Med. 2010;81(4):379–94.
17. Schauer PR, Kashyap SR, Wolski K, et al. Bariatric surgery versus intensive medical therapy in obese patients with diabetes. N Engl J Med. 2012;366(17):1567–76. https://doi.org/10.1056/NEJMoa1200225.
18. Schauer PR, Bhatt DL, Kirwan JP, Wolski K, Brethauer SA, Navaneethan SD, Aminian A, Pothier CE, Kim ESH, Nissen SE, Kashyap SR, for the STAMPEDE Investigators*. N Engl J Med. 2014;370:2002–13. https://doi.org/10.1056/NEJMoa1401329.
19. Mingrone G, et al. Bariatric–metabolic surgery versus conventional medical treatment in obese patients with type 2 diabetes: 5 year follow-up of an open-label, single-centre, randomised controlled trial. Lancet. 386(9997):964–73.
20. Ikramuddin S, Korner J, Lee W, et al. Roux-en-Y gastric bypass vs intensive medical management for the control of type 2 diabetes, hypertension, and hyperlipidemia: the diabetes surgery study randomized clinical trial. JAMA. 2013;309(21):2240–9. https://doi.org/10.1001/jama.2013.5835.
21. Kashyap SR, Bhatt DL, Wolski K, Watanabe RM, Abdul-Ghani M, Abood B, Pothier CE, Brethauer S, Nissen S, Gupta M, Kirwan JP, Schauer PR. Metabolic effects of bariatric surgery in patients with moderate obesity and type 2 diabetes. Diabetes Care. 2013;36(8):2175–82. https://doi.org/10.2337/dc12-1596.
22. Buchwald H1, Oien DM. Metabolic/bariatric surgery worldwide 2011. Obes Surg. 2013;23(4):427–36. https://doi.org/10.1007/s11695-012-0864-0.
23. Hajat C1, Harrison O. The Abu Dhabi cardiovascular program: the continuation of Framingham. Prog Cardiovasc Dis. 2010;53(1):28–38. https://doi.org/10.1016/j.pcad.2010.05.002.
24. Mofti, et al. Bariatric surgery in Saudi Arabia. Ann Saudi Med. 1992;12(5):440–5. Saudi Arabia
25. Malik M1, Bakir A. Prevalence of overweight and obesity among children in the United Arab Emirates. Obes Rev. 2007;8(1):15–20.
26. Ashy AA, et al. Laparoscopic adjustable silicone gastric banding in the treatment of super obesity in the Jeddah area, Saudi Arabia. A preliminary report. Int Surg. 1996;81(3):289–91. Review
27. Bakr AA1, Fahim T. Laparoscopic adjustable gastric banding is a safe and effective treatment for morbid obesity. JSLS. 1998;2(1):57–61.
28. Gawdat K. Gastric restrictive procedures through a mini-incision: a cost-effective alternative to laparoscopic bariatric surgery in Egypt. Obes Surg. 1999;9(5):456–8.
29. Nowara HA. Egyptian experience in laparoscopic adjustable gastric banding (technique, complications and intermediate results). Obes Surg. 2001;11(1):70–5.
30. Gawdat K. Bariatric re-operations: are they preventable? Obes Surg. 2000;10(6):525–9.
31. Taskin, et al. Laparoscopy in Turkish bariatric surgery: initial experience. Obes Surg. 2000;10(3):263–5.
32. Abdel-Galil E1, Sabry AA. Laparoscopic Roux-en-Y gastric bypass – evaluation of three different techniques. Obes Surg. 2002;12(5):639–42.
33. Abu-Abeid, et al. Resolution of chronic medical conditions after laparoscopic adjustable silicone gastric banding for the treatment of morbid obesity in the elderly. Surg Endosc. 2001;15(2):132–4.
34. Haciyanli M, Erkan N, Bora S, Gulay H. Vertical banded gastroplasty in the Aegean Region of Turkey. Obes Surg. 2001;11(4):482–6.
35. Dhafar KO. Initial experience with Swedish adjustable gastric band at Al-noor hospital. Obes Surg. 2003;13(6):918–20.
36. Gavert N1, Szold A, Abu-Abeid S. Laparoscopic revisional surgery for life-threatening stenosis following vertical banded gastroplasty, together with placement of an adjustable gastric band. Obes Surg. 2003;13(3):399–403.
37. Al-Momen A. A. Initial experience with Swedish adjustable gastric band at Saad Specialist Hospital, Al-Khobar, Saudi Arabia. Obes Surg. 2005;15(4):506–9.

38. Talebpour, et al. Laparoscopic total gastric vertical plication in morbid obesity. J Laparoendosc Adv Surg Tech A. 2007;17(6):793–8. Laparoscopic Surgical Ward, Sina Hospital, Tehran Medical University, Tehran, Iran. mmahkk@yahoo.com
39. Al-Qahtani AR1. Laparoscopic adjustable gastric banding in adolescent: safety and efficacy. J Pediatr Surg. 2007;42(5):894–7.
40. Noun, et al. Mini-gastric bypass by mini-laparotomy: a cost-effective alternative in the laparoscopic era. Obes Surg. 2007;17(11):1482–6. Department of Digestive Surgery, Hôtel-Dieu de France Hospital, Beirut, Lebanon. rnoun@wise.net.lb
41. Noun R1, Zeidan S, Riachi E, Abboud B, Chalhoub V, Yazigi A. Mini-gastric bypass for revision of failed primary restrictive procedures: a valuable option. Obes Surg. 2007;17(5):684–8.
42. Biagini J, Karam L. Ten years experience with laparoscopic adjustable gastric banding. Obes Surg. 2008;18(5):573–7. https://doi.org/10.1007/s11695-008-9470-6.
43. Hakaem, et al. Obes Surg. 2009;19(11):1491–6. Epub 2009 Jul 15. King Faisal Specialist & Res Hosp Riyadh Saudi Arabia
44. Mahdy T1, Atia S, Farid M, Adulatif A. Effect of Roux-en Y gastric bypass on bone metabolism in patients with morbid obesity: Mansoura experiences. Obes Surg. 2008;18(12):1526–31. https://doi.org/10.1007/s11695-008-9653-1. Epub 2008 Aug 21
45. Khoursheed MA, Al-Bader IA, Al-asfar FS, Mohammad AI, Shukkur M, Dashti HM. Revision of failed bariatric procedures to Roux-en-Y gastric bypass (RYGB). Obes Surg. 2011;21(8):1157–60. https://doi.org/10.1007/s11695-010-0229-5.
46. Toolabi, et al. Effects of laparoscopic Roux-en-Y gastric bypass (LRYGB) on weight loss and biomarker parameters in morbidly obese patients: a 12-month follow-up. Obes Surg. 2011;21(12):1834–42. Department of Surgery, Imam Khomeini Hospital, Tehran University of Medical Sciences, Tehran, Iran
47. Al Qahtani. Laparoscopic sleeve gastrectomy in 108 obese children and adolescents aged 5 to 21 years. Ann Surg. 2012;256(2):266–73. Department of Biostatistics, Obesity Research Chair, College of Medicine, King Saud University, Riyadh, Saudi Arabia. qahtani@yahoo.com
48. Nimeri A, Mohamed A, El Hassan E, McKenna K, Turrin NP, Al Hadad M, Dehni N. Are results of bariatric surgery different in the Middle East? Early experience of an international bariatric surgery program and an ACS NSQIP outcomes comparison. J Am Coll Surg. 2013;216(6):1082–8. https://doi.org/10.1016/j.jamcollsurg.2013.01.063. Epub 2013 Apr 23
49. Alqahtani AR, Elahmedi M, Alqahtani YA. Bariatric surgery in monogenic and syndromic forms of obesity. Semin Pediatr Surg. 2014;23(1):37–42. https://doi.org/10.1053/j.sempedsurg.2013.10.013. Epub 2013 Nov 15. Review
50. Alqahtani AR, Elahmedi M, Alamri H, Mohammed R, Darwish F, Ahmed AM. Laparoscopic removal of poor outcome gastric banding with concomitant sleeve gastrectomy. Obes Surg. 2013;23(6):782–7. https://doi.org/10.1007/s11695-013-0895-1.
51. Alqahtani A, Alamri H, Elahmedi M, Mohammed R. Laparoscopic sleeve gastrectomy in adult and pediatric obese patients: a comparative study. Surg Endosc. 2012;26(11):3094–100.
52. Alqahtani AR, Elahmedi MO, Al Qahtani A. Co-morbidity resolution in morbidly obese children and adolescents undergoing sleeve gastrectomy. Surg Obes Relat Dis. 2014;10(5):842–50. https://doi.org/10.1016/j.soard.2014.01.020. Epub 2014 Jan 28
53. Safadi BY, Shamseddine G, Elias E, Alami RS. Definitive surgical management of staple line leak after sleeve gastrectomy. Surg Obes Relat Dis. 2015;11(5):1037–43. https://doi.org/10.1016/j.soard.2015.04.017. Epub 2015 Apr 30.
54. Khoursheed M, Al-Bader I, Mouzannar A, Al-Haddad A, Sayed A, Mohammad A, Fingerhut A. Sleeve gastrectomy or gastric bypass as revisional bariatric procedures: retrospective evaluation of outcomes. Surg Endosc. 2013;27(11):4277–83. https://doi.org/10.1007/s00464-013-3038-9. Epub 2013 Jun 12.
55. Alazmi W, Al-Sabah S, Ali DA, Almazeedi S. Treating sleeve gastrectomy leak with endoscopic stenting: the Kuwaiti experience and review of recent literature. Surg Endosc. 2014;28(12):3425–8. https://doi.org/10.1007/s00464-014-3616-5. Epub 2014 Jun 20. Review
56. Al-Sabah SK, Almazeedi SM, Dashti SA, Al-Mulla AY, Ali DA, Jumaa TH. The efficacy of laparoscopic sleeve gastrectomy in treating adolescent obesity. Obes Surg. 2015;25(1):50–4. https://doi.org/10.1007/s11695-014-1340-9.
57. Alqahtani A, Elahmedi M, Qahtani AR. Laparoscopic sleeve gastrectomy in children younger than 14 years: refuting the concerns. Ann Surg. 2016;263(2):312–9.
58. Alqahtani AR, Elahmedi MO, Al Qahtani AR, Lee J, Butler MG. Laparoscopic sleeve gastrectomy in children and adolescents with Prader-Willi syndrome: a matched-control study. Surg Obes Relat Dis. 2016;12(1):100–10. https://doi.org/10.1016/j.soard.2015.07.014.
59. Alqahtani AR, Elahmedi MO. Pediatric bariatric surgery: the clinical pathway. Obes Surg. 2015;25(5):910–21. https://doi.org/10.1007/s11695-015-1586-x.
60. Al-Bader I, Khoursheed M, Al Sharaf K, Mouzannar DA, Ashraf A, Fingerhut A. Revisional laparoscopic gastric pouch resizing for inadequate weight loss after Roux-en-Y gastric bypass. Obes Surg. 2015;25(7):1103–8.
61. Nimeri A, Ibrahim M, Maasher A, Al Hadad M. Management algorithm for leaks following laparoscopic sleeve gastrectomy. Obes Surg. 2016;26(1):21–5. https://doi.org/10.1007/s11695-015-1751-2.
62. Nimeri A, Maasher A, Salim E, Ibrahim M, Al Hadad M. The Use of intraoperative endoscopy decreases postoperative stenosis in laparoscopic sleeve gastrectomy. Obes Surg. 2016;26(4):864.
63. Al-Sabah S, Al-Ghareeb F, Ali DA, Al-Adwani A. Efficacy of intragastric balloon for the manage-

ment of obesity: experience from Kuwait. Surg Endosc. 2016;30(2):424–9. https://doi.org/10.1007/s00464-015-4212-z. Epub 2015 Apr 22

64. Toolabi K, Golzarand M, Farid R. Laparoscopic adjustable gastric banding: efficacy and consequences over a 13-year. Am J Surg. 2016;212(1):62–8. https://doi.org/10.1016/j.amjsurg.2015.05.021. Epub 2015 Jul 31
65. Abu-Gazala S1, Sadot E, Maler I, Golomb I, Carmeli I, Keidar A. Laparoscopic conversion of failed silastic ring vertical gastroplasty (SRVG) and vertical banded gastroplasty (VBG) into biliopancreatic diversion (BPD). J Gastrointest Surg. 2015;19(4):625–30. https://doi.org/10.1007/s11605-014-2736-5. Epub 2015 Jan 6
66. David MB, Abu-Gazala S, Sadot E, Wasserberg N, Kashtan H, Keidar A. Laparoscopic conversion of failed vertical banded gastroplasty to Roux-en-Y gastric bypass or biliopancreatic diversion. Surg Obes Relat Dis. 2015;11(5):1085–91. https://doi.org/10.1016/j.soard.2015.01.026. Epub 2015 Feb 11
67. Khoursheed M, Al-Bader I, Mouzannar A, Al-Haddad A, Sayed A, Mohammad A, Fingerhut A. Sleeve gastrectomy or gastric bypass as revisional bariatric procedures: retrospective evaluation of outcomes. Surg Endosc. 2013;27(11):4277–83. https://doi.org/10.1007/s00464-013-3038-9. Epub 2013 Jun 12
68. Goitein D1, Feigin A, Segal-Lieberman G, Goitein O, Papa MZ, Zippel D. Laparoscopic sleeve gastrectomy as a revisional option after gastric band failure. Surg Endosc. 2011;25(8):2626–30. https://doi.org/10.1007/s00464-011-1615-3. Epub 2011 Mar 17.
69. Khoursheed M, Al-Bader I, Mohammad AI, Soliman MO. Dashti H Slippage after adjustable gastric banding according to the pars flaccida and the perigastric approach. Med Princ Pract. 2007;16(2):110–3.
70. Nimeri A, Maasher A, Al Shaban T, Salim E, Ibrahim M. Tips and tricks in converting LAGB to LRYGB in one stage Obes Surg. 2016. In press.
71. Nimeri A, Al Shaban T, Salim E, Maasher A. Internal hernia following LRYGB: prevention and tips for intra operative management. Obes Surg. 2016. In press.
72. AlSabah S, Alsharqawi N, Almulla A, Akrof S, Alenezi K, Buhaimed W, Al-Subaie S, Al Haddad M. Approach to poor weight loss after laparoscopic sleeve gastrectomy: re-sleeve vs. gastric bypass. Obes Surg. 2016;26(10):2302–7. https://doi.org/10.1007/s11695-016-2119-y.
73. Lomanto D, Lee W, Goel R, et al. Obes Surg. 2012;22:502. https://doi.org/10.1007/s11695-011-0547-2.
74. Brethauer SA, et al. Systematic review on reoperative bariatric surgery. Surg Obes Relat Dis. 10(5):952–72. 77. Moszkowicz D, Arienzo R, Khettab I, et al. Sleeve gastrectomy severe complications: is it always a reasonable surgical option? Obes Surg 2013;23(5):676–86.
75. Himpens J, Cadière G-B, Bazi M, Vouche M, Cadière B, Dapri G. Long-term outcomes of laparoscopic adjustable gastric banding. Arch Surg. 2011;146(7):802–7.
76. Suter M, Calmes JM, Paroz A, Giusti V. A 10-year experience with laparoscopic gastric banding for morbid obesity: high long-term complication and failure rates. Obes Surg. 2006;16(7):829–35.
77. Markus Weber, Markus K, Mu¨ller, Bucher T, Wildi S, Dindo D, Horber F, Hauser R, Clavien P-A. FACS laparoscopic gastric bypass is superior to laparoscopic gastric banding for treatment of morbid obesity. Ann Surg. 2004;240:975–83.
78. O'Brien PE, MacDonald L, Anderson M, Brennan L, Brown WA. Long-term outcomes after bariatric surgery fifteen-year follow-up of adjustable gastric banding and a systematic review of the bariatric surgical literature. Ann Surg. 2013;257:87–94.
79. Al-Haddad FH, Little BB, Abdul Ghafoor AG. Childhood obesity in United Arab Emirates schoolchildren: a national study. Adolescents in Arab countries: health statistics and social context, DIFI Family Research and Proceedings 2015:1 https://doi.org/10.5339/difi.2015.1 Ann Hum Biol. 2005;32(1):72–9. Makhlouf Obermeyer C.
80. World Bank Indicators – Middle East And North Africa – Population.
81. Geneva, World Health Organization. Fight childhood obesity to help prevent diabetes, say WHO & IDF [press release]. 2004. http://www.who.int/mediacentre/news/releases/2004/pr81/en/print.html. Accessed 5 Mar 2010.
82. Geneva, World Health Organization. Physical status: the use and interpretation of anthropometry. Report of a WHO Expert Committee. 1995. (WHO Technical Report Series No. 854).
83. Centers for Disease Control and Prevention. Defining childhood overweight and obesity. [website] http://www.cdc.gov/obes- ity/childhood/de ning.html. Accessed 16 June 2010.
84. Cole TJ, et al. Establishing a standard definition for child over- weight and obesity worldwide: international survey. Br Med J. 2000;320:1240–3.
85. Mirmiran R, Sherafat-Kazemzadeh S, Jalali-Farahani, Azizi F. Childhood obesity in the Middle East: a review P., Nutrition Unit, Obesity Research Centre, Research Institute for Endocrine Sciences, Shaheed Beheshti University of Medical Sciences, Tehran, Islamic Republic of Iran.
86. Al Mohaidly M, et al. Laparoscopic sleeve gastrectomy for a two-and half year old morbidly obese child. Int J Surg Case Rep. 4(11):1057–1060.
87. Noun R1, Skaff J, Riachi E, Daher R, Antoun NA, Nasr M, Khoursheed M1, Al-Bader I. One thousand consecutive mini-gastric bypass: short- and long-term outcome. Obes Surg. 2012;22(5):697–703. https://doi.org/10.1007/s11695-012-0618-z. Abu-Abeid S, Gavert N, Klausner JM, Szold A

7 Asian Experience

Muffazal Lakdawala and Aparna Govil Bhasker

Overview of Obesity Demographics

With the emergence of capitalism and rise of romantic consumerism, currently the wheels of industry are spinning faster than ever. From being a disturbed and deprived region in the past, Asia has steadily risen in the global economic growth chart. This newfound affluence has led to a lot of positive changes in the arena of healthcare in terms of increased life expectancy, a significant decrease in child mortality, and reduction in infectious diseases. The standard of living of an average Asian today is much higher as compared to 50 years ago, and the caloric intake of an ordinary Asian today is easily double or triple of those consumed by his ancestors. This has tilted the scales toward obesity, and as we battle malnutrition on one end, most Asian countries today are facing a concomitant epidemic of obesity and related disorders especially type 2 diabetes mellitus.

Obesity is emerging as one of the biggest health challenges in Asia. According to a 2015 study published in the *Lancet*, almost half the population of countries like Malaysia and Singapore is overweight or obese [1]. The rate of overweight and obese population in India and China is slated at a lower percentage of about 20–30%, but the burgeoning population of these two countries is enough to raise an alarm. China and India rank as the second and third most obese nations in the world. These two countries also have the largest number of diabetics in the world, thus making it the largest population afflicted with diabesity. Table 7.1 shows the prevalence of overweight and obese populations in some of the Asian countries.

The Impact: Obesity is responsible for 3.4 million deaths annually, 3.9% of years of life lost, and 3.8% of DALY's worldwide. Till date, no country in the world has been able to curtail this ever-growing epidemic [1].

Table 7.1 Prevalence of overweight and obese populations in men and women >20 years of age in Asian countries [1]

Countries	Men >20 years (%)	Women >20 years (%)
Singapore	44.3	32.5
Malaysia	43.8	48.6
South Korea	36.9	27.2
Taiwan	33.8	30.9
Bhutan	33.0	38.2
Thailand	32.1	39.7
Japan	28.9	17.6
China	28.3	27.4
Pakistan	27.9	38.4
Maldives	21.4	54.0
India	19.5	20.7
Indonesia		30.6

M. Lakdawala
Department of Bariatric Surgery and Lap Oncosurgery, Saifee Hospital, Mumbai, Maharashtra, India
e-mail: muffidoc@codsindia.com

A. G. Bhasker (✉)
Bariatric Surgeon, Global and Apollo Hospitals, Mumbai, Maharashtra, India

R. Lutfi et al. (eds.), *Global Bariatric Surgery*, https://doi.org/10.1007/978-3-319-93545-4_7

Surgical Landmarks in the Evolution of Bariatric Medicine and Surgery

In 1981, Prof. Kai Mo Chen and Prof. Wei Jee Lee of Taiwan were the first Asian surgeons to perform an open vertical banded gastroplasty in the region. They were followed in quick succession by Prof. Isao Kawamura of Japan. More than 35 years ago, these surgeons dared to tread on a road less travelled, into an unchartered territory when bariatric surgery was yet to find its legitimate place in the textbooks of general surgery.

Prof. Emeritus Ti Thiow Kong of Singapore in 1987, Prof. Freda Meah of Malaysia in 1996, and Dr. Shrihari Dhorepatil of India in 1999 performed the first bariatric procedures in the form of open vertical banded gastroplasties in their respective countries. Each of these leaders is special in their own way as they paved the way for an unconventional specialty in their home countries. To take that first step in societies where obesity is perceived as a sign of good health, in the midst of naysayers within their own peers in the medical fraternity, without any support from the government, and in complete absence of insurance cover called for a lot of guts and courage. They were the visionaries who recognized obesity as a disease and bariatric surgery as its treatment.

Figures 7.1 and 7.2 depict pioneer bariatric surgeons from various Asian countries.

The advent of laparoscopy in the late 1990s made bariatric surgery increasingly acceptable. Laparoscopy decreased surgical morbidity to a large extent, was less painful, and enabled the patient to get back to work much earlier. Dr. Wei Jee Lee from Taiwan was the first Asian surgeon to perform a “laparoscopic” vertical banded gastroplasty in 1998. In 2004, Dr. Muffazal Lakdawala was the first Indian surgeon to per-

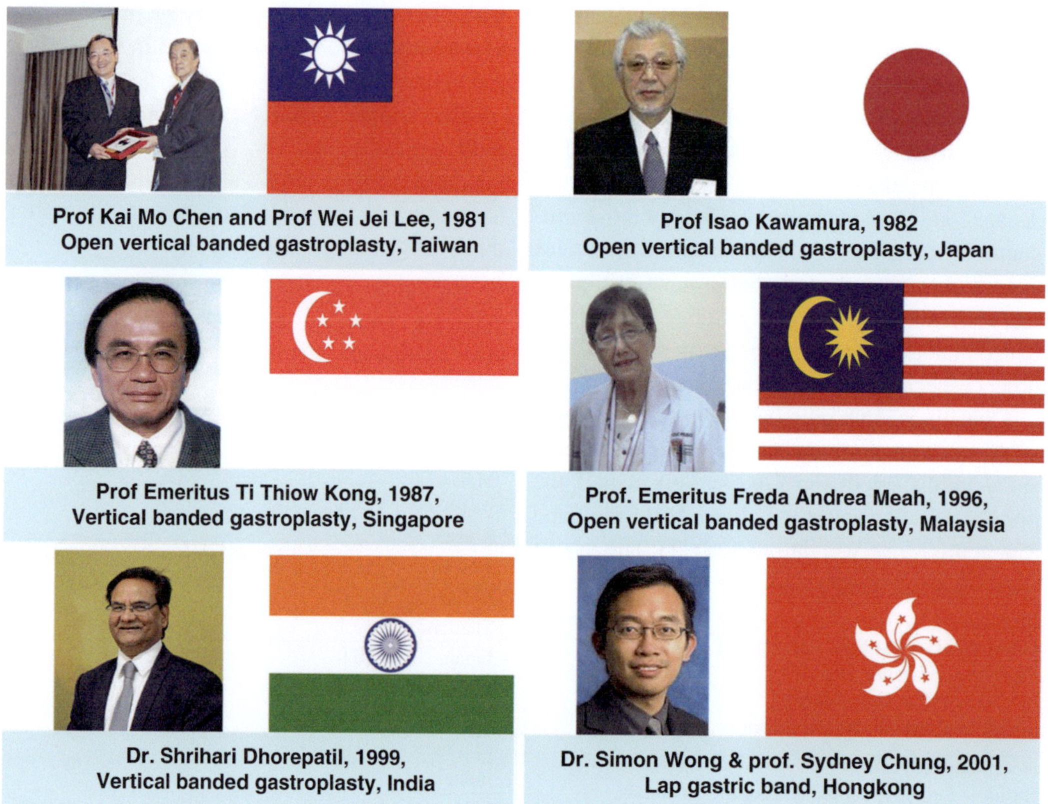

Fig. 7.1 Pioneer bariatric surgeons from various Asian countries

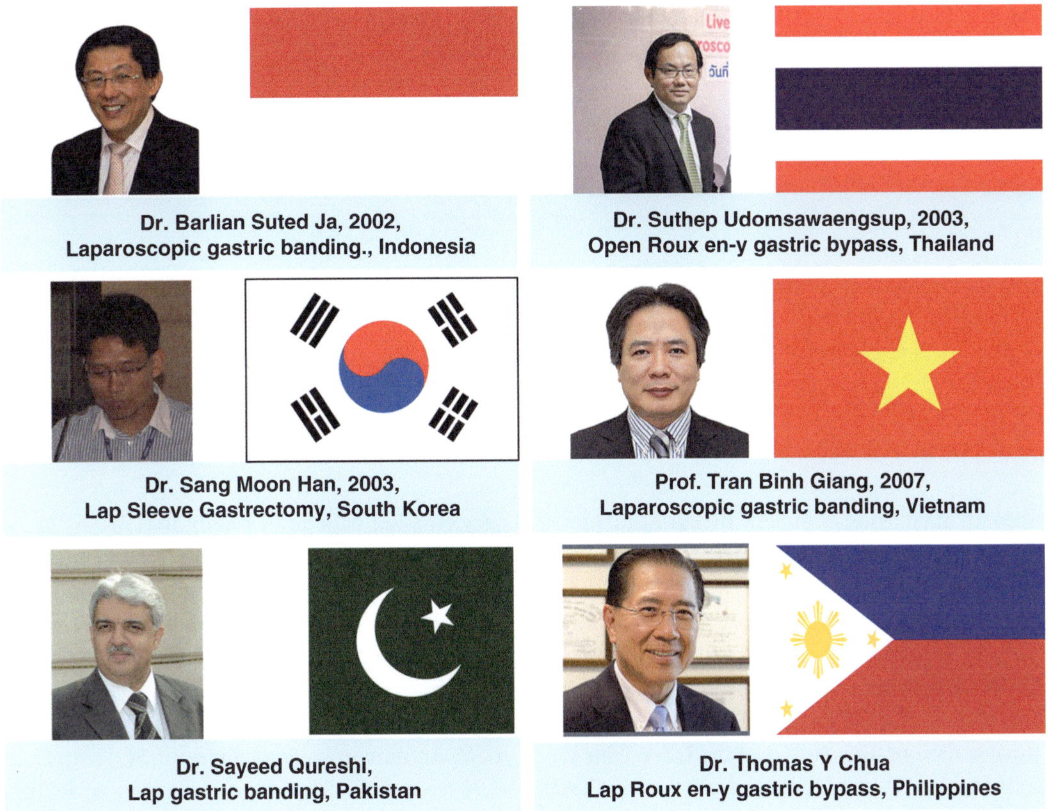
Dr. Barlian Suted Ja, 2002,
Laparoscopic gastric banding., Indonesia
Dr. Suthep Udomsawaengsup, 2003,
Open Roux en-y gastric bypass, Thailand
Dr. Sang Moon Han, 2003,
Lap Sleeve Gastrectomy, South Korea
Prof. Tran Binh Giang, 2007,
Laparoscopic gastric banding, Vietnam
Dr. Sayeed Qureshi,
Lap gastric banding, Pakistan
Dr. Thomas Y Chua
Lap Roux en-y gastric bypass, Philippines

Fig. 7.2 Pioneer bariatric surgeons from various Asian countries

form a laparoscopic Roux-en-Y gastric bypass, and in 2006, he operated on the heaviest Asian man in China weighing 285 kg. First single incision Roux-en-Y gastric bypass in Asia was performed by Dr. C. K. Huang, and first single incision sleeve was performed by Dr. Muffazal Lakdawala. Dr. Kasama Kazunori of Japan performed the first sleeve with duodenojejunal bypass, Dr. Surendra Ugale from India performed the first ileal transposition, and Dr. W. J. Lee from Taiwan performed the first omega loop gastric bypass in Asia.

By 2004, many surgeons across Asia were performing bariatric surgery. In October 2004, a group of bariatric surgeons gathered in Seoul for the "thought leader's summit" and decided to form the Asia-Pacific Bariatric Surgery Group (APBSG) which is currently known as the Asia-Pacific Metabolic and Bariatric Surgery Society (APMBSS). Dr. Wei Jee Lee was the founding president of APBSG.

The Asia-Pacific chapter of International Federation for Surgery of Obesity and Metabolic Surgery (IFSO-APC) was founded in 2008. IFSO-APC was formed with the intent of promoting multicultural transfers between the Asia-Pacific region and other national societies. Dr. Harry Frydenberg of Australia was the founding president of IFSO-APC. Dr. Muffazal Lakdawala is the current president of IFSO-APC (Fig. 7.3).

Dr. Pradeep Chowbey from India was the first president of IFSO from the region.

First bariatric and metabolic surgery guidelines were formed by ADSS led by Dr. W.J. Lee from Taiwan followed by ACMOMS guidelines published by Dr. Muffazal Lakdawala and Dr. Aparna Govil Bhasker from India [2]. Latest guidelines were published by IFSO-APC in 2011 [3]. The first bariatric nutrition guidelines for Asian patients were published by Carlyne Remedios from India [4].

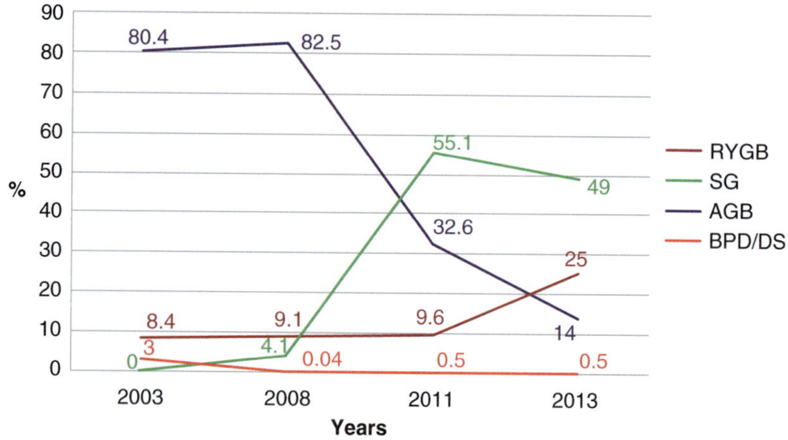

Fig. 7.3 Bariatric surgery trends in the Asia-Pacific region, 2013 [5]

With increasing numbers of bariatric procedures in Asia, a need for improving the quality of care and safety for patients was felt. In 2010, Bariatric and Metabolic International (BMI) Surgery Center of E-Da Hospital along with Dr. C. K. Huang became the first Asian Center for Excellence (COE) recognized by the Surgical Review Corporation (SRC) of the USA. This was followed in 2011 by COE accreditation of CODS (Center for Obesity and Digestive Surgery, Mumbai) along with Dr. Muffazal Lakdawala and Dr. Aparna Govil Bhasker and Max hospital along with Dr. Pradeep Chowbey. These were the first few Asian centers to be awarded the status of COE and set the benchmark for many other bariatric centers in Asia before SRC parted ways with ASMBS.

Current Situation of Bariatric Surgery

A total number of bariatric procedures in Asia have gone up from 2770 in 2003 to 46,110 in 2013 as reported by Angrisani et al. [5]. While laparoscopic gastric banding was the commonest procedure being performed in 2003, its popularity reduced manifold in the next 10 years, and by 2013, it constituted only 14% of all bariatric procedures.

Laparoscopic sleeve gastrectomy (SG) is the most widespread procedure being performed in Asia currently. Technical ease of performing surgery coupled with good weight loss results in the short term has contributed to the growth of sleeve gastrectomy in a short duration. In addition, accessibility of the stomach pouch to UGI endoscopy has rendered it to be the preferred bariatric procedure in Asian countries like Japan and Korea that are endemic for gastric cancer. While there are numerous advantages of SG, leak from a sleeve and GERD remain to be one of its biggest postoperative challenges. Lack of long-term data is a concern, and the incidence of weight regain in the future is yet unknown.

Laparoscopic Roux-en-Y gastric bypass is the second most common surgery performed in this region. Variants of gastric bypass like the banded gastric bypass and single anastomosis gastric bypass are also performed in good numbers although exact data is unavailable. BPD-DS is rarely performed in Asia owing to low protein intake by most Asians.

Laparoscopic sleeve with duodenojejunal bypass (LSG with DJB) and ileal transposition (IT) are the other procedures that are being performed by a few surgeons in Asia. LSG with DJB is an alternative to a Roux-en-Y gastric bypass in Asian countries that are endemic for gastric cancer [6]. Few cases of ileal transposition are being performed, and this procedure has not gained much popularity among the Asian surgeons. The first case of loop bipartition was reported by Dr. Wilfred Mui of Hong Kong, but again this procedure has not found much favor among the surgeons [7].

Single incision bariatric surgery (SILS) is worth a mention here. Unlike the west, SILS technique has gained a lot of popularity in Asia, especially in India and Taiwan. In 2009, the first case of SILS Roux-en-Y gastric bypass was reported by Dr. C. K. Huang from Taiwan [8]. Dr. Muffazal Lakdawala performed the first SILS sleeve gastrectomy in Asia in 2009. In 2015, the largest series of SILS sleeve gastrectomy was published by Dr. Muffazal Lakdawala and Dr. Aparna Bhasker of India [9]. SILS technique has found much favor especially among the young obese Asian women who prefer not to have any tell-tale signs of having a surgery done. It also confers the added advantage of confidentiality to a patient and is more acceptable culturally as obesity is still considered a taboo in this part of the world.

Special Consideration for Specific Geographic Population Such as Indian and Far East as Far as BMI and Diabetes Prevalence in Lower BMI

India and China are the two most populous countries in the world, and together they carry more than half of the world's diabetic burden. Environmental factors coupled with genetic predilection have predisposed Asians to develop diabetes at a younger age. Asians tend to acquire diabetes much earlier, suffer longer, develop complications earlier, and are likely to die sooner.

This high incidence can be attributed to multiple factors:

1. *Genetic factors*: In the Asian population, susceptibility to diabetes has been attributed to "thrifty" gene which conferred a survival advantage in the past but has become detrimental in these times of surplus [10].
2. *Maternal and neonatal factors*: Body composition has been shown to be influenced by adiposity levels of the mother prior to pregnancy as also by aspects of maternal nutritional intake and circulating nutrient concentrations during pregnancy. In a study conducted by KEM hospital, Pune, it was shown that low birth weight babies had higher degree of insulin resistance by the age of 8 years. Low birth weight babies also had higher adiposity levels as compared to their Caucasian counterparts. "The thin fat baby" syndrome is specific to the Asian region [11, 12].
3. *Greater adiposity levels:* It is widely known that Asians tend to develop metabolic syndrome at a BMI as low as that of 22–23 kg/m^2 [13]. Although many Asians may not classify as obese according to the standard WHO criteria, they are metabolically obese at much lower BMIs owing to high visceral obesity levels. Multiple studies have established the relationship between central obesity and hyperglycemia [13].

As Asia undergoes rapid nutritional and lifestyle transition, these genetic traits, coupled with food abundance, increasing psychosocial stress, increasing physical inactivity, and an ageing population, substantially increase the risk of obesity and diabetes in this region. As a result of this, today Asia accounts for more than 50% of the world's diabetic load, and these numbers are expected to increase in the next decade. Some countries like South Korea, China, and Taiwan are routinely performing metabolic surgeries in patients with BMI less than 30 for T2DM.

Challenges in the Region

Although the number of bariatric surgery procedures is rising in the Asian region, there are many challenges for its growth. Currently less than 1% of eligible patients are able to avail surgery. There are multiple reasons for this low penetration. Some of these are discussed as under:

1. *Lack of insurance coverage*

   Many Asian countries like India, Bangladesh, Pakistan, etc. do not have the provision of compulsory health coverage for all. Moreover even in countries with health coverage, bariatric surgeries may not be included in the insurance cover. Presently

Japan, Taiwan, and Singapore are the only Asian countries that provide insurance coverage for bariatric surgery. India, Pakistan, Bangladesh, Korea, China, Malaysia, Indonesia, Thailand, and the Philippines do not have insurance coverage. Lack of insurance coverage is a significant stumbling block as the eligible patient population is compelled to pay out of pocket. Due to the expensive nature of the surgery, it is rendered out of reach for the majority.

2. *Lack of government policy*

   The combined prevalence of overweight and obesity increased by 46% in Japan from 16.7% in 1976–1980 to 24.0% in 2000 and by 414% in China from 3.7% in 1982 to 19.0% in 2002 [14]. The figures are similar for other Asian countries. Although obesity and diabetes together have been accorded an epidemic status by the World Health Organization, most Asian countries lack a national health program to battle the scourge of these diseases. Obesity is yet to be conferred a "disease" status and is considered a taboo in most cultures. Obesity and its related diseases confer a huge economic burden on the national GDPs. In China alone, the total medical cost attributable to overweight and obesity was estimated at about 2.74 billion US dollars [15]. At the moment there is an urgent need of concerted policy action in all sectors with focus on preventive, curative, and rehabilitative aspects of obesity.

3. *National data registries*

   Registries form the precursors to formulation of national health policies. Data entered in registries is used to develop models of risk stratification and setting international standards for postoperative complications and mortality. Most of the demographic and surgical outcome data from Asia is yet unknown. In 2016, India, China, Hong Kong, and Taiwan were the only four countries to contribute data to the IFSO Global Registry. This data however is not representative as most Asian countries failed to contribute their data. Obesity and metabolic surgery society of India has taken the lead in the region by forming the first Bariatric National Registry. We hope that this is a start of a process that will be replicated by all Asian countries in the near future.

4. *Research*

   India and China together constitute more than half of the world's diabetic burden. With an increasing number of bariatric and metabolic professionals, there is a tremendous potential for clinical trials in the region. Lack of regulatory and ethical approval frameworks, hospitals with inadequate research backup, lack of trained research personnel, lack of funding, and cultural barriers are a few stumbling blocks that prevent high-quality research from being carried out. In addition to this, the inherent problems associated with surgical trials tend to increase the difficulties around bariatric surgery research. Unfortunately Asia lags behind in this arena, and till date there is only one randomized controlled trial on metabolic surgery that has been reported from the Asian region [16]. Considering that evidence-based medicine forms the cornerstone of medical therapy today, direct extrapolation of results of western studies on Asian ethnic population may not be a great idea. There is need for a more proactive approach to create a more conducive research environment and conduct world class clinical trials.

5. *Cultural factors and prejudices*

   Most Asian countries take pride in their customs of hospitality. Food forms an important component in the life of Asian people. Obesity is still not considered as a disease, and being overweight is usually considered as a sign of good health and prosperity. Bariatric surgery is still a taboo especially for younger women. Lack of awareness fuels general fear of surgery among patients, and inconsistent media reports do not help the cause. Most people continue to live in denial and fail to seek treatment at appropriate time. Although there are exceptions, most physicians, diabetologists, and endocrinologists still have a skeptical view of bariatric and metabolic surgery. More efforts need to be made to spread awareness about the benefits of bariatric/metabolic surgery among the general population as well as the medical fraternity. To add to this, most of those who have had good results with surgery prefer to deny that they have undergone surgery adding to mistrust around surgery.

6. *Infrastructure and quality control*

   Low healthcare budgets by most Asian governments have resulted into healthcare systems which are underdeveloped and overstretched. Bariatric and metabolic surgery is primarily being performed in the private and corporate setups with an exception of few government hospitals and universities. Dearth of infrastructure needed to support a bariatric practice limits its scope and is thus not offered to a vast majority in smaller towns who could potentially benefit. Quality control is another limiting factor as there are not many regulations that govern the Asian market especially in some Asian countries like India, Pakistan, Myanmar, Sri Lanka, China, Taiwan, and Bangladesh.

7. *Training*

   With an increase in the number of bariatric procedures, there is an augmented interest among surgeons to take up bariatric surgery as a specialty. Off late a few university-recognized programs have been developed and implemented in a few countries. Centers led by Dr. Muffazal Lakdawala in India and those led by Dr. C. K. Huang and Dr. W. J. Lee in Taiwan have been the international training hubs for many years in the Asian region. However training in bariatric surgery still remains haphazard with most surgeons relying on 2–3-day workshops and observerships before they start practicing bariatric surgery. There is an unmet need, and we need many more fellowships and formal programs to inculcate the bariatric culture among the surgeons and paramedical support staff like dieticians, bariatric coordinators, and psychologists.

8. *Newer procedures*

Lack of regulations is a boon and bane at the same time in the Asian region. On one hand, it provides surgeons the freedom to experiment with newer procedures and develop better and more suited surgeries for their population. Procedures like the sleeve gastrectomy with duodenojejunal bypass were designed with Japanese and Korean population in mind as they have a high incidence of gastric cancer. Unfortunately Asia has also become the breeding ground for many hybrid procedures with no supporting data.

Future of Bariatric Surgery in Asia

Rising levels of obesity and diabetes are posing a threat to the Asian growth story. Obesity is a disease, and bariatric/metabolic surgery is the only way to achieve sustained weight loss. With the world's heaviest woman Eman Abd el Aty choosing India to come for her medical treatment, the world has woken up to India and Asia as a destination for bariatric/metabolic surgery. The skillsets of Asian surgeons are at par with their western counterparts. What we need is a bit more perspective in terms of better training, more focus on research, commitment to national data registries, more governmental support, and insurance coverage for bariatric/metabolic surgery. We need better standardization of the existing procedures and more awareness campaigns to bring more physicians, diabetologists, and endocrinologists on the same page. Last but not the least, we need to focus more on prevention of obesity with special emphasis on children and adolescents.

References

1. Ng M, Fleming T, Robinson M, et al. Global, regional, and national prevalence of overweight and obesity in children and adults during 1980–2013: a systematic analysis for the Global Burden of Disease Study 2013. Lancet. 2014;384(9945):766–81.
2. Lakdawala M, Bhasker A. Asian Consensus Meeting on Metabolic Surgery (ACMOMS). Report: Asian Consensus Meeting on Metabolic Surgery. Recommendations for the use of bariatric and gastrointestinal metabolic surgery for treatment of obesity and type ii diabetes mellitus in the asian population: August 9th and 10th, 2008, Trivandrum. Obes Surg. 2010 20(7):929–36.

3. Kasama K, Mui W, Lee WJ, et al. IFSO-APC consensus statements 2011. Obes Surg. 2012;22(5):677–84.
4. Remedios C, Bhasker AG, Dhulla N, et al. Bariatric nutrition guidelines for the Indian population. Obes Surg. 2016;26(5):1057–68.
5. Angrisani L, Santonicola A, Iovino P, et al. Bariatric surgery worldwide 2013. Obes Surg. 2015;25(10):1822–32.
6. Kasama K, Tagaya N, Kanehira E, et al. Laparoscopic sleeve gastrectomy with duodenojejunal bypass: technique and preliminary results. Obes Surg. 2009;19(10):1341–5.
7. Mui WL-M, Lee DW-H, Lam KK-Y. Laparoscopic sleeve gastrectomy with loop bipartition: a novel metabolic operation in treating obese type II diabetes mellitus. Int J Surg Case Rep. 2014;5(2):56–8.
8. Huang CK, Houng JY, Chiang CJ, et al. Single incision transumbilical laparoscopic Roux-en-Y gastric bypass: a first case report. Obes Surg. 2009;19(12):1711–5.
9. Lakdawala M, Agarwal A, Dhar S, et al. Single-incision sleeve gastrectomy versus laparoscopic sleeve gastrectomy. A 2-year comparative analysis of 600 patients. Obes Surg. 2015;25(4):607–14.
10. Neel JV. Diabetes mellitus: a 'thrifty' genotype rendered detrimental by 'progress'? Am J Hum Genet. 1962;14:353–62.
11. Yajnik CS. Obesity epidemic in India: intrauterine origins? Proc Nutr Soc. 2004;63:387–96.
12. Bavdekar A, Yajnik CS, Fall CHD, et al. The insulin resistance syndrome [IRS] in eight-year old Indian children: small at birth, big at 8 years or both? Diabetes. 2000;48:2422–9.
13. Ko GTC, Tang JSF. Waist circumference and BMI cut-off based on 10-year cardiovascular risk: evidence for central pre-obesity. Obesity. 2007;15:2832–40.
14. Asia Pacific Cohort Studies Collaboration. The burden of overweight and obesity in the Asia-Pacific region. Obes Rev. 2007;8:191–6.
15. Zhao W, Zhai Y, Hu J, Wang J, Yang Z, Kong L, Chen C. Economic burden of obesity-related chronic diseases in Mainland China. Obes Rev. 2008;9:62–7.
16. Ikramuddin S, Korner J, Lee WJ, et al. Durability of addition of Roux-en-Y gastric bypass to lifestyle intervention and medical management in achieving primary treatment goals for uncontrolled type 2 diabetes in mild to moderate obesity: a randomized control trial. Diabetes Care. 2016;39(9):1510–8.

Part III

Standard Bariatric Operations

Gastric Banding

8

Jaclyn Clark, Christine Ren Fielding, and George Fielding

Introduction and History of the Procedure

The surgical management of morbid obesity now has over five decades of history. In the early 1960s, malabsorption through intestinal bypass was recognized to result in significant weight loss for obese patients [1, 2]. Paired with the restriction of a gastric pouch, the RYGB (Roux-en-Y gastric bypass) grew to become the procedure of choice for surgical weight loss. Malabsorption was the main focus of the first generation of bariatric procedures; however, in 1982 the vertical banded gastroplasty (VBG) was introduced after it became clear that gastric restriction also led to weight loss [3, 4]. Importantly, restrictive operations avoid the sequelae of malabsorption. The surgery was described by Mason in 1982 and modified in the years to follow [3, 5]. First, a 32F tube passed through the mouth defined the width of the gastric pouch. A gastrotomy was made through the anterior and posterior walls of the stomach approximately 2 cm from the gastroesophageal junction (GEJ) with a circular stapler. A linear stapler through this gastrotomy was aimed toward the angle of His and fired to create a small pouch and exclude the fundus. Finally, a band or mesh was fixed at the base of the pouch to restrict its expansion and provide a consistent-sized gastric outlet. While successful in producing weight loss, the VBG was often complicated by staple line dehiscence, migrated bands, or mesh erosion [6].

To address these complications, the first adjustable band was placed by laparotomy in 1986 and offered patients a weight loss procedure that did not involve intestinal rearrangement or staple lines [7]. The product and technique were honed through the late 1980s and early 1990s, until the first LAP-BAND™ (BioEnterics, Santa Barbara, CA) was placed in 1993 by Belachew in Belgium [8]. The system is comprised of a silicone band placed around the proximal stomach that can be filled with saline to adjust the diameter of the band and thus the gastric outlet. The band is connected to thin tubing, which is brought out of the peritoneal cavity, and connected to a port, which is then anchored to the fascia. The port is accessed by a non-coring needle, which can be used to inflate and deflate the band by injecting saline.

The procedure rose to international popularity, and the United States began clinical trials in 1995. Currently there are two FDA-approved banding devices available in the United States: the LAP-BAND system (Apollo Endosurgery, Austin, TX), as previously mentioned, approved

J. Clark (✉)
Department of Surgery, New York University Langone Medical Center, New York, NY, USA
e-mail: Jaclyn.clark@nyumc.org

C. R. Fielding · G. Fielding
Department of Surgery, NYU School of Medicine, New York, NY, USA
e-mail: Christine.ren-fielding@nyumc.org; George.fielding@nyumc.org

R. Lutfi et al. (eds.), *Global Bariatric Surgery*, https://doi.org/10.1007/978-3-319-93545-4_8

in 2001, and the REALIZE band (Ethicon, Endo-Surgery, Cincinnati, OH) [7]. Since 2010, laparoscopic adjustable gastric banding (LAGB) has been approved for body mass index (BMI) 30–35 kg/m^2 with obesity-related comorbidities, which makes it a common option for those in this BMI range. The adjustable band remains a popular option for morbidly obese patients today, as well as an option for revisional bariatric surgery [9].

Pre- and Postoperative Care

All patients undergoing evaluation for bariatric surgery are encouraged to consult with a registered dietician, mental health professional, and surgeon. After determining the patient's eligibility for bariatric surgery, the surgical options along with data on percentage of excess weight loss, complications, and required follow-up are provided to the patient. The choice to undergo LAGB is often influenced by patient preference.

The idea of an adjustable band appeals to patients who are averse to intestinal manipulation, as well as those who enjoy its reversibility. Prior to surgery, a 2-week low-fat liquid diet is recommended to both assess patient compliance and facilitate liver retraction during the operation.

At our institution, LAGB has largely become an outpatient procedure, with low postoperative morbidity. After surgery the patients are assessed and subsequently discharged from the postanesthesia care unit after tolerating slow sips of water without nausea, emesis, or pain. Patients are placed on a strict postoperative diet. The first night after surgery, patients are allowed thin liquids. For the next 10 days, patients are maintained on clear or opaque thin liquids. In the following 10 days, pureed foods are introduced, and at day 21 patients can self-advance to a regular diet.

The follow-up schedule after LAGB is rigorous. At 1 week, patients undergo a baseline esophagram and are seen for their first postoperative visit. At 4 weeks post-procedure, patients are evaluated and undergo their first band adjustment. The amount of saline injected into the band system depends on the type and size of the band. Patients are seen monthly for adjustments for the 1st year, four to six times per year for 2 years, and eventually annually. Patients have yearly esophagrams to evaluate band position. Patients are also seen by registered dieticians and are encouraged to attend monthly bariatric surgery support groups.

Technical Aspects of the Procedure

Surgical technique for LAGB has evolved since first described. The perigastric method, described by Belachew [10], involved placing the band through a tunnel located 3 cm below the gastroesophageal junction through the lesser sac. This technique had high rates of gastric prolapse and has fallen out of favor [11]. At our institution we use the presently mainstream "pars flaccida" technique, described below [12, 13]:

1. Positioning and perioperative monitoring: The patient is placed in the supine position on the operating table with both arms extended (Fig. 8.1). After intubation, an orogastric tube is placed for gastric decompression.
2. Port placement and access: OptiView technique is used to enter the peritoneal cavity under direct vision using a 12 mm OptiView trocar in the left upper quadrant, and pneumoperitoneum is established. Three additional trocars are placed: a 15 mm trocar in the midline and two 5 mm trocars in the right and left subcostal regions in the maxillary line (Fig. 8.2).
3. Liver retraction: A Nathanson liver retractor (Cook, Bloomington, Indiana) is placed through a 5 mm subxiphoid incision and is used to elevate the liver to reveal the hiatus and gastroesophageal junction (Fig. 8.3).
4. Dissection of the angle of His: The omentum above the first short gastric vessel is elevated, and the fundus is retracted inferiorly, which exposes the plane of dissection between the gastroesophageal junction and hiatus. These peritoneal attachments are divided (Figs. 8.4 and 8.5).
5. Fat pad dissection: There is reliably a small collection of fat overlying the GE junction, which should be dissected off to lessen likelihood of esophageal obstruction and optimize visualization of the stomach. The fat pad is grasped and elevated, and the fundus is

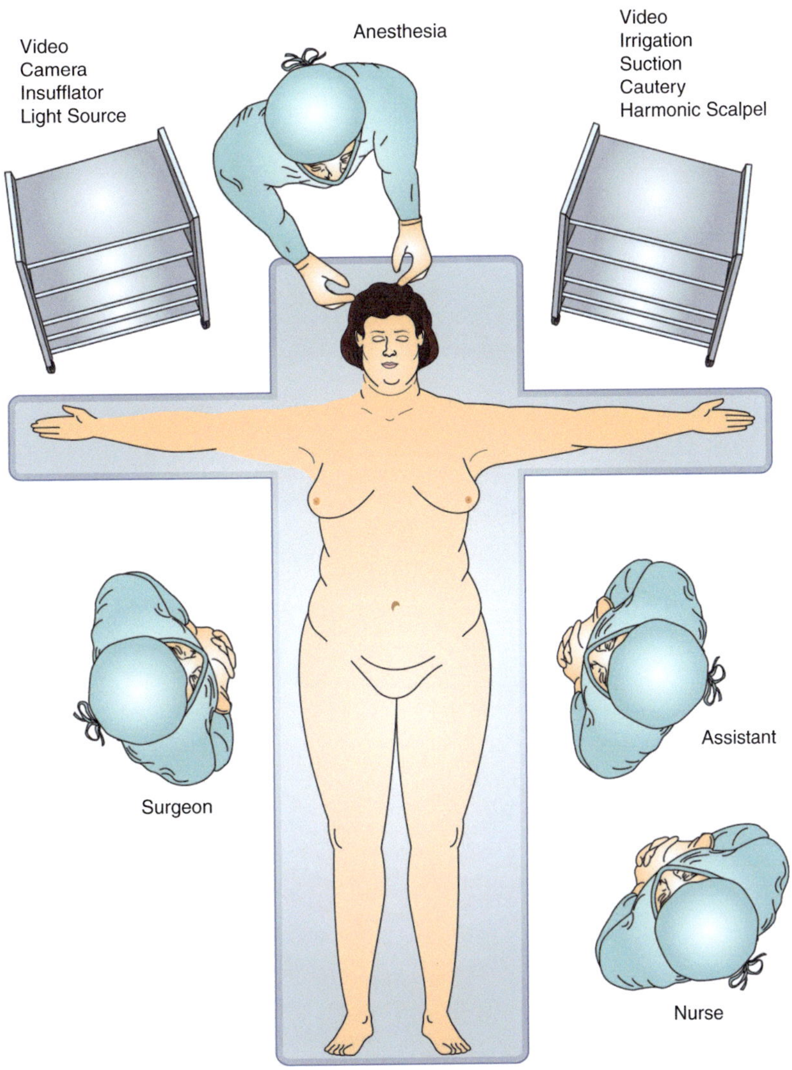

Fig. 8.1 Patient positioning: surgeon stands to patient's right with assistant to patient's left; arms out

retracted inferiorly to expose the plane of dissection, which can be taken using an energy device of surgeon preference. If the fat pad is small, this step is not necessary.

6. Pars flaccida approach: This step involves dividing the lesser omentum at its translucent aspect over the caudate lobe and carrying the dissection superiorly to the diaphragmatic hiatus. This will expose the right crus of the diaphragm, which should be grasped and elevated at its most inferior aspect. The overlying peritoneum is incised and a grasper placed through the window created, posterior to the esophagus and through to the left side via the window created in step 4. If there is resistance, more dissection is needed. This step is done without perfect visualization, and it should be noted that if the surgeon is in the wrong plane, the grasper could be dissecting into the esophagus or stomach—very little force should be used here. At this point the band is introduced into the abdomen through the 15 mm trocar and handed to the grasper that is in the window. The band is pulled into position using the grasper. The band is secured when the tubing is passed through the locking mechanism of the band, and the band is locked. The band should not be tight and should rotate with ease. This step becomes more complicated if the patient has a replaced left hepatic artery arising from the left gastric artery, as it will cross above

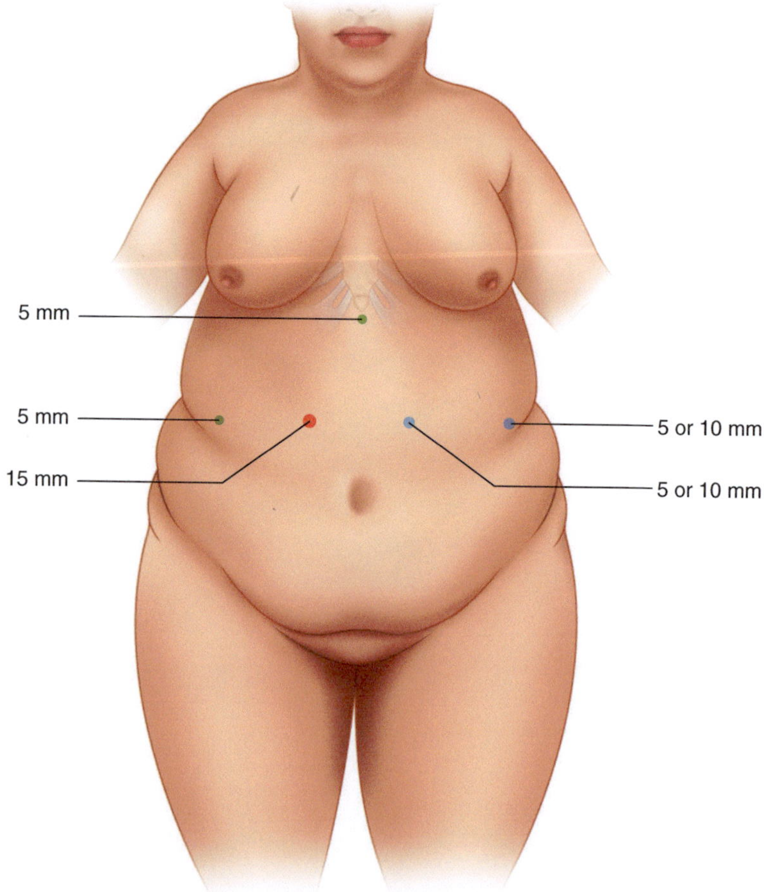

Fig. 8.2 Trocar placement

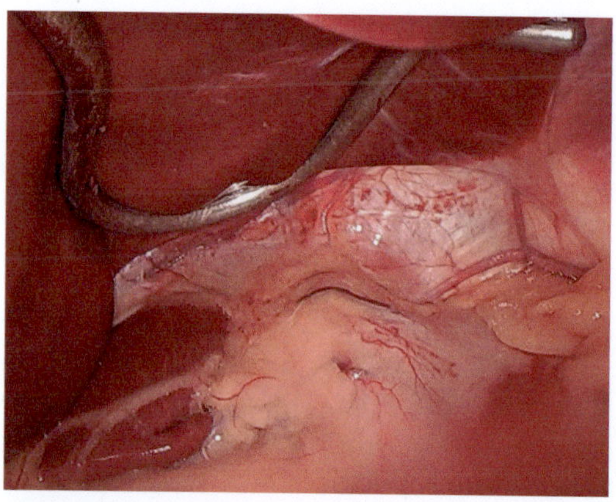

Fig. 8.3 Use of the Nathanson liver retractor to reveal the GE junction

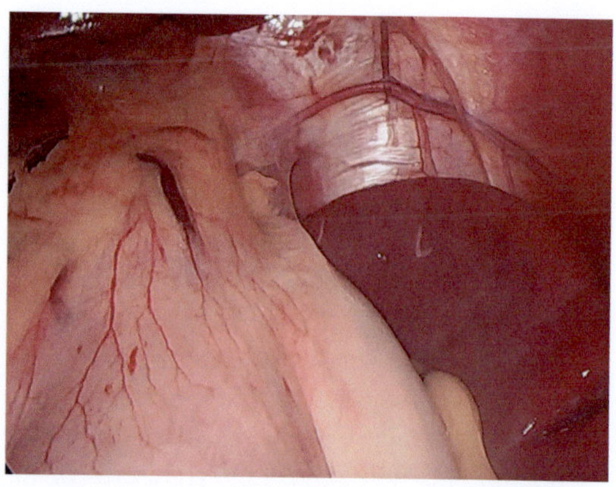

Fig. 8.4 Caudad retraction of the stomach to reveal the angle of His

the right crus in the lesser omentum and should be preserved. Additionally, it is imperative not to mistake the inferior vena cava (IVC) for the esophagus or the right crus, as the IVC will be visible next to the caudate lobe (Figs. 8.6, 8.7, 8.8, and 8.9).

7. Fundoplication: While the band is limited in its posterior movement by the extent of our

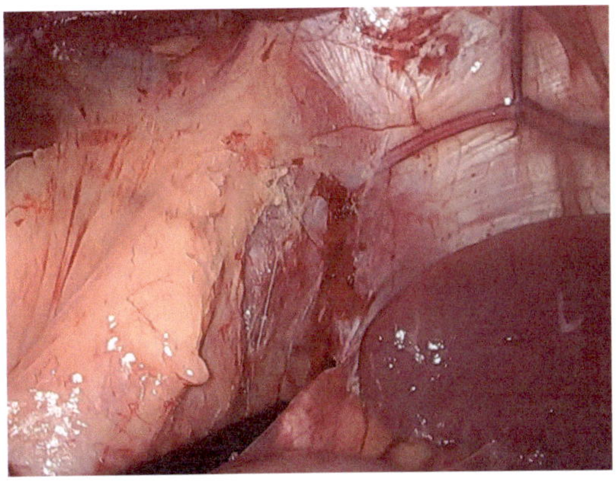

Fig. 8.5 Dissection of the angle of His

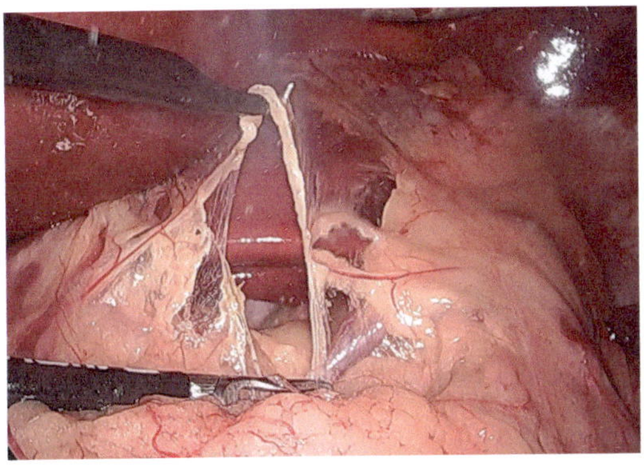

Fig. 8.6 Entry into the lesser sac via the pars flaccida

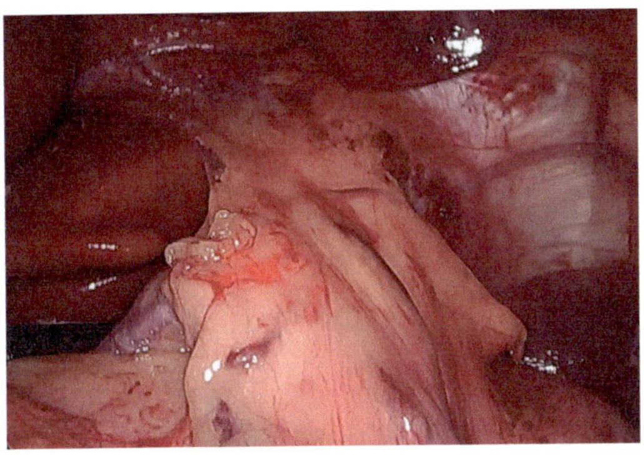

Fig. 8.7 An instrument is passed behind the esophagus at the base of the crura

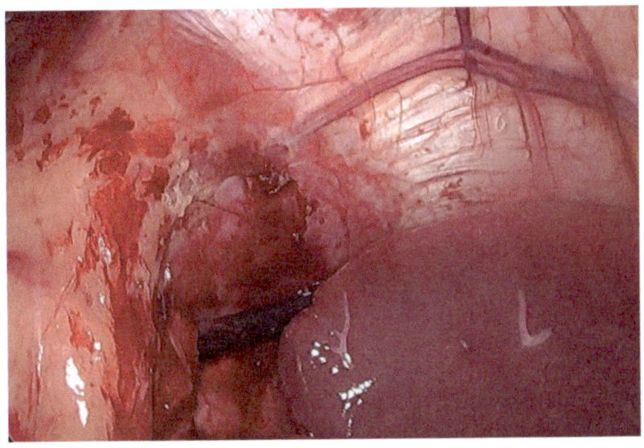

Fig. 8.8 The grasper passing through the retro-esophageal window

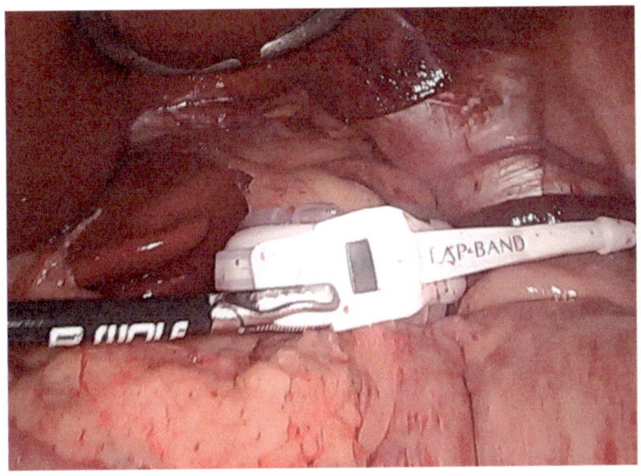

Fig. 8.9 Securing the band in place by fastening the buckle

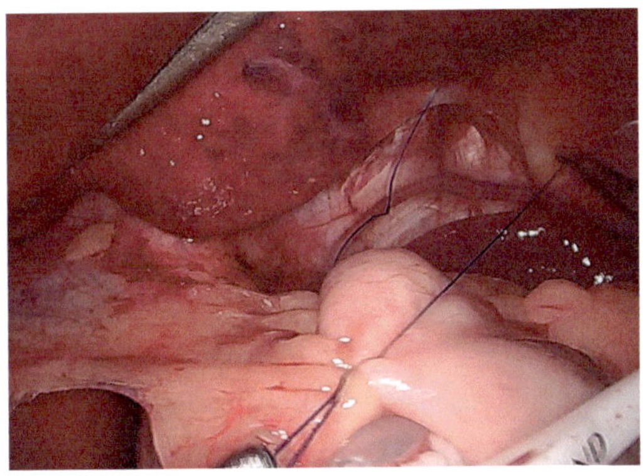

Fig. 8.10 Fundoplication securing the band's position anteriorly

dissection and the retroperitoneum, anteriorly it is unrestricted. We perform a plication of the fundus to the cardia using a nonabsorbable suture to restrict its movement without creating too much tension to risk erosion. This can be accomplished using a running or interrupted suture, to secure the stomach that is folded up and over the band (Figs. 8.10 and 8.11).

8. Access port placement: The band tubing is pulled through the 15 mm trocar, all trocars are removed, and the abdomen is allowed to col-

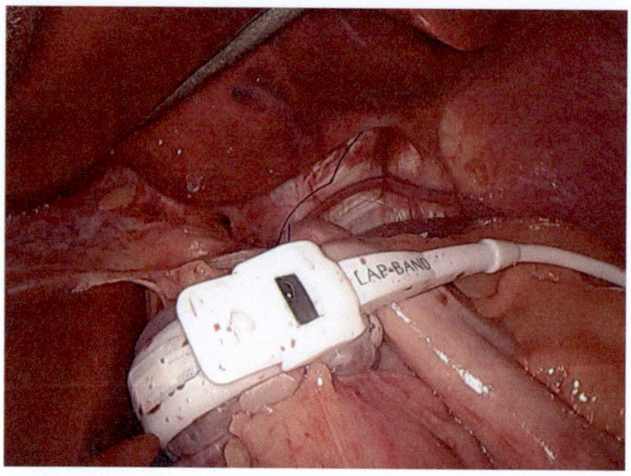

Fig. 8.11 Band in situ

lapse. The tubing is cut, left long to prevent bowel obstruction, and attached to the port. The access port is secured to the anterior fascia using nonabsorbable 0 Ethibond sutures in each corner. The band is left empty and the skin is closed.

We have also employed and studied the single-incision laparoscopic surgery (SILS) technique to place the LAGB [14]. This involves using a single 3–4 cm periumbilical incision with placement of a 12 mm trocar in the Hassan fashion. The band is introduced into the abdomen, and two 5 mm trocars are placed through the same skin incision to the left and right of the Hassan trocar. It is best if one trocar has a low profile and is short, while the other trocar is extra-long. This allows for the trocars to move easily without clashing into each other. Liver retraction is used either via the same incision or a 5 mm subxiphoid incision. Dissection proceeds as described above.

Complications

Although considered a safer alternative to other bariatric procedures, LAGB is not without complications. These can be broadly divided into problems related to the band and those related to the port [15]. Regardless of the underlying mechanism, band complications are often heralded by oral intolerance and epigastric pain.

Gastric prolapse is the most common intra-abdominal complication following LAGB [15]. Also referred to as a "band slip," this involves part of the stomach, usually the fundus, herniating superiorly through the band. Etiologies are not definitively known but are often attributed to failure of the anterior gastro-gastric plication sutures. This can either be due to breakdown or tearing, the latter exacerbated by excessive vomiting. Patients with this entity also report dysphagia and reflux. The immediate step in management of these patients is complete band deflation and observation for symptomatic improvement. This maneuver can distinguish patients with gastric prolapse from those who are simply not tolerating a recent adjustment. If symptoms are relieved with fluid removal and the patient can tolerate sips of thin liquids, no emergent imaging is needed. For those who have continued emesis and oral intolerance after band deflation, an esophagram is warranted to visualize the gastric pouch in real motion. In the event of prolapse, this study will show a large pouch with delayed emptying and rotation of the band along its anterior-posterior axis (Figs. 8.12 and 8.13). The consequences of a slipped band range from nocturnal reflux with mild irritation to gastric necrosis. This complication is managed in the operating room and can involve repositioning of the band, band removal, or most drastically gastric resection for ischemia or perforation [16].

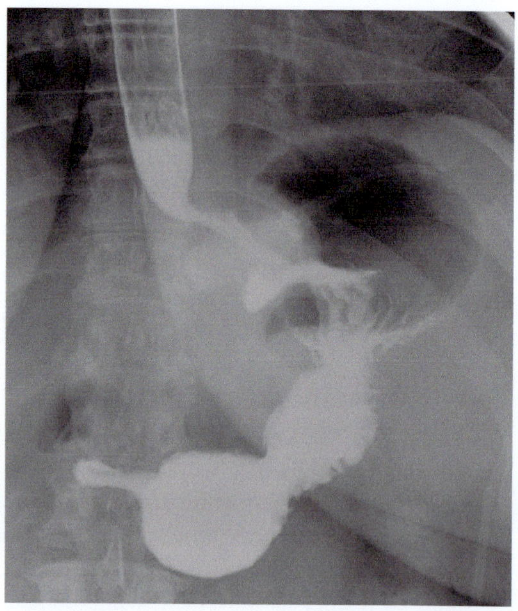

Fig. 8.12 A normal esophagram after LAGB showing the band in proper position and the passage of contrast

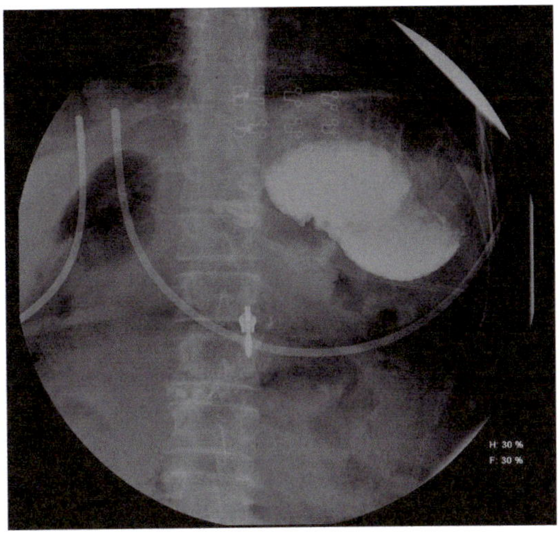

Fig. 8.13 The esophagram of a slipped band shows a complete obstruction of contrast passage at the level of the band, an overlying large gastric pouch

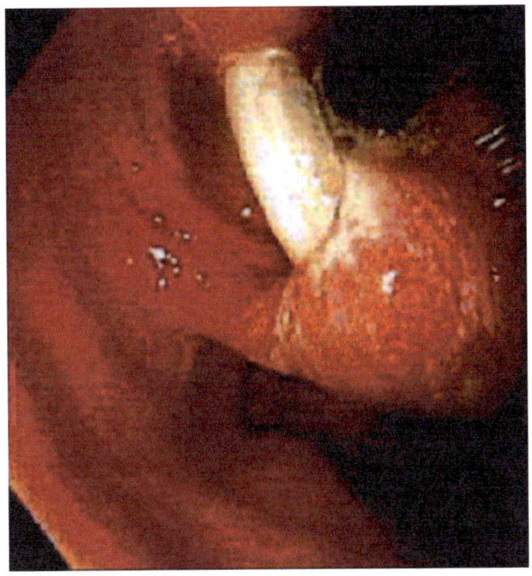

Fig. 8.14 Intraluminal band demonstrated on EGD

Often, patients will have strong feelings on removal versus repositioning, which should be taken into account if feasible.

A serious complication of LAGB is band erosion. Patients can be asymptomatic but commonly present with sudden loss of restriction and weight gain. Another presentation of band erosion is port-infection due to bacterial tracking [15]. Proposed mechanisms include serosal injury at the time of surgery, placing plicating sutures above the band locking mechanism, or mucosal injury such as chronic NSAID use. The esophagram is less useful for making the diagnosis in these patients, and esophagogastroduodenoscopy (EGD) is the modality of choice [17] (Fig. 8.14). Presentation is most often subacute, with peritonitis being rare due to healing of the stomach around the band; and the treatment is removal of the band and closure of the remaining gastrotomy.

Port-related problems include infection, leak, and difficult access [18]. These carry less morbidity; however, they are often more irritating to patients than dangerous. Port site infection, as referenced above, can herald band erosion or can simply represent local abscess or cellulitis. These entities can be treated with oral antibiotics, incision, and drainage and, if needed, port removal with delayed relocation.

A flipped or inaccessible port can be frustrating. Ports generally become inaccessible due to failure of the anchoring sutures to the anterior fascia during placement. After multiple attempts at accessing a port without success, a PA and lateral abdominal plain film can be useful in identifying a flipped port. Additionally, fluoroscopy can be used to attempt to visualize the needle entering the port [19]. These ports need to be revised and reanchored to the fascia to restore functionality.

The third port-related complication is system leakage due to tubing punctures that occur during access attempts. The point of extravasation can be located on fluoroscopy; however, as this requires replacement of the tubing, often local incision over the port site with careful examination of the tubing can identify the leak. This is performed by injecting dilute methylene blue solution into the port and evaluating for entry. Other areas of saline extravasation can be from external compression of tubing entering the abdominal wall, tubing break, or balloon section of the band. For this reason, if the port appears to be intact during surgical exploration, laparoscopy is required to evaluate the entire system (Fig. 8.15).

Data

Several studies have examined outcomes following gastric banding. In 2010, Carelli et al. examined complication rates 7 years after

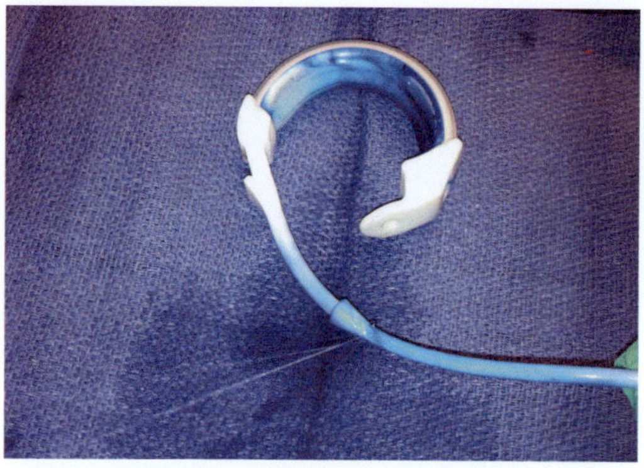

Fig. 8.15 Port leak demonstrated in the tubing by injecting saline

LAGB performed by three surgeons [20]. Data were collected on 2909 patients prospectively between 2001 and 2008 and included general outcomes along with band-related complications. Twelve percent of patients experienced a complication, most commonly slipped band at 4.5%, followed by port-related issues at 3.3%. Only seven (0.2%) patients developed band erosion. In terms of weight regain, there were nine (0.3%) reoperations, most of which were converted to RYGB.

In 2013, O'Brien et al., the authors, performed a systematic review of the literature to examine long-term weight loss data in bariatric surgery [21]. Nineteen trials were included, each with 10 years of patient follow-up. Pooled data showed 33–64% EWL with 8–60% revisional rate for LAGB.

In 2014, Xiaojun Shen and colleagues performed a systematic review of the LAGB literature in China which included 17 articles with 10-year follow-up [22]. They corroborated results showing almost 50% EWL with 36% requiring reoperation. The most common indication or reoperation was band slippage, at 15.3%. Bands were removed in 10%.

One prospective, randomized trial by Angrisani and colleagues in 2013 assigned a cohort of 51 patients to either LAGB or laparoscopic Roux-en-Y gastric bypass (LRYGB) [23]. After a decade of follow-up, 9 out of 22 LAGB patients (40.9%) required band removal, and 1 required port replacement (4.3%). The reoperation rate in the LRYGB group was 6 out of 21 (28.6%); however, 4 of these operations were cholecystectomies for gallstones. Mean excess weight loss (EWL) favored the LRYGB with 69% compared to 46% in LAGB ($p = 0.003$ at 10 years). Early complications were significantly higher in the LRYGB group compared to the LAGB group (8.3% vs 0%).

A prospective randomized study by Himpens et al. in 2006 compared LAGB to laparoscopic sleeve gastrectomy (LSG) in terms of weight loss and complication rate [24]. After 3 years, it showed percent EWL of 48% in LAGB vs 66% in LSG ($P = 0.0025$). The study included subjective measures of hunger which were lost in 2.9% of band patients vs 46.7% of LSG patients after 3 years ($P < 0.0001$). Overall, there is a paucity of data comparing LSG to LAGB.

Discussion

The LAGB is a unique and useful option among bariatric surgical procedures. As its name suggests, it provides the possibility of adjustability based on patient comfort and sustained weight loss. Data favors the RYGB for percent EWL; however, the LABG still affords patients with nearly 50% EWL. It remains the only surgical option that does not require intestinal bypass or staple lines, thus avoiding the major severe complications of RYGB and sleeve gastrectomy. These include malnourishment, leaks, and internal hernias, which often result in chronic and indolent hospital courses. LAGB is a safe outpatient procedure which appeals to patients. Lastly, it is ideal for those with a BMI of 30–40 kg/m^2 who do not need to lose a dramatic amount of weight.

As detailed above, the LAGB is not without its drawbacks. The procedure has its own set of complications that often require reoperation, including gastric prolapse, band erosion, and port inaccessibility. By understanding how to diagnose and treat these complications, patients can continue to have long-standing weight loss with LAGB. Therefore, LAGB should be performed at bariatric centers of excellence by those with experience in the procedure and managing its complications. Patient selection, rigorous follow-up, and office visits are essential for success.

References

1. Scott HW Jr, Dean R, Shull HJ, et al. Considerations in use of jejunoileal bypass in patients with morbid obesity. Ann Surg. 1973;177:723–35.
2. Shibata HR, MacKenzie JR, Long RC. Metabolic effects of controlled jejunocolic bypass. Arch Surg. 1967;95:413–28.
3. Mason EE. Vertical banded gastroplasty for obesity. Arch Surg. 1982;117:701–6.
4. Szinicz G, Muller L, Erhart W, Roth FX, Pointner R, Glaser K. "Reversible gastric banding" in surgical treatment of morbid obesity – results of animal experiments. Res Exp Med (Berl). 1989;189:55–60.
5. Harrison RA, Clark CG. Vertical banded gastroplasty: operation for morbid obesity. Ann R Coll Surg Engl. 1984;66:346–7.
6. Schouten R, Wiryasaputra DC, van Dielen FM, van Gemert WG, Greve JW. Long-term results of bariatric restrictive procedures: a prospective study. Obes Surg. 2010;20:1617–26.
7. McBride CL, Kothari V. Evolution of laparoscopic adjustable gastric banding. Surg Clin North Am. 2011;91:1239–47, viii–ix.
8. Belachew M, Legrand MJ, Defechereux TH, Burtheret MP, Jacquet N. Laparoscopic adjustable silicone gastric banding in the treatment of morbid obesity. A preliminary report. Surg Endosc. 1994;8:1354–6.
9. Vijgen GH, Schouten R, Bouvy ND, Greve JW. Salvage banding for failed Roux-en-Y gastric bypass. Surg Obes Relat Dis. 2012;8:803–8.
10. Belachew M, Legrand M, Vincenti VV, et al. Laparoscopic placement of adjustable silicone gastric band in the treatment of morbid obesity: how to do it. Obes Surg. 1995;5:66–70.
11. Elias B, Staudt JP, Van Vyne E. The technical approach in banding to avoid pouch dilatation. Obes Surg. 2001;11:311–4.
12. Fielding GA, Allen JW. A step-by-step guide to placement of the LAP-BAND adjustable gastric banding system. Am J Surg. 2002;184:26S–30S.
13. Ren CJ, Fielding GA. Laparoscopic adjustable gastric banding: surgical technique. J Laparoendosc Adv Surg Tech A. 2003;13:257–63.
14. Schwack BF, Novack R, Youn H, Fielding CR, Kurian MS, Fielding GA. Single-incision laparoscopic adjustable gastric banding is effective and safe: 756 cases in an academic medical center. Obes Surg. 2013;23:332–7.
15. Allen JW. Laparoscopic gastric band complications. Med Clin North Am. 2007;91:485–97, xii.
16. Tran D, Rhoden DH, Cacchione RN, Baldwin L, Allen JW. Techniques for repair of gastric prolapse after laparoscopic gastric banding. J Laparoendosc Adv Surg Tech A. 2004;14:117–20.
17. Owers C, Ackroyd R. A study examining the complications associated with gastric banding. Obes Surg. 2013;23:56–9.
18. Tog CH, Halliday J, Khor Y, Yong T, Wilkinson S. Evolving pattern of laparoscopic gastric band access port complications. Obes Surg. 2012;22:863–5.
19. Carucci LR, Turner MA, Szucs RA. Adjustable laparoscopic gastric banding for morbid obesity: imaging assessment and complications. Radiol Clin N Am. 2007;45:261–74.
20. Carelli AM, Youn HA, Kurian MS, Ren CJ, Fielding GA. Safety of the laparoscopic adjustable gastric band: 7-year data from a U.S. center of excellence. Surg Endosc. 2010;24:1819–23.
21. O'Brien PE, MacDonald L, Anderson M, Brennan L, Brown WA. Long-term outcomes after bariatric surgery: fifteen-year follow-up of adjustable gastric banding and a systematic review of the bariatric surgical literature. Ann Surg. 2013;257:87–94.
22. Shen X, Zhang X, Bi J, Yin K. Long-term complications requiring reoperations after laparoscopic adjustable gastric banding: a systematic review. Surg Obes Relat Dis. 2015;11:956–64.
23. Angrisani L, Cutolo PP, Formisano G, Nosso G, Vitolo G. Laparoscopic adjustable gastric banding versus Roux-en-Y gastric bypass: 10-year results of a prospective, randomized trial. Surg Obes Relat Dis. 2013;9:405–13.
24. Himpens J, Dapri G, Cadiere GB. A prospective randomized study between laparoscopic gastric banding and laparoscopic isolated sleeve gastrectomy: results after 1 and 3 years. Obes Surg. 2006;16:1450–6.

9 Sleeve Gastrectomy

Blake R. Movitz, Arsalan Salamat, and Rami Lutfi

Introduction

Laparoscopic sleeve gastrectomy (LSG) is the most commonly performed bariatric procedure in the United States, accounting for more than half of all bariatric procedures [1]. There are several factors that have led to its rapid traction since its inception. Firstly, in comparison to the laparoscopic adjustable gastric banding, which was still popular at the time, the sleeve was a simple yet a metabolic operation, activating significant hormonal pathways that lead to changes in eating behavior, glycemic control, and gut functions, all without the need for an implant. Secondly, in contrast to Roux-en-Y gastric bypass (RYGB), LSG is less technically complex and therefore more appealing to patients. Being limited to the stomach makes it simpler and evades the risk of internal hernias and malabsorption complications such as micronutrient and protein deficiency. Yet, if needed, it could always be converted to a malabsorptive operation by simply performing the intestinal part of these operations.

B. R. Movitz
General Surgery, University of Illinois at Chicago – Metropolitan Group Hospitals, Chicago, IL, USA

A. Salamat
General Surgery, Presence Health St. Joseph Hospital, Chicago, IL, USA

R. Lutfi (✉)
University of Illinois at Chicago, Chicago, IL, USA

The idea of making a tubular-shaped stomach for weight loss dates back to 1976, when Lawrence Tretbar described creating a tubular structure as an extension of the gastric fundoplication for reflux. The goal was to achieve meaningful weight loss in obese individuals with reflux disease [2]. The first version of this operation did not involve resection; it consisted of making a sleeve-shaped stomach without performing a gastrectomy. The "remnant" would remain connected through the antrum to the tubular stomach. This was first described by Johnston as a simpler, more physiologic gastroplasty that avoided the use of implant (in contrast to the vertical banded gastroplasty, VBG) [3]. It was called the Magenstrasse and Mill, alluding to a street of stomach that preserves the antral mill and the antro-pyloro-duodenal regulation of gastric emptying and secretion (Fig. 9.1).

The sleeve gastrectomy, as we know it today, was first described by Marceau and Hess. When performing the biliopancreatic diversion, Marceau performed the lateral gastrectomy as an alternative to the distal gastrectomy, described by Scopinaro [4]. The lateral gastrectomy allowed for preservation of the pylorus, limiting biliary reflux, marginal ulcers, and dumping syndrome. This came to be known as the duodenal switch modification. Later, Hess and Hess described the sleeve gastrectomy as part of their own modification of this procedure, leading to

R. Lutfi et al. (eds.), *Global Bariatric Surgery*, https://doi.org/10.1007/978-3-319-93545-4_9

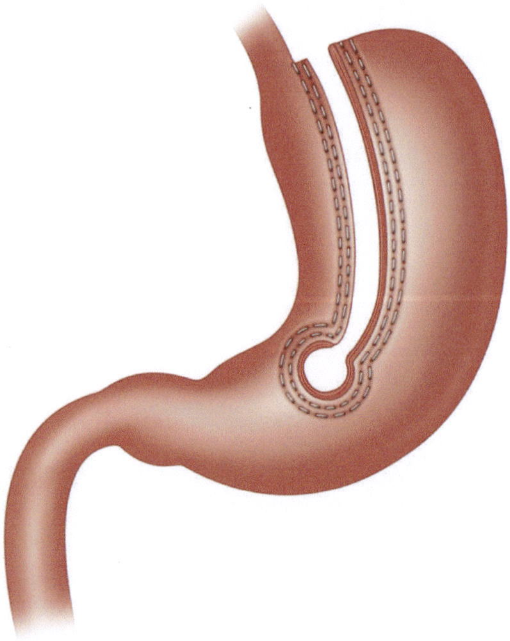

Fig. 9.1 Magenstrasse and Mill operation

the biliopancreatic diversion/duodenal switch (BPD/DS) of the modern era [5].

While highly effective operations, duodenal switch operations (and often gastric bypasses) were long procedures performed on super-obese and high-risk patients. Safety was a concern and surgeons started "staging" these operations, limiting the first-stage surgery to a sleeve gastrectomy. This allowed patients to recover, lose weight, and improve many of their comorbidities, making the "second-stage" intestinal part a safer operation with less morbidity [6–9].

Since its inception, the sleeve gastrectomy was performed laparoscopically. It was shown to have excess weight loss comparable to RYGB, significant improvement or resolution of comorbidities, and a high safety profile. In fact, many patients did not want to return for the second-stage operation as they were satisfied with the weight loss and their quality of life [10]. This earned the sleeve to be considered as a stand-alone procedure, soon to become the fastest growing and the most prevalent bariatric operation in the United States and many other countries.

Preparation for Laparoscopic Sleeve Gastrectomy

Preoperative workup for bariatric surgery is described in detail elsewhere in this book. Briefly, prior to all bariatric operations, intensive psychological, behavioral, and dietary counseling is mandatory. Medical workup is required to exclude primary causes for obesity and to diagnose and treat associated comorbidities. At the time of writing this publication, there is no consensus in the literature on the extent of preoperative evaluation of foregut pathology. However, it is our preference to routinely perform screening upper endoscopy even to asymptomatic patients, prior to sleeve gastrectomy. Many conditions that may be contraindications to sleeve gastrectomy can be asymptomatic. This includes Barrett's esophagus, Hill grade 3 or 4 hiatal hernia, and Los Angeles grade 3 or 4 esophagitis, all, if asymptomatic, may go undiagnosed unless routinely screened for. Endoscopy has the advantage over UGI to allow direct inspection of the mucosa and perform biopsy to determine pathology such as Barrett's esophagus and *H. pylori*, which may alter the surgical plan [11]. For symptomatic patients, additional studies such as 24-h pH testing, manometry, and upper GI series may be warranted.

Surgical Technique

We will describe our technique while commenting on other options for the critical steps of the operation.

Preoperatively, subcutaneous low molecular weight heparin is administered in the holding suite, and intravenous acetaminophen is initiated for auxiliary analgesia. Sequential compression devices are placed on the lower extremities bilaterally. In our practice, we avoid supplementary positioning maneuvers, such as arm tucking or lithotomy, to prevent complications related to musculoskeletal or nerve injury. The patient is placed in the supine position with a foot board to

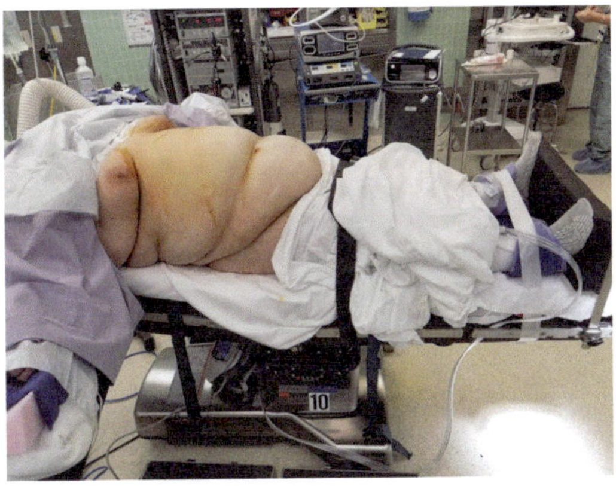

Fig. 9.2 Positioning (Note the foot board with the tape to stabilize the ankles and prevent rotation during reverse Trendelenburg positions)

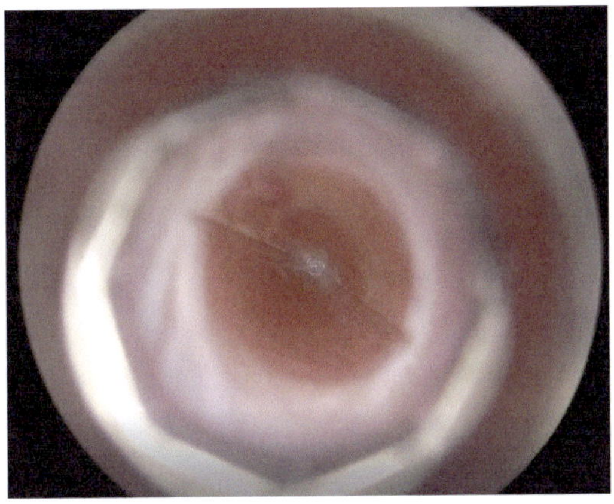

Fig. 9.3 Entering the abdominal cavity using a blunt 5-mm trocar under direct vision by 0-degree scope (Note the tip of the trocar is penetrating the peritoneum. The muscle and fascia are still visible)

prevent sliding during reverse Trendelenburg maneuvering. Special attention is made to ensure ankle stability and prevent inward rotation (Fig. 9.2).

The best technique for entering the peritoneal cavity is a controversial topic. While Veress needle and Hasson methods are acceptable, it has been our experience that the large pannus in the morbidly obese patient makes these techniques cumbersome. It is our practice to enter the abdomen under direct vision with a 0° laparoscope using a bladeless optical trocar placed immediately inferior to the left subcostal margin in the midclavicular line. Although this high positioning may add slight technical difficulty to the assistant who must work against the view of the camera when assisting near the pylorus, it has been our experience that the rib gives countertraction, while the trocar is inserted and allows for expeditious and safe penetration of the peritoneum with minimal mechanical force [12] (Fig. 9.3).

In the majority of cases, the LSG can be performed with two trocars for the surgeon and one trocar for the assistant. A single 12-mm trocar (for the stapler) is placed just lateral to the inferior aspect of the falciform ligament on the right. An additional 5-mm trocar is placed in the right upper quadrant for the surgeon's left hand (Fig. 9.4). With this distribution of ports, the first assistant can hold both the laparoscope and a retractor, obviating the need for a second assistant for the camera. The articulating capabilities of today's staplers make it possible for the surgeon to stand on the right side (instead of between the legs) and use the right-sided trocar for all stapler firings of the different parts of the stomach (Fig. 9.5).

In patients with severe visceral obesity (Fig. 9.6), a second trocar can be added for the assistant on the left to retract the omentum, optimizing exposure when dissecting the left crus.

The liver is retracted in all cases with a rigid liver retractor placed through a 5-mm incision in the sub-xiphoid area. Excellent exposure of the hiatus is mandatory for optimal sleeve construction in order to adequately inspect the hiatus for hernia and dissect the left crus to prevent retained fundus. It is more important in this operation than any other to clearly visualize the hiatus and dissect the left crus due to the "refluxogenic" nature of the sleeve gastrectomy.

The omental attachments to the greater curvature are divided beginning 3-cm proximal to the pylorus and continued along the greater curvature all the way to the left crus (Fig. 9.7).

Posterior adhesions are carefully divided, protecting the left gastric artery, splenic vessels, and pancreas from injury. While the splenic vessels are usually at a distance from the fundus, their tortuos-

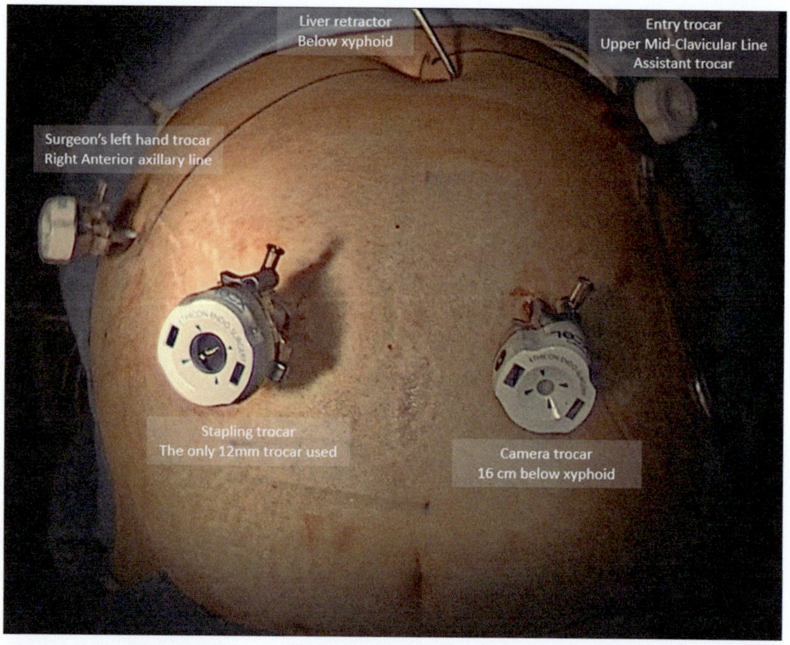

Fig. 9.4 Trocar placement for laparoscopic sleeve gastrectomy (All are 5-mm trocars except one for stapling. Using proper articulation of the stapler makes it possible to use single right-sided trocar for all stapling)

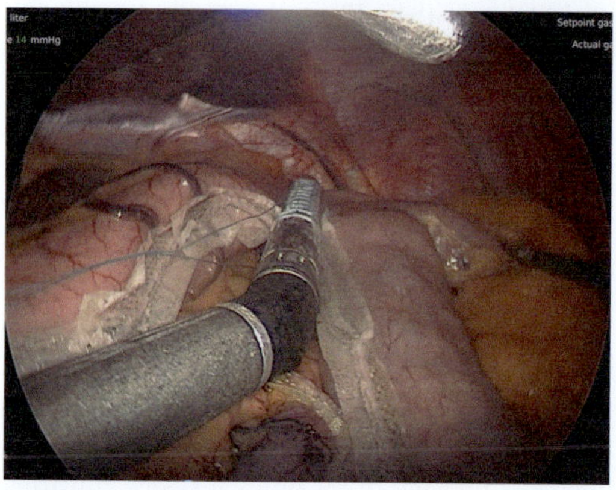

Fig. 9.5 Articulation of the stapler allows for optimal ergonomics (Here the stapler's cartridge is pointing straight up toward the angle of His, while the stapler's shaft is coming from a right-sided trocar and surgeon standing at the right side. Articulation makes it possible to do this operation without lithotomy position and to use only one 12-mm right-sided stapling trocar)

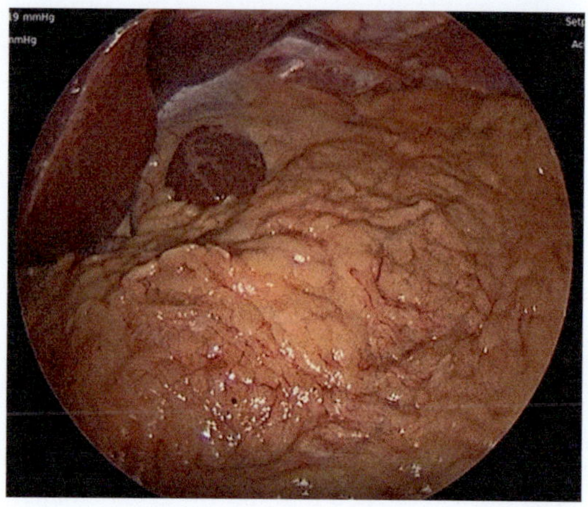

Fig. 9.6 Sea of fat (Note that the stomach cannot be seen at all due to the large amount of central fat)

ity, especially in elderly patients, may bring them in proximity to the posterior gastric dissection (Fig. 9.8a, b). Therefore, suboptimal exposure must be avoided during this part of the procedure to prevent vascular injury and massive hemorrhage. I do not clear the entire posterior wall of the stomach from its attachments as some of these adhesions help to prevent the sleeve from twisting (Fig. 9.9a–c). Care must be taken when clearing the top of the fundus and angle of His, as short gastric vessels may be present (Fig. 9.10) and could be covered with a large amount of fat that makes it difficult at times to identify them. Injury to these structures causes severe bleeding (Fig. 9.11), which is particularly challenging because the stump often retracts within the fat close to the main splenic vessels, where blind use of the energy device could result in catastrophic injury. In addition, the gastric serosa of the fundus is occasionally fused to the upper pole of the spleen (dissection leaving gastric serosa on spleen

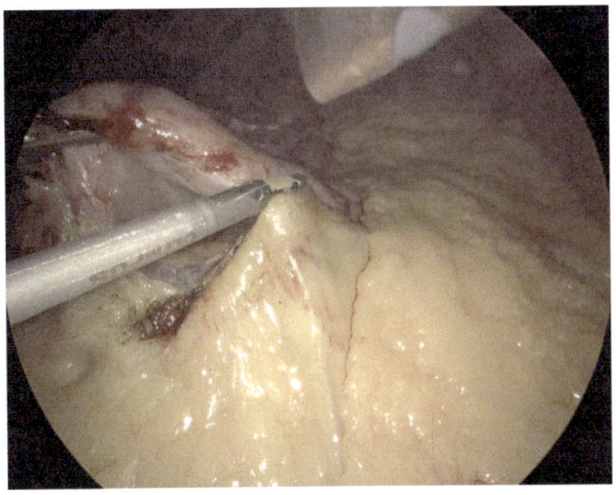

Fig. 9.7 Taking down the omental attachments off of the greater curvature

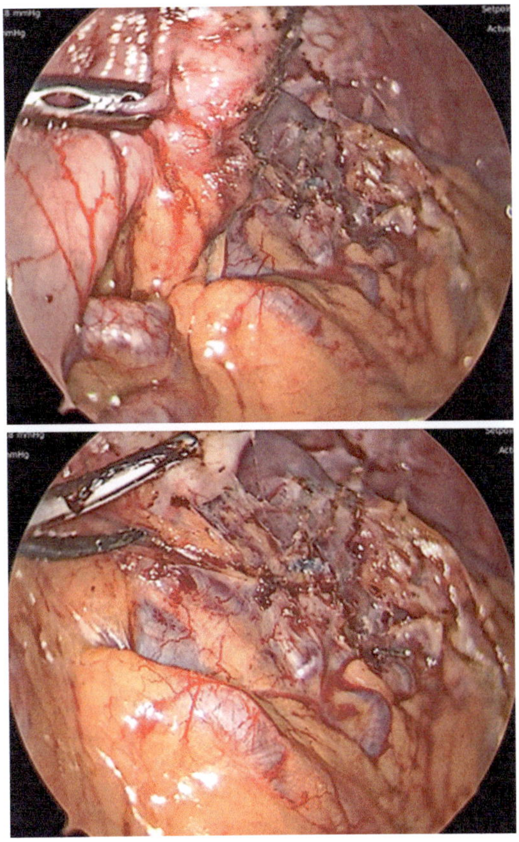

Fig. 9.8 Large tortuous splenic vessels need to be always thought of as they can get close to the stomach and be injured during posterior dissection or stapling

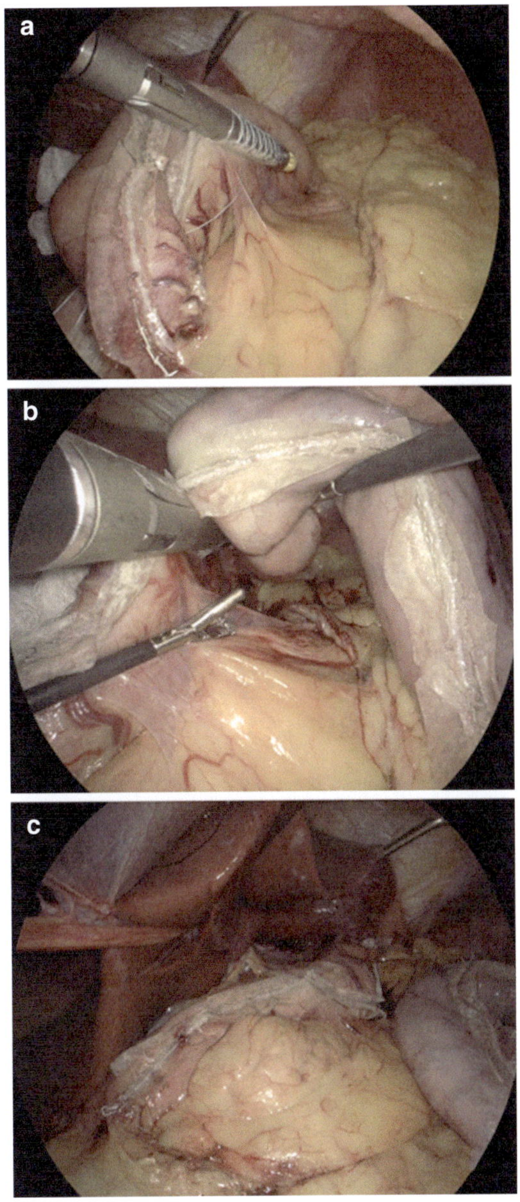

Fig. 9.9 Leaving some posterior attachments helps "fixating" the sleeve and prevent twisting and often evade the need for omentopexy. Note in (**b**) how the attachments are preventing medial twist. In (**c**) the sleeve laying flat with the attachments in place

(Fig. 9.12a)). In this case, and since this part of the stomach would eventually be resected during sleeve gastrectomy, we often find it safer to leave a thin layer of gastric serosa adherent to the splenic capsule during the release of the fundus, avoiding contact of the energy device with the spleen (Fig. 9.12b, c). Often, during this fine tedious dissection, we ask the anesthesiologist to pause respirations in order to stabilize the diaphragm and the spleen to prevent the tip of the energy device from stabbing the splenic capsule during inspiration.

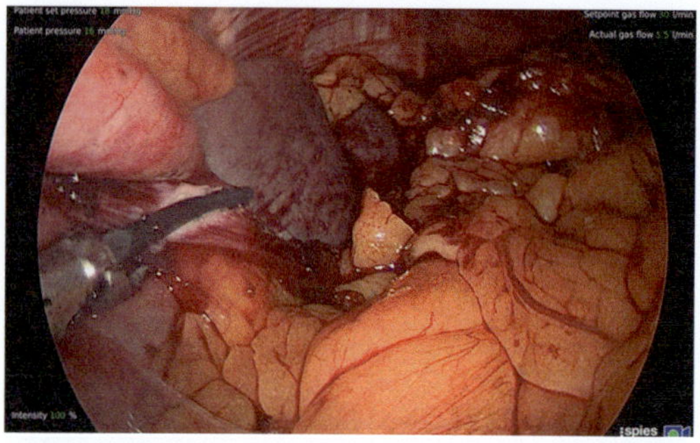

Fig. 9.10 Identifying and controlling the splenic branches going straight up to the fundus

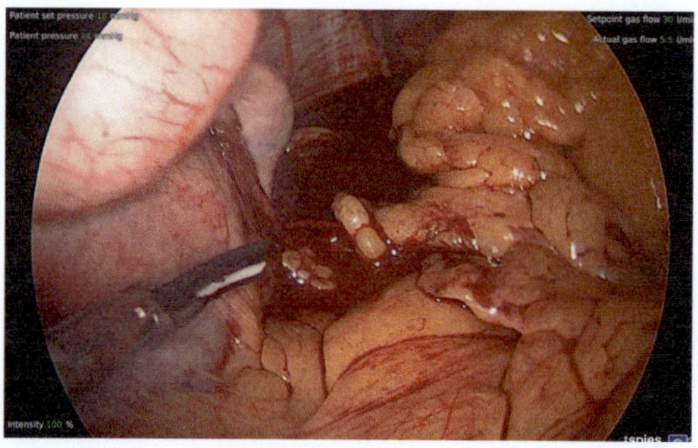

Fig. 9.11 Bleeding from a branch from the splenic vein to the fundus. Note the site of bleeding is only few millimeters above the level of the fat and could be buried easily in those with severe central obesity

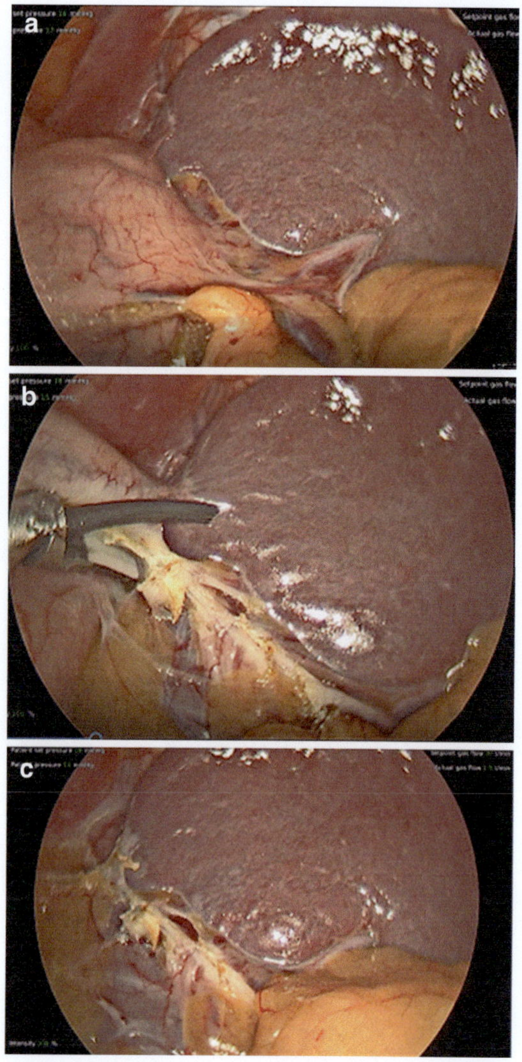

Fig. 9.12 Gastric serosa can be adherent to the splenic capsule making separation risky for splenic injury and bleeding (**a**). In these cases, leaving a thin strip of serosa adherent to the spleen decreases the risk of injury and bleeding as this part of the lateral fundus will be excised with the specimen (**b**, **c**)

The gastrophrenic ligament should be divided to expose the angle of His. It is our opinion that dissection of the left crus is the most critical step of this operation to ensure success. In the short term, a missed hiatal hernia or unresected fundus could lead to severe reflux and regurgitation postoperatively [13, 14]. In the long term, inferior weight loss can be expected as a result of unresected fundus or presence of a neo-fundus [15, 16].

We refer to the complete exposure of the left crus as the "critical view" of the sleeve gastrectomy, where the left crus is visualized posteriorly as it crosses midline and fuses with the right crus, forming the median arcuate ligament (Fig. 9.13). Inferior dissection of the left crus, and posterior exposure of the most proximal stomach, allows the surgeon to exclude hiatal hernia by visualizing the crossing fibers to the right crus and look for any defect in that area where an instrument would easily pass (Fig. 9.14). While many surgeons only inspect the hiatus anteriorly to identify a hiatal hernia, we strongly believe that posterior inspection must be performed to confidently exclude its presence. In our practice, however, routine adoption of preoperative endoscopy has been a major help in determining this issue especially in cases of super-super obesity when such high dissection could be of significant technical challenge and risk.

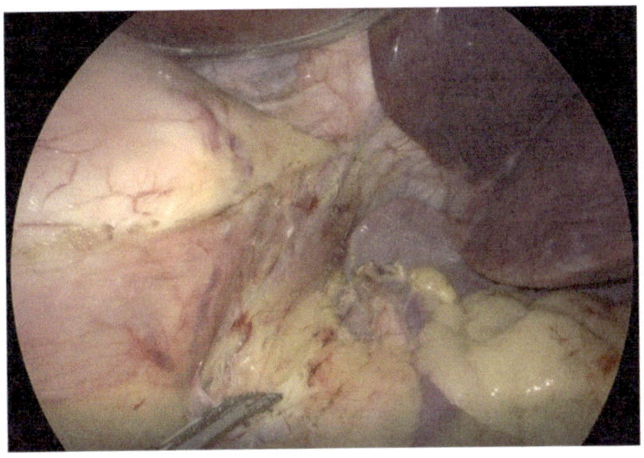

Fig. 9.13 Exposing the entire left crus. The "critical view" of VSG

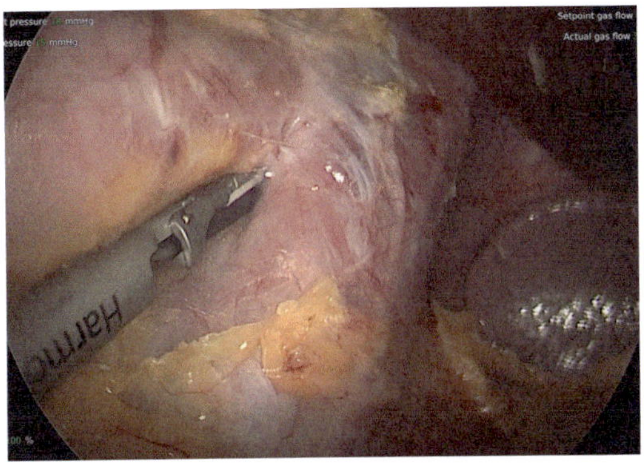

Fig. 9.14 Full exposure of the left crus. Note that a defect is being detected posterior to the upper most stomach indicating a sliding hiatal hernia. In this case, the anterior hiatus seems tight without any evidence of a hernia. Not examining the posterior hiatus, in this case, would have missed the hernia and potentially led to reflux symptoms after the sleeve gastrectomy

While conventional hiatal hernia repair is performed through the Pars flaccida by entering the hiatus at the right crus, I have modified the repair during LSG by starting at the left crus (Fig. 9.15a). The rationale is the need to routinely dissect the entire left crus to clear the fundus. At this point, simple gentle spread across the midline will create the needed retrogastric window anterior to the left crus. Once created, the assistant places an instrument, allowing for caudal retraction of the gastroesophageal junction and division of mediastinal esophageal attachments and complete reduction of the herniated fundus. Posterior vagus should be identified (with either approach) and retracted with along with the esophagus (Fig. 9.15b).

Posterior repair is performed with nonabsorbable sutures with "figure of eights" or simple stitches with slip knots for larger defect with tension. We do not see the need for calibrating bougies for this part, and we keep closing till about few millimeters away from the posterior wall of the esophagus (Fig. 9.15c, d).

This technique (left to right) for hiatal hernia repair during LSG preserves the Pars flaccida, which may decrease adhesions and make future revisional surgery, if needed, easier. As an alternative, the hiatal hernia repair may be deferred until gastrectomy is completed. We find this to be particularly helpful for patients with severe central obesity or early in the learning curve of the surgeon, as it simplifies the technical demand since the fundus will be already excised allowing for easier exposure.

Attention is then turned to resection of the stomach. A bougie is mandatory regardless of surgeon experience. It is our belief that the bougie needs to be present before any stapler firing occurs. Although bougie size remains disputed, there is evidence to support that making a very tight sleeve will only have minimal short-term weight loss advantage while risking significant postoperative complications [17]. In general, it is advisable not to go tighter than a 40-French bougie. We should note that the stapling distance from the bougie is often more important than the actual bougie size. The stapler should never be placed abutting the bougie regardless of its size; instead, the bougie should be used only for guidance. Care must be taken to avoid tension (from excessive lateral retraction by the assistant) and allow for relaxed gastric tissues, especially at the incisura and the angle of His, as creation of narrowing or ischemia in these areas may predispose to stricture or leak. Alternatively, some surgeons elect to use the endoscope as a bougie taking care to dessufflate the stomach before firing the stapler, keeping in mind the smaller diameter of the endoscope (Fig. 9.16a–c). This eliminates some extra steps as the scope would be used to decompress the stomach initially and then as a bougie when stapling, and last, it will be used to insufflate for the leak test (Fig. 9.16d).

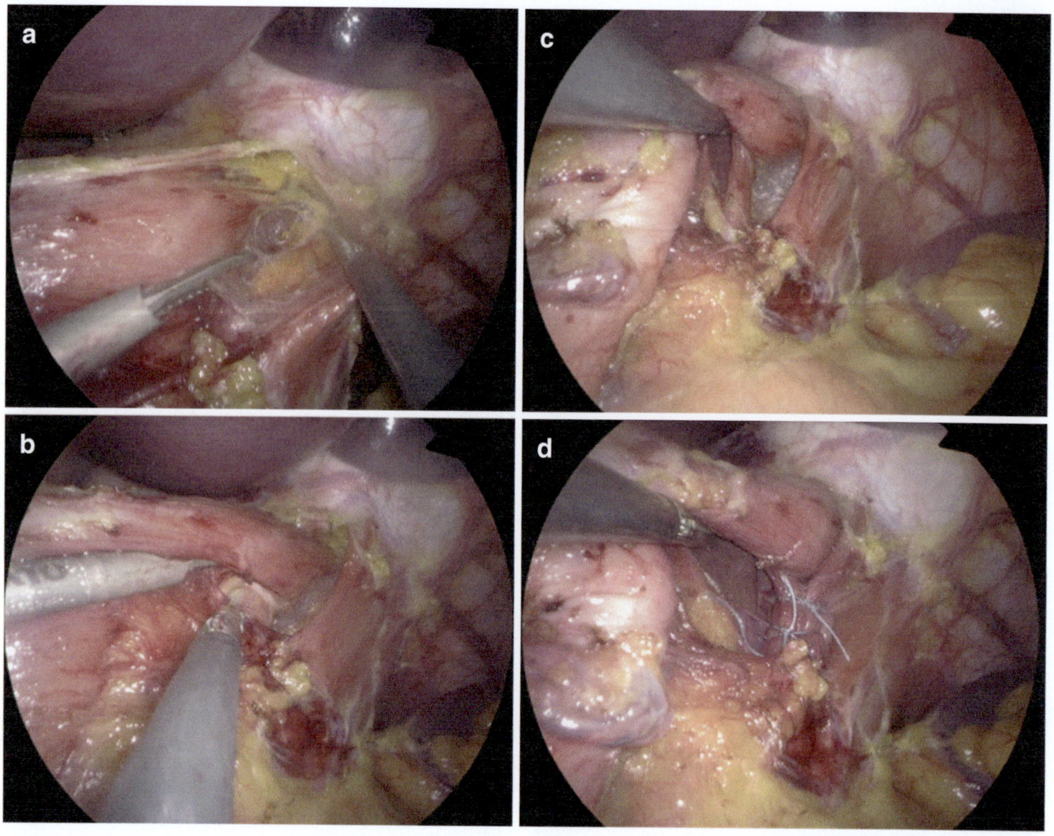

Fig. 9.15 Posterior hiatal hernia repair "left to right technique." After dissecting the left crus and achieving the "critical view," a plane is developed between the crus and the esophagus (**a**), and the hiatus is dissected on the left. The midline is crossed, and gentle spreading is made anterior to the right crus until a window is made (through which the caudate liver lobe is visualized). The posterior vagus nerve is visualized and retracted with the esophagus (**b**). The entire right crus is dissected without opening the Pars flaccida, and the circumferential dissection of the esophagus is then completed (**c**). Posterior repair is performed with nonabsorbable sutures from the left side (**d**)

As for stapling, the actual from the pylorus to begin gastric division remains controversial. Most surgeons begin the division of the antrum 2–5 cm from the pylorus to avoid postoperative enlarged antrum. Care must be taken to avoid twisting or stenosis of the sleeve at any level; however this is particularly critical when approaching the angle made by the incisura (Fig. 9.17a–c).

Although no consensus exists on choice of cartridge and staple heights, autopsies and histologic data clearly show wall thickness increases distally toward the gastric antrum. Therefore, it is our preference to choose the tallest stapler cartridge at the antrum and gradually choose shorter staplers as the division continues proximally. In revisional cases, however, the gastric tissues are typically thicker. Accordingly, in such cases, tall stapler cartridges are selected for the entire stomach even proximally. It is our technique to place the anvil anteriorly when firing, in order to inspect the staples and ensure their "B shape" formation. This will ensure the absence of any misfiring or a mismatch that could lead to staple line failure (Fig. 9.18a–d).

Discrepancy in the distance between the stapler and the lesser curvature between the anterior and posterior gastric walls risks twisting the staple line, as the stomach is fixed medially but free laterally (Fig. 9.19a–e). Therefore, gentle lateral retraction should be performed by grasping only the greater curvature in order to have equal traction on the anterior and posterior walls. It is crucial to elevate the tissues and inspect the posterior gastric wall, particularly medially, to ensure adequate tissue resection is performed. This step is most critical at the fundus, where a large volume of gastric tissue can be retained posteriorly despite an adequate appearing sleeve anteriorly (Fig. 9.20a, b).

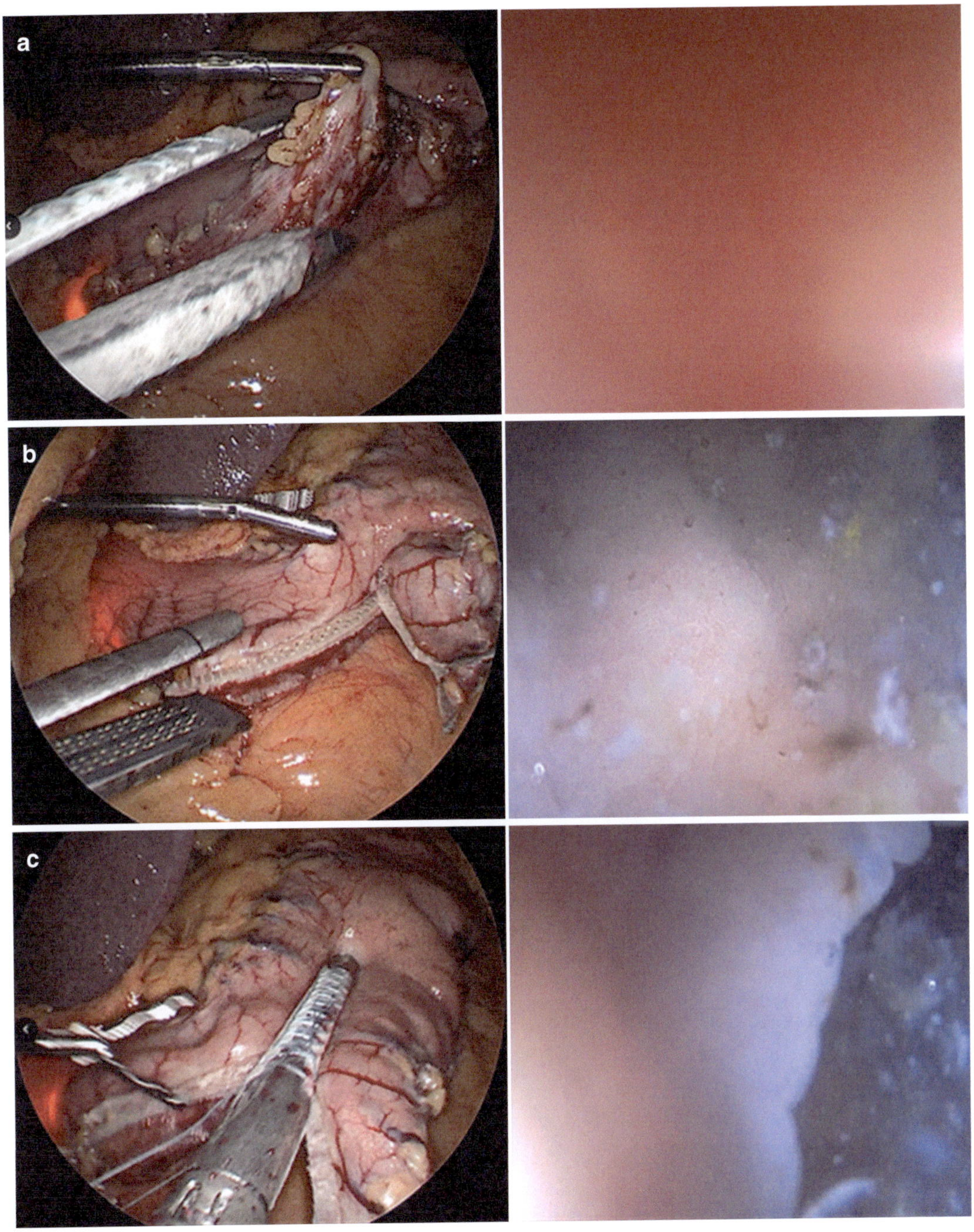

Fig. 9.16 Using the endoscope as a bougie. Note the light staying on for guidance (**a**–**c**). The endoscopic image (on the right) is blurred as the stomach is deflated and the light intensity on low (to avoid mucosal thermal injury). After completing the stapling process (**d**), the light intensity is back to high, and the scope will be withdrawn. Then, the sleeve will be insufflated for careful inspection and leak (bubble) test

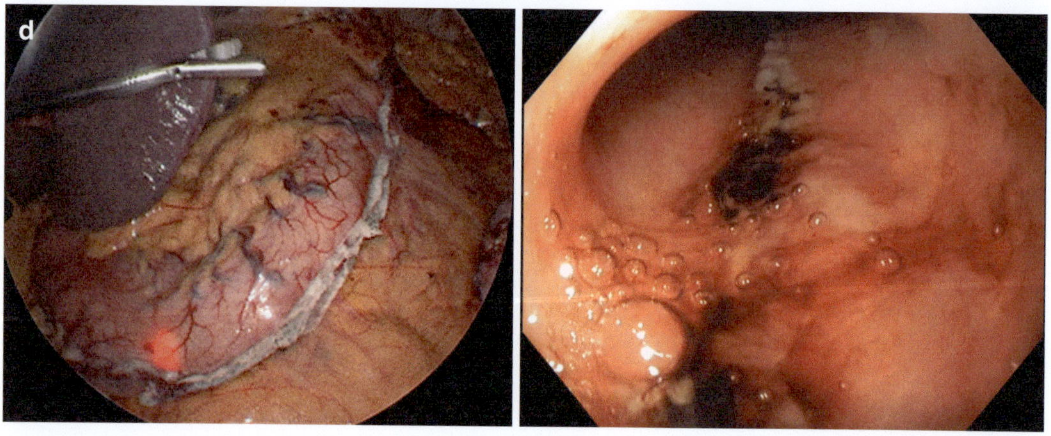

Fig. 9.16 (continued)

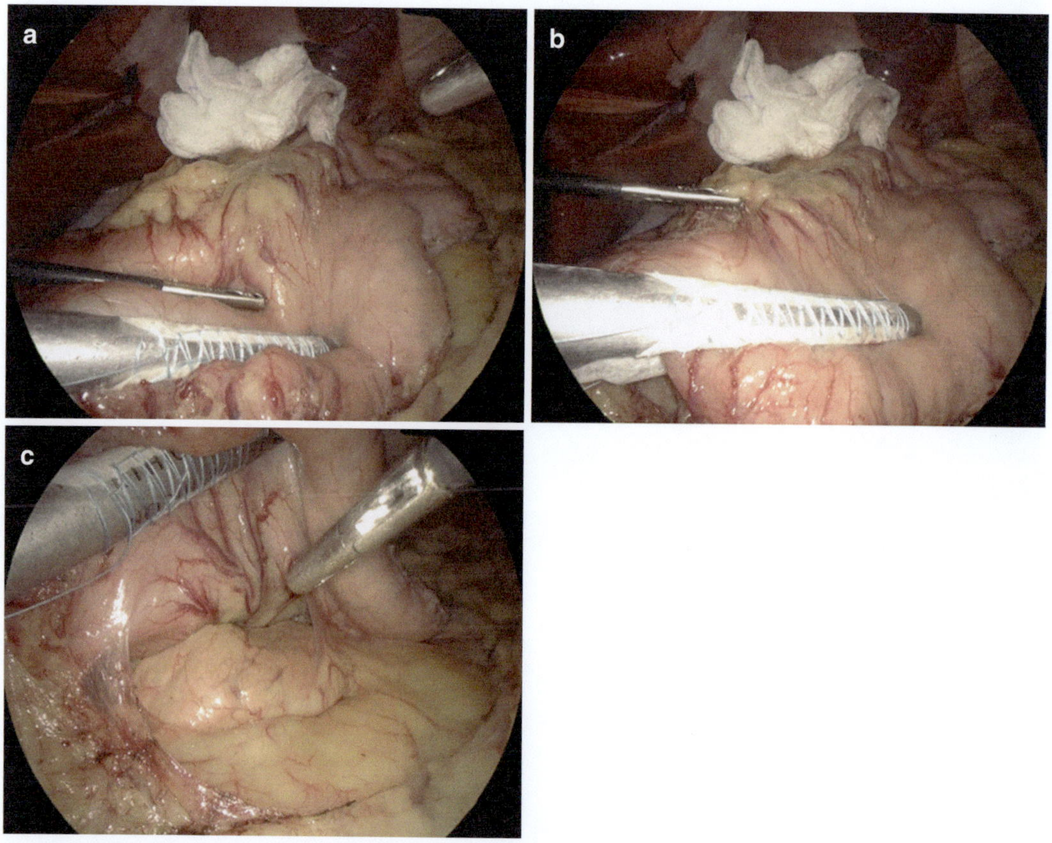

Fig. 9.17 Stapling at the level of the incisura. Note that despite the smaller bougie diameter, we are retracting the bougie medially (**a**) and stapling a few millimeters lateral to it. This guarantees adequate width in the critical area of the incisura. The stapler is articulated *away* from the incisura (**b**). Often, we retract the vessels medially to ensure adequate space before locking the jaws. It is critical to carefully examine the posterior side; the "claw foot" vessels should not be within the stapler jaws (**c**). If they are, it is almost certain that a stricture will occur

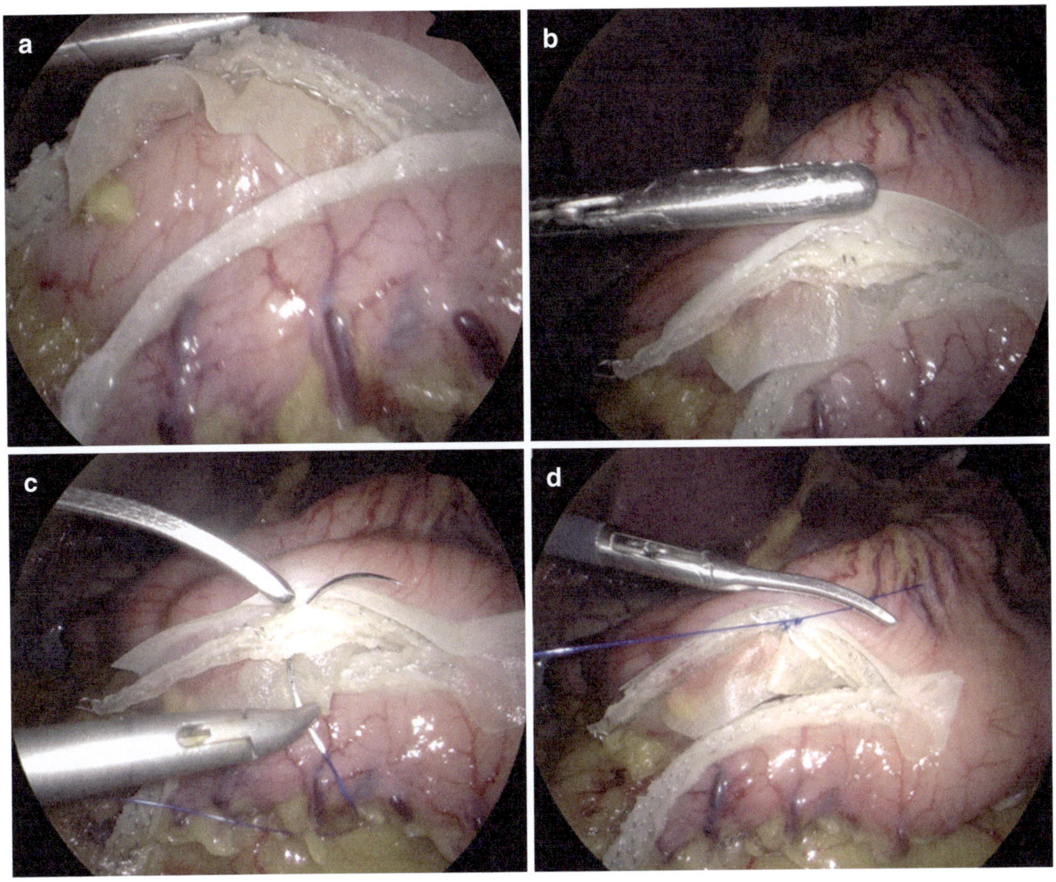

Fig. 9.18 Staple line issues. Note that while the (back) cartridge side of the staple line may look good, it is critical to examine the front (anvil) side as it may not be closed correctly (**b**). This is the reason we always place the anvil on top. In case of malalignment, we reinforce (**c**, **d**) with a superficially placed monofilament absorbable stitch (deeper stitches may narrow the lumen and should be avoided)

Approaching the proximal stomach, the stapler should be positioned a few millimeters lateral of the angle of His in order to avoid inclusion of esophageal tissue.

After complete division, inspection of the staple line is performed. We prefer to clip any area of oozing, no matter how minor. Clipping is the easier option when using staple line reinforcement due to the alignment of the tissues (Fig. 9.21). For sleeves performed without staple line reinforcement, over-sewing may be a better option.

If twisting of the sleeve is present, omentopexy is indicated to straighten the staple line. As stated earlier, the twisting or kinking is usually due to width discrepancy between the anterior and posterior walls of the sleeve, with redundancy in the posterior wall compared to the anterior wall. This results in rotation mostly around the site of the incisura medially toward the patient's right side. In that case, we tend to suture (pexy) the staple line to the matching omental edge with absorbable suture (Fig. 9.22a–c). Some surgeons perform routine omentopexy of the staple line in order to fixate the sleeve and prevent potential twisting. Although some suggest this improves postoperative nausea and vomiting, as well as decreases the risk of torsion or obstruction, no evidence exists to support these claims [18].

Due to the length of the staple line in the LSG and the high-pressure nature of the sleeve, staple line reinforcement has been adopted since the early days of performing this operation. In fact, at least half of the international experts believed

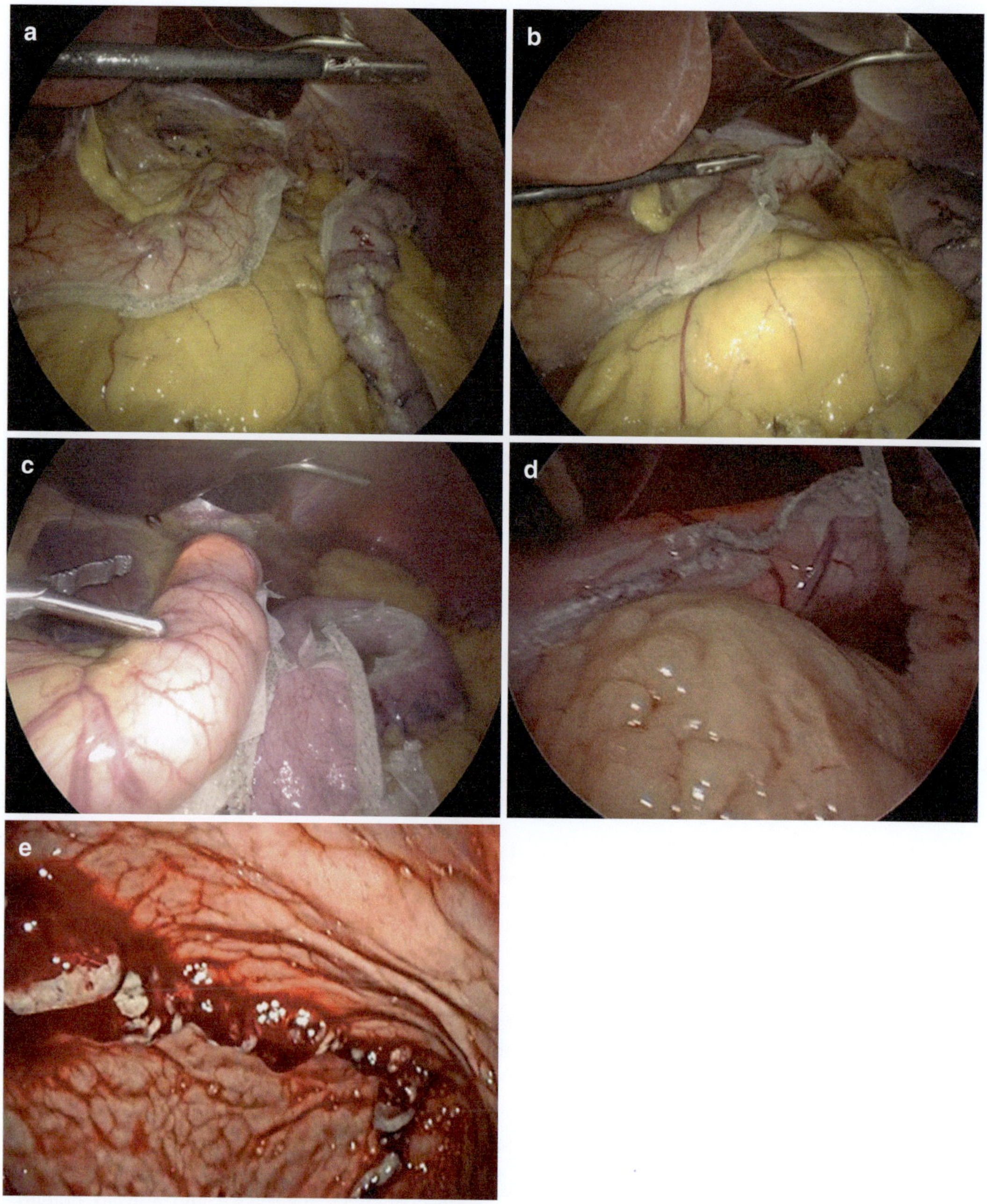

Fig. 9.19 Staple line twist. Note that this is due to the posterior wall being larger than the anterior wall. The direction of the staple line should be examined well to be sure it is "straight," as a twist could be subtle and may be missed (**a**) leading to narrowing postoperatively. Insufflating the sleeve during endoscopy generally makes it more apparent which is another benefit of intraoperative endoscopy (**b**). (**c**) shows well-aligned straight staple line with insufflation. The staple line direction should also be examined endoscopically during the leak test, and it should be a straight line and not have angulation (**d** laparoscopic view, **e** endoscopic view)

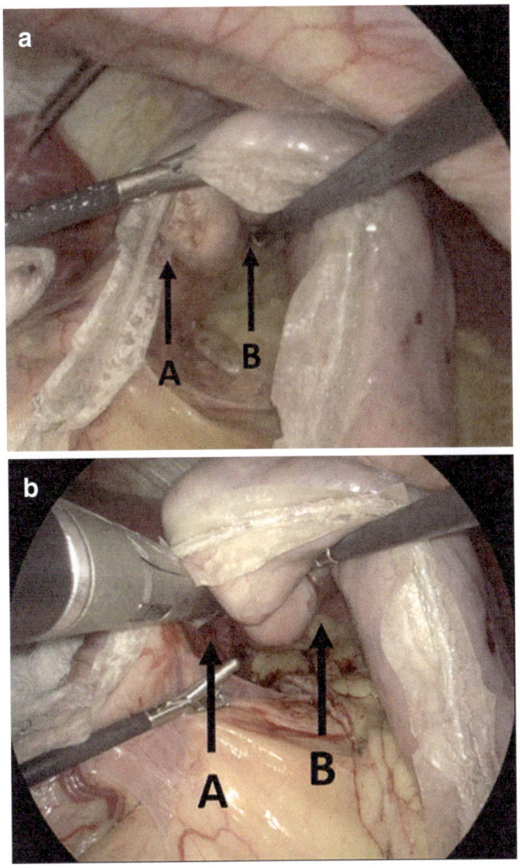

Fig. 9.20 Most proximal firing of the stapler. (**a**) Note that arrow "B" marks where inexperienced surgeons often divide the stomach, leaving a retained fundus. (**b**) Adequate lateral retraction allows inspection of the posterior fundus, so the surgeon can identify the proper line of transection, arrow "A." This prevents retained fundus which limits inadequate weight loss and post-op GERD

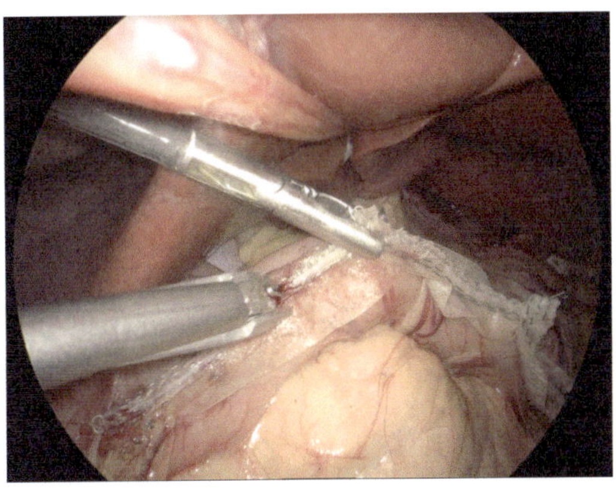

Fig. 9.21 Clipping area of hemorrhage made easier by staple line reinforcement

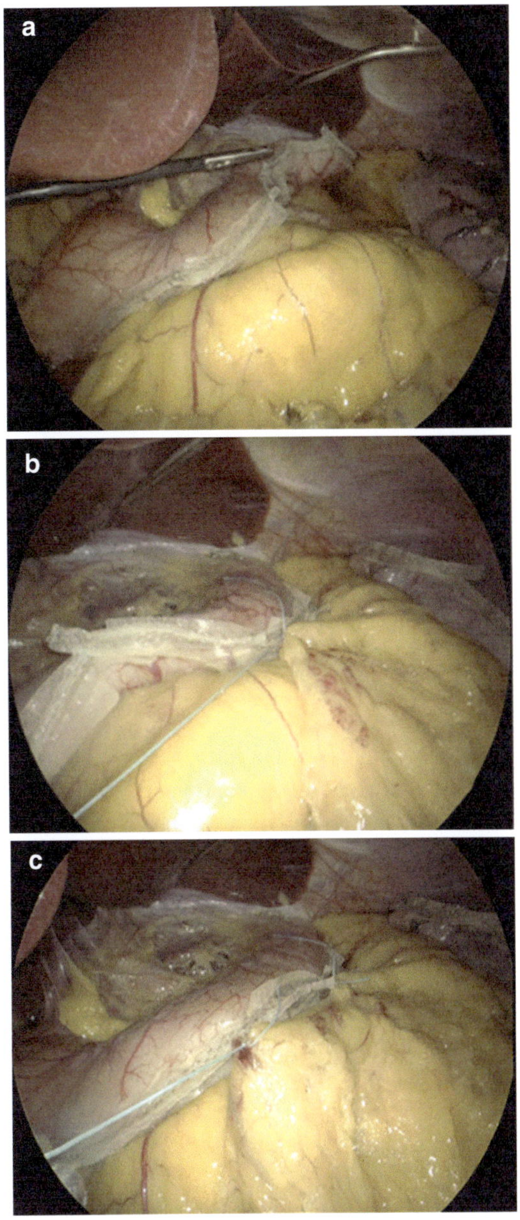

Fig. 9.22 Staple line twist (**a**) with omentopexy repair (**b**, **c**)

buttressing would decrease the risk of leaks, and nearly two-thirds suggested buttressing would be used routinely if it weren't for the cost [19]. Buttress material is used more commonly than over-sewing the staple line. There is currently no consensus for the optimal buttress material. It is generally agreed that over-sewing should be performed with nonabsorbable material. In a meta-analysis of 10,000 patients, it was found that absorbable buttress decreases the risk of leak compared to over-sewing and nonabsorbable buttressing carries the highest risk of leak when comparing both techniques [20]. Until recently, absorbable buttressing has been shown to improve rates of bleeding and leak. However, a recent analysis of MBSAQIP (Metabolic and Bariatric Surgery Accreditation and Quality Improvement Program) data showed different results. They analyzed 190,000 patients who had their sleeve gastrectomy performed by 1634 surgeons in 720 US Center of Excellence over 2 years (2012–2014). Their data showed that staple line reinforcement was used in 80% of cases and was associated with decreased risk of bleeding but was associated with increased risk of leak 0.96% vs 0.65%, odds ratio [OR] 1.20, and 95% confidence interval [CI] 1.00–1.43 [21]. The study was criticized due to the heterogeneity of the "buttress" group as far as the materials used.

Despite no solid evidence, it is generally advisable to test the anastomosis and staple lines in foregut surgery, particularly in bariatric surgery [22, 23]. Leak tests with upper endoscopy have shown higher sensitivity than using oral gastric lavage tubes [24] (Fig. 9.23). In addition, inspection of the lumen, sleeve diameter, hemostasis, and detection of an inadequately resected fundus can be achieved with upper endoscopy.

Postoperative Care

Immediate- and Short-Term Postoperative Care

Patients are admitted to the surgical floor. Patients are kept strictly NPO immediately postoperatively. Analgesia consists of scheduled alternating intravenous ketorolac and acetaminophen. Narcotic pain medications are routinely avoided and only given "as needed" after evaluation by a physician. Ambulation is mandatory on the day of surgery. Nausea is managed with ondansetron and scopolamine patch placed preoperatively.

Postoperative upper gastrointestinal series used to be standard practice to rule out a leak and assess patency. This practice, however, is now challenged due to its low sensitivity, cost, and unnecessary radiation exposure [25]. In addition, most leaks, in the case of sleeve gastrectomy, happen more than 48 h postoperatively, a time when patients in most cases have been discharged.

In our practice, patients get admitted postoperatively to a special bariatric unit. Patients ambulate and use their incentive spirometer. They stay overnight and the next day, if feeling well with normal vital signs, will be started on bariatric clear liquids and monitored for 6 h to ensure adequate intake to maintain hydration. If doing well, patients are discharged by 2 p.m. No laboratory studies or radiographic studies are

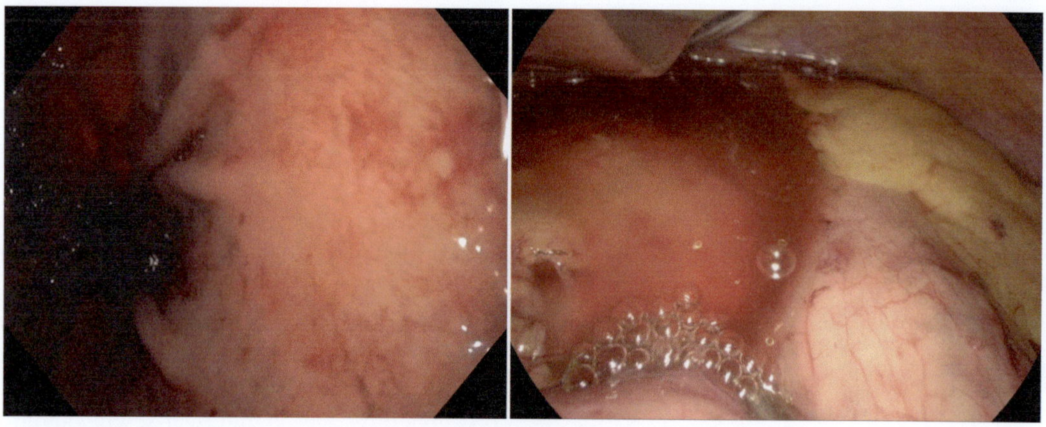

Fig. 9.23 Positive leak test with intraoperative endoscopy (after a gastric bypass)

ordered unless indicated, and over 90% of patients are discharged timely following this protocol. Historically, nausea has been the major reason for longer admissions; this problem was nearly eliminated by moving to narcotic-free postoperative care.

Long-Term Care

Long-term follow-up with a multidisciplinary team is paramount for long-term success. Assessments are made by the bariatric surgeon, registered dietician, nurse specialized in bariatric surgery, social worker, and other members of the ancillary care staff. Biochemical surveillance is performed preoperatively and yearly after surgery (or sooner if indicated). This includes complete blood count, chemical metabolic profile, iron, vitamins, and mineral level. Care is taken to evaluate, diagnose, and treat weight regain, protein malnutrition, anemia, and vitamin and mineral deficiencies [26] in a timely manner.

Results

Sleeve gastrectomy results in stable long-term weight loss in the majority of cases. The 5-year %EWL is 54.8±6.9 [27]. The weight loss is maintained even in super-obese patients was 5 years [28]. Several studies demonstrate diabetes remission rates, improvement in inflammatory markers and cardiovascular risks, and improvements in obesity-related comorbidities comparable to RYGB [29–32]. After sleeve gastrectomy, patients report improvements in several metrics for quality of life and health behaviors [33–36].

Complications

In the postoperative period, tachycardia, tachypnea, and fever deserve prompt evaluation and may indicate leak. Leaks after sleeve gastrectomy occur at a rate of 1–3% [20, 37]. Most often, gastric sleeve leaks occur along the staple line in the proximal stomach within 4 cm of the gastroesophageal junction. Most leaks present in the acute period, within 7 days of surgery. However, they may also appear as a subacute or chronic complication as well. Contributing elements comprise of tissue ischemia including reduced perfusion from sacrificed left gastric artery tributaries, elevated intraluminal pressures including stricture or stenosis, impaired healing, infection, and technical factors [38–40].

Management of postoperative leaks may involve multiple modalities including endoscopic stent, laparoscopic washout, percutaneous drainage, or open interventions. Novel approaches to this complicated problem are evolving. Early intervention with adequate drainage and nutritional access remains paramount for good outcomes when early leaks are detected [41].

Strictures after sleeve gastrectomy are often the result of narrowing at the incisura, leading to obstructive symptoms including dysphagia and vomiting. In the early postoperative period, this may be related to mucosal edema. However, stricture is frequently the result of poor surgical technique. Strictures can be avoided by keeping a safe distance from the bougie and always checking the back wall. Initial interventions to treat stricture may involve endoscopic balloon dilatations [42]. Strictures not amenable to endoscopic intervention may require surgical management with seromyotomy or longitudinal lateral gastrotomy with transverse closure. These interventions carry significant technical risks. Revision to gastric bypass remains (with anastomosis above the level of the stricture) the most effective but may be technically challenging in some cases.

Anatomic and physiologic changes resulting from LSG may exacerbate GERD symptoms or induce GERD in previously asymptomatic patients [43]. Attention should be paid to the size and diameter of the sleeve, disruption of the antropyloric pump mechanism, as well as identification and repair of hernias at the time of surgery [44]. Pharmaceutical therapy is a generally effective medical treatment option. For refractory GERD, revision to a gastric bypass would usually eliminate symptoms completely.

Conclusions

LSG is a safe and effective bariatric surgery with durable weight loss in compliant patients.

The simple concept of this operation, without the need to manipulate the intestine, is what made it popular to patients and is behind the rapid rise of its popularity to quickly become the most common bariatric surgery performed in most countries. Nevertheless, the fine details in this operation are paramount to decrease catastrophic complications and adverse outcome, and therefore they cannot be overlooked. Therefore, we believe that while this is a simple operation, it should not be called "easy" and should be performed only by surgeons trained or dedicated to bariatric surgery.

References

1. Ponce J, DeMaria EJ, Nguyen NT, et al. American Society for Metabolic and Bariatric Surgery estimation of bariatric surgery procedures in 2015 and surgeon workforce in the United States. Surg Obes Relat Dis. 2016;12(9):1637–9.
2. Tretbar LL, Taylor TL, Sifer EC. Weight reduction. Gastric plication for morbid obesity. J Kans Med Soc. 1976;77(11):488–90.
3. Johnston D, Dachtler J, Sue-Ling HM, et al. The magenstrasse and mill operation for morbid obesity. Obes Surg. 2003;13(1):10–6.
4. Marceau P, Biron S, St Georges R, et al. Biliopancreatic diversion with gastrectomy as surgical treatment of morbid obesity. Obes Surg. 1991:1381–7.
5. Hess DS, Hess DW. Biliopancreatic diversion with a duodenal switch. Obes Surg. 1998;8:267–82.
6. Ren CJ, Patterson E, Gagner M. Early results of laparoscopic bilio-pancreatic diversion with duodenal switch: a case series of 40 consecutive patients. Obes Surg. 2000;10:514–23.
7. Kim WW, Gagner M, Kini S, et al. Laparoscopic vs. open biliopancreatic diversion with duodenal switch: a comparative study. J Gastrointest Surg. 2003;7:552–7.
8. Chu CA, Gagner M, Quinn T, et al. Two-stage laparoscopic bilio-pancreatic diversion with duodenal switch: an alternative approach to super-super morbid obesity. Surg Endosc. 2002;16:S069.
9. Regan JP, Inabnet WB, Gagner M, et al. Early experience with two stage laparoscopic Roux-en-Y gastric bypass as an alternative in the super-super obese patient. Obes Surg. 2003;13:861–4.
10. Alexandrou A, Felekouras E, Giannopoulos A, et al. What is the actual fate of super-morbid-obese patients who undergo laparoscopic sleeve gastrectomy as the first step of a two-stage weight-reduction operative strategy? Obes Surg. 2012;22(10):1623–8.
11. Gomberwalla A, Lutfi R. Early outcomes of helicobacter pylori and its treatment after laparoscopic sleeve gastrectomy. Bariatr Surg Pract Patient Care. 2015;10(1):12–4.
12. Berch BR, Torquati A, Lutfi RE, et al. Experience with the optical access trocar for safe and rapid entry in the performance of laparoscopic gastric bypass. Surg Endosc. 2006;20(8):1238–41.
13. Himpens J, Dobbeleir J, Peeters J. Long-term results of laparoscopic sleeve gastrectomy for obesity. Ann Surg. 2010;252(2):319–24.
14. Laffin M, Chau J, Gill RS, et al. Sleeve gastrectomy and gastroesophageal reflux disease. J Obes. 2013;2013:741097.
15. Silecchia G, De Angelis F, Rizzello M, et al. Residual fundus or neofundus after laparoscopic sleeve gastrectomy: is fundectomy safe and effective as revision surgery? Surg Endosc. 2015;29(19):2899–903.
16. Noel P, Nedelcu M, Nocca D, et al. Revised sleeve gastrectomy: another option for weight loss failure after sleeve gastrectomy. Surg Endosc. 2013;28(4):1096–102.
17. Parikh M, Gagner M, Heacock L, et al. Laparoscopic sleeve gastrectomy: does bougie size affect mean %EWL? Short-term outcomes. Surg Obes Relat Dis. 2008;4(4):528–33.
18. Afaneh C, Costa R, Pomp A, et al. A prospective randomized controlled trial assessing the efficacy of omentopexy during laparoscopic sleeve gastrectomy in reducing postoperative gastrointestinal symptoms. Surg Endosc. 2015;29(1):41–7.
19. Rosenthal R. International Sleeve Gastrectomy Expert Panel Consensus Statement: best practice guidelines based on experience of >12,000 cases. Surg Obes Relat Dis. 2012;8(1):8–19.
20. Parikh M, Issa R, McCrillis A, et al. Surgical strategies that may decrease leak after laparoscopic sleeve gastrectomy: a systematic review and meta-analysis of 9991 cases. Ann Surg. 2013;257(2):231–7.
21. Berger E, Clements R, Morton J, et al. The impact of different surgical techniques on outcomes in laparoscopic sleeve gastrectomies: the first report from the metabolic and bariatric surgery accreditation and quality improvement program (MBSAQIP). Ann Surg. 2016;264(3):464–73.
22. Sethi M, Zagzag J, Patel K, et al. Intraoperative leak testing has no correlation with leak after laparoscopic sleeve gastrectomy. Surg Endosc. 2016;30:883–91.
23. Bingham J, Kaufman J, Hata K, et al. A multicenter study of routine versus selective intraoperative leak testing for sleeve gastrectomy. Surg Obes Relat Dis. 2017;13(9):1469–75.
24. Alaedeen D, Madan A, Ro C, et al. Intraoperative endoscopy and leaks after laparoscopic Roux-en-Y gastric bypass. Am Surg. 2009;75(6):485–8.
25. Terterov D, Leung P, Twells L, et al. The usefulness and costs of routine contrast studies after laparoscopic

sleeve gastrectomy for detecting staple line leaks. Can J Surg. 2017;60(5):335–41.
26. Caron M, Hould FS, Lescelleru O, et al. Long-term nutritional impact of sleeve gastrectomy. Surg Obes Relat Dis. 2017;13(10):1664–73.
27. Bohdjalian A, Langer FB, Shakeri-Leidenmuhler S, et al. Sleeve gastrectomy as sole and definitive bariatric procedure: 5-year results for weight loss and ghrelin. Obes Surg. 2010;20:535–40.
28. Saif T, Strain GW, Dakin G, Gagner M, Costa R, Pomp A. Evaluation of nutrient status after laparoscopic sleeve gastrectomy 1, 3 and 5 years after surgery. Surg Obes Relat Dis. 2012;8:542–7.
29. Benaiges D, Goday A, Ramon JM, et al. Laparoscopic sleeve gastrectomy and laparoscopic gastric bypass are equally effective for reduction of cardiovascular risk in severely obese patients at one year of follow-up. Surg Obes Relat Dis. 2011;7:575–80.
30. Leyba J, Aulestia S, Llopis S. Laparoscopic Roux-en-Y gastric bypass versus laparoscopic sleeve gastrectomy for the treatment of morbid obesity: a prospective study of 117 patients. Obes Surg. 2011;21:212–6.
31. Nocca D, Guillaume F, Noel P, et al. Impact of laparoscopic sleeve gastrectomy and laparoscopic gastric bypass on HbA1c blood level and pharmacological treatment of type 2 diabetes mellitus in severe or morbidly obese patients: results of a multicenter prospective study at 1 year. Updated position statement on sleeve gastrectomy. Surg Obes Relat Dis. 2012;2:21026.
32. O'Keefe K, Kemmeter P, Kemmeter K. Bariatric surgery outcomes in patients aged 65 years and older at an American Society for Metabolic and Bariatric Surgery center of excellence. Obes Surg. 2010;20:1199–205.
33. Kafri N, Valfer R, Nativ O, et al. Health behavior, food tolerance, and satisfaction after laparoscopic sleeve gastrectomy. Surg Obes Relat Dis. 2011;7:82–8.
34. Alley J, Fenton S, Harnisch M, et al. Quality of life after sleeve gastrectomy and adjustable gastric banding. Surg Obes Relat Dis. 2012;8:31–40.
35. Brunault P, Jacobi D, Leger J, et al. Observations regarding "quality of life" and "comfort with food" after bariatric surgery: comparison between laparoscopic adjustable gastric banding and sleeve gastrectomy. Obes Surg. 2011;21:1225–31.
36. D'Hondt M, Vanneste S, Pottel H, et al. Laparoscopic sleeve gastrectomy as a single-stage procedure for the treatment of morbid obesity and the resulting quality of life, resolution of comorbidities, food tolerance, and 6-year weight loss. Surg Endosc. 2011;25:2498–504.
37. Nedelcu M, Manos T, Cotirlet A, et al. Outcome of leaks after sleeve gastrectomy based on a new algorithm addressing leak size and gastric stenosis. Obes Surg. 2015;25(3):559–63.
38. Perez M, Brunaud L, Kedaifa S, et al. Does anatomy explain the origin of a leak after sleeve gastrectomy. Obes Surg. 2014;24(10):1717–23.
39. Warner D, Sasse K. Technical details of laparoscopic sleeve gastrectomy leading to lowered leak rate: discussion of 1070 consecutive cases. Minim Invasive Surg. 2017;2:4367059.
40. Aurora A, Khaitan L, Saber A. Sleeve gastrectomy and the risk of leak: a systematic analysis of 4,888 patients. Surg Endosc. 2012;26(6):1509–15.
41. Dakwar A, Assalia A, Khamaysi I, et al. Late complication of laparoscopic sleeve gastrectomy. Case Rep Gastrointest Med. 2013;2013:13153.
42. Zundel N, Hernandez J, Galvao Neto MG, et al. Strictures after laparoscopic sleeve gastrectomy. Surg Laparosc Endosc Percut Tech. 2010;20:154–8.
43. Carter P, LeBlanc K, Hausmann M, et al. Association between gastroesophageal reflux disease and laparoscopic sleeve gastrectomy. Surg Obes Relat Dis. 2011;7(5):569–72.
44. DuPree C, Blair K, Steele S, et al. Laparoscopic sleeve gastrectomy in patients with preexisting gastroesophageal reflux disease: a national analysis. JAMA Surg. 2014;149(4):328–34.

Gastric Bypass

10

Omar Ezequiel Bellorin-Marin and Alfons Pomp

History

The initial Roux-en-Y gastric bypass (RYGB) for weight loss was described by Mason and Ito in 1966 as a surgical treatment for morbid obesity after their observations that patients with antrectomy and Billroth II reconstruction remained underweight. The introduction of laparoscopic (L) RYGB by Wittgrove and Clark in 1994 [1] ushered in a new era for bariatric surgery as the numbers of operations increased tenfold from 1998 to 2003. Many modifications of the gastric bypass technique have been added since but always preserving the original concept: creation of a small gastric pouch based on the lesser curvature and bypassing the biliopancreatic secretions through a long jejunal limb in a Roux-en-Y fashion.

Preoperative Care

Every patient undergoing bariatric surgery should be assessed preoperatively by a multidisciplinary team that should include a dietitian and a primary care physician and may also include psychologists, cardiologists, pulmonologists, and gastroenterologists in order to achieve the most successful outcome following the procedure [2, 3].

Nutritional evaluation is paramount prior to weight loss surgery. Obese patients have excess stores of fat but may be deficient in protein and micronutrients as a consequence of poor eating habits. If not treated, preoperative deficiencies may worsen in the postoperative period and can manifest into significant illness with potential devastating and irreversible outcomes.

A registered dietitian (RD) or a nutritionist will perform a preoperative assessment that includes the calculation of postoperative nutritional goals and educate the patient on how to reach such goals. The RD will also assess the patient's current food choices and eating habits and will work on a preoperative weight loss program.

The patient should undergo a routine preoperative laboratory workup that includes complete blood count, comprehensive metabolic panel, liver function tests, hemoglobin A1C, albumin, TSH, Vitamin B12, thiamine, folate, calcium, 25-OH vitamin D, iron, and ferritin. When clinically indicated, levels of Vitamin A, zinc, selenium, niacin, biotin, and copper may be useful preoperatively as a baseline for postoperative follow-up. Deficiencies should be corrected with supplementation preoperatively.

O. E. Bellorin-Marin
Department of Surgery, New York Presbyterian Hospital, New York, NY, USA

A. Pomp (✉)
Department of Surgery, New York Presbyterian Hospital, New York, NY, USA

Weill Cornell Medicine, New York, NY, USA
e-mail: alp2014@med.cornell.edu

R. Lutfi et al. (eds.), *Global Bariatric Surgery*, https://doi.org/10.1007/978-3-319-93545-4_10

A psychological assessment should be considered and performed preoperatively. Eating is certainly one way to cope with stress in modern life ("comfort food"), and other eating disorders are commonly found in the morbidly obese. If these issues are not dealt with, concurrently the patient can continue the same habits after surgery that will negatively affect outcomes. Emotional concerns must be assessed and treated in conjunction with a successful weight loss surgery.

A preoperative cardiac evaluation should be considered for every patient undergoing bariatric surgery who is 50 years or older and should be a routine for those with previous cardiac history. Signs and symptoms of sleep apnea should be assessed at the initial visit (the STOP-BANG questionnaire) with preoperative pulmonary risk assessment and polysomnography testing if positive. Comorbidities such as hypertension, diabetes, and hypothyroidism should be managed and controlled preoperatively by the appropriate specialists. We think patients should undergo preoperative upper endoscopy in order to detect the presence of anatomical abnormalities like a significant hiatal hernia and other problems like cryptic esophagitis which can affect operative planning. An attempt should be made to eradicate *Helicobacter pylori* and to rule out premalignant lesions as the gastric remnant will not be amenable to endoscopic surveillance postoperatively.

Preoperative Contraindications of Gastric Bypass

- Mental illness that impairs the patient's ability to understand the risks of surgery and postoperative care
- Active neoplastic disease
- Cirrhosis with portal hypertension
- Patient unable to comply with a postoperative dietary regimen, including vitamin supplementation and follow-up
- Pregnancy
- Patient unable to participate in a postoperative exercise program due to debilitating chronic joint disease or cardiovascular limitation (relative contraindication)
- Extensive prior abdominal surgery (relative contraindication)

Postoperative Care

The postoperative care of a gastric bypass patient is focused on minimizing postoperative pain, encouraging early oral intake and early ambulation. Patients with minimal comorbidities may be safely transferred from recovery to the floor where specialized nurses are able to detect early signs of complications. Patients with cardiac or pulmonary comorbidities should remain in a continuous monitoring unit for the first 24 h. The patient can be given clear liquid diet immediately after surgery and progressed to a full liquid diet the following day.

Subcutaneous heparin injection is given prophylactically during the hospital stay and may be continued for 1 month with low molecular weight heparin for patients who do not ambulate well before the operation and have preoperative BMI >60 or those with a previous history of DVT/PE. Narcotic medications should be minimized. Our ERAS protocol consists of standing acetaminophen and ketorolac for the first 48 h and oral oxycodone for breakthrough pain. The patient is encouraged to ambulate in the early postoperative period and to use incentive spirometer for respiratory therapy.

A typical gastric bypass patient spends only one or two nights at the hospital. We make sure the patient is able to maintain hydration successfully and have adequate pain control prior to discharge in order to avoid early readmissions. Postoperative radiologic tests (esophagram, CT) are not performed routinely in our practice. They are reserved as diagnostic tests, to rule out specific complications such as leaks or pulmonary embolism when suspected.

An exception to this rule is revisional surgery to gastric bypass, when an upper gastrointestinal series with oral contrast may be performed in selected cases.

Patients remain on full liquid diet for the first week postoperatively and are progressed to pureed/soft for the following 3 weeks. During the first visit at 3 weeks, each patient is assessed by the RD, and the diet is progressed to soft diet. Each patient is routinely seen at 3, 6, and 12 months and then yearly. Follow-up visits consist of weight measurement, surgical and nutrition consultation, and blood work (including vitamin and micronutrient levels).

Procedure

Patient Positioning and Room Setup

Patients routinely receive prophylaxis for surgical site infection and deep vein thrombosis with antibiotics and sequential compression stockings combined with subcutaneous heparin injection. An anesthesiologist with experience in difficult airway and overall understanding of the physiology of the morbidly obese is recommended to minimize intraoperative complications. The operating table should be capable of supporting the weight of the patient and also able to tilt into steep reverse Trendelenburg position.

While most surgeons operate from the right side of the patient, we prefer the lithotomy position allowing the surgeon to stand between the legs (French position). Pressure points are padded, and arms and legs are secured to the table in order to avoid hyperextension. Footboards are also applied. This is the preferred position by the authors, as it allows the surgeon to stand in front of the abdomen, following the basic principles of triangulation in laparoscopic surgery. It is also ergonomic, limiting awkward positions and body turns (neck, lower back, shoulders) and avoiding possible injuries to the operating surgeon over the long term. The assistant stands on the right side of the patient and the scrub nurse on the left. An additional assistant (optional) stands on the left side in front of the scrub nurse. Laparoscopic monitors are placed at the level of the patient's head in front of the surgeon (Fig. 10.1).

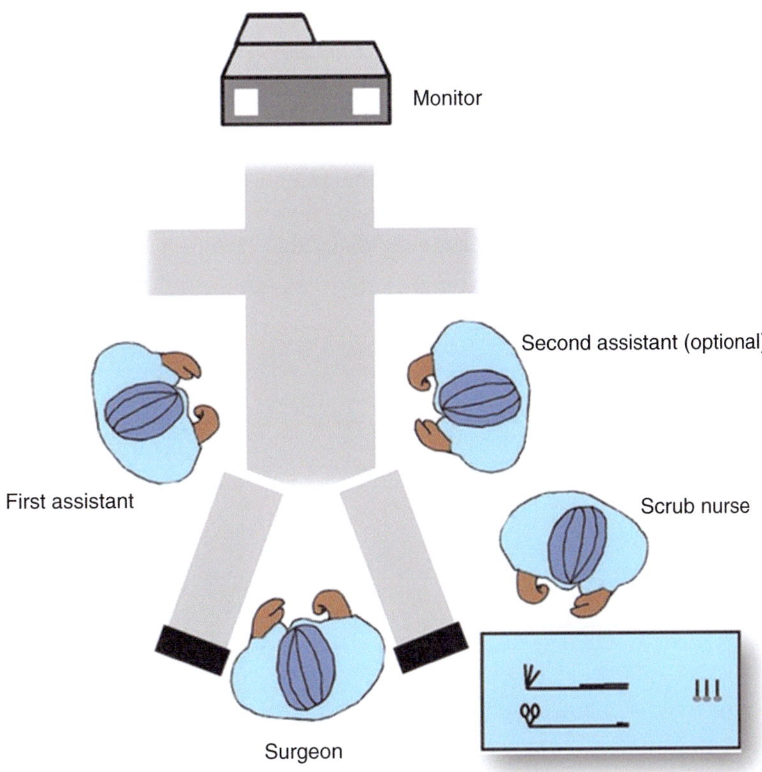

Fig. 10.1 Room setup

Trocar Placement

There are many different ways to establish pneumoperitoneum and place trocars for a LRYGB. We use a 5 mm incision in the left upper quadrant at the intersection point of the middle clavicular line and two fingerbreadths below the costal margin (Palmer's point). A 5 mm optical trocar is placed under direct vision using the dominant hand to advance the device and the non-dominant hand to hold the camera. It is important to keep in mind that there is a marked discrepancy between the external and internal circumference of the abdominal cavity in the obese patient. The surgeon must keep a 90° angle between the trocar and the abdominal wall. The pneumoperitoneum is started to a pressure of 15 mmHg. The anesthesiologist should be made aware of this step and look for any hemodynamic repercussions of the pneumoperitoneum. Once in the abdominal cavity, a 5 mm trocar is placed above the umbilicus, and the camera is switched to this trocar for a more central view. The following trocars are now placed under direct vision: a 12 mm trocar in the right upper quadrant, 5 mm trocar in the epigastrium, 5 mm trocar in the high epigastrium, and a 5 mm trocar in the left upper quadrant laterally. The initial 5 mm trocar is replaced by a second 12 mm trocar. Another 5 mm trocar is added in the left lower quadrant to assist with the jejuno-jejunum anastomosis (Fig. 10.2). An orthostatic liver retractor is placed via the high epigastric port and positioned carefully under the left lobe of the liver.

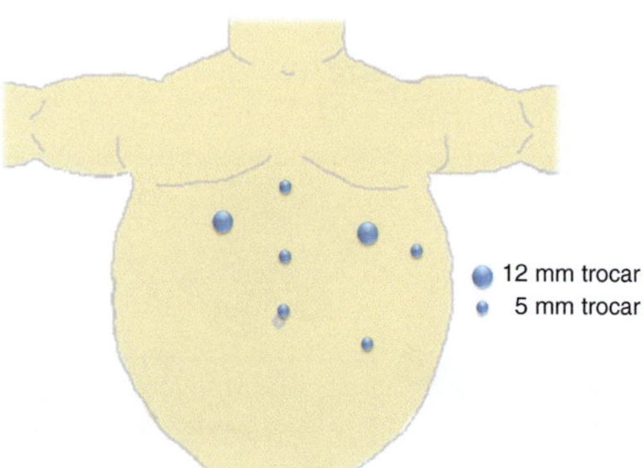

Fig. 10.2 Trocar placement

Creation of the Gastric Pouch

The objective of this step is to create a small 25 cc proximal gastric pouch that is completely separated from the distal stomach and the fundus. First, the angle of His is identified and dissected free from the left crus (Fig. 10.3). This will ease the passage of the stapler in the final division of the G-E junction off the gastric fundus. During this step, there should be careful attention to the spleen and the short gastric vessels. A common mistake is to dissect too laterally that increases the risk of bleeding.

Approximately 6–8 cm below the gastroesophageal junction on the lesser curvature, preserving the vagus nerve (perigastric technique) (Fig. 10.4a), blunt dissection is now carried out between the hepatogastric ligament and the stomach into the retrogastric space. The left hand of the surgeon should do the actual dissection maintaining a flat plane, while the right hand retracts the lesser curve of the stomach in an inverted "J" movement until the lesser sac is reached. This technique avoids injury of the pancreas and the peripancreatic vessels (Fig. 10.4b). The authors do not use the "pars flaccida technique" that consists of transection of the hepatogastric ligament at the level of the lesser curvature to gain access to the retrogastric space; while more rapid, this technique results in transection of the vagus nerve with subsequent denervation of the gastric remnant.

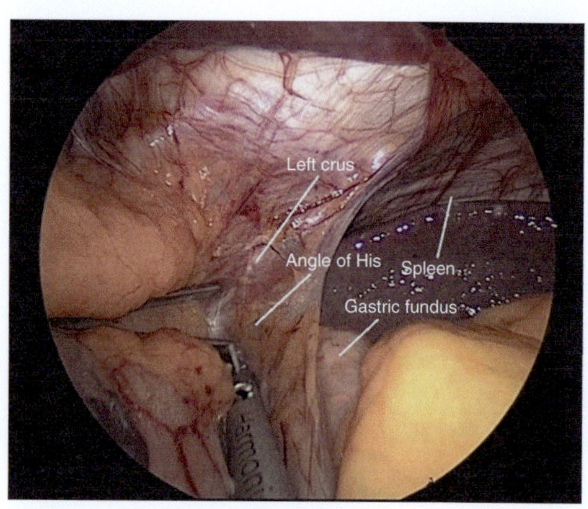

Fig. 10.3 Angle of His dissection

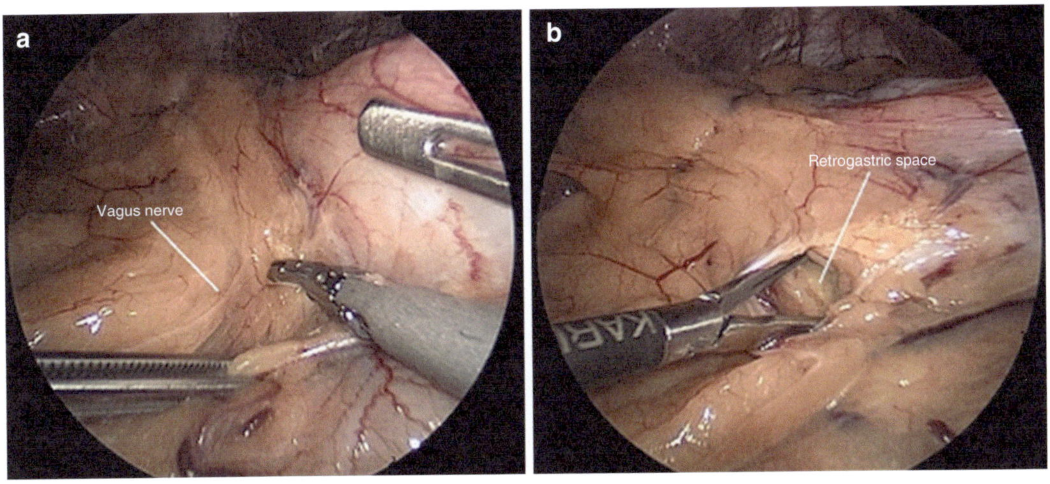

Fig. 10.4 Perigastric technique. (**a**) Identification of the vagus nerve. (**b**) Access to the retrogastric space

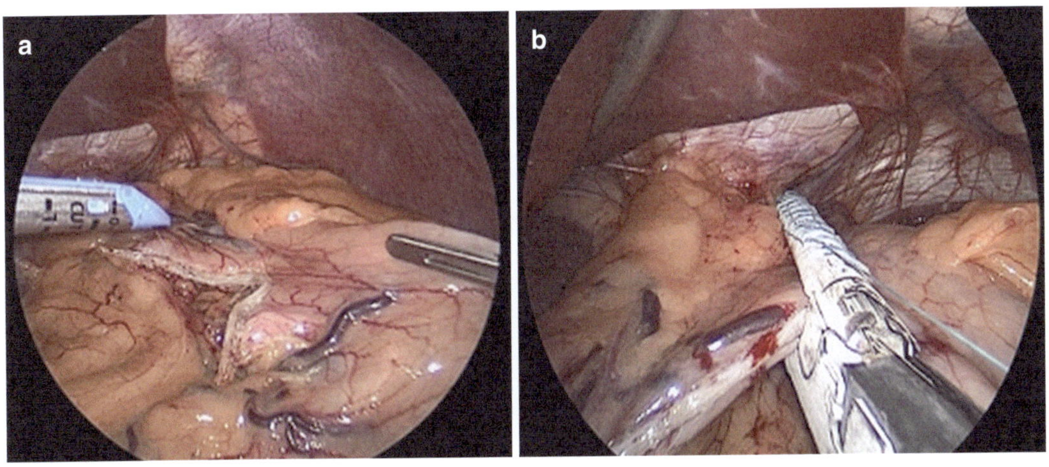

Fig. 10.5 Gastric pouch creation. (**a**) Horizonatal stapler firing without buttress - future site of anastomosis. (**b**) vertical stapler firing with bioabsorbable buttress on stapler

Once the retrogastric space is reached, a 45 mm Endo GIA stapler is used to perform a transverse transection of the stomach (Fig. 10.5a). Sequential vertical firings of 60 mm Endo GIA stapler are then used aiming toward the left crus of the diaphragm avoiding inclusion of the gastric fundus (Fig. 10.5b). A common pitfall is to aim too medial creating a "K"-shaped pouch with possible proximal narrowing or aiming too lateral which results in a larger pouch size with also risk of staple line dehiscence due to ischemia. Some surgeons advocate the use of a 34 Fr calibration tube during this part of the procedure.

Gastrojejunostomy Creation

There are three common techniques used to create the gastrojejunostomy: hand sewn, linear stapling, and circular stapling. We use that latter technique as it creates a reproducible anastomosis (and is easiest to teach). An orogastric tube armed with the anvil of an EEA 25 (Orvil, Medtronic, Minneapolis, MN) is passed by the anesthesiologist through the mouth into the proximal gastric pouch where a small opening is made. The orogastric tube is removed, leaving the anvil in place (Fig. 10.6a).

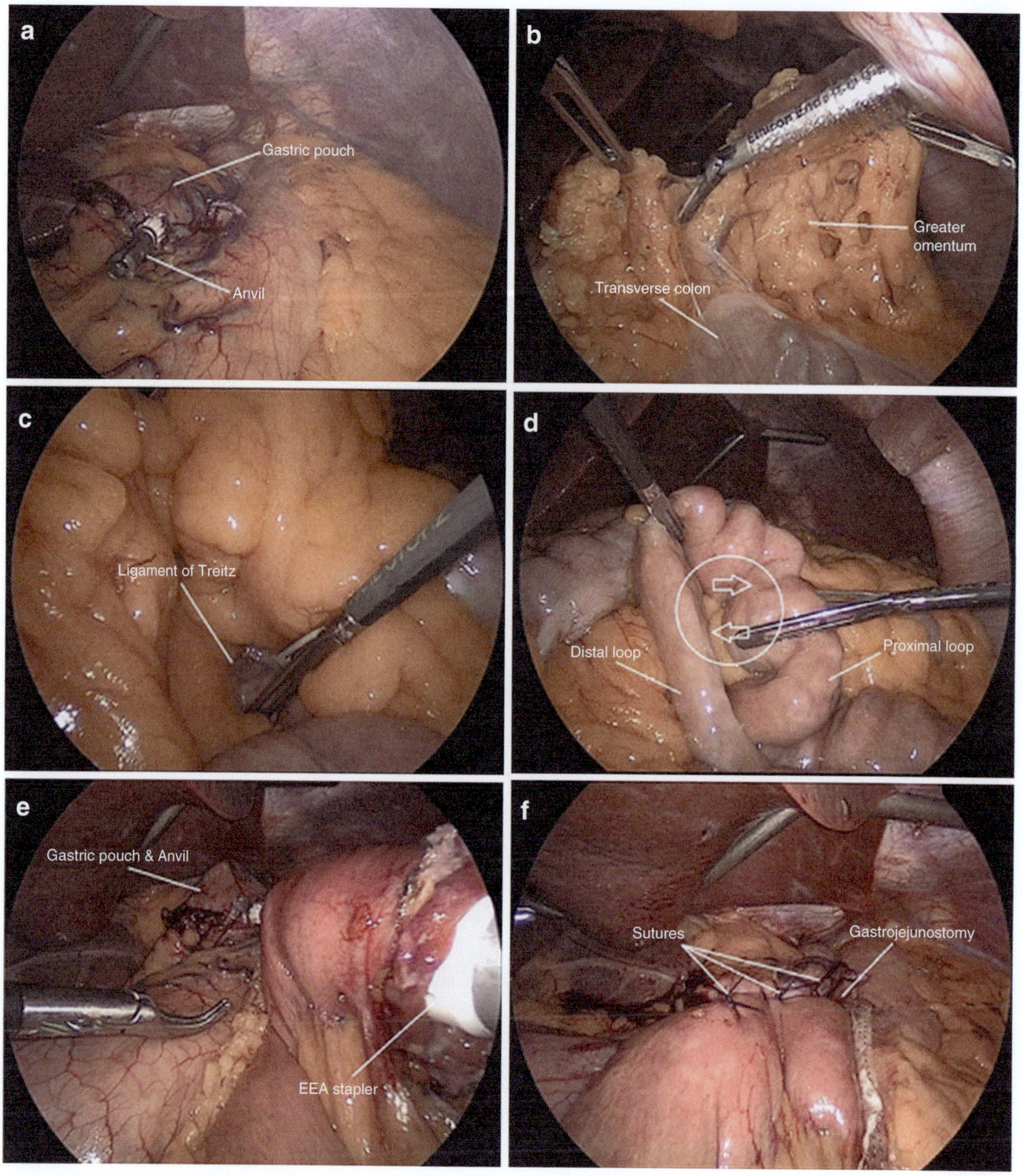

Fig. 10.6 Gastrojejunostomy creation. (**a**) Anvil in the gastric pouch. (**b**) Division of the greater omentum. (**c**) Identification of the angle of Treitz. (**d**) Clockwise bowel motion. (**e**) Introduction of the EEA 25 mm stapler. (**f**) Gastrojejunostomy

The Roux limb can be brought in an ante- or retrocolic fashion; by bringing the limb over the colon (antecolic), a potential internal hernia site is avoided. A rent is created in the greater omentum using the harmonic scalpel. This is to facilitate the cephalic advancement of the jejunal loop decreasing tension in the anastomosis (Fig. 10.6b). The ligament of Treitz is next identified and measured in a clockwise fashion caudad approximately 100 cm and transected with a 45 mm GIA stapler (Fig. 10.6c). The clockwise measurement allows the mesentery of the small bowel to remain in its natural position and untwisted (Fig. 10.6d). The staples on the distal small bowel are removed, and the left upper quadrant trocar site is enlarged to allow the introduction of an EEA 25 into the abdominal cavity. The EEA is carefully inserted into the opened distal small bowel to approximately 6 cm where the spike perforates on the antimesenteric side under direct vision (Fig. 10.6e).

The male and female parts of the EEA are drawn together to create an antecolic, antegastric, gastrojejunostomy. The EEA is fired and removed from the abdominal cavity in a sterile (camera) sheath which was previously placed on the EEA. The anastomosis is now inspected and reinforced with interrupted 2–0 absorbable sutures between the seromuscular layer of the gastric pouch and the jejunum. The opening in the small bowel is closed with a 45 mm GIA stapler (Fig. 10.6f). An orogastric tube is inserted by the anesthesiologist, and a methylene blue test is performed to rule out leaks at the gastric suture line, at the anastomosis, and at the small bowel closure. Some surgeons prefer to do this verification with an endoscope.

Jejunojejunostomy Creation

While many surgeons prefer to do this anastomosis first and then finish with the gastrojejunostomy (i.e., work in the supra-colic area to finish the case), others now do the whole surgery in the left upper quadrant (Brazilian technique). We measure the jejunum caudad from the gastrojejunostomy approximately 150 cm in a counterclockwise fashion (Fig. 10.7a). At this point, the proximal and distal jejunal loops are anastomosed by creating two small openings in the antimesenteric side of each small bowel and advancing a 60 mm GIA stapler from the right upper quadrant trocar (Fig. 10.7b). The resulting unique opening is closed in a two-layer fashion with a running 2–0 absorbable suture followed by nonabsorbable material. The opening in the mesentery under the enteroenterostomy (Fig. 10.8a) and the Petersen's defect are then closed with a running 2–0 nonabsorbable sutures (Fig. 10.8b).

Complications

In a high-volume center RYGB, morbidity typically ranges from 0.2% to 3.6% with a mortality rate of 0.1%, 1.5%, and 8% at 1, 5, and 10 years. Complications after gastric bypass may be classified as early (within 30 days) and late (more than 30 days) [4–6].

Early complications

- Anastomotic leak
- Hemorrhage
- Small bowel obstruction
- Acute gastric remnant distention
- Wound infection

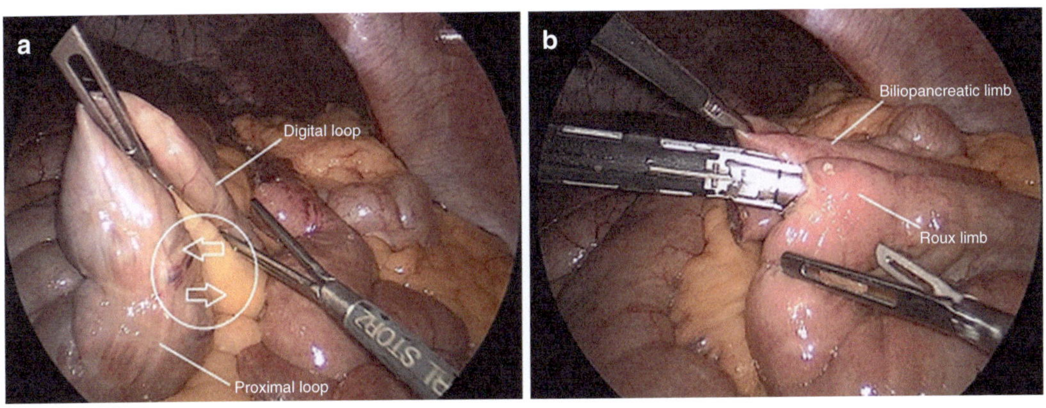

Fig. 10.7 Jejunojejunostomy creation. (**a**) Counterclockwise bowel motion. (**b**) Linear stapler anastomosis

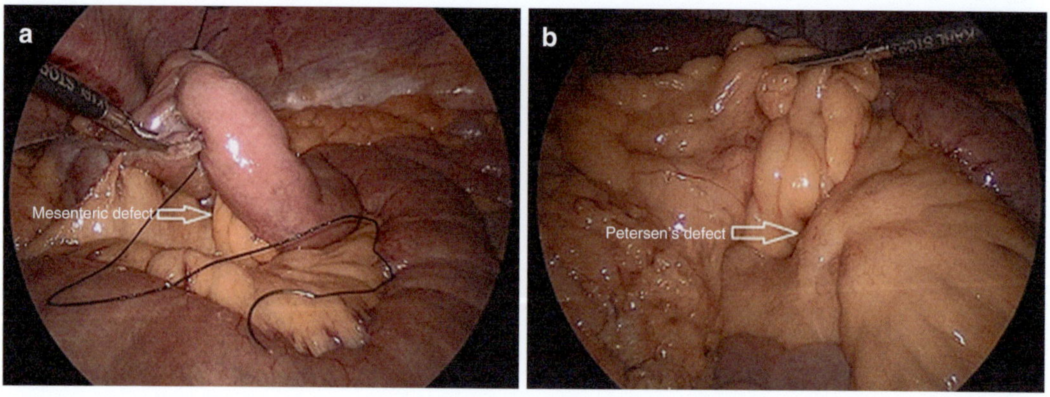

Fig. 10.8 (**a**) Mesenteric defect. (**b**) Petersen's defect

Late complications

- Marginal ulceration
- Gastrojejunostomy stricture
- Small bowel obstruction
- Pouch dilatation
- Gastrojejunostomy dilatation
- Symptomatic cholelithiasis
- Gastrogastric fistula
- Metabolic/nutritional complications

Anastomotic Leak

The incidence of anastomotic leak in contemporary series has declined and ranges from 1% to 3%, but this is still high enough in our opinion. Therefore, we recommend routine intraoperative leak tests. Leaks are a harbinger for longer hospitalization and an increase in overall complication rate. Risk factors for anastomotic leaks include surgeon experience and different factors related to patients (super obesity, uncontrolled comorbidities). The type of anastomosis and staple manufacturer do not appear to alter the risk of leak; however, the use of buttressing material may be more common in cases where leaks occurred.

Clinical Presentation

The usual presentation is within the first 7 days of the postoperative period. The patient presents with classic signs and symptoms of systemic inflammatory response (tachycardia, tachypnea, fever/hypothermia, leukocytosis/leukopenia) and abdominal pain. The presence of any of these symptoms should raise the suspicion, and immediate action must be initiated. The abdominal exam in the obese patient is unreliable, and lack of peritoneal signs does not rule out the presence of a leak. While persistent tachycardia and tachypnea are the most common signs of leak, pulmonary embolism must be also considered. The patient should be placed in a monitored unit with the initiation of intravenous fluids and broad-spectrum antibiotics. Imaging studies such as upper gastrointestinal series (UGI) and CT of the abdomen with oral contrast may help in the diagnosis. There are a significant number of false negatives in these tests, and the concerned physician should proceed with diagnostic laparoscopy if warranted by the clinical situation.

Management

Some patients can be managed nonoperatively with intravenous broad-spectrum antibiotics, nothing per mouth, total parenteral nutrition (TPN), and CT-guided drainage of any intra-abdominal collection/abscess. Most patients will require diagnostic laparoscopy with abdominal washout and drainage. Delaying laparoscopy while continuing substantial fluid resuscitation results in increasing turgor of the abdominal wall making laparoscopy more difficult and often requiring conversion to laparotomy. A gastrostomy tube placement in the remnant stomach should be considered in any reoperation to allow enteral access for medications and nutrition.

Gastrointestinal Bleeding

The incidence of gastrointestinal bleeding after RYGB ranges from 0.8% to 9.4%. Acute bleeding usually is defined as occurring within the first 72 h after surgery, but significant bleeding can also present at a later time (subacute and chronic bleeding). This classification is helpful primarily in the identification of the source. Acute bleeding is mainly located at the staple lines as a result of inadequate compression of vessels within the cut tissue or a preexisting bleeding disorder. There are three possible primary locations: the gastric pouch with gastrojejunostomy, the gastric remnant, and the jejunojejunostomy. Subacute bleeding (72 h–30 days) while possibly located at the staple line is more commonly associated with a gastric or duodenal ulcer (missed preoperatively), gastritis, NSAID gastropathy, and bleeding secondary to anticoagulation. Chronic bleeding (more than 30 days) is usually encountered as result of marginal ulceration at the gastrojejunostomy, although other causes unrelated to RYGB should be considered (malignancy, duodenal and gastric ulcers, coagulopathy).

Clinical Presentation

Tachycardia, hypotension, and low urine output may be present in a patient with hemorrhage; however, early enteric leak and pulmonary embolism should also be part of the differential diagnosis. Usually the diagnosis is made based on a drop in hemoglobin and the presence of hematemesis or melena. Bleeding at the gastrojejunostomy most commonly presents as hematemesis followed by melena. Bleeding from the gastric remnant and jejunojejunostomy usually presents as melena but can also present as bowel obstruction. Bleeding might also be extraluminal (intra-abdominal); this type of bleeding should be considered in a tachycardic patient with a drop in the hemoglobin and unusual abdominal distention and pain.

Management

The stable patient should be transferred to a monitored unit. Nonoperative treatment is reserved for patients who adequately respond to initial resuscitation and should include serial quantification of hemoglobin, closed monitoring of vitals and urine output, acid secretion reduction therapy, and discontinuation of DVT prophylaxis. An unstable patient should go to the operating room for an emergent upper endoscopy with possible diagnostic laparoscopy under full (intubated) general anesthesia (Fig. 10.9). The patient should be aggressively resuscitated with early transfusion and correction of coagulopathy if present. It is important to emphasize that interventional radiology has a minimal role in this setting; embolization of a major vessel in the stomach could lead to ischemia and potential leak. An exception is embolization of the gastroduodenal artery as the treatment of choice in patients with known duodenal ulcer.

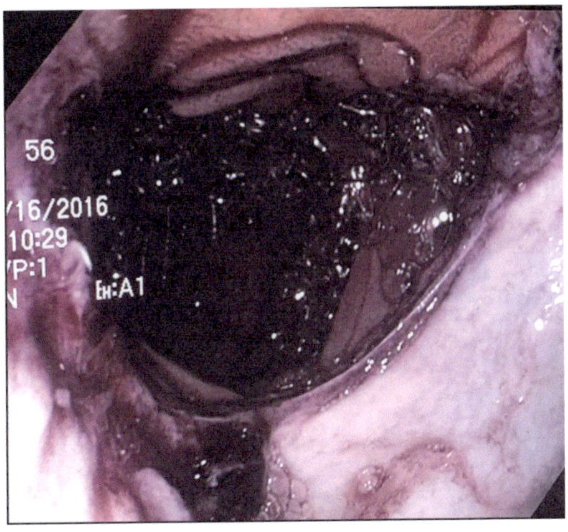

Fig. 10.9 Bleeding at the gastrojejunostomy

Intestinal Obstruction

Intestinal obstruction after RYGB ranges from 1.5% to 5.2%. Common causes include internal hernias, adhesions, and kinking at the jejunojejunostomy. This condition must be diagnosed and treated promptly due to the possibility of bowel ischemia, resulting in sepsis and even death [7].

Clinical Presentation

The landmark symptom is periumbilical or left upper quadrant pain that may radiate to the back. Nausea and emesis are less frequent due to the presence of a small pouch; however, bile emesis should raise the suspicion of obstruction at or distal to the jejunojejunostomy. Patients with an obstruction of the biliopancreatic limb may have a nonspecific clinical presentation and laboratory findings, and this diagnosis maybe missed by a healthcare provider not familiar with this type of complication. A consultation with a bariatric surgeon should be made in this setting. CT scans of the abdomen with intravenous and oral contrast is the radiologic study of choice with a sensitivity of 50–90%. The presence of a "swirl sign" is a reliable indicator of internal hernia after RYGB, and surgical treatment should be immediately initiated (Fig. 10.10). Although highly sensitive, a negative CT scan should not delay diagnostic laparoscopy in a patient with clear signs and symptoms of bowel obstruction after RYGB.

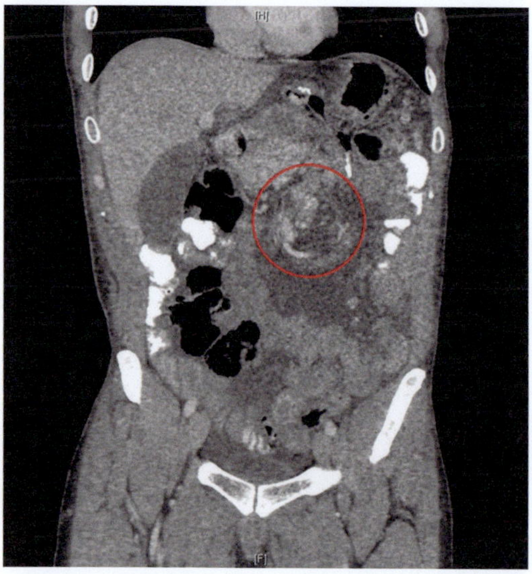

Fig. 10.10 "Swirl sign" in a Petersen's internal hernia

Management

A nasogastric tube placement should usually be avoided in a patient with RYGB, especially in the early postoperative period, due to the risk of perforation. Fluid resuscitation and continual monitoring of vital signs and urine output should be initiated. Diagnostic laparoscopy is ultimately the management of choice in this setting. The authors prefer to place the trocars in the following manner in order to systematically run the bowel in a distal to proximal fashion. A left upper quadrant 5 mm optical trocar is used for access and the initial creation of pneumoperitoneum. A second, 5 mm trocar is placed in the left lower quadrant followed by a suprapubic and a right lower quadrant 5 mm trocar. The camera is initially situated in the left lower quadrant to "run" (examine) the bowel cephalad from the ileocecal valve. Once about half of the bowel is ran, the camera is switched to the suprapubic trocar, and the surgeon will continue to assess the bowel using the right lower quadrant and the left lower quadrant trocars (Fig. 10.11). The adhesions are taken down sharply if present; the spaces of Petersen, jejunojejunostomy mesenteric defect, and the retrocolic space in the case of a retrocolic Roux limb are evaluated. If an internal hernia is found, the surgeon should

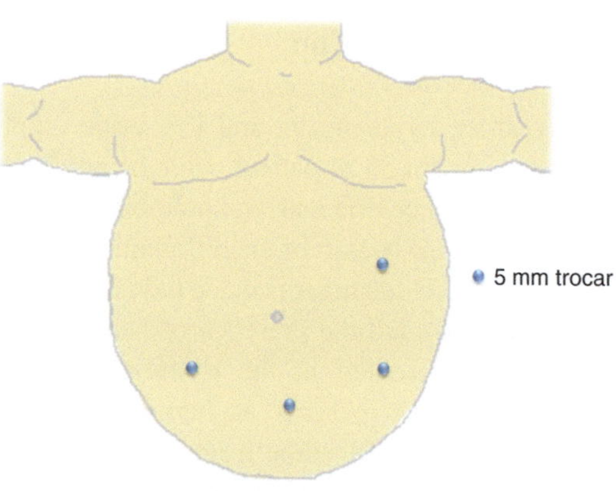

Fig. 10.11 Trocar placement for diagnostic laparoscopy

reduce the bowel in a counterclockwise fashion. The mesenteric defects should then be closed with a running nonabsorbable suture.

Retrograde intussusception is a rare cause of intestinal obstruction (0.1–0.5%). Diagnosis is difficult, and intermittent intussusception is not an uncommon finding in abdominal imaging of patients for other reasons. Pain appears to be related to vascular compromise and not to the degree of intestinal obstruction. Early diagnosis is (again) imperative to avoid mesenteric ischemia. There is no true surgical consensus on management, but intestinal resection/complete anastomotic revision appears to have a lower recurrence rate.

Marginal Ulceration

Marginal ulceration is a late complication after RYGB with an incidence of 1–4%. This almost always occurs on the jejunal side of the anastomosis due to the lack of protective mechanisms against acid exposure. The etiology of marginal ulcerations is complex and may involve a combination of factors including an increase in acid gastric secretion, weakening of the mucosal defenses, and technical aspects of the operation. Risk factors for marginal ulceration include NSAIDs, smoking, *H. pylori*, ischemia, alcohol, nonabsorbable suture, larger pouch (inclusion of more parietal cells), and gastrogastric fistula.

Clinical Presentation

Marginal ulcers most commonly present as chronic epigastric pain that, unlike classic peptic ulcer disease in a non-operated patient, exacerbates with eating. They can also present as acute or chronic gastrointestinal bleeding and less commonly as free perforation and sepsis that may require emergent surgical intervention.

Management

It is important to identify in the initial assessment any potential risk factor that may contribute to marginal ulceration. An upper endoscopy with biopsy is the initial tool of choice to characterize the size and location of the ulcer (Fig. 10.12). An UGI series is helpful to diagnose an excessively large gastric pouch and/or the presence of a gastrogastric fistula. Initial treatment consists of lifestyle modification and discontinuation of potential aggravating factors such as NSAIDs, alcohol, and especially tobacco. A trial of acid reduction therapy with proton pump inhibitors and sucralfate is initiated. Eradication of *H. pylori* if positive is warranted. A repeat endoscopy after the initial treatment is recommended to evaluate response.

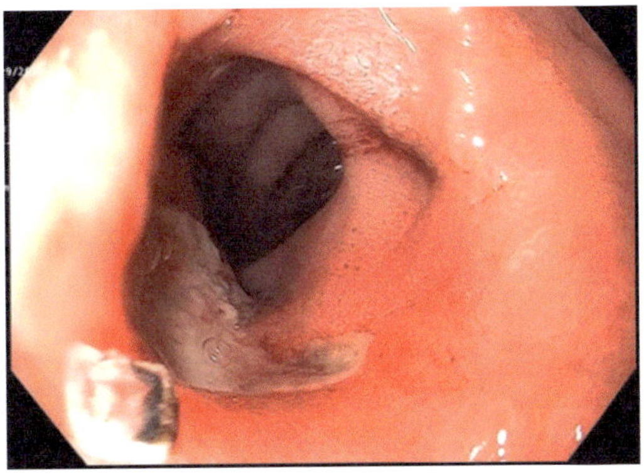

Fig. 10.12 Gastrojejunostomy ulcer

Surgical treatment is considered with acute complications (perforation, hemorrhage), recurrent ulceration, gastrogastric fistula, and the presence of debilitating symptoms such as chronic pain, dysphagia, malnutrition, and stricture. Operative intervention is tailored depending on the findings in the initial workup (UGI, EGD). This usually consists of revision of the gastrojejunostomy with reduction of the gastric pouch size and/or excision of gastrogastric fistula if present. This procedure may be combined with a remnant gastrostomy for feeding purposes in selected (malnourished) cases. In the setting of a free perforation with peritoneal contamination, the best surgical option is probably an omental patch placement.

Gastrojejunostomy Stricture

Stricture at the gastrojejunostomy anastomosis is late complication with an incidence reported between 3% and 15% depending mostly on the definition of stricture. The heterogeneity of literature concerning stricture rates related to stapler type (or hand sewn) should be interpreted cautiously [8]. Stricture development is usually multifactorial, related to tension on the anastomosis, injury from acid exposure, submucosal hematoma, and additional reinforcement of the anastomosis (perhaps worse with non-resorbable suture), all resulting in ischemia leading to scar formation. There is no perfect size for the initial gastrojejunostomy. The surgeon is challenged to perform a small anastomosis understanding that this creates the risk of developing a stricture in the future.

Clinical Presentation

The patient typically presents with history of progressive dysphagia (or odynophagia) to solids and the need to eat slowly with intermittent episodes of nausea and vomiting. The symptoms usually occur after 1 or 2 months postoperatively. It may be difficult to discern difficulty with adaptation to the gastric bypass with a pathologic stricture.

Presentation after more than 4 months suggests the presence of an associated ulcer or foreign body (suture). Patients who present in this time frame may also present with continued, inappropriate weight loss complicated with important vitamin deficiencies (thiamine and others) and protein caloric malnutrition.

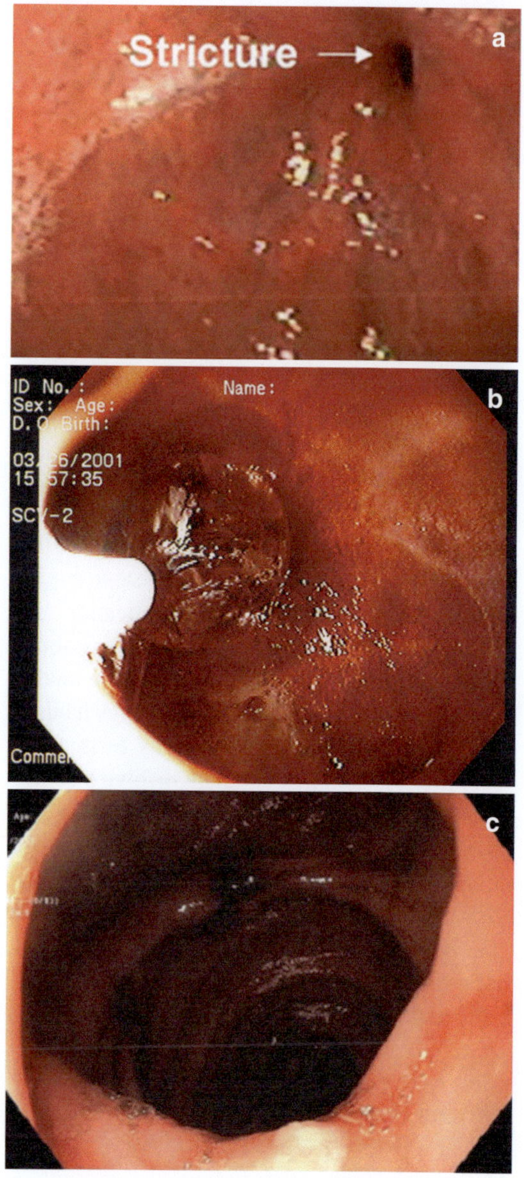

Fig. 10.13 (**a**) Gastrojejunostomy stricture. (**b**) Through the scope balloon dilator. (**c**) Status post balloon dilatation

Management

Initial management consists of upper endoscopy which can be both diagnostic and therapeutic. If the endoscope passes the anastomosis, decreasing meal size and increasing meal frequency usually help patient adapt and avoid the need for intervention. If a stenosis is present, dilatation of the stricture is the treatment of choice (Fig. 10.13a, b). This can be done via endoscopic- or fluoroscopic-guided balloon dilators. Savary-Gilliard dilators are another option but should be used with caution. The goal is to achieve a sequential dilatation up to 15–18 mm; more robust dilations increase the risk of perforation. Most patients will show resolution of symptoms after one dilatation; however, a small subset of patients will require multiple sessions. We think it is wise to start with smaller size balloons and progressively increase, if necessary, to the anastomotic size objective in more than one session.

Comorbidities Resolution and Weight Loss

Gastric bypass has demonstrated that it is a powerful tool for weight loss and resolution of comorbidities. Gastric bypass achieves improvement in most risk factors associated with obesity: cardiovascular disease, diabetes, hyperlipidemia (metabolic syndrome), and obstructive sleep apnea, decreasing the patient's overall risk of death [9]. This improvement in comorbidities usually has a direct relationship to weight loss with a median percentage of excess weight loss (%EWL) of 70% and a percentage of total weight loss (%TWL) of 30% at 1 year in most series [10, 11]. Table 10.1 shows a summary of outcomes after gastric bypass according to the most relevant literature.

Among all postoperative benefits, RYGB often results in remarkable improvements in type 2 diabetes (T2D). The alteration in the anatomy increases the delivery of food to the distal intestine stimulating the rise of insulin-regulating hormones such as glucagon-like peptide 1 (GLP-1). GLP-1 is an incretin hormone that is released postprandially from the ileum and colon. This hormone stimulates insulin secretion and decreases appetite. The overall effect is a hypersecretion of insulin with associated weight loss that improves glucose tolerance in T2D with either resolution or substantial improvement of the disease.

Randomized prospective studies have shown that RYGB is a better option than conventional medical management in the treatment of T2D. Mingrone et al. found that at 2 years, diabetes remission occurred in 75% of diabetic patients undergoing RYGB versus zero remission in the medical group [12]. More recently, Schauer et al. demonstrated that after 5 years, surgery achieved a greater mean percentage reduction from baseline in glycated hemoglobin levels than did patients who received medical therapy alone [13].

Special Considerations

Currently, there is no clear consensus in the bariatric community as to which represents the best operation in weight loss surgery. RYGB is still considered a landmark procedure, with well-described complications, and the only procedure with a plethora of data on long-term outcomes [14–20]. It is important to be able to understand the advantages and disadvantages that the operation carries and how this could affect the decision-making of the patient and the bariatric surgeon.

Advantages

- Indicated for patients with documented gastroesophageal reflux disease (GERD). Also recommended as treatment of choice in a patient with a previously failed anti-reflux procedure
- Better success rate in resolution of T2D when compared to other bariatric procedures
- Well-documented literature on the incidence and management of complications

Table 10.1 Summary of outcomes after gastric bypass

Author	No. of patients	Follow-up years	%EWL	%TWL	HTN % resolution/ improvement	DM % resolution/ improvement	OSA % resolution/ improvement
Higa et al.	242	10	57.1–68.6	28.5–34	87	83	76
Kothari et al.	1402	10	57–79	nd	59	86	nd
Peterli et al.	110	3	73.8–76.6	nd	71	77	82
Adams et al.	1156	6	nd	27.7	42	75	nd
Obeid et al.	328	10	58.9	nd	46	58	nd
Mehaffey et al.	1087	10	nd	27.7	20.4	57.3	54.7

EWL excess weight loss, *TWL* total weight loss, *HTN* hypertension, *DM* diabetes mellitus, *OSA* obstructive sleep apnea

- Well-documented long-term outcomes
- Better and more sustained weight loss achieved when compared to sleeve gastrectomy

Disadvantages

- Not recommended in the high-risk surgical candidate. RYGB is a more extensive and usually a longer procedure. This is likely to increase the chances of postoperative complications in high-risk subset of patients.
- The procedure involves more than one anastomosis with several staple lines, which increase the potential for staple-line complications such as postoperative bleeding and leak.
- Alteration of the small bowel anatomy with potential development of internal hernias
- Complex procedure that demands high level of surgical skills and learning curve concerns.
- Malabsorption of micro- and macronutrients with the potential of severe (and irreversible) nutritional deficiencies in the noncompliant patient.

RYGB confers enormous benefits to the morbidly obese patient and overall has few complications. It is of paramount importance to select the best procedure for any given patient, taking into consideration their individual risks and benefits after a complete initial assessment. It is the role of the bariatric surgeon and the multidisciplinary team to educate the patient on the perioperative course and potential complications associated to this procedure.

References

1. Wittgrove AC, Clark GW, Tremblay LJ. Laparoscopic gastric bypass, Roux-en-Y: preliminary report of five cases. Obes Surg. 1994;4(4):353–7.
2. Collazo-Clavell ML1, Clark MM, McAlpine DE, Jensen MD. Assessment and preparation of patients for bariatric surgery. Mayo Clin Proc. 2006;81(10 Suppl):S11–7.
3. Kuruba R1, Koche LS, Murr MM. Preoperative assessment and perioperative care of patients undergoing bariatric surgery. Med Clin North Am. 2007;91(3):339–51.
4. Jacobsen HJ, Nergard BJ, Leifsson BG, et al. Management of suspected anastomotic leak after bariatric laparoscopic Roux-en-y gastric bypass. Br J Surg. 2014;101(4):417–23.
5. Kruger RS, Pricolo VE, Streeter TT, Colacchio DA, Andrade UA. A bariatric surgery center of excellence: operative trends and long-term outcomes. J Am Coll Surg. 2014;218(6):1163–17.
6. Varban OA, Cassidy RB, Sheetz KH, Cain-Nielsen A, Carlin AM, Schram JL, Weiner MJ, Bacal D, Stricklen A, Finks JF, Michigan Bariatric Surgery Collaborative. Technique or technology? Evaluating leaks after gastric bypass. Surg Obes Relat Dis. 2016;12(2):264–72.
7. Felsher J, Brodsky J, Brody F. Small bowel obstruction after laparoscopic Roux-en-Y gastric bypass. Surgery. 2003;134(3):501–5.
8. Jiang HP, Lin LL, Jiang X, Qiao HQ. Meta-analysis of hand-sewn versus mechanical gastrojejunal anastomosis during laparoscopic Roux-en-Y gastric bypass for morbid obesity. Int J Surg. 2016;32:150–7.
9. Kim J, Eisenberg D, Azagury D, Rogers A, Campos GM. American society for metabolic and bariatric surgery position statement on long-term survival benefit after metabolic and bariatric surgery. Surg Obes Relat Dis. 2016;12(3):453–9.
10. Abdeen G, le Roux CW. Mechanism underlying the weight loss and complications of Roux-en-Y gastric bypass. Review. Obes Surg. 2016;26(2):410–21.
11. Ibrahim AM, Ghaferi AA, Thumma JR, Dimick JB. Variation in outcomes at bariatric surgery centers of excellence. JAMA Surg. 2017. https://doi.org/10.1001/jamasurg.2017.0542. [Epub ahead of print].
12. Mingrone G, Panunzi S, De Gaetano A, Guidone C, Iaconelli A, Leccesi L, Nanni G, Pomp A, Castagneto M, Ghirlanda G, Rubino F. Bariatric surgery versus conventional medical therapy for type 2 diabetes. N Engl J Med. 2012;366(17):1577–85.
13. Schauer PR1, Bhatt DL, Kirwan JP, Wolski K, Aminian A, Brethauer SA, Navaneethan SD, Singh RP, Pothier CE, Nissen SE, Kashyap SR. Bariatric surgery versus intensive medical therapy for diabetes – 5-year outcomes. N Engl J Med. 2017;376(7):641–65.
14. Sjöström L, Peltonen M, Jacobson P, Sjöström CD, Karason K, Wedel H, Ahlin S, Anveden Å, Bengtsson C, Bergmark G, Bouchard C, Carlsson B, Dahlgren S, Karlsson J, Lindroos AK, Lönroth H, Narbro K, Näslund I, Olbers T, Svensson PA, Carlsson LM. Bariatric surgery and long-term cardiovascular events. JAMA. 2012;307(1):56–65.
15. Higa K, Ho T, Tercero F, Yunus T, Boone KB. Laparoscopic Roux-en-Y gastric bypass: 10-year follow-up. Surg Obes Relat Dis. 2011;7(4):516–25.
16. Kothari SN, Borgert AJ, Kallies KJ, Baker MT, Grover BT. Long-term (>10-year) outcomes after laparoscopic Roux-en-Y gastric bypass. Surg Obes Relat Dis. 2016. https://doi.org/10.1016/j.soard.2016.12.011. [Epub ahead of print].

17. Peterli R, Wölnerhanssen BK, Vetter D, Nett P, Gass M, Borbély Y, Peters T, Schiesser M, Schultes B, Beglinger C, Drewe J, Bueter M. Laparoscopic sleeve gastrectomy versus roux-Y-gastric bypass for morbid Obesity-3-year outcomes of the prospective randomized Swiss multicenter bypass or sleeve study (SM-BOSS). Ann Surg. 2017;265(3):466–73.
18. Adams TD, Davidson LE, Litwin SE, Kolotkin RL, LaMonte MJ, Pendleton RC, Strong MB, Vinik R, Wanner NA, Hopkins PN, Gress RE, Walker JM, Cloward TV, Nuttall RT, Hammoud A, Greenwood JL, Crosby RD, McKinlay R, Simper SC, Smith SC, Hunt SC. Health benefits of gastric bypass surgery after 6 years. JAMA. 2012;308(11):1122–31.
19. Obeid NR, Malick W, Concors SJ, Fielding GA, Kurian MS, Ren-Fielding CJ. Long-term outcomes after Roux-en-Y gastric bypass: 10- to 13-year data. Surg Obes Relat Dis. 2016;12(1):11–20.
20. Mehaffey JH1, LaPar DJ, Clement KC, Turrentine FE, Miller MS, Hallowell PT, Schirmer BD. 10-year outcomes after Roux-en-Y gastric bypass. Ann Surg. 2016;264(1):121–6.

11 Duodenal Switch

Sébastien Blaye-Felice, Stéfane Lebel, Simon Marceau, François Julien, and Laurent Biertho

Introduction

The classical biliopancreatic diversion (BPD) was first described in 1979 by Nicola Scopinaro [1]. The goal of the procedure was to preserve the excellent long-term metabolic outcomes from the malabsorptive component of the jejunoileal bypass (JIB), while decreasing gastrointestinal side effects and risks of liver and kidney failures, which led to the abandon of the JIB a long time ago. In BPD surgery, the distal two-third of the stomach are removed, to obtain a mild gastric restriction, and the gastric pouch is connected to the distal ileum, creating a 250-cm alimentary tract and a 50-cm common channel. In the late 1980s, Hess and Marceau [2, 3] modified the type of gastrectomy to perform a large "sleeve gastrectomy, SG," keeping the same length of strict alimentary limb and common channel but connecting the alimentary limb to the first duodenum ("duodenal switch, BPD-DS"). This modification was based on animal study by DeMeester et al., who originally described duodenal switch procedure for the treatment of bile gastritis [4]. The length of the common channel was later increased to 100 cm to decrease malabsorption and side effects.

S. Blaye-Felice · S. Lebel · S. Marceau · F. Julien
L. Biertho (✉)
Department of Bariatric and General Surgery, Institut Universitaire de Cardiologie et Pneumologie de Québec – Université Laval, Quebec, QC, Canada

In summary, a BPD-DS includes three specific components: a longitudinal gastrectomy (SG) to decrease meal volumes, acid production, and appetite through ghrelin reduction; a 150-cm strict alimentary limb; and a 100-cm common channel where food bolus mixes with biliopancreatic juices, decreasing protein and fat absorption (Fig. 11.1). Significant metabolic and hormonal effects result from avoiding the mixing of food with bile and pancreatic juices, resulting in bringing undigested food in the distal ileum. Laparoscopic BPD-DS was first performed by M Gagner in 1999 [5] and has since shown a reduction in complication rates compared to open approach [6].

Perioperative Care

Preoperative Assessment

All bariatric patients are evaluated by a multidisciplinary team, including a bariatric surgeon, specialized bariatric nurse, and dietician. Consultation with a dietician qualified in BPD-DS is very important to correct eating disorders and for patient's education of the recommended diet after BPD-DS (high-protein, low-fat diet). Before surgery, a low-calorie, high-protein diet can also be used to decrease the size of the liver and the amount of intraperitoneal fat. A psychiatric evaluation is requested for patients with a history of mental health issue or when clinically

R. Lutfi et al. (eds.), *Global Bariatric Surgery*, https://doi.org/10.1007/978-3-319-93545-4_11

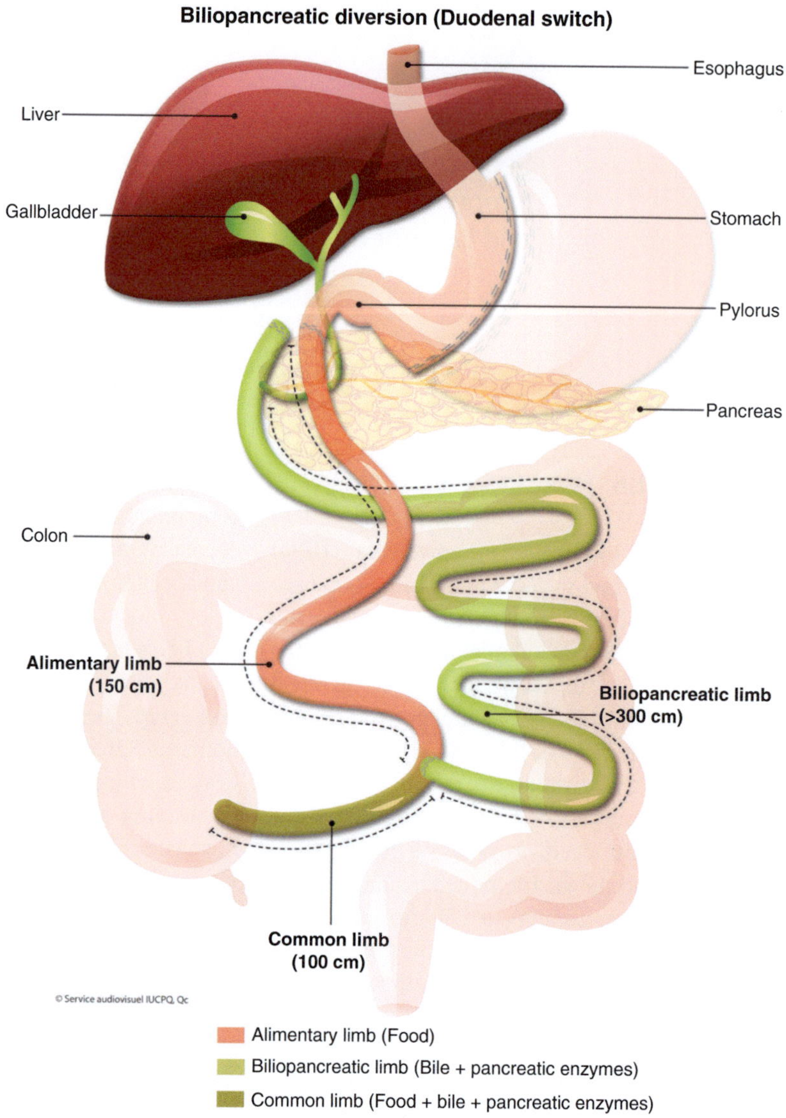

Fig. 11.1 BPD-DS: the first duodenum is anastomosed to the last 250 cm of small bowel. A 100-cm common channel is created. *Service audiovisuel, IUCPQ-UL*

indicated. Screening for diabetes, dyslipidemia, and obstructive sleep apnea is performed. These comorbidities are controlled prior to surgery. For example, if sleep apnea is detected, noninvasive positive pressure ventilation is initiated by a pneumologist before surgery.

Preoperative blood work consists of a complete blood cell count, liver enzymes, albumin, calcium, parathyroid hormone, vitamin D, vitamin A, vitamin B12, and iron panel. In our practice, all patients receive a multivitamin complex (Centrum Forte©) before surgery (usually 3 months in advance) and vitamin D3 supplementation (10,000 U per day for 1 month followed by 1000 U per day until surgery). Other vitamin and mineral deficiencies are corrected before surgery.

Surgical Technique

Patient Preparation and Positioning

The patient is positioned in a split leg position on a bariatric OR table. The patient is strapped to the operative table, and both arms are placed in abduction. Thrombo- and antibio-prophylaxis are given 2 h prior surgery (heparin 5000 s/c and cefazolin 2–3 g for patients below and above 110 kg, respectively). Pneumatic compression devices are used during the procedure and until patients are ambulatory. The surgeon stands between the patient's legs, with the assistant to the patient's left. During the surgery, the surgeon moves to the left of the patient for the ileoileal anastomosis.

The following laparoscopic instrument set is used during the surgery:

- A 5-mm or 10-mm 30° endoscope
- Nontraumatic bowel graspers, including long (45-cm) instruments
- Articulating linear stapler-cutter, 60 mm in length, with cartridges ranging from white to black loads (Echelon Flex long 60, Ethicon, Cincinnati, OH)
- Ultrasonic shear dissection device (Ethicon, Cincinnati, OH)
- Laparoscopic curved needle holder with DeBakey forceps
- 5-mm and 12-mm disposable trocars, 10 cm in length (Endopath Xcel, Ethicon), with 15-cm length trocars available
- 15-cm Veress needle
- A 5-mm liver retractor with table-mounted holding device
- V-Loc absorbable 3-0 suture (Covidien, Mansfield, Massachusetts)
- Long clip applier
- Fascia closure device

A long Veress needle (15 cm) is first inserted in the left upper quadrant to create a 15-mmHg pneumoperitoneum. A 5-mm or 10-mm optical trocar is used to enter the abdominal cavity under direct vision, two handbreadths under the xyphoid, and slightly off-midline to the left, to avoid the hepatic ligament. Two 12-mm ports are placed at the same level in the left and right flanks. A 5-mm port is placed in the epigastria area for the liver retractor, in the left upper quadrant for the assistant and in the left flank for the submesocolic part of the procedure (Fig. 11.2). If a particularly large falciform is present, a transfascial suture can be placed with a suture passer to lift the ligament up. The first step of the procedure is the gastric mobilization and creation of the SG. The duodenum is then transected 3–4 cm distal to the pylorus. The small bowel is transected 250 cm from the ileocecal valve. A handsewn duodeno-ileostomy is then created. The biliary limb is anastomosed side to side to the alimentary limb, 100 cm from the ileocecal valve.

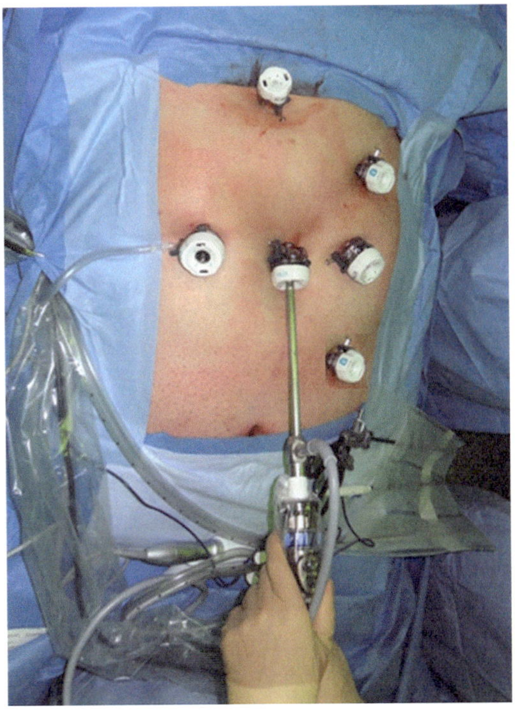

Fig. 11.2 Trocars position for a laparoscopic BPD-DS

Gastric Mobilization

The first step of the procedure is similar to a standard SG. An ultrasonic device is used to devascularize the greater curvature. Dissection of the gastrocolic ligament begins along the gastric body where the lesser omental cavity is easily entered (Fig. 11.3). The greater curvature is mobilized to the angle of His. Mobilization is completed up to the left crus of the diaphragm. Short gastric vessels can be controlled with large clips.

At that point, it is important to evaluate the feasibility of the duodenal switch. For example, in super-super obese patients with a short mesentery, dense adhesions at the level of the duodenum

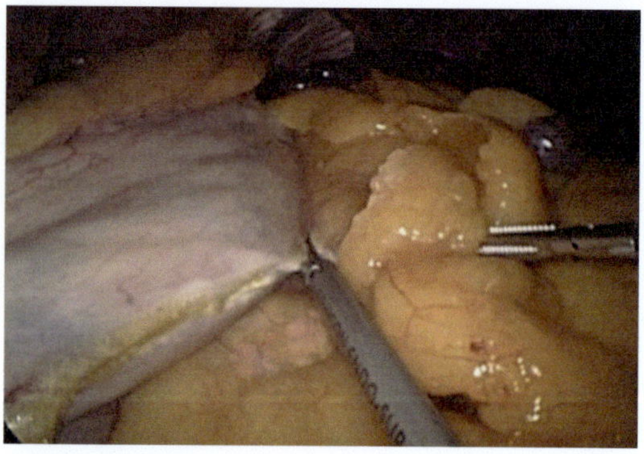

Fig. 11.3 Dissection of the gastrocolic ligament

or pelvis, or patients with high intra-abdominal pressure with limited working space, the surgery can be converted to a SG alone, as a first-stage surgery.

Duodenal Dissection

The duodenal dissection is the most specific step of the DBP-DS. The proximity of several important anatomic structures (pancreatic head, common bile duct, and gastroduodenal artery) requires precise surgical approach. The liver retractor is placed on the right liver to expose the first duodenum and pylorus. The Mayo's vein on the lower aspect of the pylorus can be useful to identify the pylorus.

The antrum is retracted to the left, which brings the first portion of the duodenum to the midline. The peritoneum is opened above and below the first duodenum. The common bile duct is often identified at the superior aspect of the duodenum and represents a good landmark for the dissection. Two different techniques can be used to mobilize the duodenum. The inferior and posterior attachments of the duodenum are mobilized for the inferior approach, and a tunnel under the posterior aspect of the duodenum is created for the posterior approach.

Inferior Approach The gastrocolic ligament is dissected using ultrasonic energy, passed the pylorus. The pyloric artery can be controlled with clips. The posterior attachments of the duodenum are dissected to mobilize the first 3–4 cm of duodenum. The gastroduodenal artery, which lies at the posterior aspect of the first duodenum, marks the distal aspect of the dissection. A window is created at the upper aspect of the duodenum, just lateral and above the common bile duct. A 15-cm Penrose drain is then passed into that window to retract the duodenum. Care is taken to avoid injury to the right gastric artery. That window is slightly enlarged to accommodate the anvil of a linear stapler. An Echelon Flex with a blue cartridge is passed through the 12-mm port in the left flank to transect the duodenum.

Posterior Approach The duodenum is retracted medially by pulling the antrum to the left. The surgeon pulls the duodenum up, and the peritoneum is opened 3–4 cm distal from the pylorus on the lower and the upper border of the duodenum. A window is created at the inferior part of the duodenum, 3–4 cm distal to the pylorus. Blunt dissection is used to identify the plane between the posterior duodenal wall and the pancreas (Fig. 11.4). A 15-cm Penrose drain is then passed into that window to retract the duodenum. The window is slightly enlarged to accommodate the anvil of the linear stapler, and the duodenum is transected (Fig. 11.5).

Sleeve Gastrectomy

A 34-Fr bougie is inserted transorally and carefully positioned under laparoscopic guidance. The first stapling is performed at the level of the crow's foot, about 5 cm proximal to the pylorus,

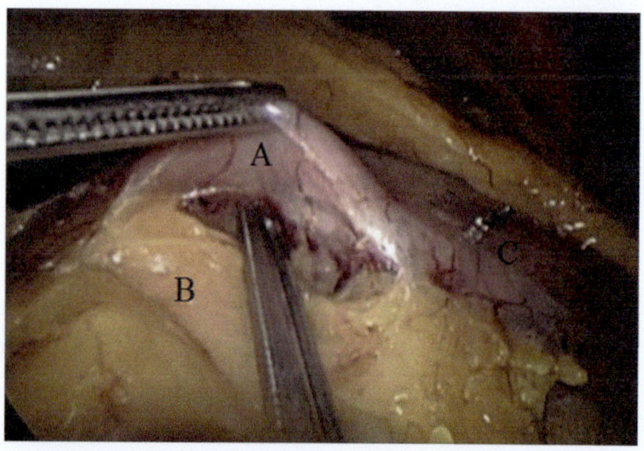

Fig. 11.4 The duodenum (A) is lifted up, and the retroduodenal window is created above the pancreatic head (B) 3 cm distal from the pylorus (C)

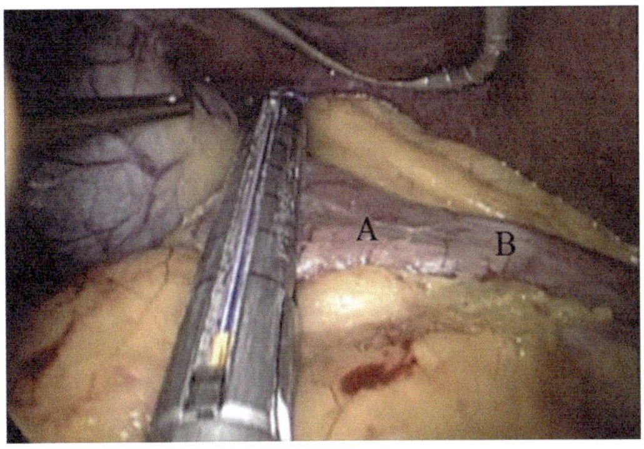

Fig. 11.5 Transection of the duodenum (A) using a 60-mm stapler with a blue load, 3 cm from the pylorus (B)

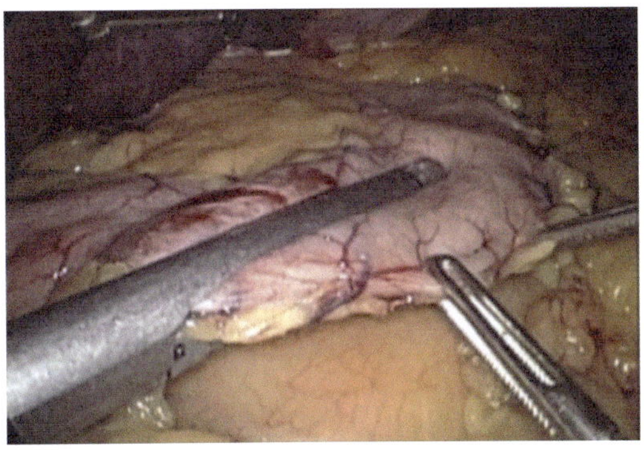

Fig. 11.6 The SG is started 5–7 cm from the pylorus

using black or green cartridges (Fig. 11.6). The length of the staples is decreased, from green to blue cartridges, as the gastric transection progresses toward the fundus. The staple line is checked for hemostasis and clips are applied if required. The gastrectomy specimen is then placed in a plastic bag and removed through the 12-mm trocar in the right flank.

Small Bowel Transection

The patient is placed in a head-down position with a slight tilt to the patient's left. The surgeon and first assistant now stand on the patient's left side, and the surgeon uses the two lower trocars in the left flank. The ileocecal junction is identified and adhesions between the ascending colon and the omentum are released. In patients with prior abdominal surgery, one should examine this area for adhesions prior to duodenal transection. The ileum is then measured from the ileocecal valve, using small bowel graspers (the length of the grasper's jaw is 5 cm). The small bowel is first marked at 100 cm from the ileocecal junction, using a large clip on each side of the mesentery to mark the site of the future ileoileostomy. The small bowel is then run another 150 cm and transected at that level to create a 250-cm alimentary limb, using a white cartridge. The alimentary limb is directly identified using a metallic clip on the mesentery to maintain orientation. The small bowel mesentery is usually opened a few centimeters to decrease tension on the duodenal anastomosis.

Duodeno-ileal Anastomosis

The patient is now placed in a slight head-up position. The surgeon goes between the patient's legs and the assistant stays on the left. The alimentary limb is brought to the right upper quadrant in an antecolic fashion and approximated to the transected duodenum. A hand-sewn end-to-side anastomosis is then created. A 23-cm 3-0 absorbable V-Loc suture is used for the first posterior layer. The antimesenteric side of the small bowel is anastomosed to the duodenum (Fig. 11.7). The intestinal lumens are opened, and the back wall of the anastomosis is created using another 23-cm 3-0 V-Loc suture. The anterior layer of the anastomosis is created using a 15-cm V-Loc suture, starting from the top of the anastomosis (Fig. 11.8). The two running sutures are crossed or attached together on the inferior aspect of the anastomosis. The anastomosis can

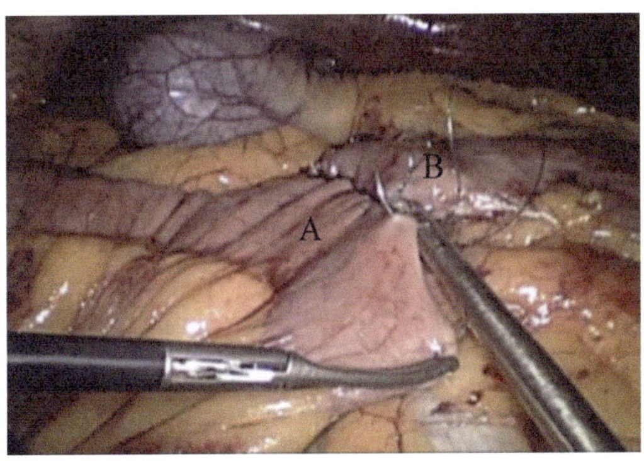

Fig. 11.7 The first posterior layer is created using 3-0 absorbable suture, to approximate the ileon (A) to the first duodenum (B)

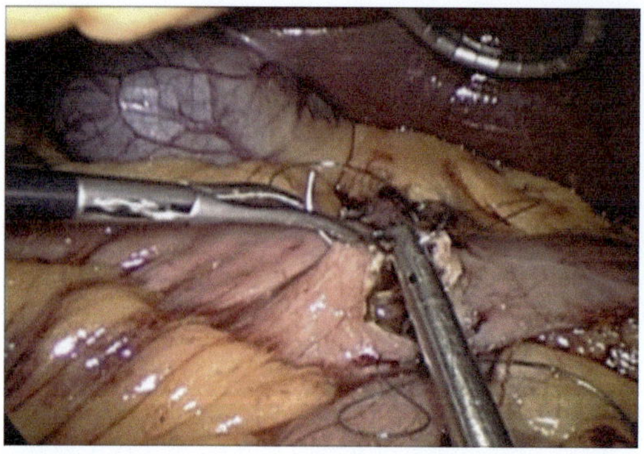

Fig. 11.8 The anterior wall of the anastomosis is created, using an absorbable 3-0 running suture

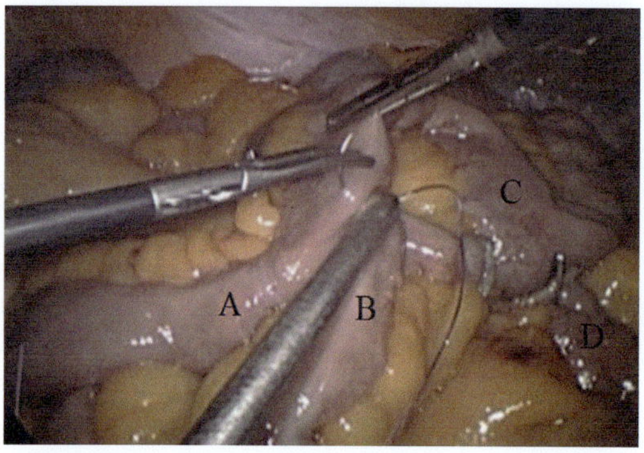

Fig. 11.9 A 2-0 Vicryl suture is placed to approximate (A) the common channel and (B) the biliary limp. (C) The alimentary limp is located in the patient's right flank and (D) proximal ileon

be tested by insufflating air through a nasogastric tube or with an endoscope. This also allows testing the patency of the anastomosis.

Ileoileal Anastomosis

The ileoileal anastomosis is then created at 100 cm from the ileocecal valve. The patient is place head-down and the surgeon moves back to the patient's left side. The biliary limb is attached to the ileon using a 2-0 Vicryl in an antiperistaltic technique (Fig. 11.9). This stitch is used to provide an adequate exposure for the anastomosis. An enterotomy is made on the antimesenteric side of the marked ileum and on the end of the biliopancreatic limb. A side-to-side anastomosis is created using another white load of a 60-mm linear stapler-cutter. The intestinal opening is closed using a single layer of 3-0 V-Loc suture,

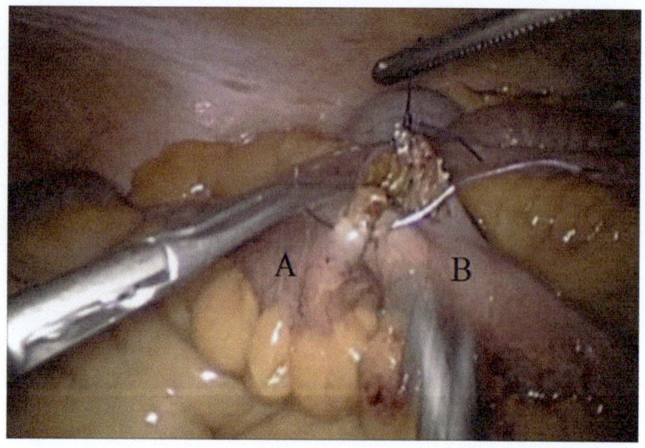

Fig. 11.10 The intestinal opening of the anastomosis is closed with a 3-0 absorbable suture. The common channel is on the left (A) and the biliary limb is on the right (B)

starting from the mesenteric side (Fig. 11.10). The small bowel is then retracted to the right upper quadrant using the 2-0 Vicryl stay suture. The mesenteric window is closed using a nonabsorbable 2-0 Prolene suture. The Petersen window is also closed using a 2-0 Prolene suture. In that purpose, the patient is placed head up, and the assistant lifts the transverse colon up. The alimentary limb is placed in the right flack to expose Petersen's defect. A routine cholecystectomy and liver biopsy are usually performed at the end of the surgery; 12-mm trocars are closed with 2-0 Vicryl using a fascia closure device, and the pneumoperitoneum is exsufflated under direct vision.

Postoperative Care

Regular or low-molecular-weight subcutaneous heparin is given the day of surgery. All patients are switched to a low-molecular-weight heparin on postoperative day 1. Pneumatic compression devices, incentive spirometry, and noninvasive airway support (C-PAP or Bi-PAP) are also used. Patients are started on water the day of surgery, followed by clear liquids on the first postoperative day and a full liquid diet on postoperative day 2. Patients are usually discharged by the third postoperative day on a liquid diet for 2 weeks. The diet is progressed to pureed diet, minced diet, and regular diet every 2 weeks. Patients who still have their gallbladder are placed on ursodiol

(Actigall, Ciba-Geigy, Summit, New Jersey), 250 mg orally, twice a day, for 6 months. Daily vitamins and mineral supplementations are started within the 1st month after surgery (ferrous sulfate, 300 mg; vitamin D, 50,000 IU; vitamin A, 30,000 IU; calcium carbonate, 1000 mg; and a multivitamin complex). These supplements are adjusted over time, and education in consuming a high-protein diet is reinforced. The patient is followed with blood analysis (similar to preoperative bloodwork) at 4, 8, and 12 months and annually thereafter. Fasting glucose, hemoglobin A1C, and lipid panel are performed every year.

Technical Tips

In this section, we will review surgical pitfalls and methods to avoid them.

Gastric Mobilization

The most important point is the dissection of the angle of His, which must be entirely freed from the left crus to facilitate subsequent stapling. Dissection follows the fat pad to avoid devascularizing the cardia. An important hiatal hernia must be reduced and repaired with permanent sutures to prevent postoperative reflux. The posterior vessels must be controlled and the fundus completely mobilized to avoid inadequate weight loss.

Duodenal Dissection

One of the reasons for the lack of popularity of BPD-DS is the specificity of the laparoscopic dissection of plane between the pancreatic head, the duodenum, and the portal triad. Poor understanding of the anatomical relationships can result in injuries to the pancreatic head, gastroduodenal artery, or bile duct. Intra-abdominal fat or adhesion can make the dissection difficult, and care should be taken to avoid any bleeding at that level, which can blur tissue planes.

For the *posterior approach*, meticulous attention to the pancreas, gastroepiploic artery, and pyloric vessels is needed to avoid pancreatic injuries or bleeding. The retroduodenal window should be created in an avascular plane, along the duodenal wall, using blunt dissection to avoid injuries of the right gastric vessels or common bile duct.

For the *inferior approach*, a tunnel, just anterior to the pancreatic head and gastroduodenal artery, is created with gentle dissection. That dissection has to be done carefully, to avoid bleedings from the small venous branches draining the duodenum to the pancreatic head and to prevent an injury to the back wall of the duodenum. The duodenum should be divided to the right of the common bile duct. Before transecting the duodenum, the nasogastric tube must be removed to avoid any risk of stapling it.

Sleeve Gastrectomy

The sleeve in BPD-DS should not be as tight as a stand-alone sleeve. The goal of the gastric resection in BPD-DS is to reduce acid secretion and to be mildly restrictive. This is in stark contrast with SG as a stand-alone procedure, in which the sleeve has to be much more restrictive due to the absence of associated small bowel bypass. It is also important to preserve the antrum to preserve the propulsion of the food bolus. In BPD-DS, the sleeve is typically started around 7 cm from the pylorus. Furthermore, stapler firings should be in the same horizontal plane to avoid creating a spiraled sleeve and, away from the incisura, to avoid a stenosis. Finally, we try to remove the whole fundus to avoid long-term dilatation at that level.

Small Bowel Transection and Anastomosis

One should be systematical to avoid confusing the alimentary limb for the biliary limb. The alimentary limb should be marked as soon as transected by placing a clip on the intestinal stump.

Duodeno-ileal Anastomosis

The duodeno-ileal anastomosis is usually performed first, to decrease tension on that anastomosis. In smaller patients however, the distal anastomosis can be performed before the duodeno-ileal anastomosis, avoiding one position change.

For the duodenal anastomosis, we prefer a hand-sewn technique. An anastomosis using a circular stapler will yield a higher risk of wound infection and leak and, in addition, will require enlarging a port site to accommodate the circular stapler. In addition, the use of a hand-sewn technique has virtually eliminated the risk of anastomotic stenosis, which occurred in an average of 10% of patients who had a circular-stapled anastomosis.

Petersen's Defect Closure

The defect is closed from the patient's left side because there is a wider space on the left and because closure from the left side permits visualization of the ligament of Treitz and helps to avoid catching proximal jejunum in the closure. The omentum is placed above the transverse colon, and the closure has to involve the whole length of the transverse mesentery and the mesentery of the ileum.

Complications

This section will review the management of the most frequent early and late surgical and nonsurgical complications.

Anastomotic Leak

Anastomotic leaks are some of the most worrisome complications, with an incidence of 1–3% [5]. In BPD-DS, anastomotic leaks occur mainly at the duodeno-ileostomy. They can also happen at the gastric staple line, the duodenal stump, or the ileoileostomy. In obese patients, clinical signs of anastomotic leak can sometimes be subtle. Sustained tachycardia (heart rate above 120 bpm for more than 0.5 h) is the most sensitive sign of leak [6]. Other signs include decreased urine output, left shoulder pain (Kehr's sign), fever, confusion, and dyspnea.

Stable patients can undergo a CT scan. However, in unstable patients or patients with a clinical suspicion of leak, a diagnostic laparoscopy should not be delayed.

In stable patients with a late leak (more than a week post-op) presenting as a contained abscess, a percutaneous drainage can be attempted. When reoperation is required, irrigation and drainage are the mainstay of the procedure. In early leaks (first 48 h post-op), primary closure of the leak can be tried. Nutritional support is provided by parenteral nutrition, naso-jejunal feeding tube or – if technically feasible during a reoperation – a jejunal feeding tube placed at the level of the Treitz angle. Most duodenal leaks will eventually close with time, drainage, and adequate nutritional support. These tend not to become chronic, in opposition to some of the leaks following sleeve gastrectomy.

Small Bowel Obstruction

The most frequent cause of small bowel obstruction following laparoscopic BPD-DS is from an internal hernia at the mesenteric window. Other potential causes include adhesions, Petersen's hernia, obstruction at the ileoileal anastomosis, and port site hernias. Like gastric bypass, the creation of mesenteric defects combined with massive weight loss predispose to internal hernias. Small bowel obstruction can present as a closed-loop obstruction with small bowel ischemia and perforation. Closure of both mesenteric and Petersen's windows with nonabsorbable sutures is recommended.

Timely recognition of clinical signs and symptoms and appropriate management are essential. Obstruction of the alimentary limb or common channel will result in typical symptoms of small bowel obstruction (vomiting, abdominal pain and bloating, absence of gas or stools). Obstruction of the biliopancreatic limb, on the other hand, can be associated with minimal clinical signs. Initially, the only clinical symptoms can be a feeling of fullness, bloating, and pain. The patient may be able to eat and pass gas, with an abdominal X-ray showing no air-fluid levels (i.e., no passage of air in the biliary limb). Later in the presentation, obstruction of the duodenum can result in increased hepatic and pancreatic enzymes. This should lead to an emergency exploration for decompression of the biliary tree, to avoid obstructive pancreatitis and cholangitis. CT scan will show the level of obstruction, and early surgical exploration is recommended when the obstruction is on the biliary limb. The cause of the obstruction is sought and repaired. All mesenteric defect should be visualized and closed if present. A feeding jejunostomy can be placed in the proximal biliopancreatic limb, initially to decompress the small bowel and, later, to be used for enteral feeding.

Cholelithiasis

The pros and cons of performing a routine cholecystectomy in bariatric surgery are still debated [7]. In our practice, we have been performing routine cholecystectomy to avoid long-term risks of cholecystitis, but especially choledocolithiasis. Even though retrograde access to the biliary tree through the jejunum has been described, a former surgical exploration, with possible Vater's ampulloplasty is often required. On the other hand, when the gallbladder is difficult to remove (i.e., steatosis with hepatomegaly), the gallbladder is left in place, and the patient is placed on ursodeoxycholic acid for 6 months.

Gastrointestinal Side Effects

A majority of patients will have increased stool frequency (a mean of three bowel movements per day), malodorous gas, and abdominal discomfort from bloating. Increased bowel movements and steatorrhea can be related to excessive fat intake and will require nutritional consult. Second line of treatment for GI side effects includes probiotics, cholestyramine, and pancreatic enzymes.

Bacterial overgrowth can also contribute to abdominal bloating, diarrhea, foul-smelling gas, and stools. Antibiotic therapy (oral metronidazole 500 mg TID for 10 days) followed by probiotics can be prescribed.

Nutritional Complications

Besides its excellent long-term outcome, BPD-DS can lead to protein malnutrition and micronutrient and fat-soluble vitamin deficiencies.

In our 10-year data with BPD-DS, 10% of patients presented with one episode of protein malnutrition, and 5% required readmission to correct this condition [8]. First line of therapy including nutritional consult and protein and vitamin supplementations, pancreatic enzymes, and nutritional support with enteral feeding can be used. Most patients will evolve favorably, but between 1.5% and 4.7% of patients will require a surgical revision [9, 10]. Surgical revision typically consists in dividing the alimentary limb proximal to the common channel anastomosis. A new anastomosis is performed more proximal on the biliopancreatic limb (typically 1–2 m). This results in increasing the length of the common channel and also the length of the alimentary limb.

Other vitamin and mineral deficiencies can develop but are usually treated with increased oral supplementations on an outpatient basis. Long-term follow-up and adjustment of iron, calcium, vitamin D, and vitamin A supplementations are, however, mandatory. This emphasizes the importance of proper selection and long-term follow-up after BPD-DS.

Clinical Outcomes

A recent survey of the International Federation for the Surgery of Obesity and Metabolic Disorders member national societies reported that the proportions of BPD-DS were 4.9% in 2008, 2.1% in 2011, and 1.5% in 2013. Even though the absolute number of BPD-DS procedures increased from 2008 to 2013, this suggests that other surgeries are performed preferentially (i.e., SG, which has now become the predominant surgery in North America). This decrease in the percentage of duodenal switch can be related to the lack of exposure of many surgical teams to the BPD-DS technique, its greater complexity, and greater concerns about gastrointestinal side effects and vitamin and protein deficiencies. In addition, BPD-DS can only be offered to supermorbidly obese patients (BMI above 50 kg/m^2) in some countries.

Only a few investigators [11–14] reported their outcomes beyond 5 years in a significant

Table 11.1 Clinical outcomes in large series of BPD-DS (>100 cases) with a minimal follow-up of 5 years

Authors	Follow-up (years)	*n*	Weight loss (%)	T2DM (% remission)	HTN (%)	Dyslipidemia (%)
Himpens [11]	10.8 ± 4.6	153	TBWL: 40.7 ± 10	87.5%	81% improved	>90
Marceau [12]	8 (5–20)	2615	EWL: 71% (55.3 kg)	93.4%	60% cured 91% improved	80
Biertho [13]	8.6 ± 4	810	EWL: 76 ± 22	92%	60% cured	–
Pata [14]	11.9 ± 3.1	874	21 points of BMI lost	67–97%[a]	>96%	>96

Legend: *yrs* years, % percentage, *TBWL* total body weight loss, *EWL* excess weight loss, *T2DM* type 2 diabetes, *HTN* hypertension

[a]Remission was 67% for patients initially on insulin and 97% when initially on oral medications

number of patients (>100 patients). These studies are summarized in Table 11.1. Overall, long-term outcomes are excellent, and BPD-DS has a marked effect on obesity-related diseases, specifically type 2 diabetes mellitus (T2DM) (remission in >90% for T2D on oral medications). Similarly, Buchwald and colleagues [15], in a meta-analysis of 32 studies with 4035 patients who underwent a biliopancreatic diversion or BPD-DS, reported that BPD-DS is the surgery offering the best long-term excess weight loss (EWL of 70%), improvement or remission of T2DM in 98%, resolution of hypertension in 81%, resolution of sleep apnea in 95%, and improvement of hyperlipidemia in 99%.

Perioperative Morbidity and Mortality

In a meta-analysis of 361 studies, including 85,048 patients published in 2007, the mean 30-day mortality after bariatric surgery was 0.28% [16]. Perioperative mortality for BPD-DS was the highest, with a rate between 0% and 2.7% for laparoscopic procedures. More recently, global mortality after bariatric surgery has been consistently reported to be approximately 0.1%. In a series of 1000 consecutive BPD-DS, including our initial experience with laparoscopic BPD-DS [5], we reported a 90-day mortality of 1/1000 (from pulmonary embolism). In that series, major complications occurred in 7.2%, including 1.5% leak from the SG and 1.5% leak from the duodenal anastomosis. The complication rate after BPD-DS is usually higher compared with restrictive or mixed procedure, such as gastric bypass [17]. This is partly due to the complexity of the technique but also to BPD-DS being specifically offered in super obese patients with a higher rate of metabolic complications. Even though there has been a significant decrease in both major and minor complications with laparoscopic approach in recent years, this rate is likely to remain slightly higher compared with other surgeries with shorter operative times and lower technical complexity.

There are, however, a number of clinical situations where BPD-DS has clear advantages over other procedures. Super obese patients and patients with weight regain following another bariatric surgery (i.e., sleeve or gastric band) are most likely to benefit from BPD-DS. Indeed, with the increased popularity of SG, it has become of increasing importance to be familiar with laparoscopic BPD-DS for the management of weight regain. A duodenal switch allows staying away from scarred tissue at the level of the sleeve gastrectomy, which can potentially reduce the risk of leak at the level of a gastrojejunostomy. Also, the safety and effectiveness of redo SG or conversion to Roux-en-Y gastric bypass for patients who have failed a SG are still debated. On the other hand, adding a duodenal switch represents an effective way to promote weight loss and to induce remission of comorbidities in these patients.

Standard DS Versus Single-Anastomosis DS (SADI or SIPS)

A variation of the standard duodenal switch technique has been described by Sanchez-Pernaute et al. in 2007 [18]. This technique involves the creation of a sleeve gastrectomy, the transection of the first duodenum, and a single end-to-side anastomosis between the duodenum and the small bowel, to create a long 250-cm common channel. This new procedure, called Single Anastomosis Duodeno-Ileostomy (SADI) or Stomach Intestine Sparing Surgery (SIPS), has the potential benefit of decreasing the complexity of the standard BPD-DS by avoiding one of the two intestinal anastomoses. This could potentially decrease the rate of perioperative complications and increase the access to this type of surgery. However, the length of the common channel (250 cm) is more than doubled compared to standard BPD-DS, which could also significantly change clinical outcomes. Indeed, the length of the common channel conditions the absorption of fat and fat-soluble vitamins. Currently, the scientific literature regarding this procedure is scarce, with only four published studies on SADI (prospective or retrospective case series) [19–22]. Weight loss seems promising, with an EWL ranging between 70% and 90%, with however persisting protein malnutrition that required surgical revision. The side effects will likely be decreased compared to standard DS (decreased number of bowel movements and risks of vitamin and protein deficiency) to the cost of reduced weight loss and remission rate of comorbidities. There are currently a number of randomized trials looking at the safety, efficacy, and durability of this procedure in comparison to the standard DS procedure.

Conclusion

In experienced hands, laparoscopic BPD-DS is only slightly more difficult technically, compared to other bypass procedures, like RYGB. The rate of major perioperative complications is low, at 3%, which is in similar ranges compared to other bariatric procedures. In addition, BPD-DS offers some of the best weight loss and cure rate of obesity-related diseases. It also allows a better eating experience, by preserving the pyloric valve and avoiding dumping syndrome. These long-term benefits come at the cost of certain gastrointestinal side effects, a risk of protein malnutrition, and long-term vitamin supplementation.

References

1. Scopinaro N, Adami GF, Marinari GM, Gianetta E, Traverso E, Friedman D, et al. Biliopancreatic diversion. World J Surg. 1998;22(9):936–46.
2. Marceau P, Biron S, Bourque RA, Potvin M, Hould FS, Simard S. Biliopancreatic diversion with a new type of gastrectomy. Obes Surg. 1993;3(1):29–35.
3. Hess DS, Hess DW. Biliopancreatic diversion with a duodenal switch. Obes Surg. 1998;8(3):267–82.
4. Ren CJ, Patterson E, Gagner M. Early results of laparoscopic biliopancreatic diversion with duodenal switch: a case series of 40 consecutive patients. Obes Surg. 2000;10(6):514–23. discussion 524
5. Biertho L, Lebel S, Marceau S, Hould F-S, Lescelleur O, Moustarah F, et al. Perioperative complications in a consecutive series of 1000 duodenal switches. Surg Obes Relat Dis Off J Am Soc Bariatr Surg. 2013;9(1):63–8.
6. Hamilton EC, Sims TL, Hamilton TT, Mullican MA, Jones DB, Provost DA. Clinical predictors of leak after laparoscopic Roux-en-Y gastric bypass for morbid obesity. Surg Endosc. 2003;17(5):679–84.
7. Plecka Östlund M, Wenger U, Mattsson F, Ebrahim F, Botha A, Lagergren J. Population-based study of the need for cholecystectomy after obesity surgery. Br J Surg. 2012;99(6):864–9.
8. Marceau P, Biron S, Hould F-S, Lebel S, Marceau S, Lescelleur O, et al. Duodenal switch: long-term results. Obes Surg. 2007;17(11):1421–30.
9. Dapri G, Cadière GB, Himpens J. Laparoscopic restoration of gastrointestinal continuity after duodenal switch. Surg Obes Relat Dis. 2008;4(3):451–4.
10. Gracia JA, Martínez M, Elia M, Aguilella V, Royo P, Jiménez A, et al. Obesity surgery results depending on technique performed: long-term outcome. Obes Surg. 2009;19(4):432–8.
11. Bolckmans R, Himpens J. Long-term (>10 yrs) outcome of the laparoscopic biliopancreatic diversion with duodenal switch. Ann Surg. 2016;264:1029–37.
12. Marceau P, Biron S, Marceau S, Hould F-S, Lebel S, Lescelleur O, et al. Long-term metabolic outcomes 5 to 20 years after biliopancreatic diversion. Obes Surg. 2015;25(9):1584–93.
13. Biertho L, Biron S, Hould F-S, Lebel S, Marceau S, Marceau P. Is biliopancreatic diversion with duodenal

switch indicated for patients with body mass index <50 kg/m2? Surg Obes Relat Dis. 2010;6(5):508–14.

14. Pata G, Crea N, Betta ED, Bruni O, Vassallo C, Mittempergher F. Biliopancreatic diversion with transient gastroplasty and duodenal switch: long-term results of a multicentric study. Surgery. 2013;153(3):413–22.
15. Buchwald H, Avidor Y, Braunwald E, Jensen MD, Pories W, Fahrbach K, et al. Bariatric surgery: a systematic review and meta-analysis. JAMA. 2004;292(14):1724–37.
16. Buchwald H, Estok R, Fahrbach K, Banel D, Sledge I. Trends in mortality in bariatric surgery: a systematic review and meta-analysis. Surgery. 2007;142(4):621–32. -635
17. Prachand VN, Davee RT, Alverdy JC. Duodenal switch provides superior weight loss in the super-obese (BMI > or =50 kg/m2) compared with gastric bypass. Ann Surg. 2006;244(4):611–9.
18. Sánchez-Pernaute A, Rubio Herrera MA, Pérez-Aguirre E, García Pérez JC, Cabrerizo L, Díez Valladares L, et al. Proximal duodenal-ileal end-to-side bypass with sleeve gastrectomy: proposed technique. Obes Surg. 2007;17(12):1614–8.
19. Sánchez-Pernaute A, Herrera MAR, Pérez-Aguirre ME, Talavera P, Cabrerizo L, Matía P, et al. Single anastomosis duodeno-ileal bypass with sleeve gastrectomy (SADI-S). One to three-year follow-up. Obes Surg. 2010;20(12):1720–6.
20. Sánchez-Pernaute A, Rubio MÁ, Conde M, Arrue E, Pérez-Aguirre E, Torres A. Single-anastomosis duodenoileal bypass as a second step after sleeve gastrectomy. Surg Obes Relat Dis Off J Am Soc Bariatr Surg. 2015;11(2):351–5.
21. Cottam A, Cottam D, Medlin W, Richards C, Cottam S, Zaveri H, et al. A matched cohort analysis of single anastomosis loop duodenal switch versus Roux-en-Y gastric bypass with 18-month follow-up. Surg Endosc. 2016;30(9):3958–64.
22. Sánchez-Pernaute A, Rubio MÁ, Cabrerizo L, Ramos-Levi A, Pérez-Aguirre E, Torres A. Single-anastomosis duodenoileal bypass with sleeve gastrectomy (SADI-S) for obese diabetic patients. Surg Obes Relat Dis Off J Am Soc Bariatr Surg. 2015;11(5):1092–8.

Part IV

Controversial and Nontraditional Bariatric Operations

Gastric Plication

12

Samuel Ordoñez Ortega, Eduardo Valdivieso Rueda, Juan Pablo Pantoja, and Mauricio Sierra

Introduction

Bariatric restrictive procedures include laparoscopic adjustable gastric band (LAGB), vertical subtotal gastrectomy or laparoscopic sleeve gastrectomy (LSG), and, more recently, laparoscopic gastric plication (LGP).

LGP is a restrictive procedure recently introduced to the armamentarium of the bariatric surgeon. The operation follows a similar principle as the LSG, which is to construct a narrow gastric tube with restricted drainage from the pylorus. While first described in 1969 by Kirk and colleagues as an experimental procedure for weight reduction in rats [1], Tretbar et al. described the procedure in humans for the treatment of morbid obesity in 1976 [2]. It was performed and proposed via a laparoscopic approach in 2007 by Talebpour and Amoli [3].

The surgical principle for LGP is to reduce the gastric capacity by folding the stomach onto itself with one or two layers of nonabsorbable sutures. No staplers are required, nor major gastric resection is performed. This makes for a less expensive approach, which in theory reduces the possibility of foreign body reaction and technical issues after implantation of a LAB. Similarly, LGP minimizes the risk of leakage, bleeding, and nutritional deficiencies: well-known complications for LSG – today's most popular approach – or laparoscopic gastric bypass (RYGB) [4].

Moreover, and because LGP is considered a reversible intervention, it has been described as an auxiliary procedure to the existing restrictive surgeries without additional resections or construction of new anastomosis.

More recently, endoluminal technology has been developed to achieve a similar restrictive effect without subjecting the patient to the risk of surgery. However, these endoscopic therapies frequently achieve restriction with only mucosal apposition of the opposing gastric walls, which likely compromises the durability of these emerging procedures.

Technique

A multidisciplinary approach is always recommended for all patients to ascertain the indication for a bariatric procedure and to prepare the patient for the operation. This may include gastroscopy, *Helicobacter pylori* treatment if present, control of comorbidities including cardiorespiratory complications, and preoperative nutritional support.

S. O. Ortega · J. P. Pantoja · M. Sierra (✉)
Division of Endocrine and Laparoscopic Surgery, Instituto Nacional de Ciencias Médicas y Nutrición, Mexico City, Mexico

E. V. Rueda
Gastrointestinal and Endoscopic Surgery, International Digestive Diseases Center/FOSCAL, Universidad Autónoma de Bucaramanga, La Sabana University, Bogotá, Colombia

R. Lutfi et al. (eds.), *Global Bariatric Surgery*, https://doi.org/10.1007/978-3-319-93545-4_12

While two basic techniques are found in the current literature, several variations have been described depending on the author. Thus, the anterior plication (AP) and the greater curvature plication (GCP) are the best-known approaches [5]. Irrespective of the selected approach, patients are placed in supine, legs spread (French) reverse Trendelenburg position.

Regarding the AP technique, the anterior gastric wall is folded medially from the fundus to the antrum using two rows of 2-0 polypropylene running suture, and entering the lesser sac or dividing the short gastric vessels is not required. The greater and lesser curvatures are thus approximated on the anterior surface to the stomach to create a tube similar to that of a LSG [5]. The GCP requires section of the gastroepiploic arcade and opening of the lesser sac (Fig. 12.1). Dissection is then carried out along the greater curvature, dividing the branches of both gastroepiploic arteries and short gastric vessels with the advanced energy device of choice. The assistant retracts the omentum laterally during this maneuver to help in exposure and reduce bleeding. The remainder of the gastrocolic ligament is sectioned distally 2–4 cm proximal to the pylorus. The gastrophrenic ligament is divided and the angle of His is exposed. This latter maneuver helps in exposure of the left crus and identifies a hiatal hernia that may need repair before completing the procedure. After the fundus and body are completely mobilized, the greater curvature is folded inward in itself with two single or running suture lines of 2-0 polypropylene to create a large intraluminal gastric fold (Fig. 12.2). This last part of the procedure may be gauged with the help of a 32 or 36 Fr bougie. The plication is started just below the angle of His and continued distally to within 2–4 cm of the pylorus (Fig. 12.3). For either procedure, seromuscular suture bites are recommended to secure the plication (Fig. 12.4). It is in this part of the procedure where the technique varies greatly according to the author and probably explains the variable results in the short, mid-, and long term as well [3, 5]. The approximate remaining volume is 100 ml.

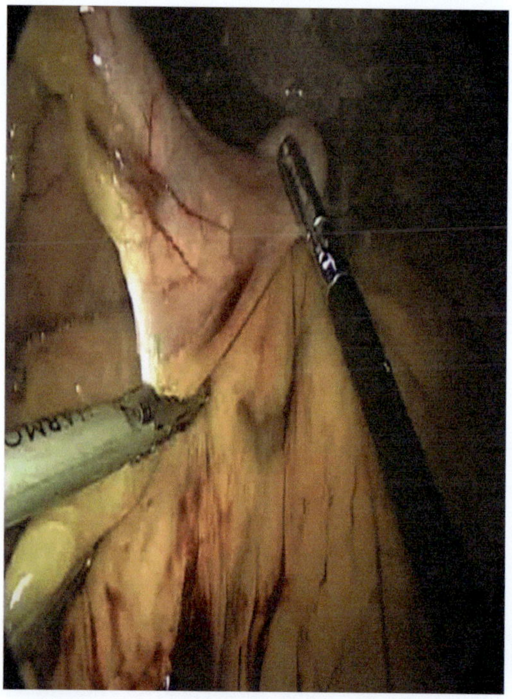

Fig. 12.1 Opening the lesser sac and mobilize the fundus

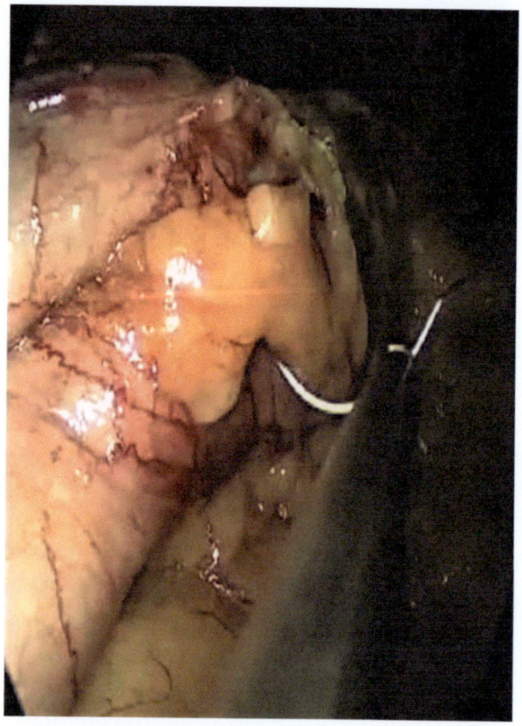

Fig. 12.2 The greater curvature is folded inward in itself with two single suture lines

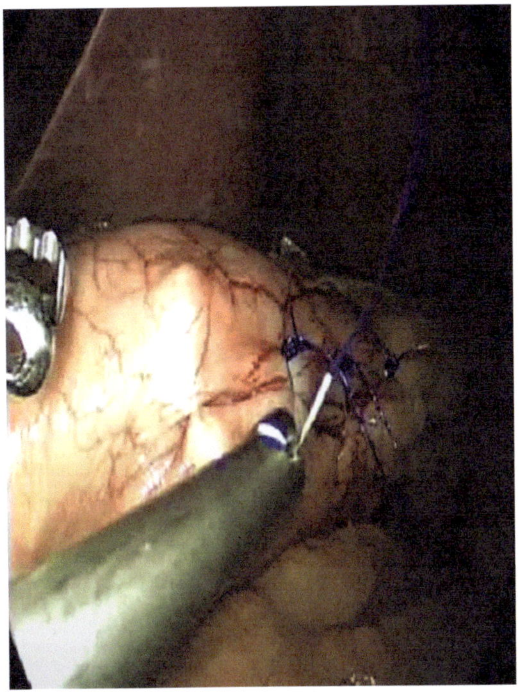

Fig. 12.3 The plication is started just below the angle of His and continued distally to within 2–4 cm of the pylorus

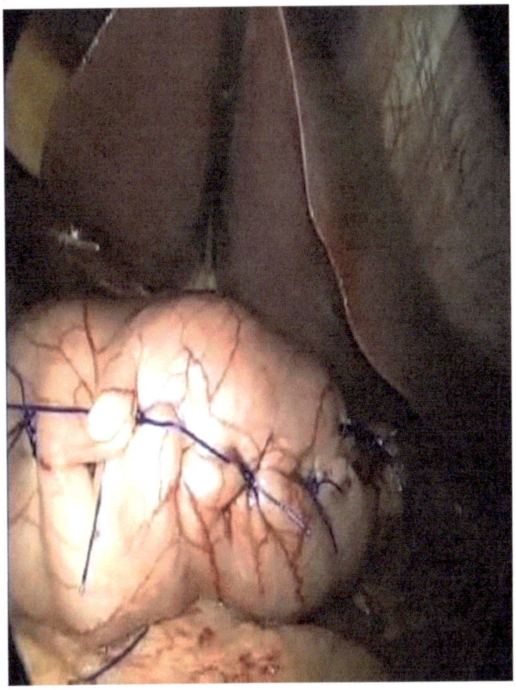

Fig. 12.4 Full-thickness or seromuscular suture bites are recommended to secure the plication

Postoperative Period

Appropriate hydration and pain and nausea control is initiated. Patients are observed for signs of leak or bleeding such as tachycardia, tachypnea, or fever. Abdominal pain and left shoulder pain are not reliable symptoms at this point, but should not be dismissed as normal. Anti-embolic stockings and intermittent sequential compression devices can be removed as soon as the patient is ready to walk. Next day, an upper gastrointestinal contrast X-ray is recommended to identify any possible leaks and assess patency. If the study is negative for leaks and shows progress of contrast, liquid diet is started, and patients may be discharged. Respiratory and existing medical therapy is reinitiated including pain management and a proton pump inhibitor for 6–8 weeks.

Results

As previously stated, large variations exist in technique which accounts for the variable results and the great difficulty in establishing comparable outcomes at the present time.

Weight Loss

While most of the data and outcomes for LGP result from studies with 6–24 months follow-up, Talebpour et al. [6] have followed and reported results for their patients for more than 10 years. Mean excess weight loss (%EWL) at 3, 4, 5, and 10 years was 66%, 62%, 55%, and 42%, respectively. All studies show a %EWL in the range of 50% at 6 months and 60% at 12 months. Skrekas et al. [7] have one of the largest series with 135 patients and an average follow-up of 22.59 months (8–31 months). The mean %EWL was 51.7% at 6 months, 67.1% at 12 months, and 65.2% at 24 months. Inadequate weight loss (defined as less than 50% of the %EWL) was observed in 21.48%, with failure (%EWL of less than 30%) in 5.9%.

Brethauer et al. [5] compared the AP vs the GCP technique and reported better weight loss with GCP than AP at 12 months (%EWL of 53.4% versus 23.3%, respectively).

Information is equally limited when searching for studies that compare LGP against other bariatric procedures. Moreover, the published studies do not count in most cases with an adequate design and population size. Verdi et al. [8] performed a retrospective study, comparing LGP vs LSG, reporting a %EWL at 3 and 6 months of 34.7% and 40.2% for the former versus 38% and 50% for the latter. However, it is important to note that in this study the rate of reintervention due to failure (EWL <50%) was 60% in LGP versus 8.8% in LSG. Abdelbaki et al. [9], in a 1 year follow-up trial comparing the same techniques, reported a total %EWL of 52.1% vs 68.1%, respectively.

With a longer follow-up, Grubnik et al. [10] reported a 3-year prospective randomized study comparing LGP vs LSG. %EWL at 6, 12, 24, and 36 months from LGP versus LSG were 49.8%, 45.8%, 42.4%, and 20.5% vs 51.8%, 59.5%, 78.9%, and 72.8%, respectively. To our knowledge, no studies that compare LGP to LGB have been published.

Only one study has addressed results from LGP and compared them to those of a mixed procedure. Talebpour et al. [11] compared LGP to mini-gastric bypass (LMGB) results. A much better weight loss with LMGB at 12 months was achieved (%EWL of 66.9% versus 60.8%, respectively). Regarding complications however and as to be expected, lower incidence of iron deficiency occurred in the LGP group (20% vs 0%).

Considering the information obtained from other trials and meta-analysis, LGP seems to be inferior as a restrictive procedure for weight loss and other malabsorptive procedures published not only in the short term but also in the long term [11].

Comorbidity Reduction

While the majority of studies address mostly the effect of the operation in weight loss, a few formal analyses have reported on results regarding improvement for comorbidities.

Wang et al. [12] published a systematic review and analysis on the metabolic effects of LGP. Resolution and improvement rate of type 2 diabetes mellitus after LGP ranged from 0% to 100% with 6–24 months follow-up. While four of the five studies reviewed demonstrated a significant improvement in this comorbid condition, only two addressed and reported significant changes in hemoglobin A1c (HbA1c) levels.

Talebpour et al. [13] in a 6-year study of 60 obese and newly diagnosed diabetes patients found that the HbA1c levels decreased from 9.8% at baseline to 5.6% at 12 months postoperative follow-up. Diabetes remission was achieved in 92% of patients and reported significant mean blood pressure improvement from 105.9 mmHg preoperative to 75.5 mmHg 12 months after surgery. Hyperlipidemia was also significantly improved. Cholesterol and triglyceride levels improved 12 months after surgery (226–150 mg/dl and 227–115 mg/dl, respectively).

In his study comparing LGP and LSG, Abdelbaki et al. [9] reported similar comorbidities remission for both techniques: hypertension remission in LGP was 60% vs 58% in LSG; DM2 remission was achieved for LGP in 50% vs 57% in LSG, joint pain remission in LGP was improved in 80% vs 70% in LSG, and dyslipidemia remission was reported in 71% of LGP patients vs 80% in LSG.

Not all studies were successful however, regarding changes in metabolic parameters. Taha et al. [14] reported no significant decrease in the HbA1c levels from 7.9% preoperatively to 7.5% in 55 patients at 12 months postoperatively. None of the patients modified dosage to stop their hypoglycemic medications.

While LGP appears to decrease the comorbidities associated with obesity in the short term, it has not been superior to other procedures (LSG or LGB), in the long term.

Complications

Laparoscopic gastric plication does not require the use of staplers, resections, or anastomosis. Thus, complication rates appear to be low. A systematic review published by Kourkoulos et al. [15] included 521 patients enrolled in prospective studies. The rate of reported complications was 15.1% with a reoperation rate of 3%. Only one conversion occurred (0.2%) due to a mesenteric injury from a faulty trocar, a rare but serious complication of laparoscopic surgery. Mortality was zero. Minor complications occurred in 10.7% of patients, with nausea, vomiting, and sialorrhea being the most common in 5.7%. Intraoperative bleeding occurred in 1.7% of patients and managed without the need for conversion or transfusions. Dysphagia or obstruction of the gastric outlet was reported in only 2.6%. All cases were managed conservatively.

Major complications presented at a rate of 4.4%. Most were managed conservatively and included upper GI bleed managed with gastroscopy or endoscopic hemostasis in 0.6% and micro-leaks requiring only observation in 0.4%.

The most common of major complications requiring reexploration (3%) were gastric outlet obstruction in 1.5% (due to fold prolapse, fold edema, adhesions, or significant accumulation of fluid within the gastric fold), leaks due to suture line disruption and herniation in 0.7%, and gastric fistula in 0.1%. Of note, none of the studies analyzed for this review reported de novo gastroesophageal symptoms or worsening of an already preexisting condition.

Despite the theoretical advantages of LGP in reducing complications, Chouillard et al. [16] published a case-control study of LGP and LSG. An overall morbidity rate reached 22.5% in the LGP group and 10% in the LSG group ($P = 0.04$). The most common complication was nausea and vomiting occurring in 20% of patients with LGP and 5% of patients with LSG, respectively. Similarly, in a meta-analysis performed by Tang et al. [17] comparing LGP and LSG involving 299 patients, LGP was associated with more major complications than LSG ($Z = 2{,}45$, $p = 0.01$) (OR = 3,3 {1,27. 8,58}.

Conclusion

While initial results of LGP may seem promising in the short and midterm, long-term studies are lacking and for the most part not encouraging. Moreover, the number of patients enrolled is small, and quality studies are scarce.

Despite the many attractive points of the plication as a simple, inexpensive, reversible, and reproducible operation, trends and published series do not reflect this. Therefore, the procedure failed to gain the attraction predicted by many. Results regarding weight loss and resolution of comorbidities can be compared with those reported earlier and in the midterm for LSG [16]. However, with the increased safety of "stapled" procedure and their improved outcome, the advantages of the plication ceased to be of much significance. This, in addition to realizing that reversing a plication is not as simple and easy as was once thought, limited adoption of this operation.

At the time of writing this chapter, gastric plication has not achieved endorsement in the United States and is not recognized by ASMBS (American Society of Metabolic and Bariatric Surgery) as a standard procedure. Moreover, due to lack of sufficient evidence, it is not considered globally as a first-line primary procedure for treatment of morbid obesity.

Acknowledgments The authors thank Dr. Antonio López Corvalá for his help and images to produce this chapter.

References

1. Kirk RM. An experimental trial of gastric plication as a means of weight reduction in the rat. Br J Surg. 1969;56(12):930–3.
2. Tretbar LL, Taylor TL, Sifers EC. Weight reduction. Gastric plication for morbid obesity. J Kans Med Soc. 1976;77(11):488–90.
3. Talebpour M, Amoli BS. Laparoscopic total gastric vertical plication in morbid obesity. J Laparoendosc Adv Surg Tech A. 2007;17(6):793–8.
4. Esteban VJ, Nguyen NT. Laparoscopic sleeve gastrectomy leads the U.S. utilization of bariatric surgery at academic medical centers. Surg Obes Relat Dis. 2015;11(5):987–90.
5. Brethauer SA, Harris JL, Kroh M, Schauer PR. Laparoscopic gastric plication for treatment of severe obesity. Surg Obes Relat Dis. 2011;7(1):15–22.
6. Talebpour M, Motamedi SM, Talebpour A, Vahidi H. Twelve year experience of laparoscopic gastric

plication in morbid obesity: development of the technique and patient outcomes. Ann Surg Innov Res. 2012;6:7.

7. Skrekas G, Antiochos K, Stafyla VK. Laparoscopic gastric greater curvature plication: results and complications in a series of 135 patients. Obes Surg. 2011;21(11):1657–63.
8. Verdi D, Prevedello L, Albanese A, et al. Laparoscopic gastric plication (LGCP) vs sleeve gastrectomy (LSG): a single institution experience. Obes Surg. 2015;25:1653–7.
9. Abdelbaki TN, Sharaan M, Abdel-Baki NA, et al. Laparoscopic gastric greater curvature plication versus laparoscopic sleeve gastrectomy: early out come in 140 patients. Surg Obes Relat Dis. 2014:1141–6.
10. Grubnik VV, Ospanov OB, Namaeva KA. Randomized controlled trial comparing laparoscopic greater curvature plication versus laparoscopic sleeve gastrectomy. Surg Endosc. 2016;30: 2186–91.
11. Darabi S, Talebpour M, Zeinoddini A. Laparoscopic gastric plication versus mini-gastric bypass surgery in the treatment of morbid obesity: a randomized clinical trial. Surg Obes Relat Dis. 2013;9:914–9.
12. Ji Y, Wang Y, Zhu J, Shen D. A systematic review of gastric plication for the treatment of obesity. Surg Obes Relat Dis. 2014;10:1226–32.
13. Talebpour M, Talebpour A, Barzin G. Effects of laparoscopic gastric plication (LGP) in patients with type 2 diabetes, one year follow-up. J Diabetes Metab Disord. 2015;14:60.
14. Taha O. Efficacy of laparoscopic greater curvature plication for weight loss and type2 diabetes: 1-year follow-up. Obes Surg. 2012;22:1629–32.
15. Kourkoulos M, Emmanouil G, Charalampos K. Laparoscopic gastric plication for the treatment of morbid obesity: a review. Minim Invasive Surg. 2012;2012:696348.
16. Aminan A, Brethauer SA, Andalib A. Can sleeve gastrectomy "Cure" diabetes? Long-term metabolic effects of sleeve gastrectomy in patients with type 2 diabetes. Ann Surg. 2016;264(4):674–81.
17. Tang Y, Tang S, Hu S. Comparative efficacy and safety of laparoscopic greater curvature plication and laparoscopic sleeve gastrectomy: a meta-analysis. Obes Surg. 2015;25(11):2169–75.

Single Anastomosis Gastric Bypass

13

Federico Davrieux, Luciano Antozzi, Mariano Palermo, and Natan Zundel

Preoperative Management

The preoperative management of the patients is important as the rest of the treatment, being considered in occasions, fundamental to fulfill the objectives of the weight loss. This management is carried out by a multidisciplinary team that has as objective that the patient arrives to the surgery of the best form. It consists of the following controls for the following specialties:

Nutrition
Psychology
Medical Clinician
Diabetology
Traumatology
Surgery

F. Davrieux
Minimally Invasive Surgery, Fundacion DAICIM, Rosario, Argentina

L. Antozzi
Department of Bariatric and Esophago-Gastric Surgery, Hospital Italiano Regional del Sur, Buenos Aires, Argentina

M. Palermo
Department of Bariatric Surgery, Centro Cien-Diagnomed, Buenos Aires, Argentina

N. Zundel (✉)
General Surgery, Fiu Herbert Wertheim College of Medicine, North Miami Beach, FL, USA

The preparatory studies to be carried out are:

Rx Torax
Abdominal ultrasound
Upper gastrointestinal series
Upper endoscopy
Spirometry
Electrocardiogram and preoperative cardiological control
The presence of *Helicobacter pylori* can also be investigated, and its treatment can be considered if it is positive.
Once the proposed goals are met, the patient is in a position to face the surgery. Prior to this, a liquid diet of 7–10 days is required.

Operative Technique

The correct location of the surgical team inside the *operating room* is essential. The patient is placed in a modified lithotomy position in an anti-Trendelenburg position at 30°, with the surgeon standing between the patient's legs, the camera operator on the right side, and a left assistant. Six trocars are used [3]: one 10 mm for the camera, two 12 mm for the surgeon, and three 5 mm for hepatic retraction, duodenal mobilization, and gastric mobilization (Fig. 13.1).

Regarding *anesthesia equipment*, a general block may be added to general anesthesia for postoperative comfort. The venous access can be

R. Lutfi et al. (eds.), *Global Bariatric Surgery*, https://doi.org/10.1007/978-3-319-93545-4_13

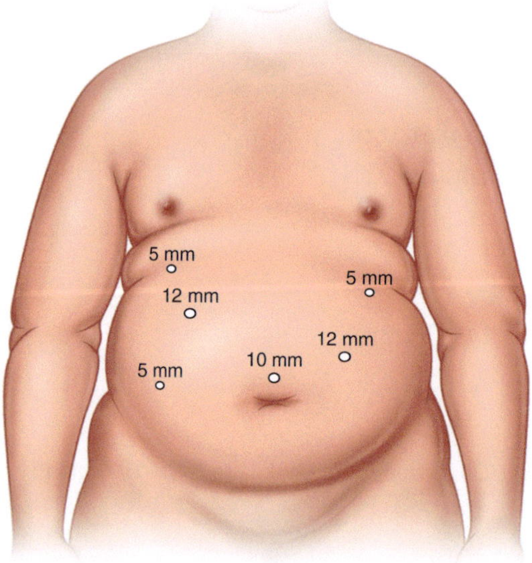

Fig. 13.1 Trocar placement

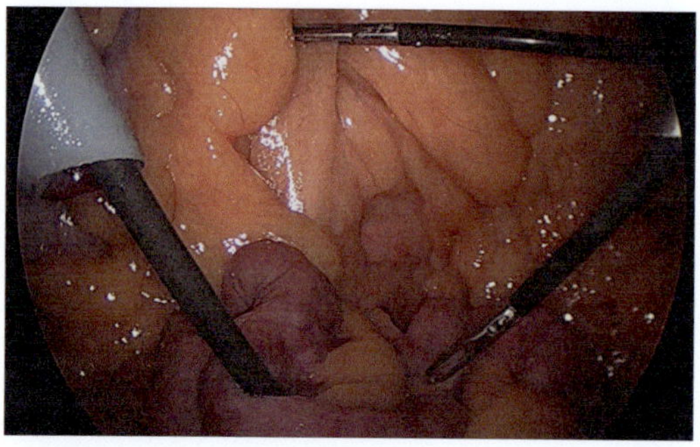

Fig. 13.2 Locate the ligament of Treitz and measure the jejunal loop to be circumvented

peripheral or central, according to availability, and the use of bladder catheter can be implemented for the correct handling of body fluids.

The *first step* is to locate the ligament of Treitz and measure the jejunal loop to be circumvented (Fig. 13.2). The small intestine can be measured routinely (Treitz to the ileocecal valve) to determine the length of the afferent and efferent loop. The middle part is selected, and therefore its lengths are usually similar (from ~250 to 350 cm).

The *second step* is to identify the angle of His and the esophageal-gastric junction (Fig. 13.3), after dissection if necessary. The aim is to visualize the left abutment of the diaphragm to position the mechanical suture correctly. If an associated hiatal hernia is found, the periesophageal adhesions and the phrenoesophageal ligament are sectioned to reduce it, and the hiatus is selectively closed.

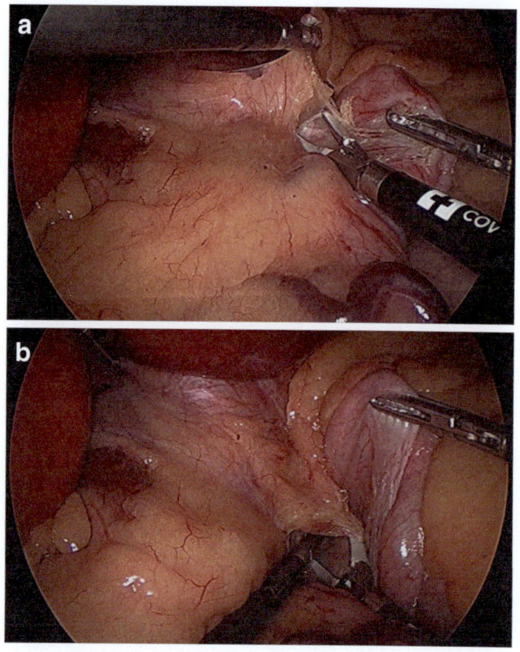

Fig. 13.3 (**a**, **b**) Identification of the angle of His and the esophageal-gastric junction

The *third step* is to work on the minor curvature. To cut the fat and blood vessels of the lower gastric curvature and correct hemostasis, different energy equipment can be used. An endoscopic stapler loaded with a 45 mm/3.5 mm cartridge is inserted through the created opening and applied, severing the stomach horizontally (Figs. 13.4a–c and 13.5). A 36-Fr double lumen orogastric tube is inserted to calibrate the gastric reservoir. Fat tissues and fibrous adhesions are dissected between the posterior gastric wall and the pancreas. An endoscopic stapler loaded with 60 mm/3.5 mm cartridges is sequentially applied, sectioning the stomach vertically and completing the gastric reservoir. The latter should be long, narrow, well vascularized, and easy to move caudally. The orogastric tube is removed, and the previously selected small intestine is mobilized upward by placing it without tension in an antecolic, antegastric position.

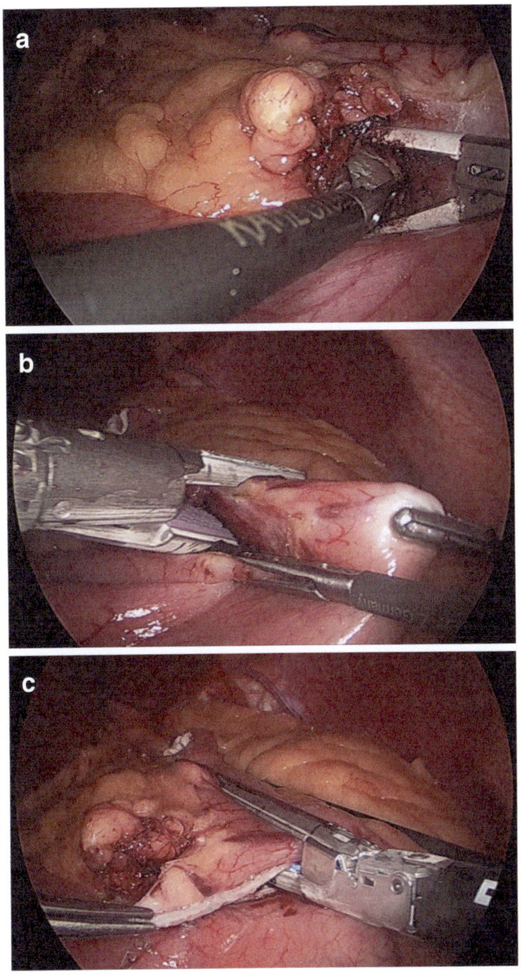

Fig. 13.4 (**a–c**) A stapler is inserted through the created opening and applied, severing the stomach horizontally

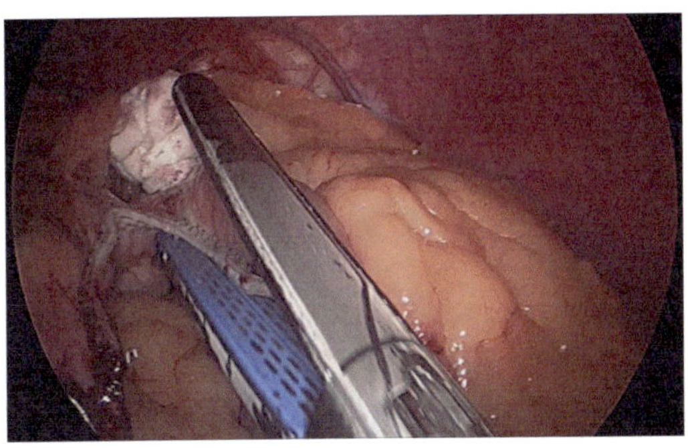

Fig. 13.5 A stapler is inserted through the created opening and applied, severing the stomach horizontally

The *fourth step* is to perform the gastroenteroanastomosis (Fig. 13.6). Enterotomy and

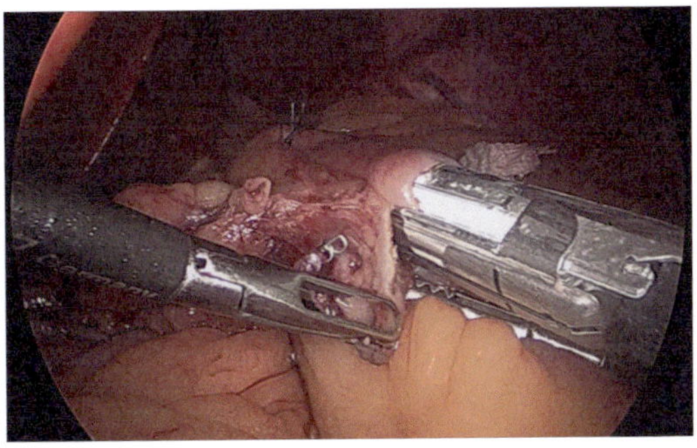

Fig. 13.6 The gastroenteroanastomosis is performed

gastrotomy (distal deposit) are performed with ultrasound shears. An endoscopic stapler loaded with a 30 mm/3.5 mm cartridge is inserted partially and applied between both, creating a gastroenteric anastomosis 2–2.5 cm long. The incisions in the anterior anastomotic wall are sutured with resorbable 2-0 continuous suture. The integrity of the anastomosis is checked by pneumatic testing (Fig. 13.7a, b). Another way to do this is to instill some dye through the orogastric probe (methylene blue). The major omentum adheres to them.

The *fifth step* is to place a Penrose drainage under the left hepatic lobe and is drawn through the right subcostal incision of 5 mm.

Postoperative Management

In the immediate postoperative period, the most important is the control of vital signs and diuretic rhythm. This can be done in a general recovery room, without intensive therapy.

Pain management can be done with intravenous analgesics of the NSAIDs or use of opioid derivatives if necessary.

At 24 h after surgery, the bladder catheter can be removed if all parameters are correct.

A hydro-soluble contrast study of the upper part of the digestive tract will be performed in order to objectify the anastomosis, to have an initial mapping of the patient's anatomy after surgery, and to rule out the presence of leaks at this level. At this time liquid diet begins with few drinks of clear liquids in a progressive way.

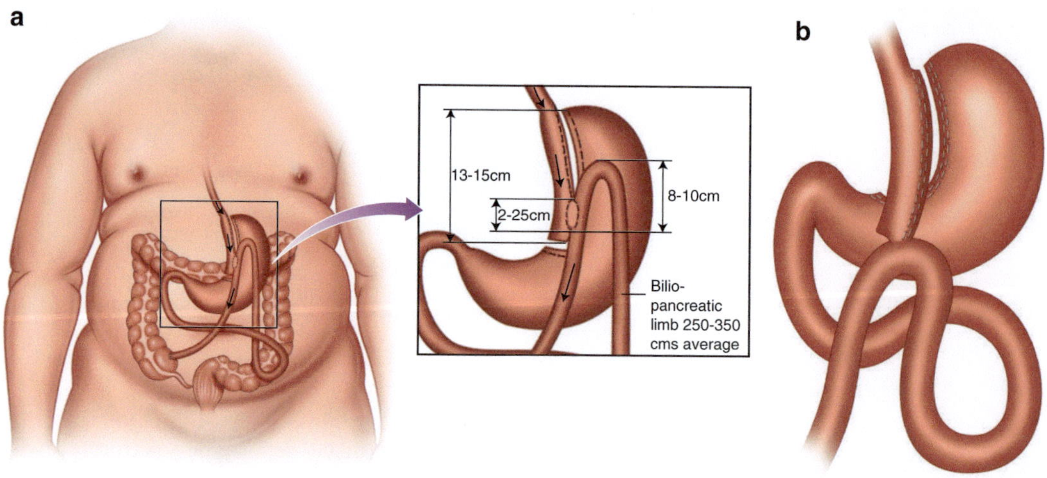

Fig. 13.7 (**a**, **b**) The final aspect of the surgery is observed

Hospital discharge with liquid diet, relative rest (not performing intense physical activity), analgesic and inhibited proton pump via oral, withdrawal of drainage, and control by office in 1 week is granted.

Office follow-up will be done at 3, 6, 12, 18, and 24 months and then annually. Weight loss, nutritional requirements, macro- and micronutrients, as well as vitamin and mineral supplements will be controlled. It is estimated that intestinal adaptation time is around 3–6 months. The reinsertion to the habitual work activity is important so that the individual feels comfortable with itself, as well as the physical activity that can realize in increasing form. At 5 years of age, a high control digestive endoscope can be performed.

Complications

Early Complications

Leaks

It is the most common complication, about 1%. More than 77% can be managed conservatively, with no need for reoperation. Given that there is no enteric cut and the entire intestinal arcade supplies the area, the blood flow in OAGB can accelerate tissue healing; also, a much longer bag and OAGB anti-reflux mechanism provide less mesenteric and vascular traction. These anastomotic features may have contributed to favorable outcomes with non-operative treatments.

Bleeding

Intra-abdominal bleeding is the second most frequent complication, with 0.9%. It can be managed noninvasively in most cases, since the trend is spontaneous cessation. It is associated with the gastric suture line, with the use of mechanical suture.

Small Bowel Obstruction

It occurs only in 0.16% of surgeries, compared to RYGB which shows 16%. This low percentage of complication is reported despite the fact that the Carbajo et al. group does not close Petersen's hernia.

Later Complications

Stomal Stenosis

It represents 0.6% of complications compared to RYGB with 27%. This may be associated with the fact that the anastomosis in the latter has a smaller diameter. When the diameter of the anastomosis exceeds 2.5 cm, no problems were found. Most of these complications can be treated with some success with endoscopic dilations and fewer percutaneously [4].

Marginal Ulcer

It can be observed in 0.6–4% of patients. It can be attributed to bilious reflux and increased gastric acid secretion, although there are no concrete studies about it. The risk factors to be treated are *H. pylori* eradication and stress and stimulate the use of sucralfate and PPIs [5]. The statistics estimate that in the RYGB this complications is confirmed between 0.6% and 25%.

Bile Reflux

Bile reflux may be one of the complications removed from this surgery. It has been found in at least 2% of patients undergoing this intervention. Symptoms may be sporadic, with or without food transgressions. They include dyspepsia, epigastric pain, heartburn, and vomiting. Follow-up can be done through endoscopy. The fear of developing this complication is that it can trigger esophagitis, GERD, and Barrett's esophagus, which may be associated with the development of GE cancer, but there is insufficient evidence to confirm this type of surgery. In the few cases in which the medical treatment is not satisfactory, a reoperation can be considered, which consists in transforming OAGB in RYGB [6].

Malabsorption and Malnutrition

The cause of malnutrition is linked to malabsorption. This can be recorded in 2% of patients [4]. It is estimated that much of this responsibility may be due to strict non-compliance with the diet offered by the working group. Despite this, when malnutrition becomes important, a solution can be to reoperate the patient, turning the surgery in laparoscopic sleeve gastric.

Anemia by iron deficiency and hair loss may also appear in the distant postoperative period, although they may be treated pharmacologically satisfactorily with supplements.

Morbidity and Mortality

The morbimortality of this procedure is quite acceptable, as demonstrated in the work of Carbajo et al. [3, 5].

Intraoperative complications (hemorrhage, esophageal perforation by the orogastric tube) can be resolved by laparoscopy or with a small left subcostal laparotomy. They account for 0.3%.

Early complications as a whole, such as bleeding, leakage of the anastomosis or gastric reservoir, or intestinal obstruction among the most frequent, represent 0.64%. Less frequently found, we found gastric necrosis [1].

Late complications include stenosis of the gastroenteroanastomosis, marginal anastomosis ulcer, gastroesophageal reflux, anemia, malnutrition, and vomiting, constituting 1.17%.

Nutritionally speaking, the main deficiencies found were vitamin D, calcium, and iron. Less important, there may be deficiency of zinc, vitamin B complex, and magnesium. With the extra contribution of these vitamins and minerals, it is usually enough to compensate these micronutrients.

Some gastrointestinal symptoms that may appear after surgery are increased generation of smelly flatulence and loose stools. They should be treated with symptomatic mediation and diet free of fats and carbohydrates.

Mortality does not exceed 0.16%.

Weight Loss

The excess weight lost with this surgery is 15–20 kg in the first month and 30–40 kg in the first trimester. Although long-term follow-up regurgitation can be observed, it is not clinically significant, according to Carbajo.

If we compare the single anastomosis gastric bypass with Roux-en-Y gastric bypass, we see that, in the long-term follow-up (2 years), the total weight loss corresponds to 44.4% and 33.4%, respectively, as the data from the work of Parmar et al.

Metabolism

The OAGB results associated with metabolism have been notable. Type II diabetes has a 94% remission. Similarly, hypertension artery has a remission of 94%, as well as hyperlipidemia, which shows values around 96%, according to Carbajo et al. and Parmar et al.

Improvements are also seen in other aspects, such as sleep apnea, osteoarthritis, and fatty liver. In the latter, the improvement sometimes reaches 100%.

Conclusions

Single anastomosis gastric bypass yields superior weight loss at 18- and 24-month follow-ups in comparison with the gold standard RYGB. There was no early major complication or mortality, and late complication rates were similar. But these findings need confirmation in larger randomized studies. Those who promote SAGB have the advantage of a longer gastric bag, compared to the standard Roux-en-Y gastric bypass, which facilitates easier reach of the jejunum, relieving the tension of the anastomosis [2]. The sensation is that OAGB has arrived to stay in the world of the bariatric surgery, not only as just a variant about RYGB, if not as a new modern and sure surgical procedure. This can be seen in the various surgical bariatrics groups that more frequently choose this technique and, furthermore, in the good results that can be shown during the postoperative times.

References

1. Guh DP, Zhang W, Bansback N, et al. The incidence of comorbidities related to obesity and overweight: a systematic review and meta-analysis. BMC Public Health. 2009;9:88. https://doi.org/10.1186/1471-2458-9-88.
2. Meydan C, Raziel A, Sakran N, et al. Single anastomosis gastric bypass-comparative short-term outcome study of conversional and primary procedures. Obes Surg. 2016;27:432–8.
3. Carbajo MA, Luque-de-León E, Jiménez JM, et al. Laparoscopic one-anastomosis gastric bypass: technique, results, and long-term follow-up in 1200 patients. Obes Surg. 2016;27:1153–67.
4. Chevallier JM, Arman GA, Guenzi M, et al. One thousand single anastomosis (omega loop) gastric bypasses to treat morbid obesity in a 7-year period: outcomes show few complications and good efficacy. Obes Surg. 2015;25:951–8.
5. Mahawar KK, Jennings N, Brown J, et al. Mini gastric bypass: systematic review of a controversial procedure. Obes Surg. 2013;23:1890–8.
6. Parmar C, Abdelhalim MA, Mahawar KK, et al. Management of super–super obese patients: comparison between one anastomosis (mini) gastric bypass and Roux-en-Y gastric bypass. Surg Endosc. 2017;31(9):3504–09.

14 Single Anastomosis Duodenal Switch (SADI-S)

Adriana Ruano, Cristina Sánchez-del-Pueblo, Andrés Sánchez-Pernaute, and Antonio Torres

History of the Procedure

Laparoscopic single-anastomosis duodenal switch or SADI-S (*single-anastomosis duodeno-ileal bypass with sleeve gastrectomy*) (Fig. 14.1) was first described in 2007 with the intention of simplifying a complex surgical technique, the biliopancreatic diversion with duodenal switch (BPD-DS) [1]. SADI-S took the one-anastomosis idea from the mini-gastric bypass and applied this concept to the duodenal switch by performing the anastomosis in the first duodenal portion, beyond the pylorus. The problems of alkaline reflux after the mini-gastric bypass should not be a problem after the preservation of the pylorus. Initially the procedure was performed with a 200 cm common limb; in this way, the alimentary channel of the duodenal switch was reduced in length, but the common limb was multiplied by 2. The initial series of 50 patients achieved very good weight loss results, with more than 90% excess weight loss in the first 2 postoperative years. However, 8% of the patients had to be submitted to reoperation for intractable diarrhoea or malnutrition. In September 2009, the common limb was changed to 250 cm, and reoperation rate decreased to 3%.

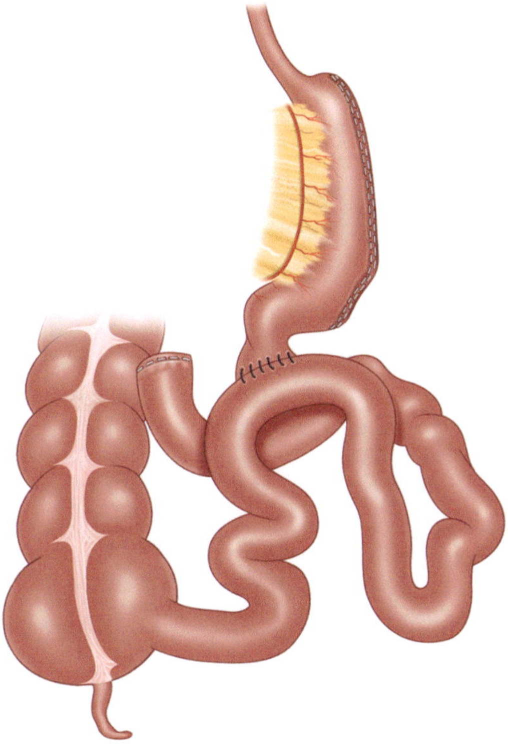

Fig. 14.1 SADI-S

Electronic Supplementary Material The online version of this chapter (doi:10.1007/978-3-319-93545-4_14) contains supplementary material, which is available to authorized users.

A. Ruano · C. Sánchez-del-Pueblo
A. Sánchez-Pernaute · A. Torres (✉)
Department of Surgery, Clinico San Carlos, Madrid, Spain

R. Lutfi et al. (eds.), *Global Bariatric Surgery*, https://doi.org/10.1007/978-3-319-93545-4_14

Pre- and Postoperative Care

All patients are thoroughly evaluated before surgery by a team of specialized endocrinologists and undergo a number of tests among which stand an upper GI endoscopy, barium swallow, chest X-ray, electrocardiogram and blood tests. Patients are recommended to follow a healthy, low-calorie diet in order to lose as much weight as possible before surgery as well as to introduce them to a fit and healthy lifestyle.

Immediately after surgery, the patient is taken to a post-anaesthesia care unit during the first hours. After 6–8 h, the patient is encouraged to start drinking small sips of water, and the next day starts with a low caloric liquid diet. The abdominal drain is usually removed in the 3rd postoperative day, and if there is no problem, the patient is discharged the following day.

Postoperatively, for the first month, patients are nourished on a low caloric diet consisting of self-prepared shakes (800 kcal/day). Multivitamin supplements, calcium and iron are initially prescribed and maintained depending upon the results of the subsequent lab tests. Follow-up is maintained for life with three to four visits/year during the first 2 years after surgery and then yearly.

Technique (Video 14.1)

The procedure can be divided into a two-step technique, starting with the sleeve gastrectomy and continuing with a one-loop duodenoileostomy:

Setting, positioning and the surgical team:
The standard laparoscopic approach is performed by placing four trocars (Fig. 14.2). This first part of the operation is performed with the operating table under forced anti-Trendelenburg position and the surgeon positioned between the legs of the patient. The first assistant is placed to the patient's left-hand side, holding the camera, and the second assistant is placed to the patient's right-hand side, holding the liver retractor.
Positioning the trocars:

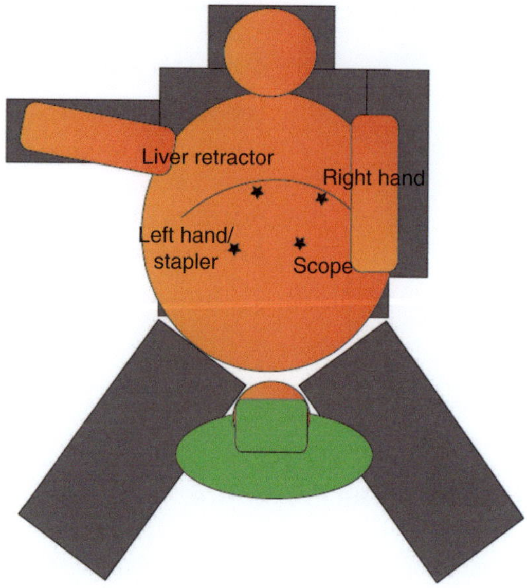

Fig. 14.2 OR position

A 10–12 mm optical trocar (Optiview) is inserted above the umbilicus, a little left from the midline. A 10–12 mm left subcostal trocar is placed for the use of the harmonic scalpel for the surgeon's right hand and for the introduction of the stapler for the duodenal section during the second step. Also, a 5 mm trocar for the surgeon's left hand initially, and subsequently for the hepatic retractor, is placed subxiphoideally. Finally, a 10–12 mm trocar is placed slightly right from the midline position for the use of the stapler during the gastrectomy.

Sleeve Gastrectomy and Duodenal Dissection

Surgery begins with complete devascularization of the greater curvature. Initially the fundus is released and dissection of the left crus is performed. Then, all vessels from the gastroepiploic arcade are divided, from the fundus to the first duodenal portion. All adhesions from the stomach to the pancreatic surface are also divided with a harmonic scalpel. The antrum is raised, and the duodenum is dissected from the pancreatic surface, held in right angles with the pancreas, until the pancreatoduodenal groove is reached and the gastroduodenal artery identified. Then, the peritoneum overlying the hepatoduodenal ligament is slightly opened, and a vessel loop is passed from behind to help later with duodenal division. Care should be taken in completing a circumferential dissection of the duodenum – up to 3–4 cm from the pylorus – removing all fat attachments to facilitate mobilization and the later anastomosis.

The sleeve gastrectomy is performed over a wide 54F bougie starting 5 cm from the pylorus, with a black cartridge linear stapler covered with Seamguard (Gore) strips as staple-line reinforcement. The suture line is searched for bleeding points, placing titanium clips where needed.

Finally, the duodenum is divided with a 60 mm blue cartridge linear stapler as far as possible from the pylorus. The stapler is introduced through the left subcostal trocar.

Duodeno-Ileal Bypass

The operating table is placed horizontally and the surgeon moves from the initial position between the legs towards the left side of the patient, as well as the camera assistant (Fig. 14.3). The ileo-cecal junction is identified and 250–300 cm are measured upwards. Measurement of the bowel is performed stretching the loops at the antimesenteric border, in 10 cm intervals, and after infusion of hyoscine butylbromide (Buscapina) to completely

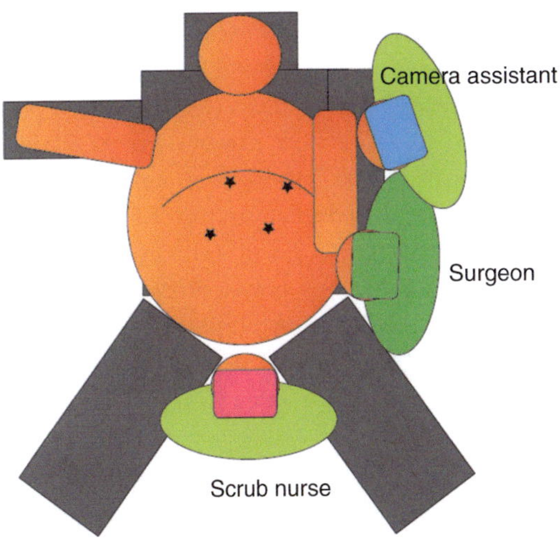

Fig. 14.3 OR position – anastomosis

relax the bowel wall and obtain the maximum possible length. The selected loop is ascended in an antecolic fashion, and an end-to-side handsewn duodeno-ileal anastomosis is completed with running sutures of PDS 3/0 (Ethicon, Johnson and Johnson) or V-Loc 3/0 (Covidien).

Both the anastomosis and the sleeve are checked for leaks with oral-tube introduction of methylene blue. A vacuum drain is left and removed when the patient resumes an oral diet.

Common Mistakes and What to Avoid

The operation involves four technical issues, i.e. the sleeve gastrectomy, duodenal dissection and division, intestinal measurement and duodeno-ileal anastomosis. Subsequent errors are insufficient fundal dissection at the sleeve, non-revision of the hiatus leaving back hiatal hernia untreated, what predisposes to a suboptimal sleeve and gastroesophageal reflux, insufficient duodenal dissection, duodenal devascularisation, errors in the intestinal measurement and technical problems with the anastomosis.

The sleeve in SADI-S is a wide one, performed over a 54 French bougie, but in spite of this, a complete fundal mobilization has to be performed to avoid building up a bicameral stomach. Hiatal hernia should be searched for with the aim of removing the whole fundus; if the hernia is not reduced, a wide fundus will be left in the mediastinum with the aforementioned problems of gastroesophageal reflux and weight regain.

The first portion of the duodenum has to be completely dissected circumferentially. The aim of this step is to mobilize it, to perform an easy and safe anastomosis. If mobilization of the duodenum is not possible, the right gastric artery should be divided at its origin in the hepatic artery (Fig. 14.4). If the artery is damaged at its entrance in the duodenal wall, the lesser curvature vascular arcade will be divided, and this could result in poor vascularization of the proximal duodenal cuff. Keeping dissection over the gastroduodenal artery avoids damage both to the right gastric artery and to the bile duct.

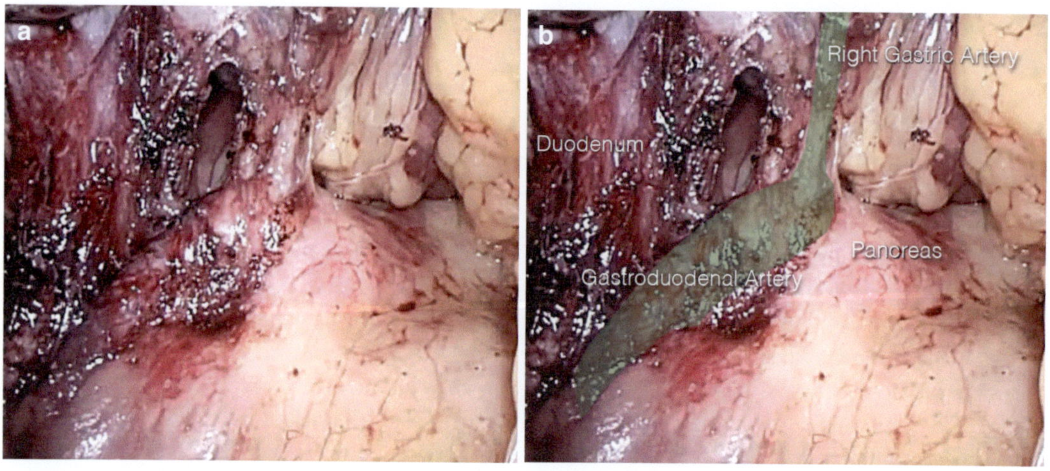

Fig. 14.4 (**a**) Gastroduodenal and right gastric arteries. (**b**) Gastroduodenal and right gastric arteries

The measurement of the common limb should be precise, as a short limb will predispose to malnutrition. It is better to obtain a less effective operation in terms of weight loss than to put the patient in danger of severe undernutrition.

The anastomosis is usually easy to perform either stapled or handsewn. No stricture has even been reported in our personal series and no problems with stomal ulcer, kinking or twisting. To avoid problems we perform a two-layer handsewn anastomosis and test it twice intraoperatively with oral methylene blue and sometimes also with gastroscopy.

Complications

Complications of SADI-S can be classified in short-term complications or postoperative complications and long-term complications.

Postoperative. Anastomotic leakage has presented in 1.9% of the patients, three treated conservatively and two reoperated, one converted into a gastric bypass due to duodenal ischemia and the other submitted to over-suture of the defect [2].

Peritoneal bleeding has occurred in one case and gastric bleeding in another patient who was endoscopically treated.

Two patients needed reoperation for incarcerated abdominal wall hernia, one in the umbilicus and another one in a 15 mm trocar orifice.

Long-term complications are usually nutritional issues. In the first series of patients with a 200 cm common limb, four patients had to be revised to a longer common channel for recurrent undernutrition and diarrhoea. In the second series with a 250 cm common channel and sometimes 300 cm (aged patients, low BMI), this initial 8% revisional rate has decreased to 2.5%. Dietary counselling and micronutrient supplementation are necessary to warrant an adequate outcome.

Results

From May 2007 to April 2017, 239 patients have been consecutively submitted to SADI-S. Thirty-three patients were submitted to SADI after a failed sleeve, 3 after a failed vertical banded gastroplasty and three were converted from a failed gastric bypass. The first 50 cases had a 2 m common limb, and in September 2009 the common limb was changed to 2.5 m; for aged patients or patients with liver or bowel diseases, 3 m has been the selected common limb length.

Surgical times ranged from 210 to 75 min, with a mean time of between 90 and 120 min. The mean age of the patients was 47 years (22–71), with a mean weight of 119 kg, and a mean BMI of 44.6 kg/m^2. Sixty percent of patients presented type 2 diabetes or had insulin resistance; among them 40% were receiving insulin treatment and had a mean duration of the disease of 9.8 years. Mean preoperative blood glucose in this group was 178.2 mg/dL, and glycosylated haemoglobin was 7.9% (5.4–13). Seventy-two percent of diabetic patients had HbA1c values above 6.5%. The preoperative mean value of peptide C was 2.12 ng/mL (0.4–7), and the mean value of the HOMA index was 7.9 (0.66–22.10). Fifty-seven percent of the patients had preoperative dyslipidemia, 27% had obstructive sleep apnea and 57% had high blood pressure undergoing treatment [3].

There were no intraoperative complications and no postoperative mortality. One patient had a gastric tube leak, and five patients suffered from anastomotic leak. Most cases were conservatively treated with the abdominal drain. One patient had an intraluminal gastric haemorrhage, which was treated endoscopically, and two patients presented an incisional hernia through a trocar defect or pre-existing umbilical hernia.

The mean excess weight loss was 95% in the first 12 months after surgery and remained at 87% at 5 years (Fig. 14.5), with 5% of the patients failing to achieve a 50% excess weight loss.

The metabolic results were excellent and comparable to the rest of the biliopancreatic diversions [4]. Mean glycemia values among diabetic patients fell to 94.7 mg/dL in the first postoperative year and to 93.1 mg/dL, 91.1 mg/dL and 79.6 mg/dL in the following 3 years, with mean HbA1c values of 5.3%, 5.2%, 5.4% and 5.0%, respectively. Eighty-five percent of the patients maintained glycosylated haemoglobin levels below 6.5%. The parameters that were associated with a worse metabolic outcome were the longer duration of metabolic syndrome before the intervention, its worse control represented by higher levels of both glycemia and glycosylated haemoglobin and preoperative insulin dependence. Dyslipidemia and obstructive sleep apnea were resolved in 73% and 88% of patients, respectively. High blood pressure was controlled in 98% of patients with complete remission in 58% of cases.

The mean daily number of bowel movements was 2.5. A small percentage of patients had more than four stools per day and were occasionally treated with oral antibiotics and colestiramine.

Major problems were hypoproteinemia, which was detected in 16% of patients, and secondary hyperparathyroidism due to deficiency of vitamin D absorption; 40% of patients presented high levels of parathormone, with a mean value of 92 pg/mL [2].

A total of nine patients, four who underwent SADI-S 200 (8% at 10 years of follow-up) and five patients who were submitted to SADI-S 250 (2.6% at 7-year follow-up), were reoperated to lengthen the common channel. The reoperation in three cases consisted on building a duodenal switch with a Roux-en-Y reconstruction by dividing the efferent loop close to the previous duodeno-ileal anastomosis and re-anastomosing this end in the afferent loop 100–200 cm proximal to the previous duodeno-ileal anastomosis

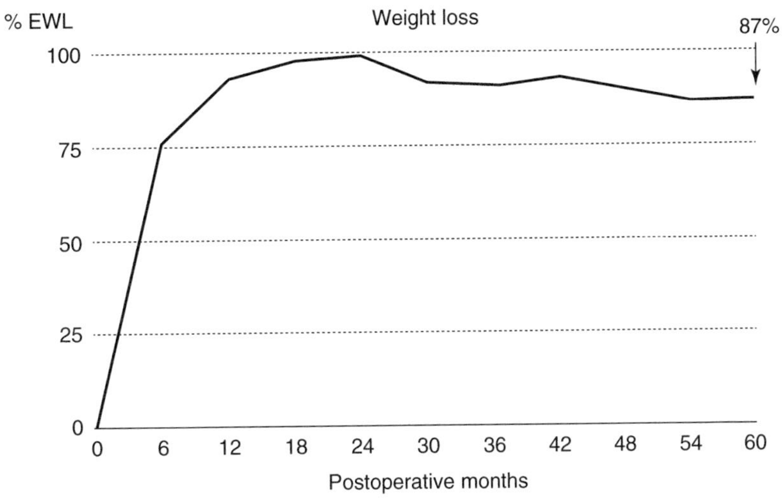

Fig. 14.5 Absolute 5-year results

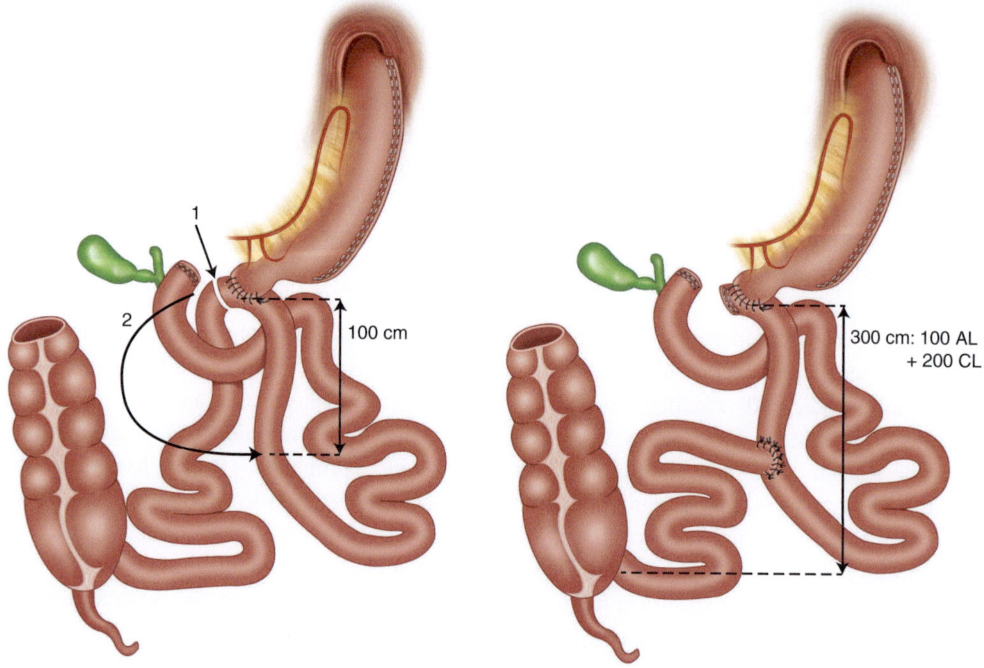

Fig. 14.6 Conversion of SADI-S into RY duodenal switch

(Fig. 14.6). In one case, a dismantling of the duodenoileostomy and a duodeno-duodenostomy was performed; in the other cases, the duodenoileostomy was divided, and a new anastomosis was performed in the same way 1 m proximally.

Our Conclusions

Advantages of SADI-S.

Over gastric bypass: Better weight loss, as a malabsorptive operation. Better metabolic results due to distal anastomosis and fat malabsorption. Easy to dismantle in case of complications. More physiologic due to pyloric preservation. No internal hernia expected, as there is no mesenteric opening. No stomal problems such as ulcers or stricture because anastomosis is in the duodenum.

Over duodenal switch: SADI-S has been shown to induce the same metabolic and weight loss results as classical DS, with a simpler procedure [3, 5]. The longer common limb decreases intestinal movements and faecal and anal problems.

References

1. Sanchez-Pernaute A, Rubio Herrera MA, Perez-Aguirre E, Garcia Perez JC, Cabrerizo L, Diez Valladares L. Proximal duodenal-ileal end-to-side bypass with sleeve gastrectomy: proposed technique. Obes Surg. 2007;17(12):1614–8.
2. Sanchez-Pernaute A, Rubio MA, Perez Aguirre E, Barabash A, Cabrerizo L, Torres A. Single-anastomosis duodenoileal bypass with sleeve gastrectomy: metabolic improvement and weight loss in first 100 patients. Surg Obes Relat Dis. 2013;9(5):731–5.
3. Sanchez-Pernaute A, Rubio MA, Cabrerizo L, Ramos-Levi A, Perez-Aguirre E, Torres A. Single-anastomosis duodenoileal by- pass with sleeve gastrectomy (SADI-S) for obese diabetic patients. Surg Obes Relat Dis. 2015;11(5):1092–8.
4. Marceau P, Biron S, Marceau S, et al. Long-term metabolic outcomes 5 to 20 years after biliopancreatic diversion. Obes Surg. 2015;25(9):1584–93.
5. Mitzman B, Cottam D, Goriparthi R, Cottam S, Zaveri H, Surve A, Roslin MS. Stomach intestinal pylorus sparing (SIPS) surgery for morbid obesity: retrospective analyses of our preliminary experience. Obes Surg. 2016;26(9):2098–104.

Vagal Nerve Control of Appetite, Energy, Regulation, and Body Weight

15

Sachin Kukreja, Mark Knudson, Katherine Tweden, Kelly Aspinwall, and Scott A. Shikora

Vagus Nerve Function

In a review article, Camilleri described the "gut" functions of the vagus nerve: "If the gut is a "puppet on a string" controlled by the brain centers, the vagus nerve may legitimately lay claim to being the string!" [1].

For all practical purposes, the only truly hardwired activity in which humans are born experts is eating. And the single most important pathway mediating this ability is the vagus nerve, connecting the brain and the gut. The vagus is also deeply connected to metabolic regulation, including, for example, endogenous gluconeogenesis.

The vagus is the 10th of the 12 cranial nerves. In Latin, the term "vagus" means "the wanderer" as the vagus is the longest of all of the cranial nerves [2]. Its distribution covers areas of the head all the way through the gastrointestinal tract to the proximal colon. It can truly be thought of as the "the spinal cord" of the parasympathetic nervous system. The vagus nerve performs many critical motor, secretory, and sensory functions in response not just to food intake but, in fact, to the sight, smell, and taste of food, the so-called cephalic phase of vagal activity [1]. This role of the vagus nerve in the regulation of food intake, processing, transit, and digestion has been described extensively [2].

At the time of food intake, vagus nerve activation results in proximal stomach relaxation or gastric accommodation in order to receive the ingested nutrient volume without increasing intragastric pressure. This accommodation permits larger nutrient intake at a single meal. Propulsive, peristaltic, antropyloric gastric contractions, also vagally mediated, triturate solid food into particulate, semifluid gastric contents, or chyme, which is then delivered during the process of gastric emptying through the pylorus into the proximal duodenum [3]. In the duodenum, pancreatic exocrine secretion (PES) occurs, providing enzymes essential for further digestion of carbohydrates, fats, and proteins. PES is also mediated by vagal input [4].

Effects of Total Vagotomy

Multiple physiologic effects are seen when both the anterior and posterior trunks of the intra-abdominal vagus are severed, intentionally, accidentally, or by a pathologic process.

S. Kukreja
Minimally Invasive Surgical Associates, Dallas, TX, USA
e-mail: sachin@texasweightlossdocs.com

M. Knudson · K. Tweden · K. Aspinwall
EnteroMedics, Roseville, MN, USA
e-mail: mbknudson@enteromedics.com; kaspinwall@enteromedics.com

S. A. Shikora (✉)
Department of Surgery, Brigham and Women's Hospital, Boston, MA, USA
e-mail: sshikora@bwh.harvard.edu

R. Lutfi et al. (eds.), *Global Bariatric Surgery*, https://doi.org/10.1007/978-3-319-93545-4_15

An early effect is loss of the gastric accommodation response initiated by food ingestion into the mouth, let alone into the stomach itself. Vagotomized individuals often experience very early satiation (sense of fullness) at mealtime with associated reduced ability to eat an adequate meal size. Accompanying this effect on satiation, there is usually an inhibition of gastric contractions which delays gastric emptying with associated prolongation of fullness and bloating (dyspepsia) after meals.

Further along the nerve's path, the effect can be even more problematic because of the inhibition of pancreatic exocrine secretion. Since, in humans, the vagal innervation of the pancreas is preganglionic, the initiation of pancreatic secretion is neutrally modulated, and the hormones known to modify pancreatic exocrine secretion act through up- or downregulation of the vagus nerve branches that innervate the pancreas. As a result, total vagotomy in humans results in long-term pancreatic insufficiency of varying degrees. This insufficiency disrupts intestinal food digestion with associated decreases in nutrient absorption. This also oftentimes results in frank or occult steatorrhea [6]. The presence of occult steatorrhea is a hallmark of patients even months or years after total vagotomy.

Historical Clinical and Preclinical Evidence for Vagotomy

A substantial body of clinical and preclinical literature describes the results of either complete or partial permanent surgical interruption of intra-abdominal vagal function by either complete truncal vagotomy or selective vagotomy. This work provides the rationale for more physiologically based interventions aimed at addressing the neural and neurohumoral mechanisms underlying the dysregulation of eating behavior and autonomic function resulting in obesity.

The lack of vagal function has a wide range of consequences in humans. Chang et al. reported a series of 120 patients with refractory duodenal ulcers who underwent either complete or highly selective (partial) intra-abdominal truncal vagotomy, along with duodenectomy [5]. The treatment goal was to reduce gastric acid secretion in order to reduce ulcer symptoms and to permit increases in body weight. Less than 50% of patients with complete interruption of the vagus nerve achieved the desired body weight gain post-vagotomy, while 94% of those with minimal vagal nerve interruption gained weight. This confirmed that vagus nerve blocking by surgery inhibits increasing body weight [5]. Indeed, this is not just an effect seen after surgery. Patients with obesity have altered autonomic function related to basic signals of satiety and satiation. Delgado-Aros and colleagues demonstrated through a series of 134 patients (BMI 17-48) a relationship between BMI, gastric volume (fasting and postprandial), and satiation. Gastric volumes were measured with single-photon emission computed tomography (SPECT). Greater BMIs and greater fasting gastric volumes were associated with reduced satiation and with greater calorie intake during a standardized liquid nutrient ingestion test [6].

This effect is not just mechanical, affecting stomach filling and emptying, it also affects digestion in the small intestine. As pointed out above, calorie absorption is disrupted even years after truncal vagotomy. This was demonstrated in a series of 48 patients admitted to a metabolic ward and studied for fecal fat absorption. Sixteen patients were studied prior to vagotomy and pyloroplasty, and the remaining 32 patients were studied at least 1-year post-vagotomy and pyloroplasty (complete truncal vagotomy, $n = 11$; selective vagotomy, $n = 9$, highly selective vagotomy, $n = 12$). Patients with highly selective vagotomies had similar fecal fat excretion to preoperative patients, while the patients with more complete vagal severance and interruption demonstrated inhibition of fat absorption (and therefore inhibition of fat-derived calories) 1 year and greater after vagotomy [7].

These effects continued after significant periods of time in patients who have undergone truncal vagotomy. In seven morbidly obese patients who underwent truncal vagotomy, at 3 and 9 months following vagotomy, body weights, as well as dietary intake of both liquids and solids (as monitored by diet diaries and urinary nitrogen levels), were significantly decreased. The authors' concluded that their study demonstrated an appetite-suppressant effect following truncal vagotomy, particularly with regard to liquid caloric intake [8].

Vagotomy as a therapy for morbid obesity has been attempted several times. Kral et al. studied 69 morbidly obese patients with a mean BMI of 47 who underwent vertical banded gastroplasty (a stomach partitioning operative procedure rarely performed anymore) either with (30 patients) or without (39 patients) truncal vagotomy [9]. They found that in patients followed for 1 year or longer, the vagotomy group had a mean excess body weight loss (EWL) of 51% as compared to 34% for the non-vagotomy patients. In the subset followed for over 5 years, the differences were even greater. The vagotomy group had a 61% EWL, while the non-vagotomy group EWL was 28% [9]. In another series reported by the same authors, 27 male patients who had undergone vagotomy alone ($n = 18$) or vagotomy and pyloroplasty ($n = 9$) for peptic ulcers were compared with matched control patients who had undergone gastrectomy alone for the same condition. At 15–20 years follow-up, no differences were observed in hematology, serum B_{12}, alkaline phosphatase, total protein, or bone density. Higher proportions of the vagotomy patients, however, continued to have decreased appetite, loss of weight, and lower serum folate levels thought possibly to be due to decreased dietary intake [10].

Interestingly, in a case report describing the treatment of obesity induced by damage to the central nervous system, a 19-year-old female with a history of resection of a craniopharyngioma developed hyperphagia and morbid obesity. She was considered not to be a candidate for gastroplasty for her obesity, so a truncal vagotomy was performed. Following the vagotomy, her body weight decreased from 106 to 76 kg over a 2-year period and stabilized at 80 kg [11].

These reports provide evidence for the key role of parasympathetic control of conscious and subconscious aspects of eating behavior underlying the problem of obesity and metabolic disease. There are substantial data from preclinical studies suggesting a potentially important role for down-regulating intra-abdominal vagal function to treat obesity and associated metabolic diseases.

A preclinical study in rats investigated the effects of truncal vagotomy, splanchnectomy, or both on body weight, as well as hypothalamic peptide Y and leptin levels. Animals with vagotomy or vagotomy plus splanchnectomy decreased food intake and lost weight, while animals that only had splanchnectomy or a sham operation did reduce food intake and lose weight. Peptide Y levels were elevated in the vagotomized rats. The authors hypothesized that the vagotomized rats lost weight either because of increased production of satiety humoral factors or because the feeding signals conducted by the vagal afferent neurons were interrupted [12].

In rats, vagal pathways mediate gastric accommodation. Both truncal vagotomy and the administration of vagolytic drugs inhibited gastric accommodation for up to 2 weeks. By 4 weeks after vagotomy, gastric accommodation returned to normal. The authors concluded the following: (1) the vagus nerve plays an important role in gastric accommodation; (2) continuous interruption of vagal function by surgical means inhibits gastric accommodation for at least 2 weeks; and (3) gastric accommodation is restored after continuous vagal interruption for 4 weeks [13].

The effects of surgical vagotomy and anticholinergic drug treatment with atropine on plasma levels of ghrelin are similar. Ghrelin is a gastrointestinal hormone that increases in the circulation with short-term food deprivation and/or weight loss and then decreases rapidly with food intake. This hormone has been hypothesized to have an anticipatory role in food intake. Vagotomy did not modify either baseline or food intake-suppressed ghrelin levels. However, vagotomy completely eliminated increased ghrelin levels induced by food deprivation. In addition, after atropine administration, food deprivation-induced elevations in ghrelin levels were substantially reduced. The authors concluded that fasting-induced increases in ghrelin are driven by vagal efferent tone [14].

Truncal Vagotomy as an Option for Weight Loss

Obesity in the USA and other developed countries has reached epidemic proportions. Treatments used to combat this disease include diet, exercise, behavior modification, drugs, and bariatric surgery [15–18]. Diets have been documented to be ineffective in the majority of long-term studies [15]. Drugs currently approved for human use in the USA have been disappointing, both in uptake and long-term efficacy and tolerance [18–20]. Adverse events reported include hypertension, abdominal discomfort, diarrhea, and fecal incontinence. In addition, the ever-worsening epidemic of obesity-related diseases and the ever-increasing number of patients undergoing surgical bariatric procedures provide strong evidence that diet and exercise programs, and even pharmacotherapy do not achieve the sustained long-term weight loss required for optimal health in many patient populations. Success rates reported for surgical approaches are dependent on the operative procedure and the patient's eating pattern [17, 18]. The most common surgical options in the USA are the Roux-en-Y gastric bypass (RYGB) and the sleeve gastrectomy (SG). These operations result in 50% or more excess weight loss that can usually, but not always, be maintained chronically. Morbidity and mortality rates of RYGB and SG, however, are dependent on the experience and annual volumes of the surgical team and center and the comorbidities of the patient [17, 18]. Banding operations are currently less popular as they result in lower degrees of weight loss and have been substantially supplanted by the RYGB and SG as the surgical procedures of choice [15, 19].

As discussed above, Kral et al. conducted several trials of vagotomy alone and vagotomy combined with a vertical banded gastroplasty to treat severe obesity with varying degrees of initial success [9, 21]. These studies followed earlier trials in humans showing initial, but not sustained, weight loss in patients with obesity who underwent a truncal vagotomy [22]. These early studies were however important in demonstrating the effectiveness of vagotomy in reducing both hunger-driven and lack of fullness-driven eating behavior in human with obesity [8].

A new, durable, mechanism-focused approach is needed. The important function that the vagus nerves play in the control of eating behavior guided the development of a new medical device [23], the vBloc® system (EnteroMedics Inc., St. Paul, MN, USA). An FDA-approved implantable device, the vBloc device, modulates vagus nerve signaling to the gut and is marketed for the treatment of obesity. This laparoscopically implantable device delivers programmable, intermittent, high-frequency electrical algorithms directly to the intra-abdominal vagus nerve through small electrodes positioned next to the anterior and posterior vagal trunks in the region of the esophagogastric junction. These algorithms reversibly block compound action potential transmission, resulting in a device with high patient satisfaction which assists with weight loss. The vBloc device and the research trials done with it will be discussed in detail below.

Overview of Maestro Rechargeable System

The Maestro Rechargeable System delivers electrical blocking signals to the anterior and posterior trunks of the intra-abdominal vagus nerve. The Maestro Rechargeable System consists of both implanted and external components (Figs. 15.1 and 15.2). Internal components include a rechargeable neuroregulator and two flexible leads, which connect the neuroregulator to the electrodes placed around the vagus nerve. The flexible electrode leads are secured around the anterior and posterior trunks (Fig. 15.3).

External components include a clinical programmer, programmer cable, mobile charger, transmit coil, and AC recharger. The mobile charger and transmit coil are used to check the charge level in the neuroregulator battery and recharge the battery when necessary. The AC recharger is used to charge the internal battery of the mobile charger. The clinician programmer is used during surgery and follow-up. It consists of a commercially available laptop computer with a proprietary software program that communicates with the mobile charger and neuroregulator. It allows clinicians to modify therapy parameters and to retrieve diagnostic information.

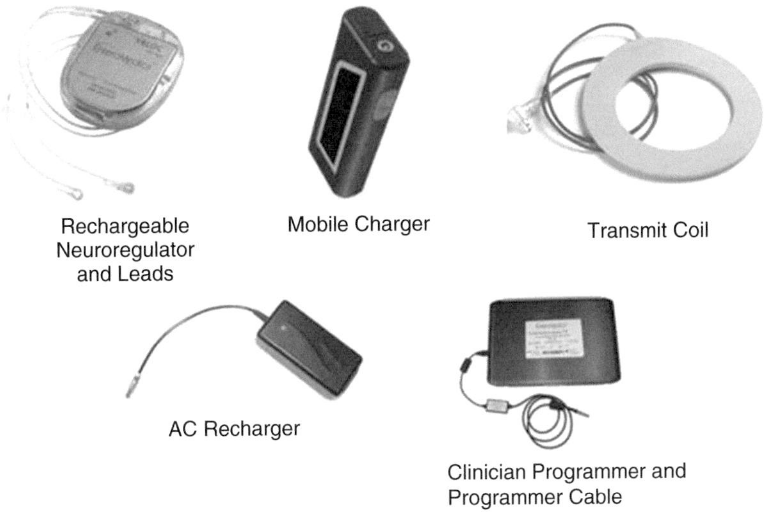

Fig. 15.1 Components of Maestro Rechargeable System

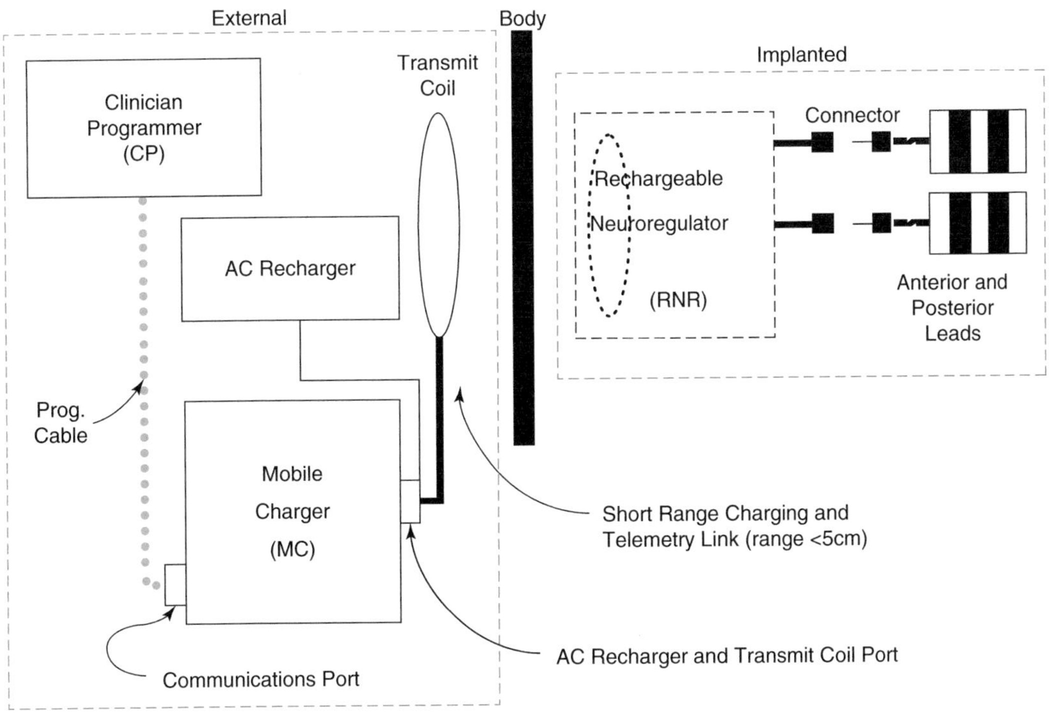

Fig. 15.2 Illustration of implanted and external components of the Maestro Rechargeable System

The Maestro Rechargeable Neuroregulator is sterile and consists of a hermetic case enclosure containing the battery and electronic circuitry surrounded by a header with an integrated coil that acts as the telemetry and recharging antenna.

The battery is an internal 2.6 AH Li-ion rechargeable battery that has been used in implantable medical devices since 1999. The battery is recharged transcutaneously using the transmit coil. The patient is instructed to recharge daily until the battery indicator on the mobile charger shows

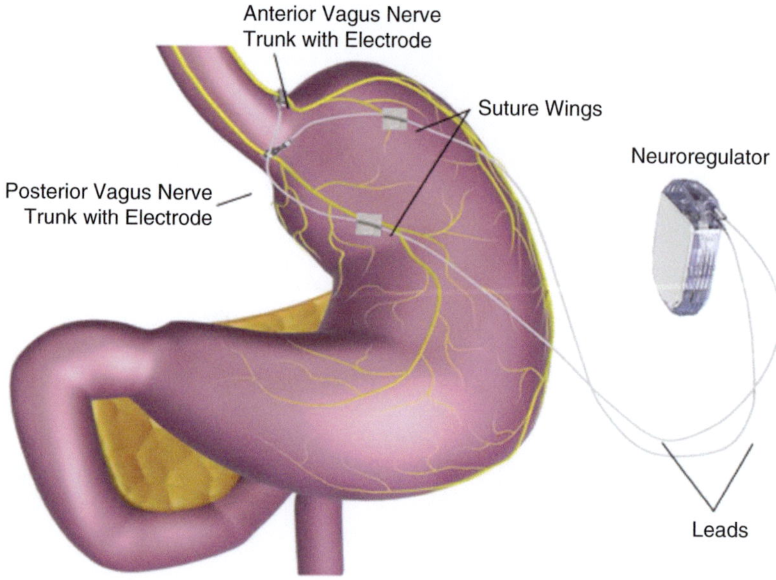

Fig. 15.3 Maestro Rechargeable System placement

that the neuroregulator battery is fully charged. Recharging takes approximately 30 min, depending on the degree of discharge of the battery.

The mobile charger and neuroregulator are designed to transfer energy and information solely between each other, up to a maximum distance of 5 cm.

Placement of the Maestro Rechargeable System Leads

The rechargeable neuroregulator is placed subcutaneously on the lower chest region in the area slightly anterior to the axial line and caudal to the axilla. The leads are implanted laparoscopically and cradle the vagus nerve at the gastroesophageal junction. Two sterile bipolar leads containing the electrodes are implanted: one lead for the anterior vagal nerve trunk and one lead for the posterior vagal nerve trunk.

The lead electrodes are placed in contact with the appropriate vagal trunk. The electrodes are not secured to the nerve but are anchored to the esophagus by the surgeon placing a suture through the superficial muscular layer of the esophagus and then through the suture hole in the suture tongue (Fig. 15.4). A nonabsorbable suture is recommended for secure attachment. No clips are used. No compression of the nerve is experienced as the electrode is of an open design and no suturing is done to the nerve. Strain relief is provided by placing two additional sutures through the suture wings along the lead in the seromuscular layer of the stomach.

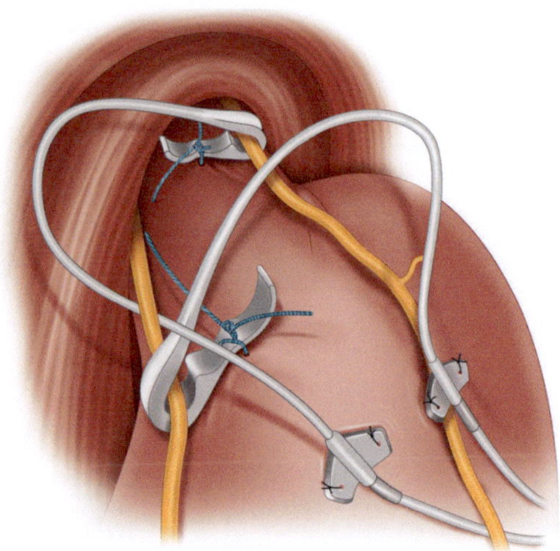

Fig. 15.4 Intra-abdominal lead placement

The neuroregulator is implanted between 2 and 3 cm deep under the skin with the flat side of the neuroregulator approximately parallel to the skin surface. Implantation at this depth produces optimal charging and telemetry link between the transmit coil and the neuroregulator.

Role in Obesity Management

The Maestro Surgical System serves to play a unique role in the care of the obese patient. Historically, the options for these patients were diet and exercise or traditional bariatric surgery. Unfortunately, the latter involved major abdominal surgery with resection of the stomach and/or re-routing of the intestine. Although considered to be the most effective and durable means of long-term weight loss, traditional bariatric surgery permanently alters the anatomy and is irreversible. Additionally, these techniques are accompanied by both short-term complications and long-term morbidities, some of which may not yet be realized due to the relative infancy of the procedures (i.e., sleeve gastrectomy). Vagal blockade helps to cover this middle ground of patients that aren't interested in permanent alterations to the anatomy or those that fear complications associated with sleeve gastrectomy or gastric bypass. At the same time, it is more aggressive and a longer-term solution than gastric balloon therapy, which may otherwise cover an overlapping patient population in terms of both BMI and patient desires and goals.

Implantation of the vBloc does not require alteration of the anatomy (with the exception of hiatal dissection with interruption of the phrenoesophageal membrane). Although the initiate iteration of the device is designed such that the battery should last 8 years, the neuroregulator can be changed without violation of the abdominal cavity if need be with little morbidity. Additionally, if the entire system needs to be removed (i.e., if the patient requires an MRI), it can be with little long-term sequelae. In fact, conversion to a traditional bariatric operation can be accomplished with little adjustment to the surgical technique. As such, future interventions should not be precluded by prior vagal blockade.

Preclinical Animal Studies

Preclinical studies evaluated vagal nerve blocking therapy for safety and to determine the appropriate algorithm to initially evaluate in humans. The studies show that application of 5000 Hz (vBloc therapy) inhibits action potential propagation, pancreatic secretions, and gastric contractions but is reversible and does not adversely affect axonal function or nerve histopathology.

A rat model was used to understand how applying 5000 Hz to the vagal nerves affected compound action potential (CAP) propagation or nerve conduction [24, 25]. In a study of nine rats, 5000 Hz was applied for 5 min which resulted in a complete inhibition of CAP propagation. When the block was terminated, the nerve recovered in about 5 min. This demonstrated that the block was reversible (Fig. 15.5).

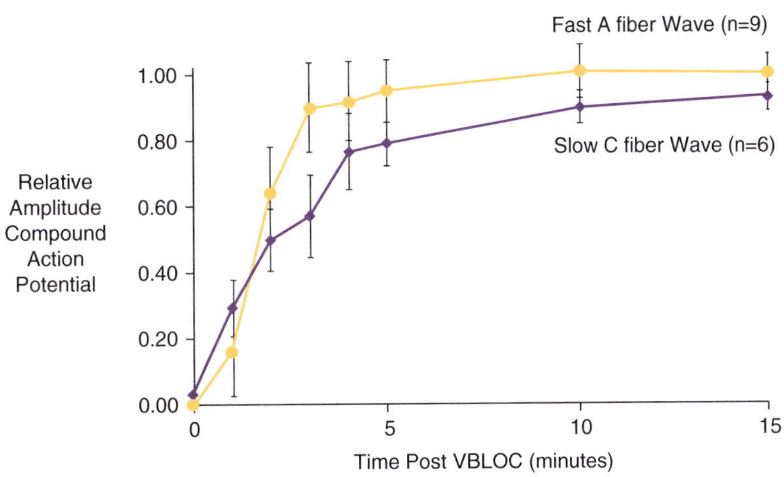

Fig. 15.5 Results of nerve function study of vBloc in rodent model

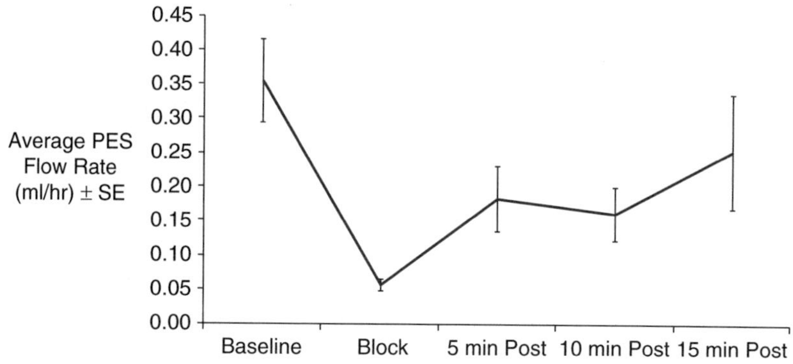

Fig. 15.6 Pancreatic exocrine secretion flow rate after vBloc in juvenile porcine model

The juvenile porcine pancreatic exocrine section model was used to understand how high-frequency algorithms applied to the abdominal vagal trunks affects gastrointestinal organ function [26]. This model utilizes juvenile pigs that are fasted for 18 h. A 5000 Hz signal was then applied to the intra-abdominal vagal trunks for 5 min which resulted in more than 80% reduction in the flow rate of pancreatic exocrine secretion. There was a statistically significant difference from baseline in the five pigs tested ($p = 0.005$). As shown in Fig. 15.6, when the block was discontinued, PES flow rate was 75% recovered by about 15 min post-block.

The same juvenile pig model was used to understand how 12 Hz, which is a stimulating frequency, and 5000 Hz, which is a blocking frequency, applied to the abdominal vagal trunks affected gastric contractions relative to baseline [27]. In this study, three pigs were used and they had a baseline contraction frequency of 5.6±1.1 contractions per minute. Relative to baseline, when vBloc therapy was applied (5000 Hz, 6 mA), the contractions were reduced by about 80% to 1.2±0.3 contractions per minute. However, when stimulating parameters are applied (12 Hz, 6 mA), the stomach contractions were shown to increase by approximately the same 80% amount. This suggests that vBloc therapy causes a relative decrease in gastric motility.

Before first use in humans, preclinical studies of vagal nerve blocking therapy were performed in a porcine model using 71 animals [27]. The algorithm used in the studies consisted of 5000 Hz up to 8 mA, 0.09 msec pulse width for 5 min "on" followed by 5 min "off" up to 24 h per day. These studies demonstrated the following:

- Ninety-one to 98% of axons were normal using axonal analysis.
- There was no evidence of necrosis or Wallerian degeneration.
- Some isolated early-stage axonal degeneration accompanied by swelling was observed. We interpret these instances as transient, since regenerating axons without inflammatory signs were observed in the same tissue samples. These changes were attributed to limitations of the animal model due to exteriorization of the leads and natural growth of the animals. Of note, the relatively mild nature of the vagally mediated adverse events seen in the clinical human studies of vBloc therapy (described in detail below) supports this conclusion.
- Cumulative histology was primarily normal fascicles.
- Fibrous capsule developed between electrode and vagus nerve was complete by 12 weeks using fibrous capsule measurements.
- Organs innervated by the vagus nerve were not adversely affected by vBloc therapy. Organs evaluated included the stomach, pancreas, gall bladder, liver, and brain.
- Conduction velocities after 12–79 days of vagal nerve blocking were consistent with those reported in the literature when controlling for similar methods and temperatures.

Overview of Maestro Rechargeable System for Clinical Use

Summary

- Maestro Rechargeable System is indicated for weight reduction in adult patients with obesity that have a BMI of 40–45 kg/m^2 or a BMI of at least 35 kg/m^2 with one or more obesity-related comorbid conditions and have failed at least one supervised weight management program within the past 5 years.
- The Maestro Rechargeable System is comprised of an implantable neuroregulator and leads and external components that are used to recharge the battery and monitor the system. It is designed to deliver vBloc therapy, which blocks conduction of the anterior and posterior trunks of the intra-abdominal vagus nerve.
- Preclinical studies evaluated the safety of vBloc therapy and the effect on nerve and target organ function. The studies show that the application of 5000 Hz with vBloc therapy inhibits pancreatic secretions and gastric contractions and inhibits action potential propagation. In addition, it has been shown to be reversible and safe.
- Clinical mechanism of action studies evaluated the effect of vBloc therapy on calorie intake and composition, pancreatic polypeptide (PPP) secretion, and maximum tolerated volume. The studies showed that vBloc therapy resulted in less calorie intake with no change in dietary composition, suppressed PPP secretion, and resulted in less volume intake (early fullness).

Clinical Mechanism of Action Studies

Clinical mechanism of action studies was performed in humans to assess calorie intake and dietary composition, inhibition of plasma pancreatic polypeptide, and maximum tolerated volume. These studies show that, compared to baseline, chronic delivery of vBloc therapy results in a reduction in food intake, inhibition of plasma pancreatic polypeptide (PP), and a reduction in maximum tolerated volume (MTV) ingested.

Calorie Intake and Diet Composition Study [28]

Ten patients (six females) with a mean BMI of 38 kg/m^2 were implanted at one center in Australia with the Maestro Rechargeable System and received vBloc therapy for 12 months. Seven-day diet diaries were taken at pre-implant and after 1, 3, 6, and 12 months of vBloc therapy to quantify changes in calorie intake and dietary composition. Each diet diary was verified during a detailed interview with a nutritionist. A validated program for determining nutrient and calorie content in food was used to quantify as percent of the total amount of intake from carbohydrates, fat, and protein. Dietary composition expressed as percent fat, carbohydrate, and protein in the daily intake was essentially unchanged throughout the follow-up period. Calorie intake decreased significantly from baseline intake of 2062 kcal/day by 45%, 48%, 37%, and 30%, respectively, at 1, 3, 6, and 12 months.

Plasma Pancreatic Polypeptide Study [29]

Twenty-five patients (20 females, BMI: 33–48 kg/m^2) at two centers outside of the USA (OUS) underwent sham feeding before implant and after 12 weeks of vBloc therapy with the Maestro RF System. Plasma pancreatic polypeptide (PP) response to sham feeding was used as a noninvasive test of vagal efferent function. Plasma PP levels were obtained in fasted patients at baseline and throughout a 20 min sham feeding. Patients avoided swallowing food or saliva to eliminate the nutrient activation of pancreatic secretion. Before Maestro System implant, sham feeding resulted in normal plasma PP response with increases above baseline of at least 25 pg/mL (mean plasma PP above baseline at 20 min, 42 ± 19 pg/mL). Following 12 weeks of vBloc therapy, plasma PP responses at 20 min were suppressed (mean plasma PP above baseline at 20 min, 20 ± 7 pg/mL).

Maximum Tolerated Volume Study [30]

Eight subjects (five females; mean BMI 40 kg/m^2) were implanted with the Maestro RF System in an open-label study at one OUS center. Subjects underwent standardized nutrient drink tests at baseline and after at least 12 months of vBloc therapy. At each evaluation, subjects ingested Ensure® (1 kcal/ml) in 120 mL volumes separated by 4-min intervals until maximum tolerated satiation. Maximum tolerated volume (MTV) was calculated as total volume ingested. The baseline MTV of 1383 ± 161 mL was significantly reduced by 246 ± 122 mL at follow-up ($p = 0.05$), representing a mean decrease of 18% in ingested volume at satiation.

Unique Surgical Candidates

In January of 2015, the US Food and Drug Administration approved vBloc therapy for severely obese individuals (BMI 35–45 kg/m^2). That approval implied that vBloc therapy would be an acceptable treatment option for patients eligible for conventional bariatric surgery. However, the unique characteristics of the vBloc system make it especially attractive for certain patient subgroups.

Extremes of age The worldwide obesity epidemic has also reached into pediatric and adolescent age groups. While there are a few surgical centers that perform conventional bariatric surgery on patients younger than 18 years of age, there are significant concerns about doing these procedures on minors. Many parents, pediatricians, and even the health insurance carriers are concerned about the operative risks, long-term consequences, and patient compliance.

Conversely, there is also a growing population of severely obese older individuals seeking treatment. Few come to surgery as many view the risks of conventional bariatric surgery to be unacceptable. Additionally, while there are no formal age limits to bariatric surgery, many surgeons set their own age cutoffs. Severely obese patients, who otherwise would be good surgical candidates, are prevented from having surgery.

Pre-existing conditions There are a number of pre-existing conditions that might render conventional bariatric surgery more complicated or even contraindicated. These would include conditions such as inflammatory bowel disease, patients taking multiple oral medications, patients dependent on nonsteroidal anti-inflammatory drugs, patients with severe iron deficiency anemia, and patients taking immunosuppressive medications such as steroids.

Previous abdominal surgery While many patients have had previous abdominal surgery, some of them may be deemed higher risk for perioperative complications that would frighten the patient away from surgery or disqualify them altogether. These conditions include patients with large ventral hernias, a history of significant adhesions, small bowel or colon resections, or liver transplantation.

Miscellaneous Miscellaneous reasons for not having conventional bariatric surgery include fear or aversion to gastrointestinal alterations, permanent dieting, and the need for lifelong vitamin supplementation.

All of the above conditions (and many others not listed) prevent many otherwise good operative candidates from having conventional bariatric surgery. Many of these patients would probably find vBloc therapy to be acceptable as it has a much more favorable safety profile and does not anatomically alter the gastrointestinal tract. Additionally, with vBloc therapy, there is no need to follow draconian dietary restrictions, and there is no need for lifelong vitamin supplementation.

Surgical Technique

Patients are prepared for surgery with a preoperative "liver reduction" diet at the discretion of the surgeon. We typically employ this for 2 weeks prior to surgery. The anticipated position of the neuroregulator should be identified in advance.

This should be done in conjunction with the patient in the supine, sitting, and standing positions. Depending on body habitus, the patient may have breast or bra-line issues that may affect placement. It is important to remember that the neuroregulator will need to be placed in a location that the charging ring can fit in the position that the patient anticipates charging. Ideal neuroregulator depth is 2 cm and typically over the ribs on the left side. Even in obese male patients, this is sometimes difficult as there may be limited subcutaneous fat over the ribs in this area. Some patients will prefer a more anterior position for their neuroregulator, while others may prefer more lateral. Additionally, depending on habitus and space issues, the neuroregulator may sit better transversely or vertically.

Details of the actual surgical technique are variable, but in general, bed position and patient positioning can be accomplished in line with other foregut and bariatric procedures. We typically place the patient supine with arms extended and utilize a Nathanson liver retractor in the subxiphoid position to expose the hiatus. Alternatively, the patients may be placed in split leg or French position, and a snake retractor could be used depending on surgeon preference.

The procedure is performed laparoscopically. Exact trocar positioning may vary, but it is most critical that an 11 mm trocar be utilized in the left anterior or left mid-clavicular line depending on planned neuroregulator position. Leads will be placed and lead tails will be extracted through this trocar.

The operation begins with identification of a hiatal hernia with an anterior inspection. If a hernia is identified, this will need to be repaired before placement of the leads. Care must be taken to preserve both anterior and posterior vagus nerves in the course of this dissection. If they are identified during dissection of the hiatal hernia, it is prudent to "tag" them with a suture to facilitate finding them later in the operation.

If no hiatal hernia is noted, the operation begins with opening of the pars flaccida to expose the length of the right crus, all the way to the apex. In incision is made at the base of the right crus, approximately 1 cm posterior to the esophagus entering the abdomen. A blunt instrument is used to spread in the direction of the esophagus. Typically, the yellow sheen of the vagus nerve is easily identified at the 6–7 o'clock position relative to the esophagus within this fatty tissue. The posterior vagus is dissected-free and encircled using a 2-0 silk tie. It is important to not "over-mobilize" either vagus nerve so when the leads are attached they can be pulled under tension into the cuff.

Dissection proceeds anteriorly through the phrenoesophageal membrane. The anterior vagus may be attached to this membrane or more intimately associated with the esophagus. With our left-handed instrument, the membrane is elevated and the space between it and esophagus is explored for the nerve. The location may be variable and it can be seen from the 11–2 o'clock position anterior to the esophagus. If necessary, the membrane can be partially divided to get a better view of the nerve. When identified, it is also encircled with a suture so it can be found later.

The anterior and posterior leads are opened and inserted into the abdomen using the 11 mm trocar. Care must be taken to insert the leads via the suture wing to minimize the possibility of damage to the leads or cuffs. The posterior lead is identified with a white line along the length of the lead while the anterior lead is clear throughout. We typically place the anterior lead first. Although it can be oriented either way, we generally orient the lead such that it is exiting toward the patient's right side. The previously placed suture is used as a handle to elevate the nerve while minimizing manipulation. The lead is sutured to the anterior esophagus with the nerve distracted and oriented 90° to the lead cuff. This is repeated with the posterior lead except it is pointing to the patient's left side.

The suture wings are then secured to the stomach, with two sutures on each lead. It is important that the wing be secured such that the lead is not arching up toward the liver but, rather, flat on the esophagus. The suture wings can be sewn to the gastrohepatic ligament if necessary for orientation. The two leads together should appear to form a "heart shape," and the leads can be brought out the 11 mm trocar.

The leads are carefully inserted into their respective spots on the neuroregulator. The ring can be brought on the field in a sterile sleeve and the neuroregulator interrogated and impedance levels checked. It is important to note that normal impedance numbers do not confirm that the tissue in the lead is indeed nerve. If everything is within appropriate ranges, the predefined subcutaneous pocket can be created and medical adhesive applied to the lead insertion points. The neuroregulator is inserted into the pocket and secured using the three sutures. The liver retractor and pneumoperitoneum can then be released and repeat impedance levels checked prior to closure. The subcutaneous depth of the device should be documented – ideal being 2–3 cm. If this is not achievable (particularly in men with limited fat in this area at time), a spacer such as a towel may be necessary to increase this distance for proper charging. If everything is acceptable, therapy can be initiated.

If impedance levels fail to be within normal range, placement issues need to be evaluated. It can be helpful to eliminate any fluid in the upper abdomen as well as release the liver and pneumoperitoneum before rechecking. Otherwise, the suture wings locations or leads may need adjusting or the equipment exchanged. Any necessary troubleshooting can usually be done from interrogation of the device with the ring and the computer programmer and should be completed before conclusion of the case.

The risks of the surgery are shared with any operation requiring general anesthesia and those in the upper abdomen. There are no staple lines to fail and no gastric or esophageal injuries reported, but they are possible. Other structures in the area include the aorta and IVC so care must be taken. Other risks include failure to properly identify either vagus nerve, most commonly the anterior vagus nerve. As such, careful, meticulous, hemostatic dissection is critical.

Patients are sent home on a full liquid diet immediately following surgery. Therapy is initiated, but the initial battery charge is sufficient to maintain them until their first postoperative visit at 2 weeks. Only at that point are patients given their mobile charger kits and are they instructed about charging technique.

Postoperative Care

Follow-Up

Patients are routinely seen at the 2-week follow-up. At this time, there are a few specific issues related to vBloc that need to be addressed. Although the patient has had therapy initiated, it is typically at too low dose for the patient to feel. As such, the computer programmer (CP) needs to be connected and the neuroregulator programmed. A typical introductory intensity is 2 mA. At default, therapy will be delivered for 5 min in 5 min intervals. A test run will be performed to ensure that the patient tolerates therapy without any untoward sensations such as heartburn, globus, dysphagia, or esophageal spasm. If they do, the intensity should be reduced. Men are often more sensitive to therapy than women and as such require lower intensity therapy. The neuroregulator can also be programmed to be active during the patient's typical schedule to ensure that all meals are blocked (i.e., it would be inappropriate to administer therapy during the day to a night worker or starting at 0800 if they eat breakfast around 0700 on most days).

The patient is given their mobile charger and needs to be taught proper charging technique. Initially, until they understand the longevity of their battery at a given therapy level, we advise our patients to check and charge their device once daily. Once a stable therapy level has been achieved and the discharge pattern of the device is understood, it is not unreasonable to charge once weekly. However, we don't encourage this typically in the first few months. If they do embrace a weekly schedule, it must be emphasized that they absolutely must not forget at that 1 week interval. If the battery level becomes too low (typically after a few months), it may not be chargeable. Because of the importance of charging, we bring the patients back again at 4 weeks to ensure they are charging properly. We interrogate the device at that time and inspect the charging history to verify the same.

Patients are enrolled in "vBloc Achieve" throughout the process. We try to enroll them preoperatively, but if by the first visit they have yet to sign up, we again encourage them. This program provides the patients with a Wi-Fi-enabled scale that transmits data to a personalized dietician and support group service. This engagement not only allows tracking of weight loss but keeps the patients engaged moving forward. If the dieticians note any issues, they notify the clinic so the patient can be returned. We routinely see the patients every 6–8 weeks and space out appointments further after 9 months if things are routine.

Because there is no malabsorptive or bypassed component to the operation, there is likely limited need to vitamin supplementation. However, bariatric patients have vitamin deficiencies at baseline; as such, we subject them to the same vitamin checks as our other bariatric surgery patients and supplement them as necessary.

Future Directions

vBloc is a new and innovative solution for the care of the obese. However, mechanisms of weight loss remain poorly understood despite our existing knowledge of vagal nerve function. Further research into the effects of vagal blockade on hormones such as ghrelin, leptin, peptide YY, and more should be undertaken moving forward. Only then will a more complete picture of this therapy be obtained. Also, given the wide-ranging influence of the vagus nerve throughout the majority of the gastrointestinal tract, hepatobiliary system, and pancreas, other applications of vagal blockade beside treatment of obesity may be adopted.

Many questions have been raised about the possibility of vBloc as a salvage operation for failed weight loss after other bariatric surgeries. At present, few surgeons offer revision of gastric bypass, either through gastrojejunostomy revision, limb lengthening, or conversion to duodenal switch, and of course, either option may be hampered by significant morbidity. Depending on surgical technique at time of initial bypass, the vagus nerves may have been partially or completely divided within the gastrohepatic ligament. Additionally, if the mechanism of action in vBloc is as believed it to be, then there may be no effect on gastric bypass. For sleeve patients, the vagus nerves are likely preserved, but the question of the role of vBloc in these patients remains as this has only been performed a handful of times to our knowledge with limited early results. Lastly, many gastric band patients may seek an operation such as vBloc; after all, they chose not to receive a stapled operation the first time. However, it is unknown if the vagus nerves could be properly and confidently identified in what is likely to be a hostile surgical field at the esophagogastric junction.

References

1. Camilleri M. Integrated upper gastrointestinal response to food intake. Gastroenterol. 2006;131:640–58.
2. Guyton AC, Hall JE. Textbook of medical physiology. 10th ed. St. Louis: W.B. Saunders Company; 2000. p. 718–63.
3. Paterson CA, Anvari M, Tougas G, Huizinga JD. Determinants of occurrence and volume of transpyloric flow during gastric emptying of liquids in dogs. Importance of vagal input. Dig Dis Sci. 2000;45:1509–16.
4. Holst JJ, Schaffalitzky de Muckadell OB, Fahrenkrug J. Nervous control of pancreatic exocrine secretion in pigs. Acta Physiol Scand. 1979;105:33–51.
5. Chang TM, Chan D, Liu YC, et al. Long-term results of duodenectomy with highly selective vagotomy in the treatment of complicated duodenal ulcers. Am J Surg. 2001;181:372–6.
6. Delgado-Aros S, Cremonini F, Castillo JE, et al. Independent influence of body mass and gastric volumes on satiation in humans. Gastroenterol. 2004;126:432–40.
7. Edwards JP, Lyndon PJ, Smith RB, et al. Faecal fat excretion after truncal, selective, and highly selective vagotomy for duodenal ulcer. Gut. 1974;15:521–5.
8. Gortz L, Bjorkman AC, Andersson H, et al. Truncal vagotomy reduces food and liquid intake in man. Physiol Behav. 1990;48:779–81.
9. Kral JG, Gortz L, Hermansson G. Gastroplasty for obesity: long-term weight loss improved by Vagotomy. World J Surg. 1993;17:75–9.
10. Johnson HD. The late nutritional and haematological effects of vagal section. Brit J Surg. 1969;56:4–9.

11. Smith DK. Truncal vagotomy for hypothalamic obesity. Lancet. 1983:1330–1. (letter)
12. Furness JB, Koopmans HS, Robbins HL, et al. Effects of vagal and splanchnic section on food intake, weight, serum leptin and hypothalamic neuropeptide Y in rat. Autonom Neurosci. 2001;92:28–36.
13. Takahashi T, Owyang C. Characterization of vagal pathways mediating gastric accommodation reflex in rats. J Physiol. 1997;504:479–88.
14. Williams DL, Grill HJ, Cummings DE, et al. Vagotomy dissociates short- and long-term controls of circulating ghrelin. Endocrinol. 2003;144:5184–7.
15. Yanovski SZ, Yanovski JA. Obesity. New Engl J Med. 2002;346:591–601.
16. Snow V, Barry P, Fitterman N, Qaseem A, Weiss K. Pharmacologic and surgical management of obesity in primary care: a clinical practice guideline from the American College of Physicians. Ann Intern Med. 2005;142:525–31.
17. Flum DR, Patchen E. Impact of gastric bypass operation on survival: a population-based analysis. J Am Coll Surg. 2004;199:543–51.
18. Nguyen NT, Paya M, Melinda C, et al. The relationship between hospital volume and outcome in bariatric surgery at academic medical centers. Annals Surg. 2004;240:586–94.
19. Thomas CE, Mauer EA, Shukla AP, Rathi S, et al. Low adoption of weight loss medications: a comparison of prescribing patterns of antiobesity pharmacotherapies and SGLT2s. Obesity. 2016;24:1955–61.
20. Krentz AJ, Fujioka K, Hompesch M. Evolution of pharmacological obesity treatments: focus on adverse side-effect profiles. Diab Obes Metab. 2016;18:558–70.
21. Gortz L, Wallin G, Kral JG. Vertical banded gastroplasty with and without truncal vagotomy. Clin Nutr. 1985;5(suppl):79.
22. Kral JG. Vagotomy as a treatment for severe obesity. Lancet. 1978;1:307.
23. EnteroMedics Inc. 2800 Patton Rd, St. Paul, MN. (n.d.).
24. Tweden KS, Anvari M, Bierk MD, Billington CJ, Camilleri M, Honda CN, Knudson MB, Larson DE, Wilson RR, Freston JW. Vagal blocking for obesity control (VBLOC): concordance of effects of very high frequency blocking current at the neural and organ levels using two preclinical models. Gastroenterology. 2006;130:A148.
25. Waataja JJ, Tweden KS, Honda CN. Effects of high frequency alternating current on axonal conduction through the vagus nerve. J Neural Eng. 2011;8:056013. https://doi.org/10.1088/1741-2560/8/5/056013.
26. Tweden KS, Toouli J, Kow L, Herrera M, Pantoja JP, Bierk MD, Knudson MB, Anvari M. Vagal blocking for obesity control (VBLOC): studies of pancreatic function and safety in the porcine model. Obes Surg. 2006;16:988.
27. Tweden KS, Sarr MG, Camilleri M, Kendrick ML, Moody FG, Bierk MD, Knudson MB, Anvari M. Vagal blocking for obesity control (VBLOC): studies of pancreatic and gastric function and safety in a porcine model. Surg Obes Relat Dis. 2006;2:301.
28. Wray N, Kow L, Collins J, Tweden KS, Toouli J. Reduced calorie intake and weight loss during vagal blocking in subjects with obesity-related type 2 diabetes mellitus. Obesity. 2011;19:S190. (presented at annual meeting The Obesity Society, Orlando, Florida, October 2011)
29. Camilleri M, Toouli J, Herrera MF, Kulseng B, Kow L, Pantoja JP, Marvik R, Johnsen G, Billington CJ, Moody FG, Knudson MB, Tweden KS, Vollmer MC, Wilson RR, Anvari M. Intra-abdominal vagal blocking (VBLOC therapy): clinical results with a new implantable medical device. Surgery. J Soc Univ Surg. 2008;143:723–31.
30. Herrera MF, Burton D, Pantoja JP, Sanchez-Leenheer S, Bachmann B, Valdovinos M, Bhole D, Prindle S, Tweden KS, Vollmer MC, Wilson RR, Camilleri M. Intermittent vagal blocking with an implantable device reduces maximum tolerated volume (MTV) during a standardized nutrient drink test in obese subjects. Gastroenterology. 2009;136:A386. (presented at Annual Meeting, Digestive Disease Week, Chicago, IL, 30 May – 4 June 2009)

Part V

Revisional Bariatric Surgery

Revision After Gastric Banding

16

Andres Giovannetti and Rami Lutfi

Goals

- Describe proper evaluation and workup of a patient with weight loss failure after adjustable gastric band (AGB).
- Discuss the factors involved in the selection of the adequate procedure for revision.
- Discuss up-to-date opinions regarding main controversies in revision surgery.
- Describe the critical differences between one-stage and two-stage revision surgery after AGB.
- Describe essential steps during laparoscopic AGB revision surgery to laparoscopic sleeve gastrectomy (LSG) and laparoscopic Roux-Y gastric bypass (LRYGB).
- Review and compare the outcomes regarding weight loss and complications between LSG and LRYGB when done for revision after AGB.

Introduction

Laparoscopic adjustable gastric banding (LAGB) was described in 1993 and approved by the FDA to be used in the USA in 2001. It is a purely restrictive procedure designed to confront obesity. By 2010 these operations accounted for 46% of all the bariatric surgeries performed in American College of Surgeons accredited centers [1].

Since its introduction, LAGB placement has been considered as a safe, reversible, and low-risk procedure with promising short-term outcomes as reported by many of the initial studies [2–4]. However, more recent investigations reviewing long-term outcomes showed high rate of reoperation and revision for complications like band erosion, slippage, and gastric pouch enlargement as well as weight loss failure [1, 5–8].

Based on the National Inpatient Sample (NIS) database, between 2005 and 2014, 159,890 morbidly obese individuals underwent LAGB insertion. Utilization of this procedure started with around 14,000 in 2005, peaking in 2008 at 35,000 cases to decrease to 1170 in 2014. Interestingly the number of procedures for removal and revision during the same period increased progressively from a total of 1405 in 2005 to 7240 in 2014 (an increase of 432%) [1].

There are multiple potential reasons for failed weight loss following LAGB. These include complications related to the adjustable gastric band prosthesis, lack of compliance with dietary

A. Giovannetti
Department of Surgery, Mercy Hospital Medical Center, Chicago, IL, USA

R. Lutfi (✉)
University of Illinois at Chicago, Chicago, IL, USA

R. Lutfi et al. (eds.), *Global Bariatric Surgery*, https://doi.org/10.1007/978-3-319-93545-4_16

advice or adjustment regimens, or low resting energy expenditure [5].

In general, AGB have inferior results compared with stapling procedures due to lack of metabolic effect. However, when minimal weight loss or recurrence of obesity occur, a comprehensive evaluation of the patient needs to be done by the team (including dietitian and psychologist) before blaming the AGB. It is our practice to look at the compliance and the number of adjustments done before going forward with further workup.

The current literature shows that up to 60% of patients required revision of the primary surgery between 30 and 80 months after placement, being the most common indication insufficient weight loss [5, 8, 9].

The goal of this chapter is to provide a review of the outcomes after different conversion options available LAGB as well as describe the essential surgical steps during these procedures.

Adjustable Gastric Band Revision

Conversion from AGB to sleeve gastrectomy (SG) or Roux-Y gastric bypass (RYGB) is safe and feasible. The selection of the procedure will depend mainly on the characteristics of the patient including BMI, comorbidities, previous surgeries, preoperative studies (EGD, upper GI), and patient preference. It is necessary to consider the risk/benefit ratio of the surgery during the evaluation of the patient by a multidisciplinary patient care program [9, 10].

The authors consider that during the evaluation of a patient with an AGB for a revisional surgery, it is critical to differentiate those that present because they did not do well with the band (suboptimal response) from those with complication related with the band (erosion, slippage). In our practice, we tend to believe that the first group of patients would fail with another restrictive procedure in a long term if they never responded at any time or were not compliant. Every patient with an AGB with suboptimal response undergoes an extensive evaluation by our team of dietitians, psychologists, and nurses, paying attention to details like how many band adjustments were done, compliance with the follow-up and progression of the weight (Fig. 16.1 illustrates our detailed approach).

In our institution, EGD is the study of choice we use routinely to evaluate patients before bariatric surgery. For the workup of "failed" band

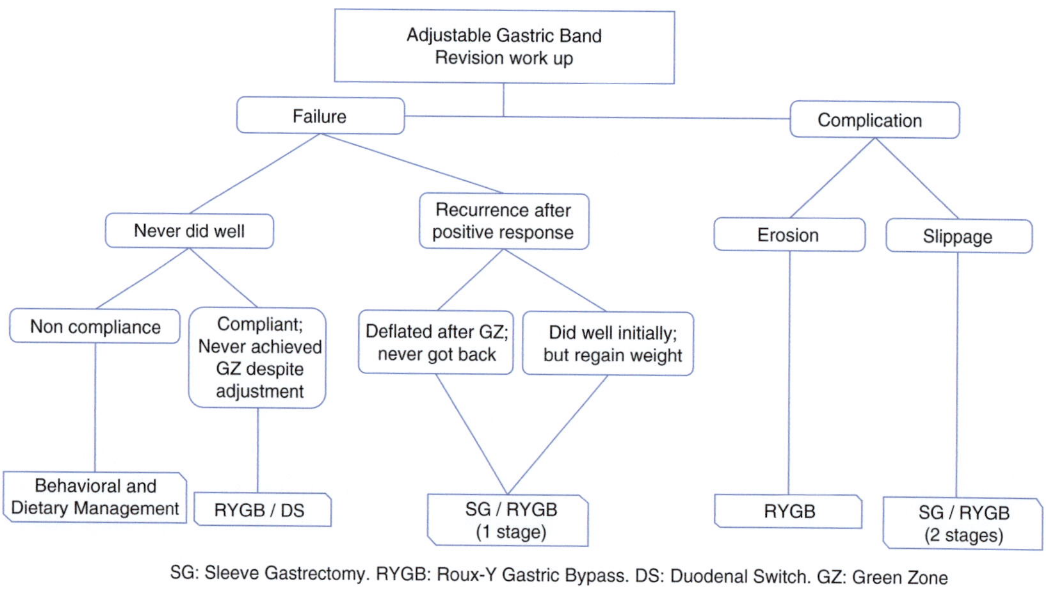

Fig. 16.1 Work up of failure after Lap-Band

and revisions, we include both, upper GI study and endoscopic evaluation (EGD). In the presence of a band, an upper GI study will evaluate the esophagus and the gastric pouch above the band to rule out anatomical problems such as band slippage or esophageal dilation. This helps deciding between one- and two-stage approaches.

The removal of the gastric band constitutes the first step of any revision surgery. It can be done simultaneously with the second surgery (one-stage revision) or as a separate procedure (two-stage revision) 3–6 months before the second surgery. The selection of the approach will depend on each surgeon and center experience as we will discuss later in this chapter.

One-Stage Versus Two-Stage

In the contrary to many, we feel that one-stage conversion from LAGB to either LSG or LRYGB is technically easier as opposed to the general belief. The band is deflated 2 weeks before the surgery to decrease the inflammation caused by pressure of the balloon and allow the gastric pouch to decrease in size.

The trocar positioning used is the same for one- or two-stage approach, using the same position as it was a primary LSG or LRYGB (this is described in detail in the Gastric Sleeve chapter). Briefly, the abdomen is accessed using a 5 mm bladeless trocar just inferior to the left costal margin in the midclavicular line; once inside, we use an angled scope and place the remaining trocars, including a 5 mm trocar 16 cm from the xiphoid and 3 cm to the left side of the midline to obtain a better angle to approach the hiatus. The umbilical region is avoided because of its inconsistent position in obese patients. A 12 mm bladeless trocar is placed on the right side near the inferior aspect of the falciform ligament and an additional 5 mm in the right upper quadrant. Unique for a one-stage procedure is a 15 mm trocar instead of the 12 mm trocar in order to remove the adjustable band.

Lysis of adhesion constitutes the initial and, occasionally, a complex portion of the procedure, but it is common for both one- and two-stage approaches. This step is performed using electrocautery close to the left lateral lobe of the liver, with the help of a liver retractor to reach the esophageal hiatus (Figs. 16.2 and 16.3).

We feel that having the band in place facilitates the dissection and preparation for the stapling process. The body of the band can be followed once the adhesions are removed to identify the gastro-gastric plication suture line. The band is kept locked and the anterior capsule is identified (Fig. 16.4).

The band tubing is retracted to the right side of the patient, and with the use of electrocautery initially and laparoscopic scissors without cautery,

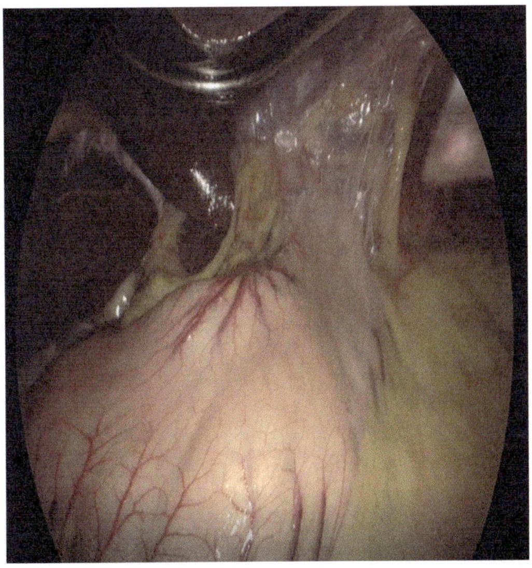

Fig. 16.2 Adhesions to the liver after the band was removed (second stage)

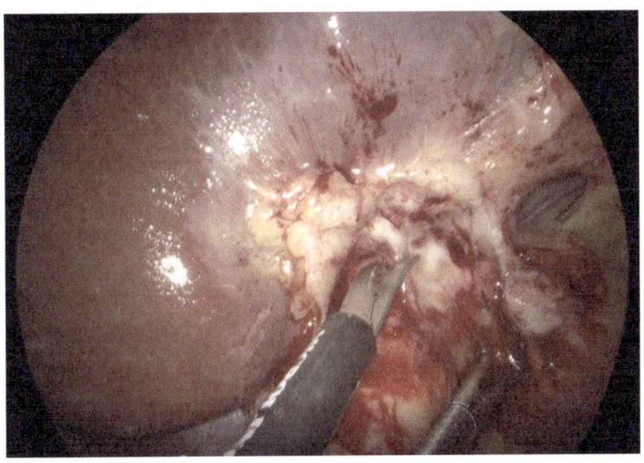

Fig. 16.3 Taking down the adhesion between the stomach and the liver (second stage)

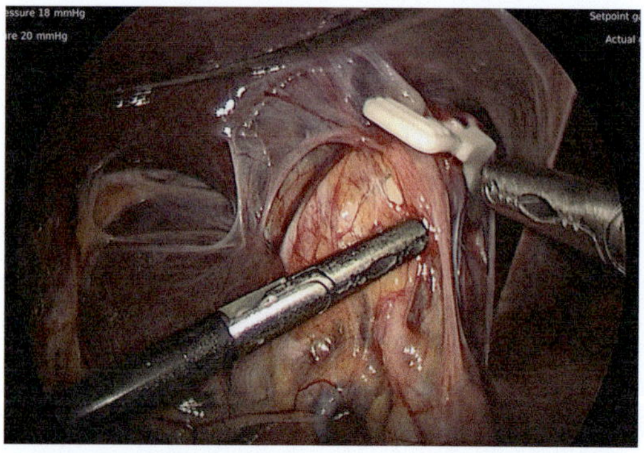

Fig. 16.4 Separating the band from the liver

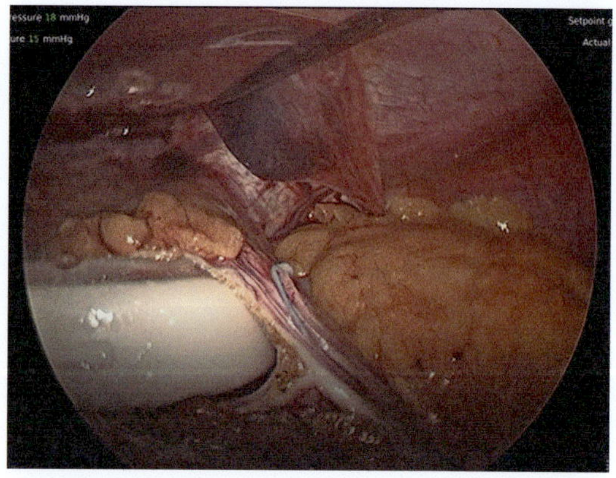

Fig. 16.6 Having the band in place makes the plane easy to visualize

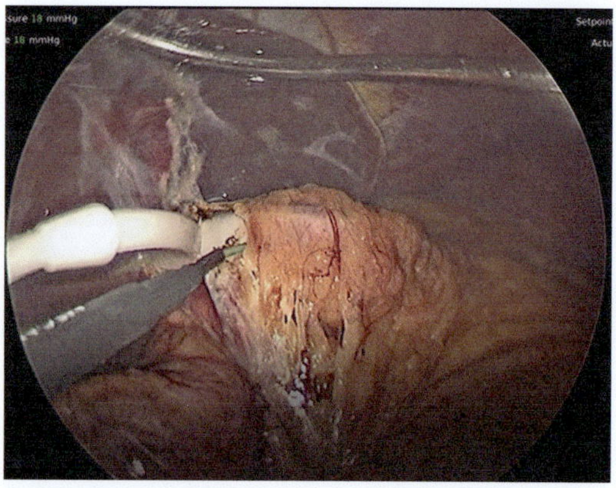

Fig. 16.5 Using the body of the band for guidance to undo the plication

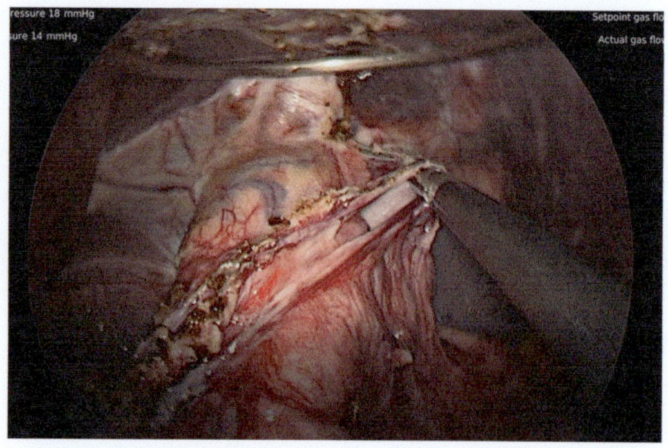

Fig. 16.7 In one-stage operation, after band removal the tunnel is easy to find

the plication line is divided to separate the two portions of the stomach from medial to lateral (Figs. 16.5 and 16.6).

When approaching to the left side of the stomach, the band is unlocked and removed (Fig. 16.7); the surgeon retracts the gastric pouch superiorly and the assistant the remaining stomach down, exposing the rest of the plication suture line which is divided with scissors until the plication is undone (Fig. 16.8).

During revisional surgery from LAGB, it is critical to clear the left crus completely like it is done during primary LSG and LRYGB. Two-stage revision has the advantage of fewer adhesions to the liver, but the plane of plication can be difficult to identify months after band removal (Fig. 16.9).

During the two-stage revision, a trick used to find the correct plane and dissect it is to use the suture previously placed in the initial surgery as a

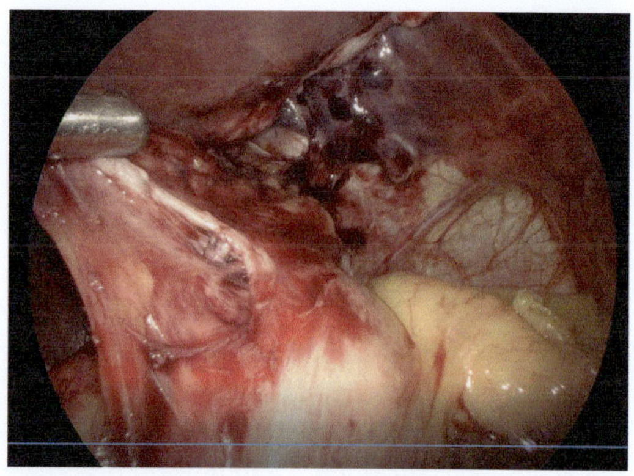

Fig. 16.8 Second stage could be tricky. Retracting the pouch up will usually lead to the separation plane

guide for the dissection of the plane and proceed as described above (Figs. 16.10 and 16.11).

Removal of the capsule in the band site is still a subject of controversy among bariatric

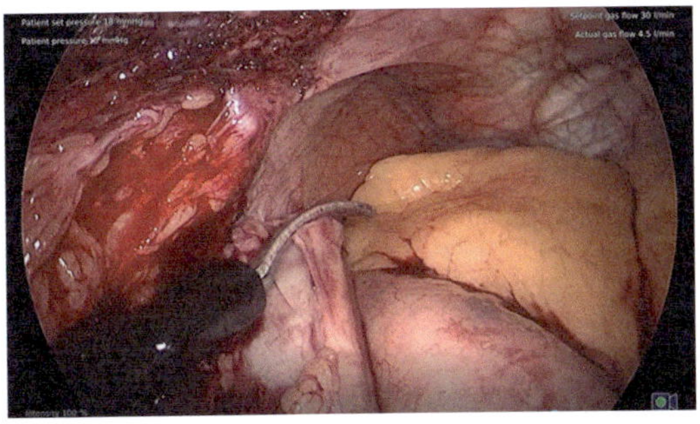

Fig. 16.9 Taking down the adhesions to the left crus is critical

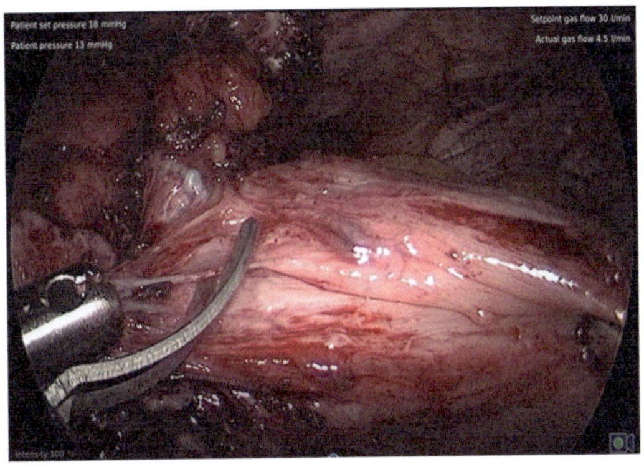

Fig. 16.10 Dividing the plane sharply in the second stage

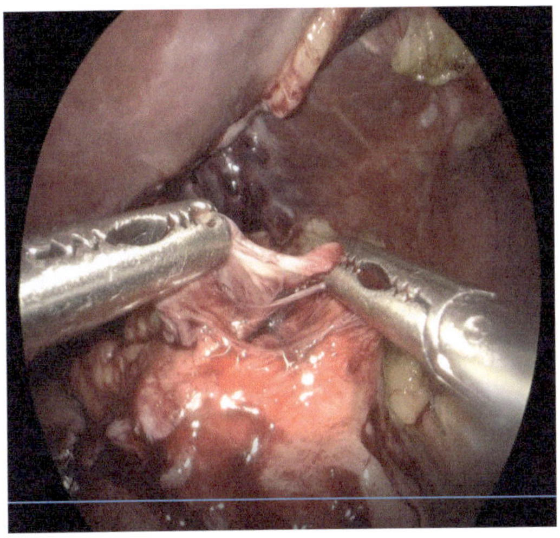

Fig. 16.11 Traction and countertraction facilitates identifying the plane in second stage

surgeons, but the authors of this chapter strongly recommend the removal of the anterior portion without the need of removal of the entire cap-

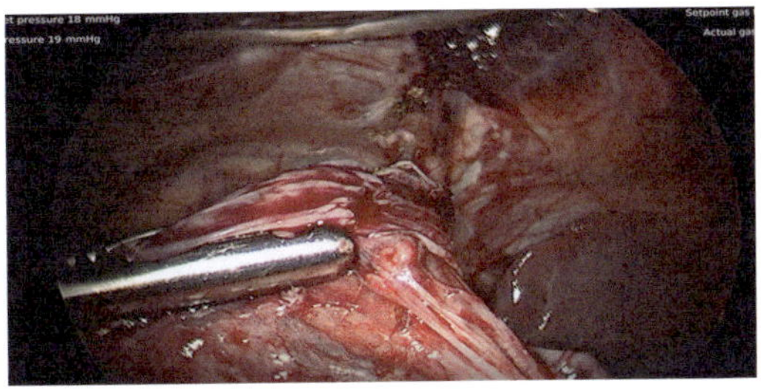

Fig. 16.12 Identifying the capsule

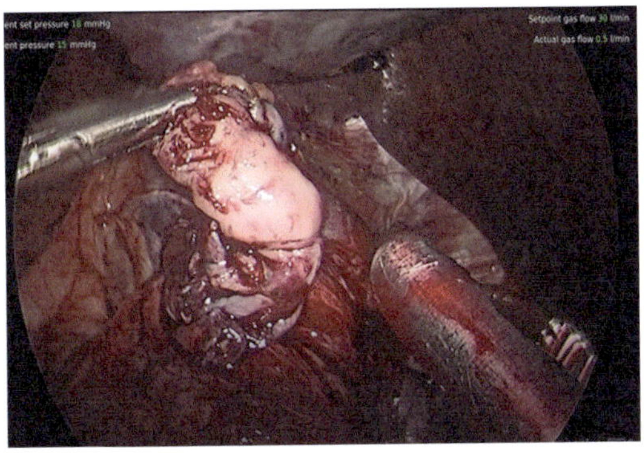

Fig. 16.13 Excising the anterior part of the capsule

sule in order to prevent gastric constriction (Figs. 16.12 and 16.13).

At the time of the revisional operation, thicker staple cartridges are used to perform the entire gastric stapling, compared with primary LSG or LRYGB where a mixture of staple heights is generally used. It is of critical importance to assure when staples are placed that no previous stitches are inside the staple line and also that the stomach has to be flat without any folds (Fig. 16.14).

Authors use a 34 Fr bougie to guide the stapling for both, revisional and primary procedures. They consider the size of the bougie not to be of critical importance. Instead, the distance between the stapler and the bougie is most critical as this could be fired "too tight" against the bougie increasing the risk of stricture or leak, even with larger bougies. Keeping a small distance is of most importance at the area of the incisura and at the top to avoid firing esophageal tissues (Fig. 16.15a, b).

It is mandatory, especially in one-stage revisions, to perform posterior dissection of the

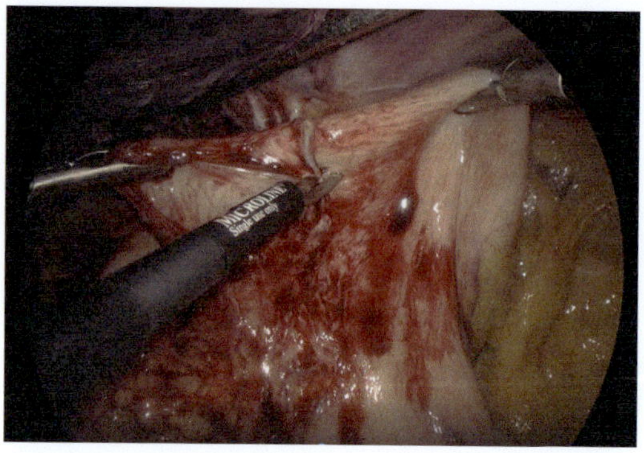

Fig. 16.14 After undoing the plication, finding all sutures could lead to settle remaining fold that need to be taken down

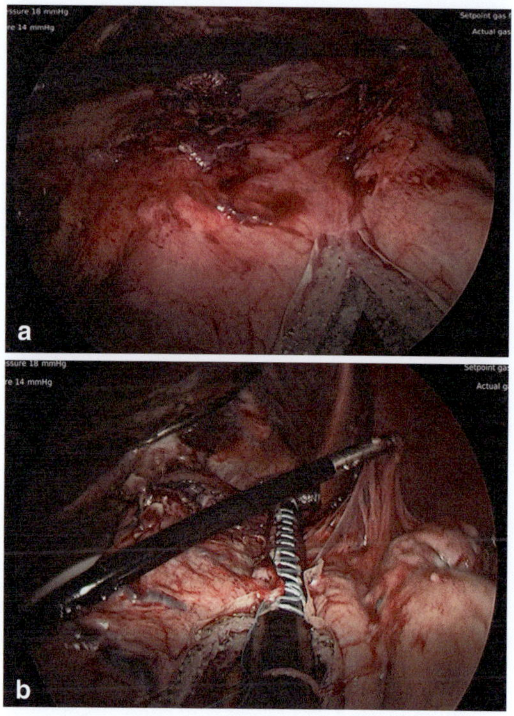

Fig. 16.15 (**a**) Preparing flat, unfolded stomach as a "landing zone" for next firing of the stapler. (**b**) Ensuring the absence of any fold before firing the stapler

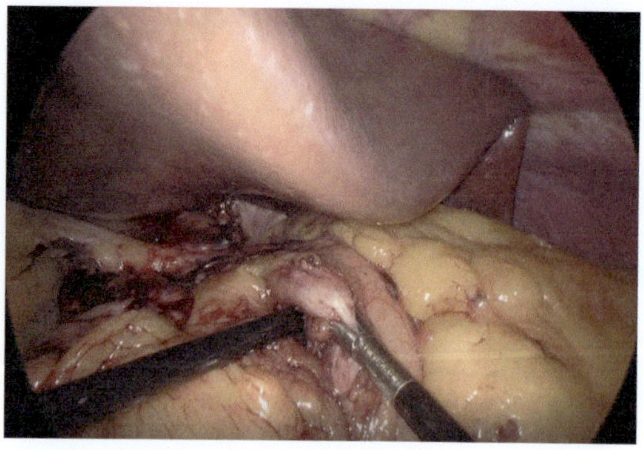

Fig. 16.16 In LRYGB creating the window for transection inferior to the prior band location

stomach superiorly to rule out a hiatal hernia, which cannot be diagnosed during preoperative EGD due to the presence of the band (Fig. 16.16). If a two-stage approach is considered, then a preoperative EGD should be performed before the second surgery looking for the presence of a hiatal hernia during the retroflection maneuver. Bariatric surgeons need to be aggressive in diagnosing and managing hiatal hernias in order to reduce the factors that may lead to failure of the procedure or persistence of the patient reflux symptoms. After the entire stomach is dissected, the surgery proceeds as a routine LSG or LRYGB with the considerations mentioned before.

The only aspect that differs in the way the LRYGB is performed in our institution is the fact that when dealing with revisional surgery the dissection of the stomach is done first as opposed to the jejunojejunostomy. This is to ensure feasibility before commitment.

Usually, the band location is very high in the stomach; the transverse gastric transection to create the pouch in LRYGB is done below the band site and below the capsule. The authors use absorbable staple reinforcement routinely in revisional surgery (Fig. 16.17).

The advantage of the one-stage approach is limiting the process to one operation which limits cost and the need for patients to undergo general anesthesia twice and recover twice as well as limiting days off work. Also, once the band is removed, the patients tend to gain weight despite strict follow-up and counseling.

While economically the one-stage approach results favorable for the health system compared with the two-stage approach, two separate stages are more profitable for the surgeon from a billing and collection standpoint.

Regardless of preference for routine revisions for failure of weight loss, the presence of dyspha-

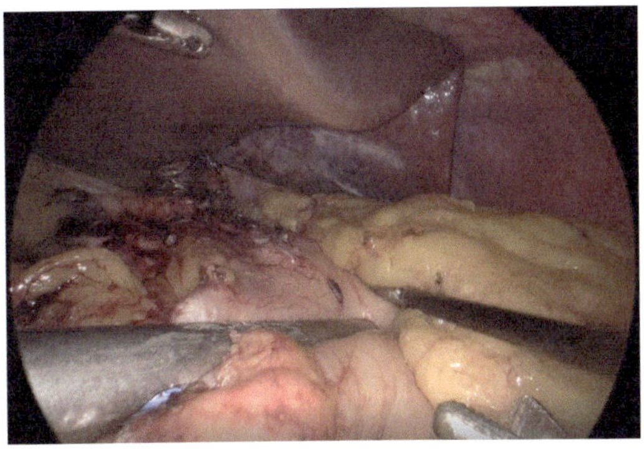

Fig. 16.17 Transecting the stomach below the capsule to create the gastric pouch

gia, slippage, erosion, or severe gastroesophageal reflux despite band deflation all mandates two-stage revisions. These patients will benefit from band removal followed by an observation period to allow improvement of symptoms before the second surgery. If no improvement of the symptoms is observed, additional workup is done.

When severe esophagitis (grade C or D) from chronically tight band is found on endoscopy, we would recommend LRYGB instead of LSG unless symptoms resolve after band removal. Repeat endoscopy can always be performed to ensure healing before a final decision is made.

Sleeve Gastrectomy Versus Roux-Y Gastric Bypass

Laparoscopic Roux-Y gastric bypass has been considered as the procedure of choice for revision for weight loss failure after AGB for many years, partially due to the short experience with other bariatric procedures like LSG. Nowadays the selection of the procedure is more complex and is usually based on patient preference, comorbidities, and response to previous surgery [11, 12].

According to recently published literature, the main reasons for band revision are weight loss failure (45–71%), band slippage (14–32%), erosion (9%), and GERD (12%) among others [13, 14]. Timing from the initial surgery varies widely ranging from 2 months after AGB placement up to 8 years without changes in outcomes or complications [14, 15].

As far as the procedure of choice, a study based on the analysis of data from the Metabolic and Bariatric Surgery Accreditation and Quality Improvement Program (MBSAQIP) published in 2017 included 2708 patients that underwent adjustable gastric band (AGB) removal with one-stage conversion to laparoscopic sleeve gastrectomy (LSG) or laparoscopic Roux-Y gastric bypass (LRYGB). Groups were closely matched. They found that conversion to LSG has better safety profile in the short term compared with conversion to LRYGB. The latter was associated with higher 30-day reoperation, 30-day readmission rates, bleeding, and more cases of leakage. At the same time, this study showed that revision surgery to either LSG or LRYGB can be done safely in 99% of patients [16].

An Italian study analyzed a single-center 5-year outcome of conversion from LAGB to LSG or LRYGB. They studied 51 patients equally distributed. All revisions were performed in one-stage fashion. No perioperative complications were present. No statistical difference was found regarding %EWL between patients that underwent LSG and those who underwent LRYGB. Patients of both groups present remission of the comorbidities (hypertension and type II diabetes after 1 year of the revisional surgery) [9].

Carr et al. did a retrospective study of 89 patients that underwent conversion from LAGB to LSG or LRYGB in the same center where the band was placed. Consideration was to convert to LSG in patients with multiple adhesions at the time of surgery that interfere with performing a LRYGB as well as in patients with multiple comorbidities that required shorter surgical time. LSG was recommended in patients who had good experience with restrictive procedures. In this study patients that underwent band removal for insufficient weight loss receive a LRYGB more often than LSG (93% vs 60%). Overall there were no statistically significant differences between the two conversion options regarding length of stay, %EWL, and complications after 2 years of follow-up [11].

Yeung et al. in a retrospective study of 72 patients undergoing conversion from LAGB to LSG and 32 patients to LRYGB found that those who underwent LRYGB had longer operative times than LSG (224 min vs 156 min); the %EWL was not significantly different at 6-month and 12-month follow-up (50.2 vs 30.6) for LRYGB and LSG, respectively. The complication rate was 18% for LRYGB and 12% for LSG. Overall, there was no statistically significant difference in the outcome between the two procedures [13].

Surgeons that favor revision to LSG after AGB consider this as a safe procedure that can be performed faster compared with LRYGB (140–160 min vs 218–224 min) which helps when patients are not able to tolerate longer operative times due to severe comorbidities and offers similar benefits compared with LRYGB regarding recovery time, %EWL (up to 60% in LSG vs up to 70% for LRYGB), and length of stay (2–3 days). Multiple studies have shown no statistically significant differences in outcomes and complications between the LSG and LRYGB as a revisional surgery after AGB [9–11, 16–18].

Complications after both procedures, considering the higher complexity and challenges encountered, are minimal when done by experienced surgeons working in centers of excellence. The ones reported are mainly leakage, infection, and bleeding with the former one being the most common [15, 19–21]. Many surgeons opt to perform a LRYGB instead of a LSG in those patients that did not respond well to a previous restrictive procedure [12].

Controversy still exists in regard to which approach must be adopted during the conversion process, performing either the band removal and conversion at the same time (one-stage approach) or removal of the band with a later conversion to LSG or LRYGB (two-stage approach). The studies supporting the use of one-stage approach for either LSG or LRYGB claim that patients will benefit of having only one surgery, will not carry the risk of gaining more weight during the interval between the procedures, and will have the same risk for complications than when a two-stage approach is used like it is shown in the meta-analysis done by Dang et al. and other studies [6, 9, 11, 17, 22].

Noel et al. compared 300 patients that underwent LSG as a revisional procedure after AGB with 1060 patients that underwent primary LSG. Reasons for conversions were the same as other studies. The complication rate was 4.5% for the primary LSG group and 2% for the conversion group, with a leak rate of 1.6% and 1%, respectively. The %EWL reported was 75.9 ± 21.4% in the primary LSG group and 62.6 ± 22.2% in the conversion group. All conversion patients underwent a two-stage procedure. They are in favor of the two-stage approach with a minimum interval of 3 months after band removal [21].

In the opposite to this study, the group from Cleveland Clinic showed same outcomes and minimal complication rate with one-stage conversion to LSG on their 209 patients compared with 3268 primary LSG. In the conversion group, one patient had a successfully stented leak. In the primary LSG group, three leak cases were reported and managed successfully through endoscopic stenting, one patient had pulmonary embolism that responded to standard treatment, and three patients had postoperative bleeding. No other major complications occurred, and there was no mortality in either group [20].

Recommendations for the use of a two-stage approach are mainly in patients with complications from the AGB like erosion, esophageal dilation, severe comorbidities that limits the operative time, and intraoperative findings during the band removal that could increase the risk of complications if a second procedure is performed at the same time and also is critical to consider patient desire during the decision process [11, 14, 15, 21].

The myth about the benefit of the two-stage approach in relation to the reduction of the inflammatory component in the previous band site has been refuted by Tan et al. when they analyzed the histology of the stomach changes after band removal and concluded that the inflammatory changes do not experience a significant change for at least 3 years after band removal [23].

The capsule formed around the band may interfere with the stapling of the stomach, some authors recommend the removal of the entire capsule before proceeding with the revisional surgery in order to avoid staple line failure and possible leak, but it is not mandatory for LRYGB. Surgeons should consider to perform the gastrojejunostomy above or under the band capsule [9, 17].

The authors of this chapter recommend removal of the anterior aspect of the capsule and careful dissection on the anterior surface of the stomach in order for it to regain its original shape, facilitating this way the stapling process. A widespread recommendation is to use thicker stapler cartridges during the stomach stapling in order to reduce the risk of leakage [9, 20].

Conclusions

Adjustable gastric band was introduced and remained as a safe and effective procedure for weight loss until long-term outcomes studies showed an increased rate of complications and reoperations, leading to a search for more permanent procedures with sustainable results.

Revisional surgery is technically challenging and generally carries inferior results than primary bariatric operations. Suboptimal results to banding should be investigated, and failure should not be simply blame on the band. Those patients should be carefully evaluated by the comprehensive bariatric team to ensure their compliance before a surgical revision is decided.

The choice of the procedure and timing should be made after extensive discussion with the patient to understand their goals and expectations as no level 1 evidence exists today to guide toward the optimal operation or its timing. These operations should only be performed by experienced surgeons in specialized center of excellence.

References

1. Rudnicki M, Giovannetti A, Bueltmann K. Have we reached the end of the lifespan of laparoscopic banding for morbid obesity? In: Poster presented at digestive disease week 2017. Chicago; 2017.
2. O'Brien P, et al. Lap-band: outcomes and results. J Laparoendosc Adv Surg Tech. 2003;13(4):265–70. https://doi.org/10.1089/109264203322333593.
3. Ren CJ, Horgan S, Ponce J. US experience with the LAP-BAND system. Am J Surg. 2002;184(6):S46–50. https://doi.org/10.1016/S0002-9610(02)01180-7.
4. Angrisani L, Alkilani M, Basso N, et al. Laparoscopic Italian experience with the Lap-Band®. Obes Surg. 2001;11(3):307–10. https://doi.org/10.1381/096089201321336656.
5. Smith MD, Patterson E. The ASMBS textbook of bariatric. Surgery. 2014;1:283–93. https://doi.org/10.1007/978-1-4939-1197-4.
6. Kowalewski PK, Olszewski R, Kwiatkowski AP, Paśnik K. Revisional bariatric surgery after failed laparoscopic adjustable gastric banding – a single-center, long-term retrospective study. Wideochirurgia i inne Tech maloinwazyjne = Videosurgery Other miniinvasive Tech. 2017;12(1):32–6. https://doi.org/10.5114/wiitm.2017.66671.
7. Mendes-Castro A, Montenegro J, Cardoso JF, et al. Laparoscopic adjustable gastric band: complications, removal and revision in a Portuguese highly differentiated obesity treatment center. Acta Med Port. 2015;28(6):735–40. https://doi.org/10.1007/s11695-016-2348-0.
8. Altieri MS, Yang J, Telem DA, et al. Lap band outcomes from 19,221 patients across centers and over a decade within the state of New York. Surg Endosc Other Interv Tech. 2016;30(5):1725–32. https://doi.org/10.1007/s00464-015-4402-8.
9. Angrisani L, Vitiello A, Santonicola A, Hasani A, De Luca M, Iovino P. Roux-en-Y gastric bypass versus sleeve gastrectomy as revisional procedures after adjustable gastric band: 5-year outcomes. Obes Surg. 2017;27(6):1430–7. https://doi.org/10.1007/s11695-016-2502-8.
10. Kassir R, Lointier P, Tiffet O, et al. Revision bariatric surgery: what technical choices should be taken depending on the first intervention? Int J Surg. 2017;44:7–8. https://doi.org/10.1016/j.ijsu.2017.05.075.
11. Carr WRJ, Jennings NA, Boyle M, Mahawar K, Balupuri S, Small PK. A retrospective comparison of early results of conversion of failed gastric banding to sleeve gastrectomy or gastric bypass. Surg Obes Relat Dis. 2015;11(2):379–84. https://doi.org/10.1016/j.soard.2014.07.021.
12. Marin-Perez P, Betancourt A, Lamota M, Lo Menzo E, Szomstein S, Rosenthal R. Outcomes after laparoscopic conversion of failed adjustable gastric banding to sleeve gastrectomy or Roux-en-Y gastric bypass. Br J Surg. 2014;101(3):254–60. https://doi.org/10.1002/bjs.9344.
13. Yeung L, Durkan B, Barrett A, et al. Single-stage revision from gastric band to gastric bypass or sleeve gastrectomy: 6- and 12-month outcomes. Surg Endosc Other Interv Tech. 2016;30(6):2244–50. https://doi.org/10.1007/s00464-015-4498-x.
14. Patel S, Eckstein J, Acholonu E, Abu-Jaish W, Szomstein S, Rosenthal RJ. Reasons and outcomes of laparoscopic revisional surgery after laparoscopic adjustable gastric banding for morbid obesity. Surg Obes Relat Dis. 2010;6(4):391–8. https://doi.org/10.1016/j.soard.2009.12.010.

15. Sergio C, Maldonado P, Rivkine E, Valenti A, Polliand C, Barrat C. Revisional surgery after failed laparoscopic adjustable gastric banding. Comparison between roux-en-y gastric bypass and gastric sleeve. Obes Surg. 2013;23(8):1184.
16. Janik MR, Rogula TG, Mustafa RR, Alhaj Saleh A, Khaitan L. Safety of revision sleeve gastrectomy compared to roux-Y gastric bypass after failed gastric banding. Ann Surg. 2017;XX(Xx):1. https://doi.org/10.1097/SLA.0000000000002559.
17. Gonzalez-Heredia R, Masrur M, Patton K, Bindal V, Sarvepalli S, Elli E. Revisions after failed gastric band: sleeve gastrectomy and Roux-en-Y gastric bypass. Surg Endosc Other Interv Tech. 2015;29(9):2533–7. https://doi.org/10.1007/s00464-014-3995-7.
18. Spaniolas K, Bates AT, Docimo S, Obeid NR, Talamini MA, Pryor AD. Single stage conversion from adjustable gastric banding to sleeve gastrectomy or Roux-en-Y gastric bypass: an analysis of 4875 patients. Surg Obes Relat Dis. 2017;13(11):1880–4. https://doi.org/10.1016/j.soard.2017.07.014.
19. Dang JT, Switzer NJ, Wu J, et al. Gastric band removal in revisional bariatric surgery, one-step versus two-step: a systematic review and meta-analysis. Obes Surg. 2016;26(4):866–73. https://doi.org/10.1007/s11695-016-2082-7.
20. Alqahtani AR, Elahmedi MO, Al Qahtani AR, Yousefan A, Al-Zuhair AR. 5-year outcomes of 1-stage gastric band removal and sleeve gastrectomy. Surg Obes Relat Dis. 2016;12(10):1769–76. https://doi.org/10.1016/j.soard.2016.05.017.
21. Noel P, Schneck AS, Nedelcu M, et al. Laparoscopic sleeve gastrectomy as a revisional procedure for failed gastric banding: lessons from 300 consecutive cases. Surg Obes Relat Dis. 2014;10(6):1116–22. https://doi.org/10.1016/j.soard.2014.02.045.
22. Chansaenroj P, Aung L, Lee WJ, Chen SC, Chen JC, Ser KH. Revision procedures after failed adjustable gastric banding: comparison of efficacy and safety. Obes Surg. 2017;27(11):2861–7. https://doi.org/10.1007/s11695-017-2716-4.
23. Tan MHL, Yee GYW, Jorgensen JO, et al. A histologic evaluation of the laparoscopic adjustable gastric band capsule by tissue sampling during sleeve gastrectomy performed at different time points after band removal. Surg Obes Relat Dis. 2014;10(4):620–5. https://doi.org/10.1016/j.soard.2014.02.037.

17 Revision After Sleeve Gastrectomy

Daniel Cottam, Hinali Zaveri, Amit Surve, and Austin Cottam

Background

Laparoscopic sleeve gastrectomy (LSG) is a partial gastrectomy of the fundus and body to create a sleeve or tubular stomach along the lesser curve of the stomach. Although it is considered restrictive procedure, weight loss results from restrictive as well as endocrine mechanism.

LSG was first reported as a part of two-stage approach for high-risk patients undergoing laparoscopic Roux-en-Y gastric bypass (LRYGB) [1]. Soon, it was recognized safe and effective as a stand-alone procedure with the weight loss superior or equivalent to laparoscopic adjustable gastric banding (LAGB) and LRYGB [2, 3]. Today, it has become the most popular bariatric procedure in the world [4] and the most commonly performed bariatric procedure at US academic medical centers [5]. Technical simplicity compared to LRYGB, short operating room time, avoidance of a foreign body compared to LAGB, high safety profile; its ability to convert, revise, or use as a staged procedure, immediate calorie intake restriction, better insurance coverage, and superior weight loss compared to LAGB explain the increasing demand for LSG [2, 6]. The safety and effectiveness of LSG have been established in three international consensus summits [7–9]. In 2012, the American Society for Metabolic and Bariatric Surgery (ASMBS) recognized LSG as an acceptable primary bariatric procedure [4].

However, there are several disadvantages of this procedure, such as the potential for weight regain or inadequate weight loss; poor results in patients with body mass index (BMI) over 50; increased complications linked to stapling, like leaks; nonreversibility; and the paucity of long-term data (>10 years).

Overview of Results of Sleeve Gastrectomy

Multiple studies have shown LSG results an average of 55% excess weight loss (EWL) during midterm follow-up [10]. However, the durability of LSG has been an important concern during the past 5 years. There are very limited studies that show the long-term (>5 years) weight loss results. Most of these studies have shown an excess weight loss ranging between 53% and 69% [4] with the tendency for some weight regain. Himpens et al. [11] reported 77% EWL at 3 years and 53% EWL at 6 years with primary LSG. Bohdjalian et al. reported 55% EWL with 19.2% weight regain and 15.4% revision rate required at 5 years [12]. Similarly, in a research article by Alvarenga et al., it showed that EWL at 8 years was only 52% [13]. This means half of all LSG patients met the standard definition of weight loss failure at most long-term follow-up.

D. Cottam (✉) · H. Zaveri · A. Surve · A. Cottam
Bariatric Research, Bariatric Medicine Institute, Salt Lake City, UT, USA

R. Lutfi et al. (eds.), *Global Bariatric Surgery*, https://doi.org/10.1007/978-3-319-93545-4_17

Sanchez-Santos et al. [14] reviewed 540 patients who had undergone LSG as a primary or staged procedure, using the Spanish national registry for bariatric surgery. At 3 years, mean %EWL was excellent; however, 15% of the patients were considered a failure because of weight regain in the first 3 years with 3.3% of patients requiring a second bariatric procedure. Younger age, lower BMI (<50 kg/m^2), and thinner bougie size (32–36 Fr.) were recommended for better outcomes. That means, in spite of the promising outcomes, LSG has poor results in patients with BMI over 50 and has a larger standard deviation [6], meaning that many patients do well with the sleeve but just as many do not. D'hondt et al. [15] observed decreasing %EWL at annual intervals; 81.5% EWL at 1 year was dropped to 55.9% EWL at 6 years.

With such sobering long-term data, it is necessary for bariatric surgeons to come up with a more acceptable approach for the patients who fail sleeve or who has weight regain.

Predictor for Outcomes of Sleeve Gastrectomy

Since it's hard to predict optimal outcomes after LSG, there are several predictor models that predict the outcomes after LSG [16–28]. Table 17.1 summarizes the outcomes of predictive models for weight loss after LSG.

Table 17.1 Outcomes of predictive models for weight loss after sleeve gastrectomy

Authors	Number of patients	Primary endpoints	Predictor outcomes
Gomberawalla et al. [16]	100	%EWL at 1 year	Preoperative BMI <50 – better weight loss
Abd Ellatifa et al. [17]	1395	%EWL	Smaller bougie size (<36F), close application of staple line to the pylorus – higher % EWL
Cottam et al. [18]	613	>55% EWL at 1 year	Preoperative diabetes, sleep apnea, % EWL at 1 month and 3 months
Andersen et al. [19]	160	%EBMIL at 2 years	Female sex, higher preoperative BMI, nonsmoking – lower %EBMIL
			For men – higher age and no diabetes – lower %EBMIL
			For women – unemployment, anxiety, and depression – lower %EBMIL
Martin et al. [20]	292	%EWL at 2 years	Lower baseline BMI, absence of HTN, and greater clinical attendance – better %EWL
Hansen et al. [21]	30	%EWL at 7 months	Preoperative increase in distance traveled in 6-minute walk test – early postoperative weight loss
Goitein et al. [22]	99	%EWL at 1 year	Delayed contrast passage on swallow study on POD 1 – better weight loss
Figura et al. [23]	64	%EWL at 20 months	An active coping style –higher %EWL
Manning et al. [24]	538	Maximal %WL	Weight loss velocity at 3–6 months predicts maximal %WL
Sioka et al. [25]	110	%EWL	Binge eating and emotional eating – lowest %EWL
			Normal eating and snacking – highest %EWL
Philouze et al. [26]	128	%EBMIL at 24 months	%EBMIL>20.1 at 3 months – success of SG at long term
Ortega et al. [27]	100	%EWL at 1 year	Young age with low BMI but higher WC and lower HbA1c and TG – higher %EWL and success
Gras-Miralles et al. [28]	7	Weight loss at 1 year	Higher calorie intake capacity had poor outcomes

EWL excess weight loss, *WL* weight loss, *EBMIL* excess BMI point lost, *BMI* body mass index, *HTN* hypertension, *POD* postoperative day, *SG* sleeve gastrectomy, *WC* waist circumference, *HbA1c* glycosylated hemoglobin, *TG* triglyceride

Causes for Sleeve Gastrectomy Failure

The most common cause of weight recidivism is the failure of adherence to dietary and lifestyle regimen as outlined by the multidisciplinary team [29]. Modifiable risk factors for LSG have been identified such as lack of nutritional behavior, lack of physical activity, or lack of follow-up [30, 31]. A frequent cause of failure of restrictive surgery is said to be sweet eating, appearing de novo or persisting despite the procedure [32].

The typical pattern seen in several articles in regard to SG failure has been long-term gastric pouch dilation [33]. There are many reasons for the gastric pouch dilatation, including technical error during the operation. The superior pouch dilation may occur because of an incomplete release of the posterior gastric fundus or preservation of a part of the fundus to avoid injury of the esophagogastric junction or when the last stapler is fired >1 cm away from the gastroesophageal (GE) junction. On the other hand, an inferior pouch dilatation may rise due to antral preservation, which may occur due to the misplacement of the bougie or misidentification of the pylorus [34]. Another possibility for antrum dilation is when the stomach is resected >4 cm distance from pylorus [35]. Another factor to consider is noncompliance with diet regimen leading to mechanical stretching of the gastric pouch due to the consistent intake of larger meals [29]. Baltasar et al. [36] reported two cases of pouch dilation following primary LSG resulting in weight regain. Both these cases required revisional surgery. A case report by Gagner et al. [37] reported dilated gastric pouch as a culprit for weight regain 2 years after a staged procedure combining SG and biliopancreatic diversion with duodenal switch (BPD-DS). Despite all these anecdotal papers, the only prospective study by Langer et al. [38] could not correlate the radiographic evidence of pouch dilation with postoperative weight regain at 1 year after LSG. Thus, while we believe pouch dilation is the culprit in weight regain, the answer remains equivocal.

The other common motif associated with failure of LSG is smaller bougie size with smaller volume gastrectomies and high residual gastric volume postoperatively. The International Sleeve Gastrectomy Expert Panel Consensus Statement for best practice guidelines [39] concluded that a bougie not wider than 32–36F should be used for LSG. Deguines et al. [31] demonstrated that high residual gastric volume (>255 cc) at 2 years was related to LSG failure. Similarly, Weiner et al. [40] reported a 13% failure rate, with a resected gastric volume of less than 500 cc being a predictor for such failure. However, recent analysis of the MBSQUIP data set suggests that larger bougie size not smaller results in better weight loss. This is counterintuitive and suggests there is still much to learn about weight loss success and failure.

By now we know that weight loss from SG is not only attributed to restrictive component but also endocrine/hormonal component [6]. There are over 40 hormones that control appetite and satiety in the human. Recently a large amount of attention has been focused on the LSG and ghrelin. The gastric fundus and body produce ghrelin, an appetite-stimulating hormone. LSG involves resecting the fundus and body; this reduces ghrelin levels, increases the paracrine effects of incretins, and decreases insulin resistance. It is hypothesized that weight regain after LSG may be attributed to increasing the body adapting to the LSG changes and increasing plasma ghrelin level [12]. Himpens et al. [32] showed that loss of appetite was seen in 75% of patients 1 year after LSG. At 3 years lack of appetite was only was seen in 46.7%. Currently there is no agreement on which hormones affect the postoperative anorexia and what happens to cause the return of hunger seen in some patients.

Work-Up of Failure of Optimal Weight Loss

The best way to approach the patients with weight loss failure or weight recidivism is to perform a full history and assess their BMI and their alimentary habits. Any patient with the maladaptive eating disorder should first undergo psychological and dietary evaluation and should be treated before considering the surgical revision. The next step is to document their anatomy with radiographical tools (upper gastrointestinal (UGI series), barium swallow, or esophagogastroduodenoscopy (EGD)) to look for the evidence of dilation [41].

If dilation is seen, then the best way to manage this patient is to perform a laparoscopic re-sleeve gastrectomy (LRSG). If no dilation is seen and the patient is still regaining weight or has not achieved optimal weight loss (>50% EWL), malabsorptive intervention should be considered (Fig. 17.1).

Management of Sleeve Gastrectomy Failure

Medical Management with Behavioral and Dietary Changes

Psychological factors need to be addressed in a patient first presenting with weight regain, as it is directly correlated psychiatric comorbidities [42]. There is limited data available on behavioral and psychological predictors of weight loss outcomes after bariatric surgery. The fac-

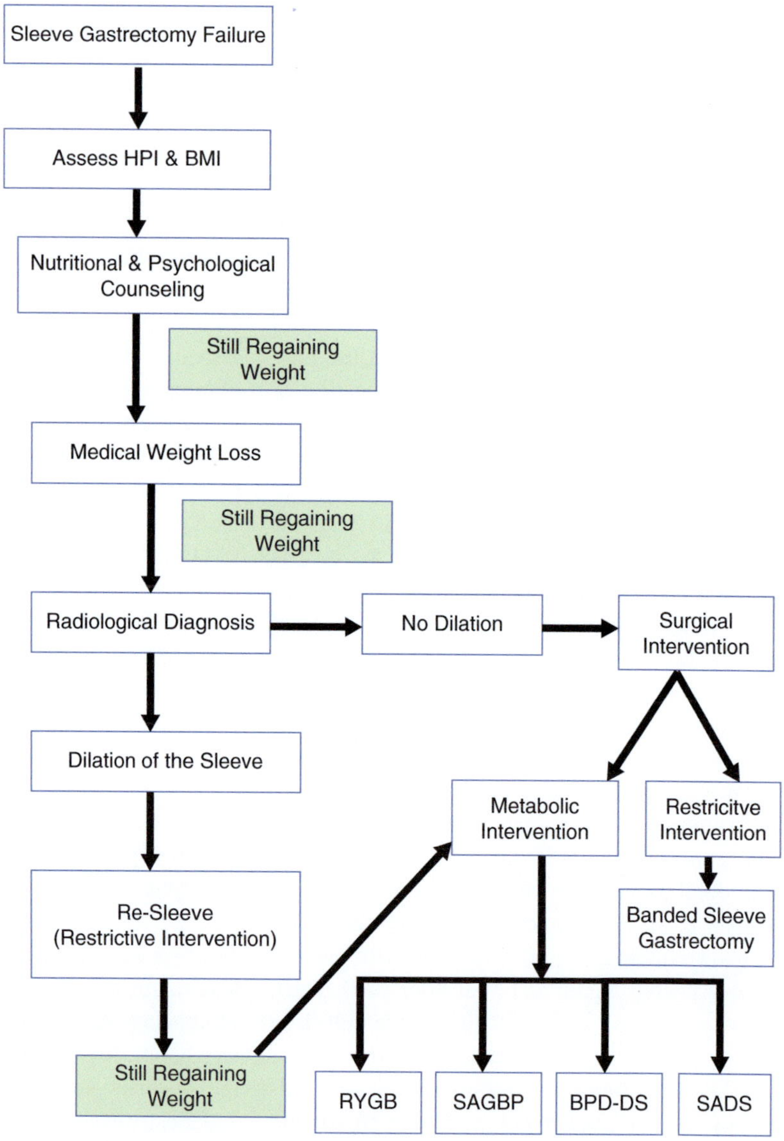

Fig. 17.1 Algorithm showing work-up of failure of sleeve gastrectomy

tors that can cause weight regain after bariatric surgery includes lack of control over food urges, decreased well-being, and concerns regarding addictive behavior [42]. Conversely, excellent self-reported well-being and self-monitoring predict freedom from regaining. The behavioral treatment is effective in nonsurgical and surgical weight loss management because it tailors therapy to the specific concerns and behavioral patterns of patients [43].

The importance of proper nutritional counseling after bariatric surgery has been supported by the literature. It has been shown that patient who maintain their food record are associated with more weight loss, while the lack of nutritional counseling follow-up is significantly associated with weight regain [44]. Collectively, these strategies are essential in helping patients prevent weight regain. In spite of above changes, if patient is still not able to reach their desired weight loss or comorbidity resolution, medical management should be considered.

Currently in the US, there are different medications, approved by FDA, that are being used for weight management (Table 17.2). These medications work on a variety of pathways, and the patient should be told that if one of the meds is successful in controlling appetite or urges, that therapy should be instituted for a lifetime. Most patients should think of weight loss not as a temporary treatment but more like treatment of high blood pressure. If you find a medication or combination of medications that keep blood pressure under control, then you should stay on them forever. It is exactly the same for weight management. While there have been several studies documenting the effectiveness of weight loss medication administered prospectively after LAGB, there currently are no papers documenting pathways or algorithms for medication use after LSG for poor weight loss results [45]. If the patient is unwilling or unable to try medications after surgery, then consideration should be given to performing a surgical revision.

Surgical Management for Failed Sleeve Gastrectomy

Restrictive Intervention

Re-sleeve Gastrectomy

A redo or LRSG is usually indicated in the event of insufficient weight loss or weight regain due to isolated gastric dilatation. Care must be taken when performing this operation as the gastric tissue around the old staple line is denser because of the scar's healing and remodeling. The new staple line should be created within the old staple line to prevent an area of ischemia. The surgeon must take into consideration important surgical revision complications when advising their patient for this option [33]. There is also increased risk of leak at the angle of His. This risk is even more in patient who had a previous LAGB.

Gagner et al. [23] first proposed LRSG for insufficient weight loss after a BPD-DS and later by Baltasar et al. [36] as a revisional operation for a failed LSG. The LRSG have shown favorable outcome in terms of excess weight loss at 1 year with the caveat that it also increases the risk of gastric stenosis and risk of fistula development [46–49].

There are several reports on the increased rate of gastroesophageal reflux disease (GERD) after LSG [32, 50–52]. GERD is described as either de novo or as being caused by aggravation of preexisting symptoms. Some authors have gone as far as saying that any patient with reflux should have a gastric bypass. However, the latest literature shows that GERD can be successfully treated in most patients with aggressive searching and repairing of hiatal hernia defects [41, 53]. In conclusion, LRSG has several advantages compared with malabsorptive procedures such as increasing the restriction and decreasing the gastric output, lessening dumping syndrome by preserving the pylorus, reducing protein and vitamin deficiency, and requiring shorter operative times [41].

It is important to remember that repeating a LSG does not protect the patient from occurrence of gastric dilation, and long-term weight regains.

Table 17.2 List of medications for weight loss

Name	Mechanism	Weight maintenance	Side effects
FDA-approved drugs			
Long-term approval drugs			
Orlistat (Xenical or Alli)	Lipase inhibitor that causes excretion of 30% of ingested TG in stools	5% WL in 1 year	GI symptoms
Lorcaserin HCI (Belviq and Belviq XR)	Selective serotonergic 5-HT2C receptor agonist causing appetite suppression	7% WL in 1 year, D/C if WL <5% after 12 weeks	Headache, dizziness, fatigue, nausea, dry mouth, upper respiratory tract infection
Naltrexone HCI + bupropion HCI (Contrave)	Inhibitor of dopamine and noradrenaline reuptake+ an opioid antagonist	5–10%WL in 1 year, D/C if WL <5% after 12 weeks on max dose	Nausea, constipation, headache, dry mouth, vomiting, and dizziness
Phentermine-topiramate ER (Qsymia)	Noradrenergic + GABA-receptor activator, kainite/AMPA glutamate receptor inhibitor causing appetite suppression	14.4%WL in 1 year, D/C if WL <5% after 12 weeks on max dose	Dry mouth, constipation, dizziness, insomnia, constipation, tachycardia, memory or cognitive changes, birth defects, and pins and needle feeling in extremities
Liraglutide injection (Saxenda)	GLP-1 analogue. It suppresses the appetite and delays gastric emptying	5–10% WL in 1 year	Nausea, vomiting, diarrhea, and constipation. High risk for thyroid cell tumor
Short-term approval drugs			
Phentermine (Adipex-P or Suprenza) (high dose)	Noradrenergic causing appetite suppression	4–5% WL in 1 year, D/C when tolerance occurs	Dry mouth, taste alteration, sleeplessness, tachycardia, increase blood pressure, dizziness, GI distress, tremors, anxiety, restlessness, headache
Phentermine (Lomaira) (low dose)			
Diethylpropion (Tenuate)	Noradrenergic causing appetite suppression	D/C if no response within 4 weeks or when tolerance occurs	Same as phentermine
Phendimetrazine (Bontril)	Noradrenergic causing appetite suppression	D/C when tolerance occurs	Same as phentermine
Benzphetamine (Didrex Regimex)	Noradrenergic causing appetite suppression	D/C when tolerance occurs	Same as phentermine
Dextroamphetamine (Dexedrine, ProCentra, Zenzedi)	Sympathomimetic		Same as phentermine, along with high abuse potential, sudden death
Amphetamines (Evekeo)	Sympathomimetic		Same as dextroamphetamines
Methamphetamines (Desoxyn) (used only when other Rx is ineffective)	Sympathomimetic		Same as dextroamphetamines
Non-FDA-approved drug for weight loss			
Topiramate (Topamax) (approved for migraine and epilepsy)	GABA-receptor activator, kainite /AMPA glutamate receptor inhibitor causing appetite suppression		Vision impairment, acidosis, kidney stones, cognitive problems, insomnia, decreased sweating, pins and needle feeling in extremities. It can cause birth defects

Table 17.2 (continued)

Name	Mechanism	Weight maintenance	Side effects
Topiramate XR (Trokendi XR) (approved for migraine and epilepsy)	GABA-receptor activator, kainite /AMPA glutamate receptor inhibitor causing appetite suppression		Vision impairment, acidosis, kidney stones, cognitive problems, insomnia, decreased sweating, pins and needle feeling in extremities. It can cause birth defects
Exenatide (approved for T2DM) (Byetta, Byduren)	GLP-1 analogue		Nausea, diarrhea, headache, nephrotoxicity
Metformin (approved for T2DM and PCOD) (Glucophage, Fortamet)	Hypoglycemia agent		Diarrhea, nausea, lactic acidosis, hepatotoxicity
Pramlintide (approved for T2DM) + metreleptin (approved for leptin deficiency)	Amylin synthetic analogue + leptin receptor agonist		Nausea and increase risk of lymphoma
Cetilistat (approved in Japan)	Pancreatic lipase inhibitor		GI symptoms
Tensofesine	Norepinephrine, dopamine and serotonin reuptake inhibition		Dry mouth, nausea, constipation
Bupropion SR + zonisamide SR (Emapatic)	Dopamine and norepinephrine reuptake inhibitor+ antiepileptic causing enhancement of dopamine and serotonin neurotransmission	6–7% WL	Nausea, headache, and insomnia
Gelesis 100	Made from food-grade material that expands in the stomach and slows gastric emptying		

WL weight loss, *GI* gastrointestinal, *TG* triglyceride, *GLP-1* glucagon-like peptide 1, *T2DM* type 2 diabetes mellitus, *D/C* discharged

If weight regain still occurs after a longer follow-up post-LRSG, patients should undergo further counseling about the possibility of malabsorptive operations.

Band Over Sleeve Gastrectomy

In LSG failure patients where the inadequate restriction is a cause of failure, a safe and efficient option will be to increase restriction by placing an adjustable gastric band below GE junction. The food will pass slowly across the proximal part of the stomach that will help in achieving satiety. At the same time, the ileal break mechanism will be triggered due to fast transit of food bolus into the small intestine. Greenstein et al. [54] first introduced this idea of adding an adjustable gastric band to SG patients to increase gastric restriction. Initial LSG was performed over 60 Fr bougie; thus enough gastric tissue was available to allow gastric plication over the band (which is not the case with all SG). Banded sleeve gastrectomy (BSG) can also be used as preventative means to avoid SG failure in the first place [55]. Agarwal et al. [56] reported the first case report of BSG as a primary procedure on the superobese patient. The patient showed favorable outcomes.

The potential advantage of placing band over sleeve is that it is relatively simple to perform and it avoids the additional staple lines associated with revisional bariatric surgery. However, the theoretical drawbacks of the procedure include band erosion and slippage. Karcz et al. [57] published an article where he matched 25 patients of BSG with LSG. The results showed that additional band implantation did not increase weight loss in the first year but increased the rate of vomiting after the first year. Thus, in certain patient populations with failed LSG, the insertion of a gastric band into its normal anatomic position proximal to the staple line of the sleeve is feasible, but the long-term effects are unknown.

Malabsorptive Interventions

Historically, SG was originally the first step in a scheduled two-step operation, where patients experienced significant additional EWL following conversion to either duodenal switch (DS) or RYGB [58]. Therefore, it is easier to revise patients with LSG weight loss failure to the second unscheduled bariatric procedure. Adding malabsorption to the already restrictive SG has been proven to be an effective means for further weight loss [33, 58]. The main concern with revising SG to a malabsorptive procedure is the significant increase of complication rates when compared to primary surgery. The safety of the revisional procedure is still debatable in the literature. Therefore, such high-risk revisional surgeries should only be performed by experienced bariatric surgeons to ensure maximum patient safety and procedural success.

There are multiple malabsorptive surgical revisional options for failed LSG- RYGB, BPD-DS, single-anastomosis gastric bypass (SAGB), and recently popularized single-anastomosis duodenal switch (SADS) operation.

Roux-en-Y Gastric Bypass

The main indications for conversion of SG to RYGB are insufficient weight loss and significant weight regain. Beside weight regain, severe reflux is also seen in some SG patients [32]. Modification of the gastric anatomy may impair the antireflux barrier. High-dose proton pump inhibitor (PPI) medications might not achieve relief of GERD symptoms in these patients and conversion to RYGB can serve as a definitive surgical option. Langer et al. [59] first reported series of patients who underwent RYGB for severe reflux or weight regain after primary LSG. Postoperatively, all the patients with GERD discontinued the PPI medications. Significant weight reduction of 33 lbs was achieved in patients with weight regain within a median follow-up of 33 months. Gautier et al. [60] reported 61.7% EWL at 15 months after the second step, whereas Alexandrou et al. [61] reported a 71.9% long-term EWL for superobese patients.

Insufficient resolution of comorbidities is another reason for SG failure. RYGB is slightly superior to SG in controlling diabetes mellitus (T2DM) [60]. Secretion of incretins and their effect on insulin secretion is mainly due to duodenal exclusion seen in RYGB [62]. Although weight loss post revision is comparable to primary RYGB, the complication rate might vary between 0% and 47% [33].

One limitation of conversion of SG to RYGB is the weight regain, which is also seen primarily after RYGB. Therefore, many debate that conversion to RYGB is not effective [63]. In fact, 25% of the patient who had a RYGB also fail to maintain their weight loss [64, 65]. In addition, the patients who regain their weight after LSG might be more susceptible to regain weight following conversion to RYGB [59]. Therefore, conversion to RYGB might be preferred in the case of dysphagia and GERD but might not be the best option for weight loss failure after SG, especially since other malabsorptive procedures show favorable weight loss results [66, 67].

Single-Anastomosis Gastric Bypass

Single-anastomosis gastric bypass (SAGB) has gained popularity and reported to have excellent weight loss and weight maintenance with a very low rate of complication [68–70]. The long-term results of SAGB have been equal or better than those of standard RYGB [69, 71]. It has been proposed as a revision surgery after LAGB or LSG because of its combined restrictive and malabsorptive effects [72–74].

Chevallier et al. [75] first reported short-term outcomes of three patients who underwent conversion of SG to SAGB for inadequate weight loss. In his series, the excess BMI loss (%EBMIL) was 51.6% at 24 months; however, the 30-day morbidity was 9.5%. Chevallier et al. [73] then published his 5-year outcomes on revisional SAGB where he observed that SAGB was well tolerated and effective in the long-term. However, quality of life and upper gastrointestinal function were lower after revisional surgery compared with primary surgery. In conclusion, although the preliminary result of revision SAGB is encouraging and is simpler and an effective operation compared to RYGB, long-term outcome with larger series is necessary.

Biliopancreatic Diversion with Duodenal Switch (BPD-DS)

BPD-DS is the feasible surgical revision option for patients who failed LSG because of insufficient weight loss or weight regain. However, there are several factors that need to be addressed before offering patients this revision option such as demonstration of good follow-up patterns and addressing vitamin and mineral deficiencies preoperatively. Compared to RYGB, conversion to BPD-DS yields higher weight loss [63, 76] as and comparable weight loss as compared to single-stage DS [77]. Sovik et al. [78] observed a 26% failure rate after RYGB versus a 0% after BPD-DS and Prachand et al. [79] also 16% failure rate after BPS-DS in superobese patients; however this rate was less when compared to RYGB (40%).

BPD-DS has been difficult to perform with high risk of postoperative complications and malnutrition. Any preoperative low levels of vitamins are predictive of postoperative insufficiencies; BPD-DS should be completely avoided in patients with preoperative vitamin deficiency not corrected on repeated labs. Iannelli et al. [77] performed BPD-DS on 25 patients after failed LSG. He observed an EWL of 59% at 30 months; however, 82% of the patients were diagnosed with vitamin or mineral deficiency. One of the other biggest concerns after BPD-DS in terms of nutrition is the development of protein deficiencies, which can be as high as 32% [80]. However, care must be taken when interpreting these results as there are many different common channel and Roux limb lengths in these papers and bowel length correlates with the level of micronutrient deficiencies.

Single-Anastomosis Duodenal Switch (SADS)

Modification of DS, a single-anastomosis duodenal switch (SADS), also known as the single-anastomosis loop duodenal switch (LDS), single-anastomosis duodenoileal bypass with sleeve gastrectomy (SADI-S), and stomach intestinal pylorus sparing surgery (SIPS), have emerged and became increasingly popular [81]. These are technically simpler surgery as compared to BPD-DS or RYGB. Juan Antonio Torres and Anders Sanchez in Spain first described the SADI-S technique in 2007 [82]. They performed LSG over 54 Fr bougie, preservation of pylorus, and a longer 200 cm common channel (later modified to 250 cm because of an unacceptably high rate of hypoalbuminemia) [83]. The SADI-S procedure has also been described as a second-step revisional procedure primarily for insufficient weight loss after SG (over a 42F–54F bougie) [84]. SADI-S showed satisfactory weight loss of 72% at 2 years and 88% complete remission of diabetes after the second-step surgery with minimal complications. Cottam et al. [85] also have used SADS as a second stage after failed LSG. Patients lost similar amount of weight as compared to primary surgery is performed within 1st year after primary SG. Similarly, nutritional complications were less than BPD-DS and similar to RYGB [86, 87].

The conversion from LSG to SADI-S or SIPS is technically simpler and less demanding than LSG to RYGB or BPD-DS. Additionally, when a loop approach is taken over a Roux approach, the long-term one-percent incidence per year of internal hernias found in Roux surgeries disappears [88]. However, SADS is still considered under investigation by many surgeons, and long-term data would help confirm how truly robust this procedure is and may show a better side effect profile.

Summary

- LSG shows promising weight loss during short-term and midterm outcomes. However, in the long-term follow-up, it has failure rate. LSG also has high failure rate in superobese patients.
- Patient selection is key for successful revisional surgery. A more intense preoperative

evaluation should be implemented for patients who are considering revisional surgery for poor weight loss or weight regain.

- Nutritional and psychological evaluation should be recommended for all the patients with weight regain or insufficient weight loss.
- Medical management should be considered in selected patients.
- Gastric dilation is one of the most common causes of LSG failure. LRSG is the best initial treatment for these patients. However, it carries the risk of leak, stricture, stenosis, or weight regain.
- If no dilation is seen then malabsorptive interventions are required.
- Revision RYGB is the optimal treatment for patients who has weight regain or insufficient weight loss long with GERD or dysphagia. However, weight regain is an important issue after this surgery.
- SAGB is alternative to RYGB after LSG and has better safety profile. However, long-term results are lacking.
- LSG is a part of staged BPD-DS. BPD-DS after failed LSG have shown excellent weight loss in superobese patients, but there is high risk of nutritional and postoperative complication when compared to RYGB.
- SADS after LSG is an excellent alternative to BPD-DS and RYGB with less malnutrition and postoperative complications. Long-term data are needed to prove these benefits.

References

1. Regan JP, Inabnet WB, Gagner M, Pomp A. Early experience with two-stage laparoscopic Roux-en-Y gastric bypass as an alternative in the super-super obese patient. Obes Surg. 2003;13(6):861–4.
2. Boza C, Salinas J, Salgado N, et al. Laparoscopic sleeve gastrectomy as a stand-alone procedure for morbid obesity: report of 1,000 cases and 3-year follow-up. Obes Surg. 2012;22(6):866–71.
3. Hutter MM, Schirmer BD, Jones DB, et al. First report from the American College of Surgeons Bariatric Surgery Center Network: laparoscopic sleeve gastrectomy has morbidity and effectiveness positioned between the band and the bypass. Ann Surg. 2011;254(3):410–20. discussion 420–2
4. ASMBS Clinical Issues Committee. Updated position statement on sleeve gastrectomy as a bariatric procedure. Surg Obes Relat Dis. 2012;8(3):e21–6.
5. Varela JE, Nguyen NT. Laparoscopic sleeve gastrectomy leads the U.S. utilization of bariatric surgery at academic medical centers. Surg Obes Relat Dis. 2015;11:987–90.
6. Brethauer SA, Hammel J, Schauer PR. Systematic review of sleeve gastrectomy as a staging and primary bariatric operation. Surg Obes Relat Dis. 2009;5:469–75.
7. Deitel M, Crosby RD, Gagner M. The first international consensus summit for sleeve gastrectomy (SG), New York City, October 25–27 2007. Obes Surg. 2008;18(5):487–96.
8. Gagner M, Deitel M, Kalberer TL, et al. The second international consensus summit for sleeve gastrectomy, March 19–21, 2009. Surg Obes Relat Dis: Off J Am Soc Bariatric Surg. 2009;5(4):476–85.
9. Deitel M, Gagner M, Erickson AL, et al. Third international summit: current status of sleeve gastrectomy. Surg Obes Relat Dis: Off J Am Soc Bariatric Surg. 2011;7(6):749–59.
10. Clinical Issues Committee of American Society for Metabolic and Bariatric Surgery. Sleeve gastrectomy as a bariatric procedure. Surg Obes Relat Dis. 2007;3(6):573–6.
11. Himpens J, Dobbeleir J, Peeters G. Long-term results of laparoscopic sleeve gastrectomy for obesity. Ann Surg. 2011;252:319–24.
12. Bohdjalian A, Langer FB, Shakeri-Leidenmuhler S, et al. Sleeve gastrectomy as sole and definitive bariatric procedure: 5-year results for weight loss and ghrelin. Obes Surg. 2010;20:535–40.
13. Alvarenga ES, Lo Menzo E, Szomstein S, Rosenthal RJ. Safety and efficacy of 1020 consecutive laparoscopic sleeve gastrectomies performed as a primary treatment modality for morbid obesity. A single-center experience from the metabolic and bariatric surgical accreditation quality and improvement program. Surg Endosc. 2016;30(7):2673–268.
14. Sanchez-Santos R, Masdevall C, Baltasar A, et al. Short and midterm outcomes of sleeve gastrectomy for morbid obesity: the experience of the Spanish National Registry. Obes Surg. 2009;19:1203–10.
15. D'Hondt M, Vanneste S, Pottel H, Devriendt D, Van Rooy F, et al. Laparoscopic sleeve gastrectomy as a single-stage procedure for the treatment of morbid obesity and the resulting quality of life, resolution of comorbidities, food tolerance, and 6-year weight loss. Surg Endosc. 2011;25:2498–504.
16. Gomberawalla A, Wilson T, Lufti R. Predictors of success after laparoscopic sleeve gastrectomy. Bariatric Surg Pract Patient Care. 2015;10(2):45–8.
17. Abd Ellatif ME, Abdallah E, Askar W, et al. Long term predictors of success after laparoscopic sleeve gastrectomy. Int J Surg. 2014;12:504–8.
18. Cottam A, Billing J, Cottam D, et al. Long term success and failure with sleeve gastrectomy is predictable by three months. A multivariate model using simple office markers. Surg Obes Relat Dis. 2017;13:1266.

19. Andersen JR, Aadland E, Nissen RM, Vage V. Predictors of weight loss are different in men and women after sleeve gastrectomy. Obes Surg. 2014;24(4):594–8.
20. Martin DJ, MY Lee C, Rigas G, Tam CS. Predictors of weight loss 2 years after laparoscopic sleeve gastrectomy. Asian J endosc Surg. 2015;8:328–32.
21. Hansen N, Hardin E, Bates C, Bellatorre N, Eisenberg D. Preoperative change in 6-minute walk distance correlates with early weight loss after sleeve gastrectomy. JSLS. 2014;18(3):e2014.
22. Goitein D, Zendel A, Westrich G, Zippel D, Papa M, Rubin M. Postoperative swallow study as a predictor of intermediate weight loss after sleeve gastrectomy. Obes Surg. 2013;23(2):222–5.
23. Figura A, Ahnis A, Stengel A, et al. Determinants of weight loss following laparoscopic sleeve gastrectomy: the role of psychological burden, coping style, and motivation to undergo surgery. J Obes. 2015;626010:2015.
24. Manning S, Pucci A, Carter N, et al. Early postoperative weight loss predicts maximal weight loss after sleeve gastrectomy and Roux-en-Y gastric bypass. Surg Endosc. 2015;2996:1484–91.
25. Sioka E, Tzovaras G, Oikonomou K, et al. Influence of eating profile on the outcome of laparoscopic sleeve gastrectomy. Obes Surg. 2013;23(4):501–8.
26. Philouze G, Voitellier E, Lacaze L, et al. Excess body mass index loss at 3 months: a predictive factor of long-term result after sleeve gastrectomy. J Obes. 2017;2017:2107157.
27. Ortega E, Morinigo R, Flores L, et al. Predictive factors of excess body weight loss 1 year after laparoscopic bariatric surgery. Surg Endosc. 2012;26:1744–50.
28. Gras-Miralles B, Haya JR, Moros JM, Delgado-Aros S. Caloric intake capacity as measured by a standard nutrient drink test helps to predict weight loss after bariatric surgery. Obes Surg. 2014;24(12):2138–44.
29. Zundel N, Hernandez JD. Revisional surgery after restrictive procedures for morbid obesity. Surg Laparosc Endosc Percutan Tech. 2010;20:338–43.
30. Snyder B, Nguyen A, Scarbourough T, Yu S, Wilson E. Comparison of those who succeed in losing significant excessive weight after bariatric surgery and those who fail. Surg Endosc. 2009;23:2302–6.
31. Deguines JB, Verhaeghe P, Yzet T, Robert B, et al. Is the residual gastric volume after laparoscopic sleeve gastrectomy an objective criterion for adapting the treatment strategy after failure? Surg Obes Relat Dis. 2006;9:660–6.
32. Himpens J, Dapri G, Cadière GB. A prospective randomized study between laparoscopic gastric banding and laparoscopic isolated sleeve gastrectomy: results after 1 and 3 years. Obes Surg. 2006;16:1450–6.
33. Switzer NJ, Karmail S. The sleeve gastrectomy and how and why it can fail? Surgery: Curr Res. 2014;4:3.
34. Al Khalifa K, AlSaad F, Al Musaifer B, Al Mansoor A, Al Ansari A. Superior and Inferior gastric pouch dilation post-sleeve surgery: does revision work? A systemic review and case report. Surg Sci. 2014;5:491–500.
35. Abdallah E, El Nakeeb A, Yousef T, Abdallah H, Ellatif MA, et al. Impact of extent of antral resection on surgical outcomes of sleeve gastrectomy for morbid obesity (a prospective randomized study). Obes Surg. 2014;24:1587–94.
36. Baltasar A, Serra C, Perez N, Bou R, Bengochea M. Re-sleeve gastrectomy. Obes Surg. 2006;16:1535–8.
37. Gagner M, Rogula T. Laparoscopic reoperative sleeve gastrectomy for poor weight loss after biliopancreatic diversion with duodenal switch. Obes Surg. 2003;13:649–54.
38. Langer FB, Bohdjalian A, Felberbauer FX, Fleischmann E, Reza Hoda MA, et al. Does gastric dilatation limit the success of sleeve gastrectomy as a sole operation for morbid obesity? Obes Surg. 2006;16:166–71.
39. Rosenthal RJ. International sleeve gastrectomy expert panel consensus statement best practice guidelines based on experience of > 12000 cases. Surg Obes Relat Dis. 2012;8:8–19.
40. Weiner RA, Weiner S, Pomhoff I, et al. Laparoscopic sleeve gastrectomy: influence of sleeve size and resected gastric volume. Obes Surg. 2007;17(10):1297–305.
41. Nedelcu M, Noel P, iannelli A, Gagner M. Revised sleeve gastrectomy (re-sleeve). Surg Obes Relat Dis. 2015;11:1282–8.
42. Odom J, Zalesin KC, Washington TL, Miller WW, Hakmeh B, et al. Behavioral predictors of weight regain after bariatric surgery. Obes Surg. 2010;20:349–56.
43. Hsu LK, Benotti PN, Dwyer J. Non-surgical factors that influence the outcome of bariatric surgery: a review. Psychosom Med. 1998;60:338–46.
44. Freire RH, Borges MC, Alvarez-Leite JI, Toulson Davisson Correia MI. Food quality, physical activity, and nutritional follow-up as determinant of weight regain after roux-en-y gastric bypass. Nutrition. 2012;28:53–8.
45. Schwartz J, Chaudhry UI, Suzo A, et al. Pharmacotherapy in conjunction with a diet and exercise program for the treatment of weight recidivism or weight loss plateau post-bariatric surgery: a retrospective review. Obes Surg. 2016;26(2):452–8.
46. Cesana G, Uccelli M, Ciccarese F, Carrieri D, Castello G, Olmi S. Laparoscopic re-sleeve gastrectomy as a treatment of weight regain after sleeve gastrectomy. World J Gastrointest Surg. 2014;6(6):101–6.
47. Iannelli A, Schneck AS, Noel P, Ben Amor I, Krawczykowski D, et al. Re-sleeve gastrectomy for failed laparoscopic sleeve gastrectomy: a feasibility study. Obes Surg. 2011;21:832–5.
48. Hong JS, Han SM. Re-sleeve gastrectomy for failure of weight loss after primary sleeve gastrectomy; 3 cases. J Metabolic Synd. 2015;4:182.
49. Dapri G, Cadiere GB, Himpens J. Laparoscopic repeat sleeve gastrectomy versus duodenal switch

after isolated sleeve gastrectomy for obesity. Surg Obes Relat Dis. 2011;7(1):38–43.
50. Soricelli E, Iossa A, Casella G, Abbatini F, Calì B, Basso N. Sleeve gastrectomy and crural repair in obese patients with gastroesophageal reflux disease and/or hiatal hernia. Surg Obes Relat Dis. 2013;9:356–61.
51. Braghetto I, Csendes A, Korn O, Valladares H, Gonzalez P, Henríquez A. Gastroesophageal reflux disease after sleeve gastrectomy. Surg Laparosc Endosc Percutan Tech. 2010;20:148–53.
52. Stenard F, Iannelli A. Laparoscopic sleeve gastrectomy and gastroesophageal reflux. World J Gastroenterol. 2015;21(36):10348–57.
53. Parikh M, Gagner M. Laparoscopic hiatal hernia repair and repeat sleeve gastrectomy for gastroesophageal reflux disease after duodenal switch. Surg Obes Relat Dis. 2008;4(1):73–5.
54. Greenstein AJ, Jacob BP. Placement of a laparoscopic adjustable gastric band after failed sleeve gastrectomy. Surg Obes Relat Dis. 2008;4:556–8.
55. Alexander JW, Martin Hawver LR, Goodman HR. Banded sleeve gastrectomy – initial experience. Obes Surg. 2009;19:1591–6.
56. Agarwal S, Dessel EV, Akin F, Cauwenberge SV, Dillemans B. Laparoscopic adjustable banded sleeve gastrectomy as a primary procedure for the super-super obese (body mass index > 60 kg/m^2). Obes Surg. 2010;20(8):1161–3.
57. Karcz WK, Karcz-Socha I, Marjanovic G, et al. To band or not to band—early results of banded sleeve gastrectomy. Obes Surg. 2014;24(4):660–5.
58. Langer FB, Shakeri-Leidenmühler S, Bohdjalian A, Schoppmann S, Zacherl J, et al. Strategies for weight regain after sleeve gastrectomy. Surg Laparosc Endosc Percutan Tech. 2010;20:159–61.
59. Langer FB, et al. Conversion from sleeve gastrectomy to Roux-en-Y gastric bypass—indications and outcome. Obes Surg. 2010;20(7):835–40.
60. Gautier T, Sarcher T, Contival N, Le Roux Y, Alves A. Indications and mid-term results of conversion from sleeve gastrectomy to Roux-en-Y gastric bypass. Obes Surg. 2013;23:212–5.
61. Alexandrou A, Felekouras E, Giannopoulos A, Tsigris C, Diamantis T. What is the actual fate of the super-morbid-obese patients who undergo laparoscopic sleeve gastrectomy as the first step of a two-stage weight-reduction operative strategy? Obes Surg. 2012;22:1623–8.
62. Lee WJ, et al. Gastric bypass vs sleeve gastrectomy for type 2 diabetes mellitus: a randomized controlled trial. Arch Surg. 2011;146(2):143–8.
63. Weiner RA, Theodoridou S, Weiner S. Failure of laparoscopic sleeve gastrectomy- further procedure? Obes Facts. 2011;4(Supple 1):42–6.
64. Zaveri H, Dallal RM, Cottam D, et al. Indications and operative outcomes of gastric bypass reversal. Obes Surg. 2016;26(10):2285–90.
65. Dykstra MA, Switzer NJ, Sherman V, Karmali S, Birch DW. Roux en Y gastric bypass: how and why it fails? Surgery Curr Res. 2014;4:165.
66. van Wezenbeek MR, van Oudheusden TR, de Zoete JPJGM, et al. Conversion to gastric bypass after either failed gastric band or failed sleeve gastrectomy. Obes Surg. 2017;27(1):83–9.
67. Homan J, Betzel B, Aarts EO, van Laarhoven KJ, Janssen IM, Berends FJ. Secondary surgery after sleeve gastrectomy: Roux-en-Y gastric bypass or biliopancreatic diversion with duodenal switch. Surg Obes Relat Dis. 2015;11(4):771–7.
68. Kular KS, Manchanda N, Rutledge R. A 6-year experience with 1,054 mini-gastric bypasses—first study from Indian subcontinent. Obes Surg. 2014;24:1430–5.
69. Rutledge R, Walsh W. Continued excellent results with the mini-gastric bypass: six-year study in 2,410 patients. Obes Surg. 2005;15:1304–8.
70. Musella M, Sousa A, Greco F, De Luca M, Manno E, Di Stefano C, Milone M, Bonfanti R, Segato G, Antonino A, Piazza L. The laparoscopic mini-gastric bypass: the Italian experience: outcomes from 974 consecutive cases in a multi-center review. Surg Endosc. 2014;28:156–63.
71. Georgiadou D, Sergentanis TN, Nixon A, Diamantis T, Tsigris C, Psaltopoulou T. Efficacy and safety of laparoscopic mini-gastric bypass. A systematic review. Surg Obes Relat Dis. 2014;10:984–91.
72. Greco F. Conversion of vertical sleeve gastrectomy to a functional single-anastomosis gastric bypass: technique and preliminary results using a non-adjustable ring instead of stapled division. Obes Surg. 2017;27(4):896–901.
73. Bruzzi M, Voron T, Zinzindohoue F, Berger A, Douard R, Chevallier JM. Revisional single-anastomosis gastric bypass for a failed restrictive procedure: 5-year results. Surg Obes Relat Dis. 2015;25:571.
74. Fobi M, Lee H, Igwe D, Felahy B, James E, Stanczyk M, Fobi N. Band erosion: incidence, etiology, management and outcome after banded vertical gastric bypass. Obes Surg. 2001;11(6):699–707.
75. Moszkowicz D1, Rau C, Guenzi M, Zinzindohoué F, Berger A, Chevallier JM. Laparoscopic omega-loop gastric bypass for the conversion of failed sleeve gastrectomy: early experience. J Visc Surg. 2013;150(6):373–8.
76. Carmeli I, Golomb I, Sadot E, Kashtan H, Keidar A. Laparoscopic conversion of sleeve gastrectomy to a biliopancreatic diversion with duodenal switch or a Roux-en-Y gastric bypass due to weight loss failure: our algorithm. Surg Obes Relat Dis. 2015;11(1):79–85.
77. Iannelli A, Schneck A, Topart P, Carles M, Hébuterne X, Gugenheim J. Laparoscopic sleeve gastrectomy followed by duodenal switch in selected patients versus single-stage duodenal switch for superobesity: case-control study. Surg Obes Relat Dis. 2013;9(4):531–8.

78. Sovik TT, Taha O, Aasheim ET, et al. Randomized clinical trial of laparoscopic gastric bypass versus laparoscopic duodenal switch for superobesity. Brit J Surg. 2010;97:160–6.
79. Prachand VN, DaVee RT, Alverdy JC. Duodenal switch provides superior weight loss in the super-obese (BMI 4 50 kg/m^2) compared to gastric bypass. Ann Surg. 2006;244:611–9.
80. Dolan K, Hatzifotis M, Newbury L, Lowe N, Fielding G. A clinical and nutritional comparison of biliopancreatic diversion with and without duodenal switch. Ann Surg. 2004;240:51–6.
81. Kim J. Position statement on single-anastomosis duodenal switch. Surg Obes Relat Dis. 2016;12:944–5.
82. Sánchez-Pernaute A, Rubio Herrera MA, Pérez-Aguirre E, et al. Proximal duodenal-ileal end-to-side bypass with sleeve gastrectomy: proposed technique. Obes Surg. 2007;17(12):1614–8.
83. Sánchez-Pernaute A, Rubio MA, Pérez-Aguirre E, et al. Single-anastomosis duodenoileal bypass with sleeve gastrectomy: metabolic improvement and weight loss in first 100 patients. Surg Obes Relat Dis. 2013;9(5):731–5.
84. Sánchez-Pernaute A, Rubio MA, Conde M, et al. Single-anastomosis duodenoileal bypass as a second step after sleeve gastrectomy. Surg Obes Relat Dis. 2015;11(2):351–5.
85. Cottam D, Surve A, Zaveri H, Cottam A. SIPS is quickly becoming an option for surgical revision of failed sleeve gastrectomy. Bariatric Times. 2016;13(11 Suppl B):B23–4.
86. Cottam A, Cottam D, Medlin W, et al. A matched cohort analysis of loop duodenal switch versus Roux-en-Y gastric bypass with 18 month follows up. Surg Endosc. 2015;30(9):3958–64.
87. Surve A, Zaveri H, Cottam D, Belnap L, Cottam A, Cottam SA. Retrospective comparison of Roux-en-Y duodenal switch with single anastomosis duodenal switch (SIPS-stomach intestinal pylorus sparing surgery) at a single institution with two year follow-up. Surg Obes Relat Dis. 2017;13(3):415–22.
88. Stenberg E, Szabo E, Ågren G, et al. Closure of mesenteric defects in laparoscopic gastric bypass: a multicentre, randomised, parallel, open-label trial. Lancet. 2016;387(10026):1397–404.

Resleeve Gastrectomy

18

Patrick Noel and Marius Nedelcu

Introduction and History

Laparoscopic sleeve gastrectomy (LSG) has rapidly become a preferred surgical procedure for morbid obesity due to its efficacy and low complication rates, as well as the technical ease of performing it. The past few years have seen significant growth in procedure numbers, and LSG has achieved becoming the most frequently performed bariatric procedure in France in 2011 and in the USA in 2013 [1, 2]. In 2013, 42.815 bariatric procedures were performed in France of which 56% were sleeve gastrectomy. According to the French National Health Insurance Fund, this figure has tripled in 7 years.

This growth can be attributed to the better outcome and quality of life of the sleeve compared to adjustable gastric bands [3], in addition to the several advantages that LSG carries over more complex bariatric procedures, such as LRYGB or DS from a technical standpoint, as well as to the absence of the side effects of bypasses procedures specifically dumping syndrome, marginal ulcers, malabsorption, small bowel obstruction, and internal hernia, and a better quality of life over gastric banding.

P. Noel (✉)
Bariatric Department, Emirates Specialty Hospital, Dubai, UAE

M. Nedelcu
Centre Chirurgical de l'Obesite, Clinique Saint Michel, Toulon, VAR, France

The rising numbers of LSG procedures now being performed (France: 480 cases in 2005 vs. 13,557 cases in 2011 and 23,976 in 2013, up to 56% of all bariatric procedure) will likely be followed by increasing numbers of patients who will experience weight loss failure (insufficient weight loss or weight regain) or will develop certain complications, such as gastroesophageal reflux disease (GERD), and will seek conversion to another bariatric procedure. A second intervention, such as revisional sleeve gastrectomy (ReSG) [4–9], LRYGB [10], or biliopancreatic diversion with DS (BPD-DS) [11–13] can be proposed for inadequate weight loss or weight regain. Single-anastomosis duodenoileal (SADI) bypass with sleeve gastrectomy represents a new alternative to standard DS, but limited results are present in the literature [14], and this new bariatric procedure must be validated over time (this procedure is discussed in detail in another chapter).

Regardless of the revisional surgery of choice, it is also necessary to know the reasons for failure or suboptimal outcome. Behavioral and dietary reasons should be ruled out before deciding to take patients for a higher-risk revisional surgery.

The concept of the resleeve (ReSG) was introduced back in 2003 by Gagner [4] for a patient with poor weight loss after biliopancreatic diversion with duodenal switch. Later on, Baltasar et al. [5] have reported two patients who underwent a resleeve. A complete review of the literature is summarized in Table 18.1. Up until now,

R. Lutfi et al. (eds.), *Global Bariatric Surgery*, https://doi.org/10.1007/978-3-319-93545-4_18

the largest resleeve series [6] of patients included 61 patients, but no long-term results regarding the follow-up are available. This chapter will present the preliminary results of a 5-year follow-up along with the decisional algorithm of treatment for revisional surgery following LSG.

Indication and Algorithm

In our experience, the requirements for revisional surgery were insufficient weight loss at 18 months after the surgery (<50% of excess weight loss [EWL]) and progressive weight regain after an initial successful weight loss (defined as EWL >50%) or symptomatic GERD (persistent heartburn despite maximum proton-pump inhibitor [PPI] treatment with mild esophagitis on upper endoscopy). A multidisciplinary team that includes a nutritionist, endocrinologist, psychologist, and surgeon routinely evaluates each patient according to a standardized protocol. Only patients cleared by the psychologist and dietitian ruling out compliance, behavioral, and dietary reasons for failure are considered for the standard algorithm for revisional bariatric procedure (Fig. 18.1). ReSG is proposed as a revisional strategy if the barium swallow shows an upper gastric pouch dilatation, a large, unresected fundus, or severe universal dilation. If the barium swallow test is negative for the upper-part sleeve dilatation or inconclusive, a CT scan volumetry is obtained. The residual gastric volume is measured by filling the gastric remnant with carbon dioxide, as follows: The patient is given a sodium bicarbonate solution (4 g in 10 cl of water) to drink, followed by a tartaric acid solution (4 g in 10 cl of water). Following the tartaric acid intake, low-dose CT acquisitions are made at 30 and 60 s. Volume is measured using Myrian® software (Microsoft Inc., Redwood City, CA, USA) and expressed in cubic centimeters (cc).

If the volumetry exceeds 250 cc, ReSG is considered. If it is less than 250 cc, resleeve is not offered as an option for revision, and the presence of GERD is investigated. Depending on whether pathologic reflux is diagnosed, in addition to many patients-related factors (such as compliance, employment, support), a decision

Table 18.1 Literature review for ReSG

Author	Journal	Cases	Morbidity (%)
Gagner and Rogula	Obes Surg (2003)	First	0
Baltasar	Obes Surg (2006)	2	0
Himpens	SOARD (2011)	7	1 leak (14.3%)
Verhaeghe	Obes Surg(2012)	15	2 leaks (13.3%)
Iannelli	Obes Surg (2011)	13	0

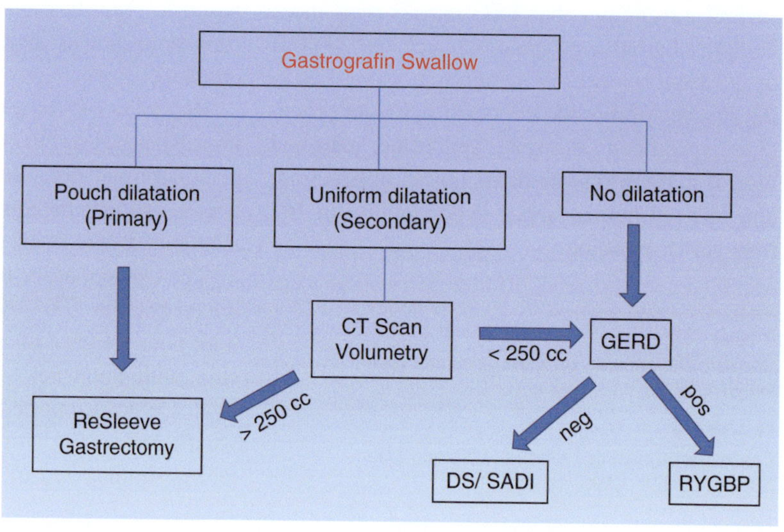

Fig. 18.1 Algorithm of treatment for revisional surgery following LSG

is made to proceed with either gastric bypass or duodenal switch.

Sleeve dilatation is classified as primary or secondary. Primary dilation is defined as an upper posterior gastric pouch incompletely dissected during the initial procedure due to the learning curve or the difficult nature of the cases (super-super obesity) with poor posterior exposure and incomplete visualization of the left crus (Fig. 18.2). A secondary dilation is defined as a homogeneous dilated gastric tube of more than 250 mL in volume in the CT scan volumetry, usually seen later during follow-up. The mechanisms involved are the narrowing of the gastric incisura during the primary operation with consequent upstream dilation of the sleeve, the natural history of LSG, the use of a large calibration bougie, a patient's eating habits, a planned second procedure, or a combination of these mechanisms (Fig. 18.3).

Surgical Technique

The pneumoperitoneum is created using a Veress needle inserted in the left hypochondrium. Only three trocars were used. The initial LSG was performed in a similar manner with a three-port approach [15]. Any intraperitoneal attachment between the left lobe of the liver and the anterior gastric surface was carefully dissected. The greater curvature was dissected next to expose the previous staple line. All adhesions between the stomach and the pancreas were divided, taking care not to injure the splenic artery. Once the mobilization of the stomach was completed, the anesthesiologist inserted a 37F orogastric bougie (we prefer the MIDSLEEVE®) to reach the pylorus and different applications of a linear stapler 60–4.1 mm were fired. A methylene blue test was performed. A non-systematic drain was left in place along the staple line only for difficult cases. Nasogastric (NG) tubes were not used in the postoperative period.

A complete detailed video that illustrates all the technical aspects of this procedure can be found at [16]:

http://www.soard.org/article/S1550-7289(13)00183-4/fulltext#mmc1

The most important technical detail during ReSG, similarly to primary LSG, is to avoid stenosis at the level of the incisura angularis.

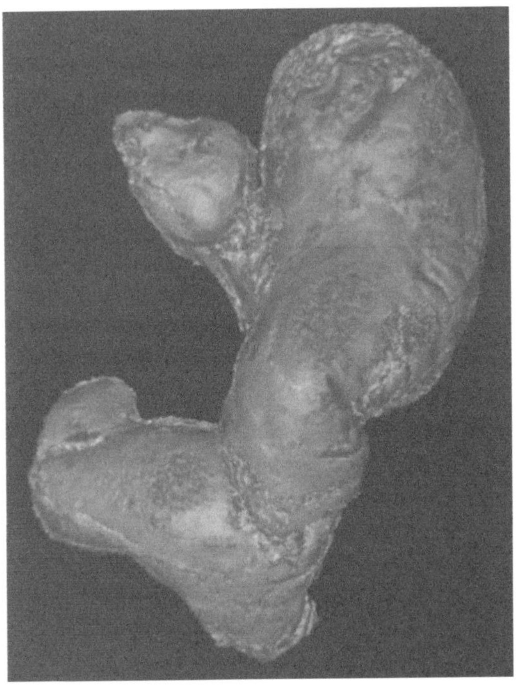

Fig. 18.2 Primary dilatation (pouch)

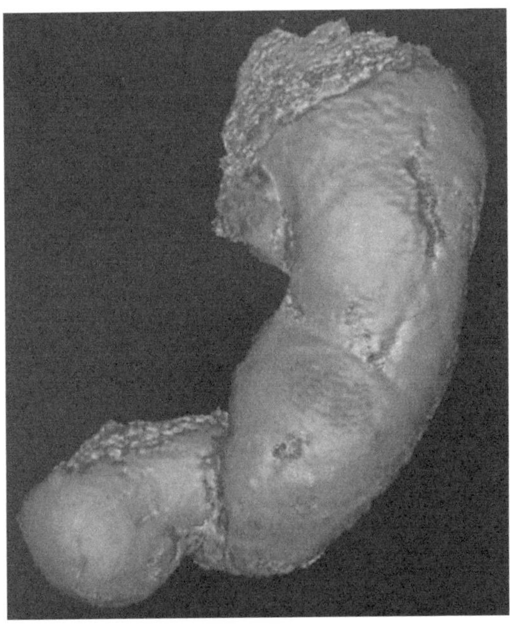

Fig. 18.3 Secondary dilatation

During the primary procedure, the first two staplers must be carefully fired in order to avoid a twist at the incisura.

For ReSG with primary dilatation (pouch), the resection of the stomach at the level of the incisura should be avoided, and the new staple line should start proximal to the incisura angularis. At the beginning of our experience, in an attempt to further reduce the diameter of the stomach, a complete sectioning was performed. At that time, we recorded up to 4% of stenosis at the level of the incisura angularis. Since we limited the resection in primary dilation to the gastric pouch, no such complication was recorded.

Another technical tip is represented by the placement of the ports, which are slightly displaced toward the left hypochondrium. The posterior approach is regularly used, and the placement of the optical port to the left side of the midline will facilitate the exposure of the posterior part of the stomach where the dilated pouch is always found.

Results and Personal Experience

Seventy patients (63 women, 7 men; mean age 40.7 years), with an average body mass index (BMI) of 39.4 kg/m^2 (+/− 1.32), undergoing ReSG in our department were enrolled in the current study. Twenty-eight patients (40%) had their original LSG surgery performed at another hospital and were subsequently referred for weight loss failure. The remaining 42 patients' primary procedures were performed in our department.

Prior to the primary LSG, 44 patients (62.8%) out of 70 had already had a laparoscopic adjustable gastric banding (LAGB) with weight loss failure. Six patients had multiple gastric band procedures for technical failures. Twenty-two patients (31.4 %) were super obese (BMI >50 kg/m^2) before LSG, and 5 patients (7.1%) were super-super obese (BMI >60 kg/m^2).

The median BMI prior to the SG was 46.2 kg/m^2 (+/− 1.29; range 35.4–77.9). After the initial LSG, a median BMI of 39.4 kg/m^2 (+/− 1.43; range 21.9–48.2) was achieved. Revision was performed after a median period of 37.4 months (range 9–80 months).

The indications for ReSG were insufficient weight loss for 36 patients (51,4%), weight regain for 34 patients (48.6%), and symptomatic GERD for 4 patients (5.7%).

The analysis of the barium swallow showed primary dilatation (upper gastric pouch) in 51 cases, and in the remaining 19 cases, the radiological findings were compatible with a secondary dilatation (gastric tube dilatation). The CT scan volumetry (38 cases) revealed a mean gastric volume of 436.3 cc (range 275–1056 cc).

All cases were completed by laparoscopy with no intraoperative complications. The mean operative time was 39 min (range = 29–70 min), and the mean hospital stay was 3.5 days (range = 3–16 days). In the immediate postoperative period, one complication was recorded—patient #12 developed a perigastric hematoma identified by CT scan with vomiting on postoperative day (POD) 2. An endoscopic stent was inserted, and the patient was discharged on liquid diet. At 4 weeks, the CT scan and upper endoscopy were normal, and the stent was removed.

In two other cases (patients 39 and 51) at 1 and 2 weeks postoperative, respectively, the patients developed progressive dysphagia. An upper endoscopy revealed the same finding—a stenosis of the midpart of the gastric sleeve—and the decision of stent deployment was made in both cases. In one case, the stenosis was rectified/cured after 4 weeks when the stent was removed. The other patient needed two additional endoscopic pneumatic dilatation sessions of the stenosis. The procedure was performed with an achalasia balloon (Rigiflex® balloon 30–35 mm) over a stainless steel or super stiff guidewire with stepwise increments in dilation pressure from 15 to 25 psi. Inflating the balloon under radiological guidance enables correction of the axis of the gastric tube. To be efficient, the treatment must be aggressive, and in our experience, we have not had any cases of iatrogenic staple line disruption.

Five-Year Results

Thirteen patients (12 women; mean age—41.6 years) with a BMI of 39.1 kg/m^2 underwent ReSG between October 2008 and June 2011. The mean interval time from the primary LSG to the ReSG was of 29.6 months (11–67 months). The indication for ReSG was insufficient weight loss for eight patients (61.5%), weight regain for four patients (30.7%), and gastroesophageal reflux disease (GERD) for one patient. In nine cases, the Gastrografin swallow results were interpreted as primary dilatation and in the remaining four cases as secondary dilatation. One patient died from a gynecological cancer. Of the remainder, one patient underwent a SADI at 33 months after ReSG for a BMI of 39.2, and one patient underwent ReSG for reflux. The rest of the ten patients had available data at 5-year follow-up. The mean excess weight loss (EWL) was 58.2% (range 3.3–100%). Of the ten patients, seven patients had >50% EWL at 5 years. All the three patients with failure of EWL (<50%) were the first three cases of our series, and two out of them had secondary dilatation. All cases were completed by laparoscopy with no intraoperative incidents. One case of gastric stenosis was recorded. No other complications or mortality were recorded.

Discussions and Literature

LSG is considered to be a technically straightforward procedure, but the surgical technique is one of the major determinants of the success of this procedure, to reduce the complication rate and to improve the long-term results. The removal of the entire gastric fundus is a key point emphasized by many bariatric surgeons and probably misunderstood at the beginning of the procedure. The left crus of the diaphragm must systematically be visualized. Our technique includes the following particularity regarding the removal of the gastric fundus. The posterior aspect of the fundus is grasped repeatedly with a forceps operated by the right hand, while the left hand releases the stapler and pulls laterally before the stapler is definitively clamped and fired [15]. The technical aspect can be incriminated in the mechanism of weight regain after LSG, but other causes are also important to be considered: nutritional noncompliance, hormonal/metabolic imbalance, mental health, and physical inactivity [17].

Recent studies comparing LSG to LRYGB show equal efficacy of both procedures in terms of weight loss and improvement of comorbidities [18–21]. As bariatric procedures are performed more frequently, the number of revisions will also rise. The need for a specific definition of weight regain and a clear algorithm is more than obvious in these cases. We found that the best way to approach these patients is to first fully assess their history and then to assess their BMI and their alimentary habits. All patients with a history suggestive of maladaptive eating disorders because of their bariatric surgery underwent further psychological evaluation and were treated prior to consideration for surgical revision. The next step was to document their anatomy with a barium swallow to look for evidence of primary or secondary dilatation of the gastric sleeve. For nonconclusive results on upper GI series, a volumetric CT scan was done.

Revisional bariatric surgery after LSG is becoming more common due to the rapid increase of patients undergoing this procedure as treatment for morbid obesity. The problem of the insufficient weight loss and weight regain after LSG is an issue as for other bariatric procedures. Possible explanations for LSG failure include the following: dilatation of the residual stomach, calibration of the stomach with an excessively large gastric bougie [22], and incomplete resection of the gastric fundus (where ghrelin is secreted) [23].

For the LSG, the risk of dilatation in time with weight loss failure was a constant source of debate. Facing 51 patients with primary dilatation (upper gastric pouch), this question came up rapidly among the authors: *Has this part of the stomach undergone secondary dilatation or was it incompletely dissected from the beginning?* The answer remains unknown. With the development of CT scan gastric volumetry, it will be easier to differentiate between secondary and primary dilation, as it provides useful details such as the position of the staple line and the 3D shape of the upper stomach.

Braghetto et al. [24] reported data on 15 LSG patients undergoing CT scan gastric volumetry on POD 3 and, repeatedly, at 24–36 months after surgery; they found that the mean gastric volume

Table 18.2 Long-term results after LSG

Author/year	Number of patients	Rate follow-up (years)	Mean EWL
Himpens/2010 [27]	30	78% (6 years)	53.3%
Rawlins/2012 [28]	49	100% (5 years)	86%
Braghetto/2012 [29]	60	11% (5 years)	57.3%
Catheline/2013 [30]	45	82% (5 years)	50.7%
Eid/2012 [31]	21	93% (8 years)	46%
Peterli/ 2013 [32]	54	91% (5 years)	57.4%
Noel—current series	99	70.7% (8 years)	71.6%

had increased from 108 to 250 mL. None of these patients experienced weight regain, and the authors concluded that the gastric capacity increased after LSG sleeve gastrectomy even when a narrow gastric tubulization was performed.

They concluded that despite enlargement with time, weight loss remained stable. This conclusion about the absence of correlation between volume increase and weight regain must be interpreted cautiously as their follow-up was limited to 3 years, while weight regain in enlarged sleeve tends to happen at 3–5 years post-op (Table 18.2).

Langer et al. [25] prospectively studied 23 patients (15 morbidly obese, 8 super obese) via UGI contrast studies and found that the dilation occurred in only 1 patient, while weight regain after initial successful weight loss occurred in 3 more patients, at a mean follow-up time of 20 months. Also in our experience, we see many patients with negative UGI studies for dilatation and CT scan volumetry <250 cc who have weight regain.

Yehoshua et al. [26] investigated the role of the intraluminal pressure in the process of dilation of the gastric tube. The preoperative mean volume of the entire stomach was 1 553 cc (600–2000 cc) and that of the sleeved stomach 129 cc (90–220 cc). Results showed that the sleeve has a higher mean pressure of 43 mmHg when filled with saline (range = 32–58 mmHg) compared to the removed stomach that had a mean pressure of 26 mmHg (range = 12–47 mmHg). The study concluded that the notably higher pressure in the sleeve reflects its markedly lesser distensibility compared to that of the whole stomach and that of the removed fundus.

The literature data is sparse regarding long-term follow-up after LSG, and the results illustrated in the Table 18.2 are highly variable. Himpens et al. [27] reported 3-year follow-up %EWL of 77.5% and a 6-year %EWL of 53.3% after LSG. They concluded that weight regain and de novo GERD symptoms (21%) appear between the third and the sixth postoperative year. In our opinion, undissected fundus or upper gastric dilatation explain many of the failures. We must mention that this study was conducted on patients operated between November 2001 and October 2002 early in the learning curve for LSG when limited left crus exposure and incomplete posterior fundus dissection were common.

Unfortunately, there is a paucity of significant data to help the surgeon decide which revisional procedure to choose in case of weight loss failure after LSG. Nonetheless, most bariatric centers advocate LRYGB as standard revisional procedure despite no long-term follow-up data and no convincing results [33]. DS (duodenal switch) or the more recent SADI (single-anastomosis duodeno-ileostomy) represents other promising options for sleeve revisions because of the superior weight loss seen with the DS when compared to other bariatric procedures.

The ReSG has already been described as a revision of LSG/DS itself. Although the operation seems to be technically easier, without conversions and acceptable complication rates, the follow-up was too short to conclude on its efficiency (Table 18.2). To date, no prospective trial has been done to adequately determine which revisional bariatric procedure should be carried out in the setting of inadequate weight loss or excessive weight regain after LSG. Considering our results and the data available in the literature, a new algorithm has defined our activity [34]. A staged approach of morbid obese patient must be considered when a LSG is proposed first. In case of weight regain, associated or not with comorbidities recurrence, multiple options are possible and future treatment must be adjusted to patient's compliance. In case of weight regain associated with pouch dilatation and no recurrence of comorbidities, a ReSG could be proposed with good results. In case of comorbidities recurrence with acceptable follow-up after the primary procedure, a SADI can be proposed. The RYGBP represents another option especially for patients with GERD. In our experience, SADI is preferred to RYGBP, because the effect of the duodenal switch on T2D remains present 20 years later in >90% of patients, as reported by Marceau et al [35]

In our opinion, the weight loss after both ReSG and primary LSG depends on the learning curve and is technically dependent. For primary LSG, the incomplete removal of the gastric fundus seems to be the most valid hypothesis for weight regain. In some cases of incomplete removal of the fundus, a small unrecognized hiatal hernia may be associated. A transthoracic stomach may be missed while performing LSG in the presence of a hiatal hernia. Intraoperative exploration of the esophageal hiatus is advised whenever a hiatal hernia is suspected. That should prevent a missed undissected fundus as per Basso [36]. To avoid unnecessary dissection, Heacock et al. [37] attempted to improve the preoperative diagnostic accuracy of hiatal hernia by using right anterior oblique (RAO) esophagogram technique rather than the commonly used upright technique. He compared the two techniques by analyzing a total of 388 patients who underwent preoperative esophagograms (69 upright, 388 RAO). Routine upright esophagogram had sensitivity of 50% and specificity of 97%, while ROA had a higher sensitivity of 70% with 77% specificity.

The undissected fundus is a risk factor for GERD, and the ReSG with hiatal hernia repair represents a valid treatment option as shown by Parikh and Gagner [38]. In our experience reported earlier, we had four patients who had complete remission of the reflux symptomatology after ReSG.

Sillechia et al. [39] reported good results in terms of GERD symptoms control after ReSG for 19 cases of a residual fundus/neofundus. Literature data on the effect of LSG for GERD are contradictory. Petersen et al. [40] have reported on 37 patients who underwent LSG showing significant increase in lower esophageal sphincter pressure after surgery, independently of the weight loss. The preoperative stationary esophageal manometry of the lower sphincter showed a preoperative pressure of 11 mmHg, increasing significantly to 24 mm Hg postoperatively.

Compared to the malabsorptive procedures, ReSG offers several advantages, including shorter operative time, regain of the early postoperative restriction, avoidance of dumping syndrome, and the different conditions resulting from malabsorption such as anemia, osteoporosis, and protein and vitamin deficiency (except B12 and thiamine level).

Conclusions

ReSG is a feasible and safe surgical approach for weight regain post-LSG and is best applied when the gastric pouch is too large after the original LSG. In the long-term, this dilatation may be responsible of weight regain, weight loss insufficiency, or GERD. Five years postoperatively, the ReSG as a definitive bariatric procedure remained effective in over half of the patients (58.3%). The results appear to be particularly more favorable for the non-super obese patients and for primary dilatation. ReSG is a generally well-tolerated procedure with low rate of long-term complications. Further prospective clinical trials are required to compare the outcomes of ReSG with those of LRYGB or DS for weight loss failure after LSG.

Take-Home Message

1. In case of primary dilatation, only the gastric fundus should be removed to avoid stenosis at the level of incisura angularis.
2. ReSG can be proposed for GERD based on the dynamic aspect of UGI studies.
3. A good selection for ReSG (mostly with primary dilatation) to improve the long-term results.
4. The urgency for a standardized weight regain definition.
5. New decisional algorithm for revisional surgery.
6. A careful evaluation of comorbidities recurrence is important in the decisional process.

References

1. Lazzati A, Guy-Lachuer R, Delaunay V, Szwarcensztein K, Azoulay D. Bariatric surgery trends in France: 2005–2011. Surg Obes Relat Dis. 2014;10(2):328–34.
2. Buchwald H, Oien DM. Metabolic/bariatric surgery worldwide 2011. Obes Surg. 2013;23(4):427–36.
3. Fezzi M, Kolotkin RL, Nedelcu M, et al. Improvement in quality of life after laparoscopic sleeve gastrectomy. Obes Surg. 2011;21(8):1161–7.
4. Gagner M, Rogula T. Laparoscopic reoperative sleeve gastrectomy for poor weight loss after biliopancreatic diversion with duodenal switch. Obes Surg. 2003;13:649–54.
5. Baltasar A, Serra C, Pérez N, Bou R, Bengochea M. Re-sleeve gastrectomy. Obes Surg. 2006;16:1535–8.
6. Nedelcu M, Noel P, Iannelli A, Gagner M. Revised sleeve gastrectomy (re-sleeve). Surg Obes Relat Dis. 2015;11(6):1282–8.
7. Dapri G, Cadière GB, Himpens J. Laparoscopic repeat sleeve gastrectomy versus duodenal switch after isolated sleeve gastrectomy for obesity. Surg Obes Relat Dis. 2011;7(1):38–43.
8. Iannelli A, Schneck AS, Noel P, Ben Amor I, Krawczykowski D, Gugenheim J. Re-sleeve gastrectomy for failed laparoscopic sleeve gastrectomy: a feasibility study. Obes Surg. 2011;21(7):832–5.
9. Rebibo L, Fuks D, Verhaeghe P, Deguines JB, Dhahri A, Regimbeau JM. Repeat sleeve gastrectomy compared with primary sleeve gastrectomy: a single-center, matched case study. Obes Surg. 2012;22(12):1909–15.
10. Regan JP, Inabnet WB, Gagner M, Pomp A. Early experience with two-staged laparoscopic Roux-en-Y gastric bypass as an alternative in the super-super obese patient. Obes Surg. 2003;13:861–4.
11. Iannelli A, Schneck AS, Topart P, Carles M, Hébuterne X, Gugenheim J. Laparoscopic sleeve gastrectomy followed by duodenal switch in selected patients versus single-stage duodenal switch for superobesity: case-control study. Surg Obes Relat Dis. 2013;9(4):531–8.
12. Gumbs AA, Pomp A, Gagner M. Revisional bariatric surgery for inadequate weight loss. Obes Surg. 2007;17:1137–45.
13. Gagner M, Boza C. Laparoscopic duodenal switch for morbid obesity. Expert Rev Med Devices. 2006;3:105–12.
14. Sánchez-Pernaute A, Rubio MÁ, Pérez Aguirre E, Barabash A, Cabrerizo L, Torres A. Single-anastomosis duodenoileal bypass with sleeve gastrectomy: metabolic improvement and weight loss in first 100 patients. Surg Obes Relat Dis. 2013;9(5):731–5.
15. Nedelcu M, Eddbali I, Noel P. Three-port sleeve gastrectomy: complete posterior approach. Surg Obes Relat Dis. 2016;12:925.
16. Noel P, Nedelcu M, Nocca D. The revised sleeve gastrectomy, technical considerations. Surg Obes Relat Dis. 2013;9(6):1029–32.
17. Karmali S, Brar B, Shi X, Sharma AM, de Gara C, Birch DW. Weight recidivism post-bariatric surgery: a systematic review. Obes Surg. 2013;23(11):1922–33.
18. Karamanakos SN, Vagenas K, Kalfarentzos F. Weight loss, appetite suppression, and changes in fasting and postprandial ghrelin and peptide-YY levels after Roux-en-Y gastric bypass and sleeve gastrectomy: a prospective, double blind study. Ann Surg. 2008;247(3):401–7.
19. Peterli R, Borbély Y, Kern B, Gass M, Peters T, Thurnheer M, Schultes B, Laederach K, Bueter M, Schiesser M. Early results of the Swiss Multicentre Bypass or Sleeve Study (SM-BOSS): a prospective randomized trial comparing laparoscopic sleeve gastrectomy and Roux-en-Y gastric bypass. Ann Surg. 2013;258(5):690–4.
20. Kehagias I, Karamanakos SN, Argentou M, et al. Randomized clinical trial of laparoscopic Roux-en-Y gastric bypass versus laparoscopic sleeve gastrectomy for the management of patients with BMI<50 kg/m^2. Obes Surg. 2011;21(11):1650–6.
21. Leyba JL, Aulestia SN, Llopis SN. Laparoscopic Roux-en-Y gastric bypass versus laparoscopic sleeve gastrectomy for the treatment of morbid obesity. A prospective study of 117 patients. Obes Surg. 2011;21(2):212–6.
22. Weiner RA, Weiner S, Pomhoff I, et al. Laparoscopic sleeve gastrectomy—influence of sleeve size and 120 resected gastric volume. Obes Surg. 2007;17:1297–305.
23. Lin E, Gletsu N, Fugate K, et al. The effects of gastric surgery on systemic ghrelin levels in the morbidly obese. Arch Surg. 2004;139:780–4.
24. Braghetto I, Cortes C, Herquiñigo D, et al. Evaluation of the radiological gastric capacity and evolution of the BMI 2–3 years after sleeve gastrectomy. Obes Surg. 2009;19:1262–9.
25. Langer FB, Bohdjalian A, Falbervawer FX, et al. Does gastric dilatation limit the success of sleeve gastrectomy as a sole operation for morbid obesity? Obes Surg. 2006;16:166–71.
26. Yehoshua RT, Eidelman LA, Stein M, et al. Laparoscopic sleeve gastrectomy—volume and pressure assessment. Obes Surg. 2008;18:1083–8.
27. Himpens J, Dobbeleir J, Peeters G. Long-term results of laparoscopic sleeve gastrectomy for obesity. Ann Surg. 2010;252(2):319–24.
28. Rawlins L, Rawlins MP, Brown CC, Schumacher DL. Sleeve gastrectomy: 5-year outcomes of a single institution. Surg Obes Relat Dis. 2013;9(1):21–5.
29. Braghetto I, Csendes A, Lanzarini E, Papapietro K, Cárcamo C, Molina JC. Is laparoscopic sleeve gastrectomy an acceptable primary bariatric procedure in obese patients? Early and 5-year postoperative results. Surg Laparosc Endosc Percutan Tech. 2012;22(6):479–86.
30. Catheline JM, Fysekidis M, Bachner I, Bihan H, Kassem A, Dbouk R, Bdeoui N, Boschetto A, Cohen R. Five-year results of sleeve gastrectomy. J Visc Surg. 2013;150(5):307–12.

31. Eid GM, Brethauer S, Mattar SG, Titchner RL, Gourash W, Schauer PR. Laparoscopic sleeve gastrectomy for super obese patients: forty-eight percent excess weight loss after 6 to 8 years with 93% follow-up. Ann Surg. 2012;256(2):262–5.
32. Sieber P, Gass M, Kern B, Peters T, Slawik M, Peterli R. Five-year results of laparoscopic sleeve gastrectomy. Surg Obes Relat Dis. 2014;10(2):243–9.
33. Carmeli I, Golomb I, Sadot E, Kashtan H, Keidar A. Laparoscopic conversion of sleeve gastrectomy to a biliopancreatic diversion with duodenal switch or a Roux-en-Y gastric bypass due to weight loss failure: our algorithm. Surg Obes Relat Dis. 2015;11(1):79–85.
34. Noel P, Nedelcu M, Gagner M. Impact of the surgical experience on leak rate after laparoscopic sleeve gastrectomy. Obes Surg. 2016;26(8):1782–7.
35. Marceau P, Biron S, Marceau S, Hould FS, Lebel S, Lescelleur O, Biertho L, Simard S, Kral JG. Long-term metabolic outcomes 5 to 20 years after biliopancreatic diversion. Obes Surg. 2015;25(9):1584–93.
36. Soricelli E, Iossa A, Casella G, Abbatini F, Calì B, Basso N. Sleeve gastrectomy and crural repair in obese patients with gastroesophageal reflux disease and/or hiatal hernia. Surg Obes Relat Dis. 2013;9(3):356–61.
37. Heacock L, Parikh M, Jain R, Balthazar E, Hindman N. Improving the diagnostic accuracy of hiatal hernia in patients undergoing bariatric surgery. Obes Surg. 2012;22(11):1730–3.
38. Parikh M, Gagner M. Laparoscopic hiatal hernia repair and repeat sleeve gastrectomy for gastroesophageal reflux disease after duodenal switch. Surg Obes Relat Dis. 2008;4(1):73–5.
39. Silecchia G, De Angelis F, Rizzello M, Albanese A, Longo F, Foletto M. Residual fundus or neofundus after laparoscopic sleeve gastrectomy: is fundectomy safe and effective as revision surgery. Surg Endosc. 2015;29(10):2899–903.
40. Petersen WV, Meile T, Küper MA, Zdichavsky M, Königsrainer A, Schneider JH. Functional importance of laparoscopic sleeve gastrectomy for the lower esophageal sphincter in patients with morbid obesity. Obes Surg. 2012;22(3):360–6.

Part VI

Complications and Adverse Outcomes

19 Complications of Gastric Bands

Bradley F. Schwack, Christine Ren Fielding, and Jaime Ponce

Abbreviations

%EWL	Excess weight lost
LAGB	Laparoscopic adjustable gastric banding

Introduction

Laparoscopic adjustable gastric banding (LAGB) is a restrictive bariatric operation. The procedure involves the placement of a gastric band around the upper part of the stomach, just below the gastroesophageal junction. This device is adjustable, and the procedure is devoid of any resection—no staples used at all. The procedure is unique in the fact that it requires strict follow-up with subsequent "fills" of the band in order to attain the proper level of satiety. These fills are performed in the office with a non-coring Huber needle. A patient's success with a LAGB is directly proportional to the patient's ability to follow up and the surgeon's availability to provide such follow-up.

The LAGB is a safe option in the world of bariatric surgery. The weight loss is a bit slower and a bit less dramatic than seen with the other restrictive procedures. Nevertheless, with proper follow-up, one can expect a weight loss of 0.5–1 kg a week over a 1.5–3 year period. With proper care and follow-up, a LAGB patient can successfully lose 40–55% excess weight (%EWL). There are many studies assessing long-term outcomes of the band. The results of the studies are quite varied—ranging from 25% to 70% EWL [1]. Overall, LAGB can provide a patient nearly 50% EWL—results comparable to the more aggressive stapled bariatric procedures.

Anyone who has ever taken care of a bariatric surgery patient can attest that no operation is devoid of its unique complications and pitfalls. Benefits of the gastric band lie in the fact that there is no permanent alteration to the gastrointestinal anatomy, as there are no anastomoses, no staple lines, and no creation of defects in the enteric mesentery. However, as this is an implantable device, complications are related to the device itself and its relationship to the gastric anatomy.

This is a discussion of the most common gastric band complications with modalities of managing these issues. The most common complications are gastric band "slippage" (gastric prolapse), gastric band erosion, pouch dilation, and gastric band access port and tubing problems.

B. F. Schwack (✉)
Department of Surgery, New York University School of Medicine – NYU Langone Medical Center, New York, NY, USA
e-mail: bradley.schwack@nyumc.org

C. R. Fielding
Department of Surgery, NYU School of Medicine, New York, NY, USA
e-mail: Christine.ren-fielding@nyumc.org

J. Ponce
CHI Memorial Hospital, Chattanooga, TN, USA

R. Lutfi et al. (eds.), *Global Bariatric Surgery*, https://doi.org/10.1007/978-3-319-93545-4_19

The data regarding frequency of such complications is quite varied. The reason for this is multifactorial. First of all, since about 2006 a more modern version of the gastric band has been the predominate device in use. Furthermore, in the last decade and a half, there has been a transition from a perigastric to a *pars flaccida* technique for LAGB placement. This evolution has permitted a significant reduction in the number of gastric band prolapses.

The rates of gastric band prolapse (resulting in subsequent operative intervention) currently range from about 1.8% to 6.2%. Furthermore, the number of gastric band erosions range, historically, from 0% to 7%. Pouch dilation, as a major complication, occurs approximately 1.7–5.1% of the time [2, 3]. In 2013, Paul O'Brien assessed 15 years of gastric band data. His work showed a significant decrease in the number of complications with the evolution toward the modern gastric band being placed by the *pars flaccida* technique. Looking at data since this evolution, gastric band revisional surgery for "pouch enlargement" above the band itself (slips/operative pouch dilations) was 6.4%. The rate of gastric band erosion was noted to be 0.8% with the modern technique. Port and tubing complications were noted to occur in approximately 5.9% of patients. Overall, since the modern technique and device have been used since 2006 in Australia, he described a 2.2% rate of band explanation [4]. Rates of explanation are variable based on surgeon, reasons for explanation, region, and type of band and technique used.

Overall, the gastric band is a very safe and effective procedure for weight loss. Nevertheless, there are varying reports on the rate of complications. Regardless of any controversy, it is important to understand how to diagnose and manage these issues so that a patient can go on to be healthy and have success with their chosen bariatric procedure.

Band Slippage (Gastric Prolapse)

The most common complication described related to the gastric band is slippage—also known as gastric prolapse. Slippage occurs when part of the stomach, most often the fundus or the greater curvature, abnormally migrates through the gastric band (Fig. 19.1).

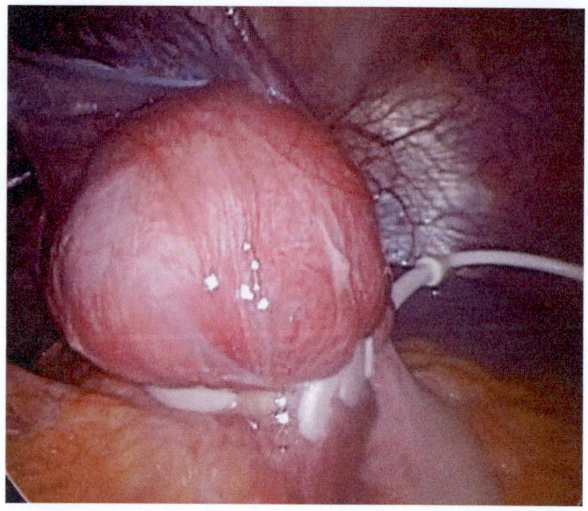

Fig. 19.1 Operative image of gastric prolapse

Clinical Presentation

A patient who is experiencing a band slippage often presents with vomiting and reflux symptoms. They often become intolerant to solid foods and, in more severe cases, to liquids as well. This can result in dehydration. In the most severe cases, patients experience severe abdominal pain (peritonitis) related to ischemia and eventual necrosis of the herniated portion of the stomach. When a slippage occurs, there is an excess of gastric tissue cephalad to the band. Unexpectedly, this condition can result in weight gain at times because this larger pouch allows more receptive relaxation, decreases the sensation of satiety, and allows more food to be consumed.

Pathophysiology

The main cause of gastric prolapse is excessive gagging or vomiting. The retro-propulsion of the stomach during subsequent fits of vomiting causes these more caudal aspects of the stomach to herniate upward through the gastric band. As this herniation occurs, the device itself migrates caudally on the stomach—thus giving the description of a "slip." This results in a greater amount of gastric tissue above the band.

When performing the LAGB procedure, a gastrogastric plication (suturing distal fundus to the gastric pouch over the band itself) is performed to keep the band in its appropriate orientation and to avoid this complication. More often than not, band slippage is the result of patient noncompliance—overeating to the point of vomiting. Either from a failed gastrogastric plication or due to excessive emesis breaking down this plication, the plication breaks down, and the stomach more easily herniates. As this prolapse occurs, there is now a preferred pathway for food to travel into the growing pouch instead of down through the gastric band itself. When a slippage occurs due to the above-described mechanism, it can be anatomically described as an anterior gastric prolapse.

Today, the LAGB is placed via the *pars flaccida* technique—the retrogastric tunnel is created at the level of the confluence of the crura through an avascular plane approximately 2 cm below the gastroesophageal junction. However, the older, perigastric technique involved the placement of the gastric band through a lower retrogastric tunnel with a wider dissection plane which often went below the confluence of the crura with frequent breaching of the lesser sac. In bands placed via the perigastric technique, the posterior wall of the stomach had a tendency to herniate through the band during episodes of emesis. Such a herniation was known as a posterior gastric prolapse. This presented in a similar manner. However, with most LAGB placement performed via the *pars flaccida* technique over the past decade and a half, this complication is mainly of historical significance.

Diagnosis

Band slippage is best diagnosed with an esophogram—a limited upper gastrointestinal swallow study assessing the area of the distal esophagus and upper stomach. Esophogram findings include the visualization of excess stomach cephalad to the band, often hanging over the band itself (Fig. 19.2). Furthermore, the band loses its normal diagonal (approximately 45°) orientation and becomes horizontal in orientation. Often, one can make out the circular shape of the band itself ("O" sign) on an esophogram with a large slippage. As the slippage becomes more severe, there can be failure of oral contrast to pass distal to the band itself—resulting in an apparent gastric outlet obstruction.

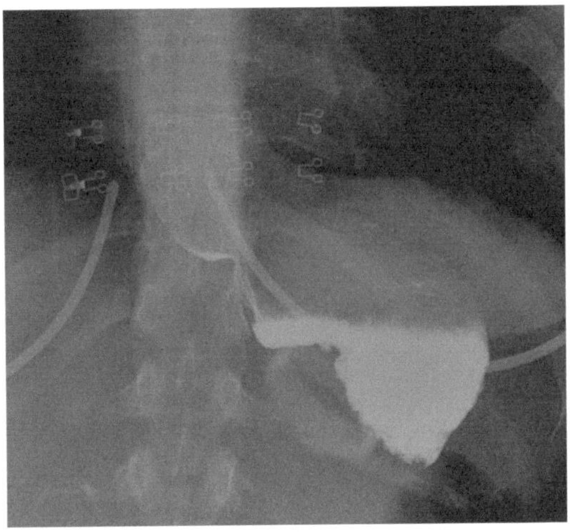

Fig. 19.2 Esophogram of a gastric prolapse (anterior)

Treatment

The first step in treating a symptomatic gastric band slippage is to remove all of the fluid from the gastric band reservoir using a Huber needle. This will alleviate symptoms of gastric outlet obstruction. If the patient can begin to tolerate liquids, sometimes, eventually, the stomach will reduce by itself. If the patient is comfortable after removal of fluid and can self-hydrate orally, the surgeon can re-image the patient in 2 weeks to assess if the slippage has corrected itself. More often than not, removing fluid simply alleviates symptoms, and surgery is necessary to repair the gastric band prolapse.

Gastric band slippage is most often treated by a laparoscopic operation—a LAGB revision or a complete replacement of the device. To revise a slipped LAGB, the patient is taken to the operating room. Due to the large pouch and tendency for vomiting and reflux, it is important for the patient to be induced in a rapid sequence manner to avoid potential aspiration.

When in the operating room, the first thing to assess for is necrosis or ischemia of the herniated pouch. Once this is ruled out, one can proceed with revisional surgery. Should there be any signs or concerns for ischemia, the gastric band and port should be immediately removed from the patient. Any necrotic gastric tissue need be resected. Wide drainage is often required in these situations, especially where there is any contamination. When a patient with a slippage presents with an acute abdomen or with pain out of proportion, emergent laparoscopy is lifesaving and essential.

The first step in a LAGB revision is to direct the anesthesiologist to place an orogastric tube under direct laparoscopic vision. The point of this is to decompress the large pouch cephalad to the band. Due to the possibility that the gastric wall may be quite thin, it is best to carefully observe the placement of this tube to avoid perforation.

The next step of a LAGB revision is to use electrocautery to open the scar capsule over the medial aspect of the band. This should be continued all the way down to the right crura of the diaphragm with adequate visualization of the caudate lobe. After this, it is important to take down the gastrogastric plication. This should be done carefully using endoshears. Care should be taken not to create a gastrostomy. This plication need be taken down all the way to the left crura of the diaphragm. Additional scar tissue at the angle of His and scarring of the fundus to the diaphragm need be carefully lysed with endoshears or cautery. Once all of this is freed completely, the gastric band should be opened, and the herniated stomach should be reduced caudally so that the band can sit, as it originally did, 2 cm below the gastroesophageal junction at a 45° angle.

Prior to placing new gastrogastric plication stitches, it is suggested to perform an air leak and a dilute methylene blue test via the orogastric tube. This helps rule out the presence of any gastrostomy created during the dissection. Should a defect be found with no intraperitoneal contamination, it can be repaired with a running nonabsorbable suture. If there is a large amount of gastric spillage, one should consider removal of the entire LAGB system to avoid infection.

During a revision of a gastric band, it is imperative to evaluate for any hiatal hernias or crural defects. It is helpful to dissect the right and left crural pillars and assess for any defect. Should one be present, it may be repaired, anteriorly or posteriorly, with nonabsorbable size 0 sutures. Aggressive repair of crural defects and hiatal hernias may result in a decreased number of postoperative complications—including slippage, chronic reflux, and pouch dilation [5, 6].

Sometimes, when beginning a gastric band revision, it is clear that the herniated pouch is extremely thickened and edematous. This may result in difficulty in reducing the prolapse. If this is the situation, if there is excessive scar tissue, or if one is not comfortable revising the band at that time, a surgeon can simply unbuckle the gastric band widely, assuring there is no compression on the stomach. This relieves the obstruction and, more often than not, the slippage symptoms. Then, either that surgeon or one more experienced in gastric band revisional surgery can perform a proper revision a few months down the line.

If the band slippage results in a band that is quite distally displaced, if it is impossible to reduce the prolapsed portion of stomach, or if the gastrogastric plication is so thick and scarred that it is nearly impossible to safely take down (at the risk of entry into the gastric lumen), it may be best to remove the gastric band and place a new band (via the *pars flaccida* technique) at the appropriate level 2 cm distal to the gastroesophageal junction.

Gastric Band Erosion

In gastric band erosion, the LAGB erodes through the serosa (and eventually mucosa) of the stomach resulting in part of or the entire device becoming intragastric. This is a very rare complication (Fig. 19.3).

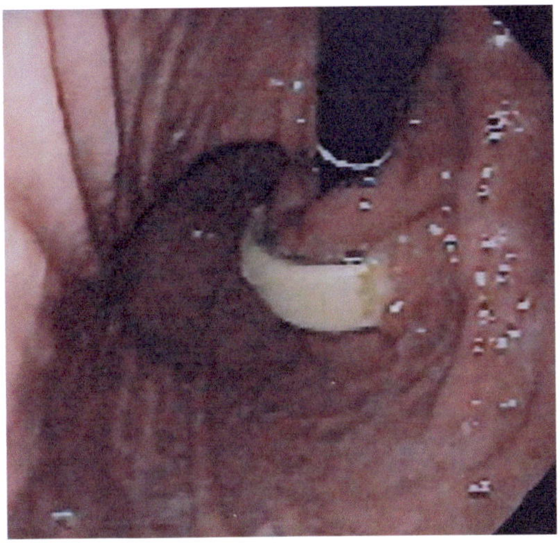

Fig. 19.3 Endoscopic view of a gastric band erosion

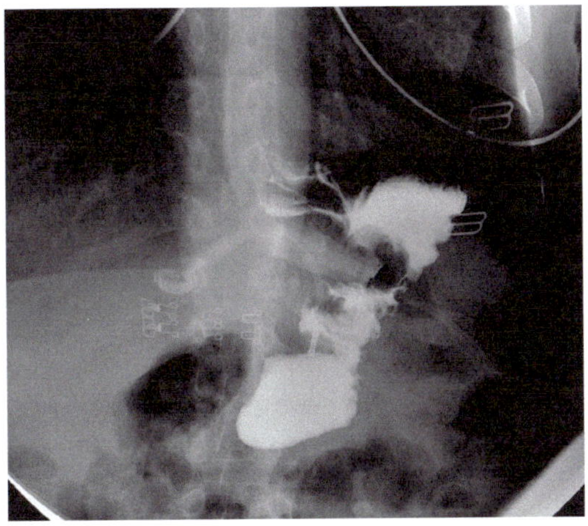

Fig. 19.4 Esophogram indicative of a gastric band erosion

Clinical Presentation

Often, there are no acute signs or symptoms of gastric band erosion. It most frequently presents as an eventual loss of satiety over time, as there is less extrinsic compression on the upper stomach. Another sign of possible band erosion is a subcutaneous port site cellulitis. As the band becomes intraluminal, it comes into contact with the intragastric microbiome. Bacteria can migrate along the band tubing to the port itself. Occasionally, at the site of erosion, a patient may develop an abscess and experience signs of an intra-abdominal collection (fever, dull abdominal pain, leukocytosis). Such findings can be diagnosed by a CT scan.

Pathophysiology

This complication is believed to be the result of one of two mechanisms. Often, it is hypothesized that this happens as a result of serosal injury at the time of band implantation. Overtime, the band slowly erodes into the wall of the stomach. Another theory as to how this occurs is due to over-tightening of the band. In these situations, excessive extrinsic pressure from the band's balloon causes an eventual serosal injury providing a site of erosion. In any event, there is no clear etiology that has been shown to definitively cause band erosion.

Diagnosis

The definitive diagnosis of gastric band erosion is obtained by an upper endoscopy with direct visualization of the gastric band (partially or completely) within the lumen of the stomach. Sometimes, albeit it is subtle, one can see signs of erosion on an esophogram. In such cases, the contrast takes a path from the proximal to distal stomach around the band itself, not passing through the central stoma (Fig. 19.4). This, once again, is very subtle, is often not seen, and is often not picked up on the film itself. It can be confirmed by endoscopy. It is suggested that one perform an endoscopy to rule out erosion whenever there is a late port site infection or when a patient suddenly begins to gain weight with an apparent change in their level of satiety (assuming the band is holding the appropriate amount of fluid in its reservoir).

Management

The definitive management of gastric band erosion is removal of the gastric band and port. This is most often done via a laparoscopic procedure. Often, there is an excessive inflammatory reaction due to this complication, and an extensive lysis of adhesions need be performed. The best way to find the site of entry is to trace the gastric band tubing upward toward the site of entry. The band tubing is cut with endoshears, the band is unbuckled from around the stomach, and it is removed through a port site using an Endocatch bag. Usually, the site of erosion (gastrostomy) is closed and sealed over by the time of operation. Sometimes, this is not the case. If a gastrostomy is found, it is best closed primarily with nonabsorbable sutures with an omental plication placed over the repair. In such situations, it is often wise to leave a temporary drain to assure there is no breakdown of the suture line or drainage at the site of the gastrostomy. It has been described, particularly when the band becomes completely intraluminal, that the device can be removed endoluminally with an endoscope by cutting the tubing endoscopically and removing the band through the mouth with the endoscope. In such cases, the port still must be removed surgically. Nevertheless, one must remain vigilant that there is no leftover gastrostomy that can result in intraperitoneal contamination.

Complications of the repair can be an intra-abdominal abscess or scar tissue related to the previously eroded band. These would be managed with interventional radiology drainage or surgical drainage of a collection.

Pouch Dilation

There are times a patient develops symptoms suggestive of a slippage; nevertheless, the band has not moved, and the pouch cephalad to the band has simply expanded. The normal "pouch" in a LAGB procedure should be no larger than, at most, 15 cc. There should also be normal flow of swallowed material through the band without a significant delay. Sometimes, a patient develops a concentric dilation of this pouch. This often presents with an associated dilated esophagus.

Clinical Presentation

A patient with a concentric dilation of the pouch often presents with dysphagia, nausea, vomiting, and reflux. An associated complaint can be a nighttime cough. Due to the ability to accommodate more food like in a slippage but perhaps a bit more dramatic, patients often describe increased hunger and increased tolerance of a larger volume of food. This can result in weight gain.

Pathophysiology

Concentric pouch dilation is often the result of over-eager tightening of a gastric band. It also sometimes results for a long-standing very tightly adjusted band complicated by a patient's over indulgence in food. The gastric pouch dilates, and this often is accompanied by an associated dilation of the esophagus. This is further complicated by the fact that the pouch is unable to rapidly empty through the tight stoma.

Diagnosis

This condition is often diagnosed by an esophogram. The patient presents with the abovementioned complaints. An esophogram is usually performed, most often to diagnose a slippage. The findings on the esophogram are a very large pouch proximal to the band with little contrast traveling distally in the setting of esophageal dilatation (Fig. 19.5).

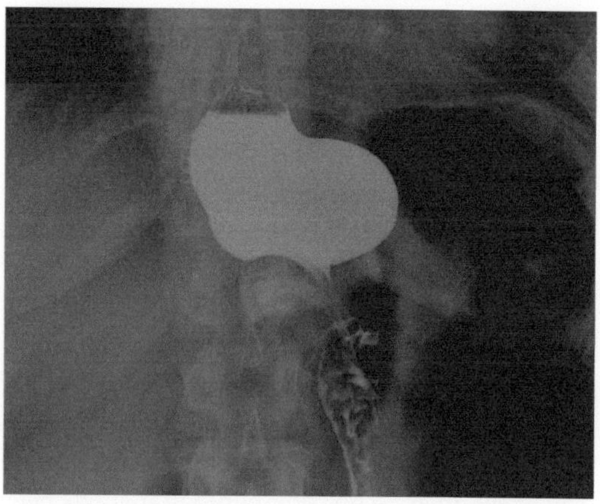

Fig. 19.5 Esophogram of a gastric band pouch dilation

Treatment

This condition is more often than not simply treated with removing a fair amount of the fluid from the reservoir of the band. Often, the patient experiences relief of the nausea, vomiting, and reflux within a day. A repeat esophogram done in a week or two will likely appear normal. Sometimes, if emptying all of the fluid fails to alleviate the symptoms, a patient may need surgical replacement of the band—often to a larger-sized band. Such band replacement is essential when this complication occurs within days to weeks after initial band placement—often before even the first fill of the band.

Port and Tubing Problems

Port Site Infection

A patient may present with cellulitis and localized infection in the area of the gastric port. If this happens in the first few days to weeks after surgery, it is likely an infectious complication of the operation. In such cases, it is important to perform a local incision and drainage of the port site with removal of the port itself. The tubing is gently replaced into the abdominal cavity. The site is often left open to heal by secondary intention with packing. Furthermore, antibiotics are often given to cover normal skin flora. If this occurs, a few months after resolution of the infection, it is safe to replace the port. In these situations, a diagnostic laparoscopy is performed, the tubing is externalized, a new flushed mediport is attached to the tubing and attached to the anterior rectus fascia in the usual technique—with mesh or with nonabsorbable size 0 sutures. It is imperative that the port location is different than the original site as to avoid any chance of recurrent infection.

If a port site infection occurs later on, as described in the discussion of band erosion, one must perform an endoscopy to rule out erosion as a possible cause of a latent port site infection. If band erosion is ruled out, one can manage the port site infection as described above.

Flipped Port

As a patient loses weight, there is often a change to the contour and laxity of the abdominal wall. In these situations, the port itself may turn over or move. If such port migration occurs in a way that LAGB adjustments become painful, difficult, or impossible, it is necessary to reposition the port. This is often done by reopening the port site incision, removing any mesh or sutures which are present, and suturing the port with four size 0 nonabsorbable sutures flush to the anterior rectus sheath.

Defect in the LAGB Tubing

The silastic material that makes up the tubing of the LAGB port travels from gastric band itself to the port. A rupture anywhere in this tubing can result in leakage of saline material from the gastric band system. This, ultimately, results in a loss of restriction, a loss of satiety, and weight gain. The best way to assess for leakage is to access the port with a Huber needle and draw back the fluid—if the amount of fluid in the band is inappropriate (based on the amount that should be present), a leak must be suspected.

To manage this issue, the patient should be taken to the operating room. The first place to rule out a tubing leak is near the port—as it is most common that a leakage is the result of failed attempts at accessing the port causing a needle hole in the distal tubing (Fig. 19.6). The patient is taken to the operating room and the port site incision is opened. The port should be removed from the anterior sheath by either cutting the sutures or removing the mesh adhering it to the anterior rectus sheath (depending on how it was initially placed). The port and tubing should be pulled out as far as it can from the abdominal cavity, without too much tension. Diluted methylene blue is injected into the mediport. If the hole is noted in the distal tubing, one can cut the tubing proximal to the defect and attach a new gastric band port (with associated tubing). Then, the port can be reattached to the anterior rectus sheath in the usual manner. Should no defect be found

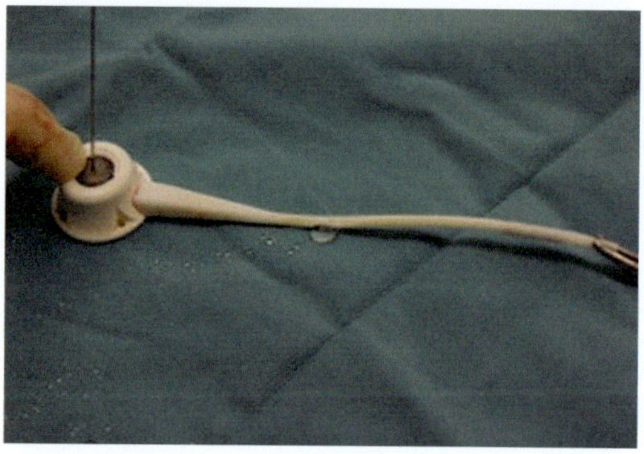

Fig. 19.6 Distal defect in gastric band tubing (proximal to the port)

this way, it is necessary to perform a diagnostic laparoscopy. Diluted methylene blue is once again instilled through the port. With direct laparoscopic visualization of the proximal tubing and gastric band's balloon itself, one can see if there is any leakage of blue dye. Should a tubing or balloon defect be present, the entire device need be replaced.

Other Concerns

As with all bariatric procedures, there will be a subset of the population who do not achieve adequate weight loss. Furthermore, perhaps unique to the gastric band, there will be patients who choose that the follow-up is too taxing on their way of life, that they cannot tolerate the adjustments to the band, or that they cannot manage the dietary modifications necessary for successful weight loss with the band. In these situations, the patient, with the help of the bariatric surgeon, may choose to remove the device and undergo a different weight loss procedure. Nevertheless, assessing the possible causes for weight loss failure or negative symptoms, it may be an option to assess radiographically if one of the abovementioned problems exists. Fixing these problems, many times, may result in renewed successful weight loss with the gastric band. A LAGB revision or replacement may very well be an option, particularly in those patients who remain opposed to a more aggressive bariatric procedure.

Conclusion

The LAGB is an important procedure with which all bariatric surgeons should be familiar. On the one hand, it provides an alternative means of surgical weight loss for a population of patients who do not wish to undergo any drastic anatomical modifications—no staples, no anastomoses. However, even if a bariatric surgeon chooses not to include this operation as part of his or her primary surgical management of obesity, she or he should be aware of the complications of this device and offer options for surgical repair of the device.

References

1. Ponce J, Dixon JB. 2004 ASBS consensus conference. Laparoscopic adjustable gastric banding. Surg Obes Relat Dis. 2005;1:310–6.
2. Fielding GF, Ren CR. Laparoscopic adjustable gastric band. Surg Clin N Am. 2005;85:129–40.
3. Cunneen SA. Review of meta-analytic comparisons of bariatric surgery with focus on laparoscopic adjustable gastric banding. Surg Obes Relat Dis. 2008;4:S47–55.
4. O'Brien PE, MacDonald L, Anderson M, Brennan L, Brown WA. Long term outcomes after bariatric surgery: fifteen-year follow-up of adjustable gastric banding and a systematic review of the bariatric surgery literature. Ann Surg. 2013;257:87–94.
5. Gulkarov I, Wetterau M, Ren CJ, Fielding GA. Hiatal hernia repair at the initial laparoscopic adjustable gastric band operation reduces the need for reoperation. Surg Endosc. 2008;22:1035–41.
6. Ponce J, Fromm R, Paynter S. Outcomes after laparoscopic adjustable gastric band repositioning for slippage or pouch dilation. Surg Obes Relat Dis. 2006;2:627–31.

Acute and Subacute Leaks

20

Ricardo Funke, Camilo Boza, and Fernando Muñoz

Overview

Anastomotic and staple line leaks remain a feared complication after laparoscopic Roux-en-Y gastric bypass (LRYGB). Although the incidence of leaks has declined over time, recent studies still suggest rates as high as 1–3% [1].

The most frequent site of leak in patients with RYGB is the GJ anastomosis, followed by the gastric pouch, and jejunojejunal anastomosis, whereas, in a vast majority of patients with SG, the location of the leak is proximal, near the esophagogastric junction (EGJ).

In sleeve gastrectomies, the most common location of staple line leak is the proximal third of the stomach, occurring at the level of the cardiac notch in approximately 75–87.5% [2].

According to the UK Surgical Infection Study Group, a leak was defined as "the leak of luminal contents from a surgical join between two hollow viscera." Fistulas are the abnormal communication between two different epithelia. A fistula could be secondary to a leak or a collection, for example, a gastric-cutaneous fistula [3–4].

This can be a result of stapler misfire, wrong staple size for the tissue, or tissue trauma. This produces a suture dehiscence which alters the normal cicatrization. A leak can also be produced by a tissue lesion near the suture point.

Different leak risk factors have been described like ischemia, infection near the suture, tension, and heat damage by electrocauterization [5].

Leaks can be classified based either on the time of onset, clinical presentation, site of leak, radiological appearance, or mixed factors.

Leaks are classified according to the time of occurrence: acute <7 days, early 1–6 weeks, late 6–12 weeks, chronic >12 weeks.

Most post-bariatric leaks occur early and usually require surgical cleansing with external drainage and should be associated with basic conservative management, such as fasting, total parenteral nutrition, and administration of intravenous antibiotics [6].

In cases of late or delayed leaks, nonsurgical management, such as percutaneous or internal drainage using the GI tract rather than surgical debridement, is the most used option [7].

Presentation

Most leaks are due to local factors at the site of the staple line, such as inadequate blood supply and oxygenation, which impede the healing process.

Leaks can also be due to gastric intestinal wall ischemia, a consequence of the heat gener-

R. Funke (✉) · C. Boza · F. Muñoz
Department of Digestive Surgery, Clinica Las Condes, Santiago, Chile
e-mail: rfunke@clc.cl; cboza@clc.cl

R. Lutfi et al. (eds.), *Global Bariatric Surgery*, https://doi.org/10.1007/978-3-319-93545-4_20

ated by the electrocautery used during dissection. Although the blood supply to the stomach is robust, the gastroesophageal junction tends to be an area of decreased vascularity and thus more liable to leaks. SG produces high intragastric pressure which can affect the healing process and lengthen the amount of time for a leak to close.

Patients with LGBYR could present leaks in the gastric pouch and the jejunojejunal anastomosis. The most common site is the GJ anastomosis. There is no difference reported if the anastomosis is mechanic or manual, and the causes are similar to the leaks at SG.

Mostly the diagnosis of a leak is produced post discharge. Sometimes it only manifests with tachycardia, so a high diagnostic suspicion is required. Symptoms may vary from tachycardia, tachypnea, left shoulder pain, nausea, vomiting, fever, abdominal pain, poor blood tension, or shock. It depends on the patient comorbidities, the amount of the leak, and the time of detection. If a patient presents any of these symptoms at the postoperative time, a leak must be discarded because of the high morbidity and mortality of this complication.

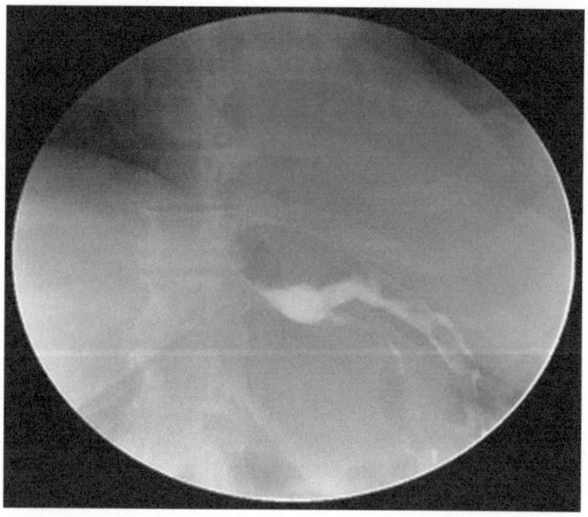

Fig. 20.1 Leaks are usually identified with an esophagram/limited UGI series

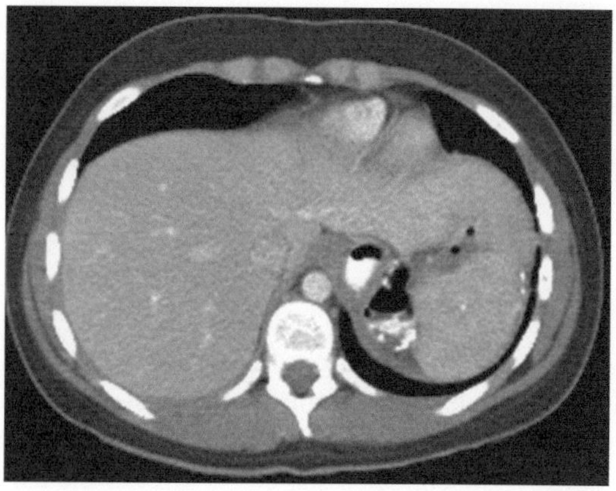

Fig. 20.2 A leak can generally be identified as an extraluminal contrast

Diagnosis

Leak diagnosis should be supported with images to evaluate the size, complications, and the leak site. In many centers, postoperative radiographic imaging studies following bariatric surgical procedures are routinely indicated to identify early leaks, although there is no consensus as to whether imaging should be performed routinely or selectively following bariatric surgery [8].

Leaks are usually identified with an esophagram/limited UGI series (Fig. 20.1). If a leak is suspected, and the UGI is negative, a CT scan can be obtained. If an abscess or fluid collection is suspected, CT of the abdomen and pelvis will provide the most useful information. Chronic leaks usually are accompanied with complications like fistulas or abscess, so a CT may be more useful [9].

A leak can generally be identified as an extraluminal contrast material (Fig. 20.2). The clinical condition of the patient should be evaluated along with the image to plan the management. If the imaging is negative, but the clinical condition of the patient makes us suspect of the presence of a leak or a fistula, action should be taken [10].

If an abscess or a collection is suspected, the most useful procedure is an interventional scanner so that percutaneously CT-guided aspiration or drainage of an abscess or fluid collection can be performed (Fig. 20.3).

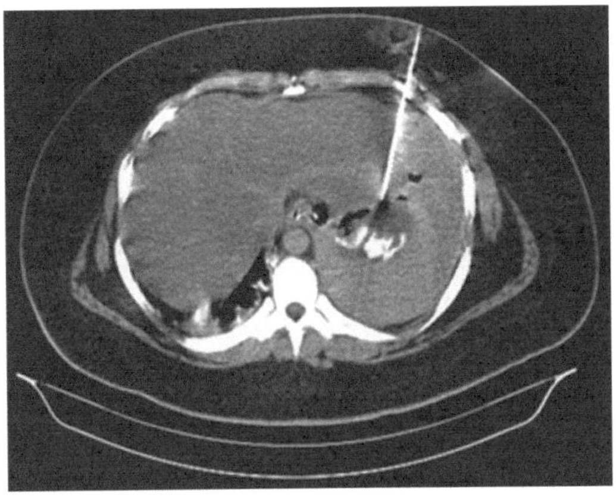

Fig. 20.3 If an abscess or a collection is suspected, the most useful procedure is an interventional scanner so that percutaneously CT-guided aspiration or drainage of an abscess or fluid collection can be performed

Management

Because of the low rate and high mortality of leaks in bariatric surgery, management has many controversies and difficulties in the adoption of a standard algorithm.

The management must ensure:

- A correct sepsis control
- An adequate drainage
- To handle and prevent secondary obstruction
- To administrate an adequate nutritional support

Based on the First International Summit for Sleeve Gastrectomy, the treatment may include:

- Early over sewing
- Drainage (open or laparoscopic)
- Endoscopic clipping
- Stenting or using fibrin glue
- Roux limb or total gastrectomy as the last resort

The adoption of a more conservative approach for intermediate-late leaks in clinically stable patients is more reasonable with adequate hydration, proton-pump inhibitors, nutritional support, percutaneous drainage of any collection, and broad-spectrum antibiotherapy, with a follow-up by upper gastrointestinal series to ensure healing. With any concern about healing, more invasive approaches may be considered [11].

Unstable patients, upon presentation, justify prompt surgical intervention by laparoscopic or open means for washout and drainage at least. That may be coupled with debridement and suturing of the orifice if the condition of the patient and the tissues and the skills and experience of the surgeon permit.

The minimally invasive approach can be used initially in septic patients or with poor nutritional conditions in order to leave the emergency and then propose the use of more invasive techniques. For example, percutaneous drainage can be used initially to stabilize and manage the infection focus, while antibiotics and nutritional support are administrated; later, the patient could be in optimal conditions for a more invasive approach [12].

The endoscopic modalities can be divided on the following.

Closure Techniques

Endoclips were used initially for hemostasis, later, on trials to treat esophageal, colonic, and duodenal mucosal defects and perforations. They were extrapolated to be used in post-sleeve gastrectomy leakage. Now the new over-the-scope clips (OTSC) have more promising results (Fig. 20.4).

OTSC®System (Ovesco Endoscopy, Tübingen, Germany) with the potential ability to achieve full-thickness apposition has been used with more success. Mercky et al. [13] reported an 89% success rate among 18 patients with post-sleeve gastrectomy leaks [13]. Keren et al. also reported a series of 26 patients after sleeve gastrectomy leakage treated with OTSCs after a median of 8 days. Sixteen patients were successfully managed by OTSC treatment alone [14]. These data suggest that OTSCs should be considered as an alternative endoscopic treatment for early leakage.

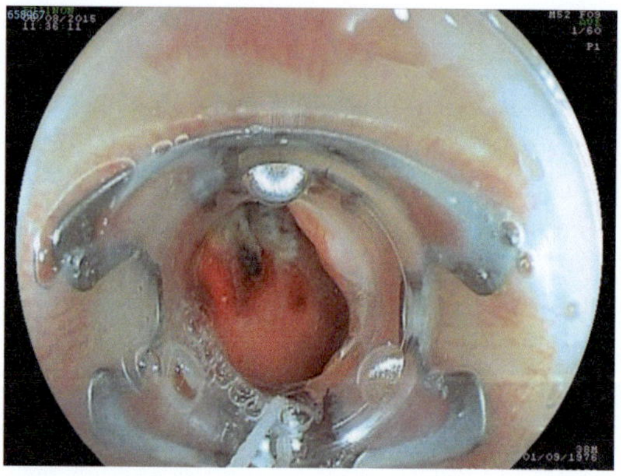

Fig. 20.4 OVESCO ™ device using in GI fistula after Sleeve Gastrectomy

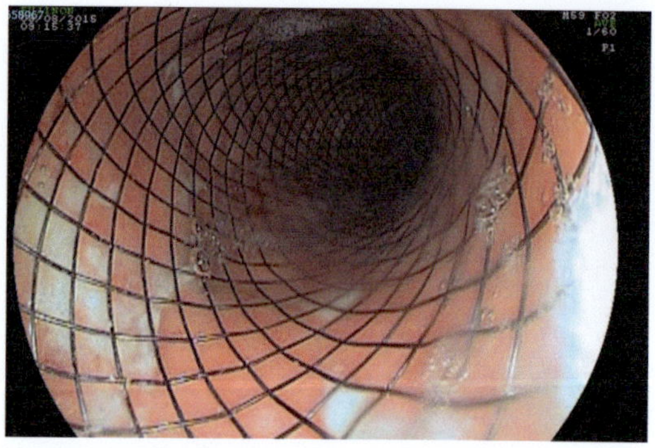

Fig. 20.5 Endoscopic view of stent

Sealant Materials The endoscopic injection of two sealant materials, fibrin glue and cyanoacrylate, has been used to occlude the leak orifice.

Fibrin glue acts by dual effect, as a plug directly occluding the defect and as a troflobroblast promoter to enhance wound healing. Thus, it is absorbed after 4 weeks and replaced by connective scar tissue. There is limited evidence about its use.

Exclusion Techniques

Endoprosthesis Initially stents were used to treat stenosis. It was shown that they decrease the intraluminal pressure, which may be part of the pathophysiology of the gastric leak post-sleeve, so its use gained a widespread in the management of proximal and middle gastric leak due to the advantage of the ability to resume patients feeding and discharge the patient home [15] (Figs. 20.5 and 20.6).

To cover the defect, endoscopic stent insertion has been widely performed. In particular, newly developed, partially or fully covered SEMS are flexible and maintain patency of a narrow GI lumen, combined with a delivery system for through-the-scope (TTS) placement via a working channel, enabling endoscopists to insert stents under direct inspection of the target area.

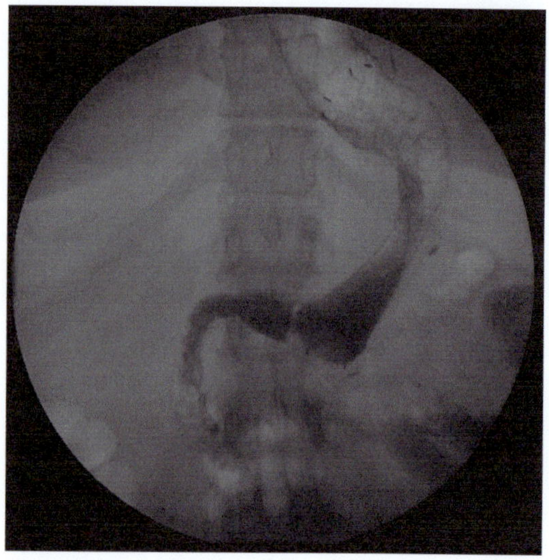

Fig. 20.6 Use of covered stent after SG leak

Recently, the use of tailored stents for post-bariatric surgery patients has been introduced, with some published results. These stents were specially designed for the treatment of post-SG leak; both ends of the stent had high profile edges allowing a more firm anchorage and longer length (23–24 cm) than conventional esophageal stents, enabling the stent to bypass the entire gastric sleeve or wider diameter (40 mm) to facilitate sufficient sealing of the leaks. Large-scale, randomized, prospective studies to compare conventional and tailored stents are needed.

Gastric sleeve leaks usually take more than 6 weeks to heal (average of 45 days) compared to healing time in laparoscopic Roux-en-Y gastric

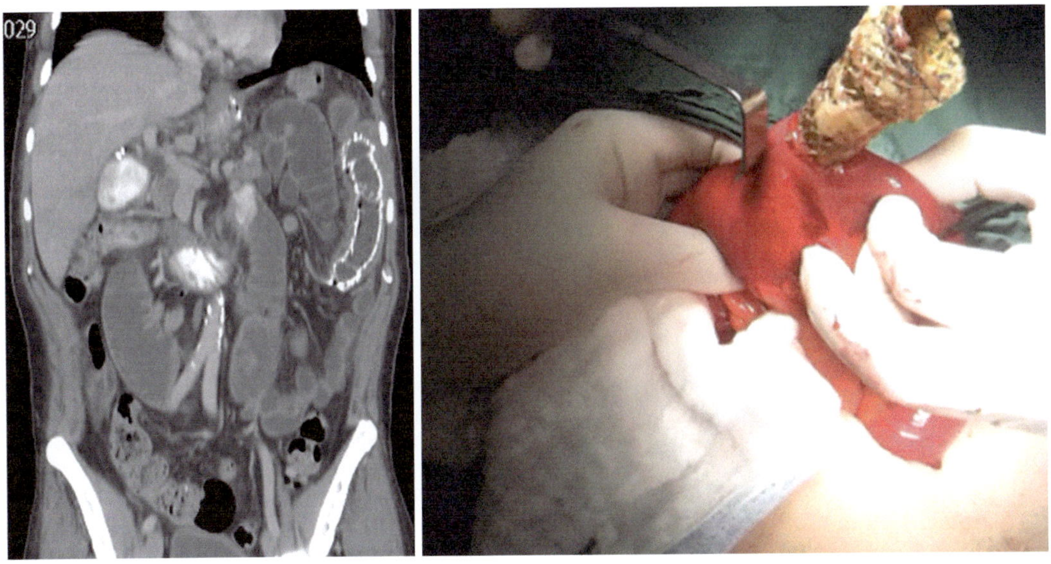

Fig. 20.7 Small bowel stent migration

bypass leaks (30 days), at the same time, keeping the stents for long period risks to damage the underlying mucosa, especially with uncovered stents. Ideally, most authors agree that 6–8 weeks is the optimal removal time, but these prosthesis should be observed closely with the possibility to remove them after 4 weeks [14].

In terms of complications, stent migration occurs most frequently (Fig. 20.7). Its reported rate of occurrence varies widely, from 5% to 62%, and more serious complications, such as perforation, have also been reported. A previous meta-analysis regarding the use of SEMS in the treatment of post-bariatric surgery leaks reported an 88% clinical success rate, and successful endoscopic stent removal was achieved in 92% of cases, while stent migration was observed in 17% of cases.

Partially covered SEMS might be superior to fully cover SEMS for prevention of migration because mucosal hypertrophy at both uncovered ends of the stent may reduce the risk of migration. However, embedding of both ends of stents due to mucosal hyperplasia may cause difficulty in stent removal, which can be resolved by a "stent-in-stent" strategy.

The clinical success rate of the procedure, which indicates complete closure of leak or fistular opening, has been acceptable, ranging from 65% to 95% [16–18]. Overall, the clinical success of stent insertion is significantly associated with shorter delay between bariatric surgery and stent insertion because delayed stenting may lead to fibrous change and chronic fistula formation from acute leaks and eventually to a higher failure rate of closure of leaks. Another important factor is larger leak size (≥10 mm) [15].

Several factors are important in its success. A shorter delay between the initial bariatric surgery. A larger leak size (>10 mm) was also reported as being more likely to be associated with difficult healing after stenting than smaller leaks.

The management of post-bariatric leaks is challenging and requires a multidisciplinary approach. Frequently, endoscopic treatment is an adjunct to surgery although a complete endoscopic approach is also feasible.

References

1. Tringali A, et al. Treatment of post-laparoscopic sleeve gastrectomy leaks using a specially designed metal stent. Endoscopy. 2017;49(1):64–8.
2. Rached AA, Basile M, Hicham E. Masri gastric leaks post sleeve gastrectomy: review of its prevention and management. World J Gastroenterol. 2014;20(38):13904–10.

3. Delko T, Hoffmann H, et al. Patterns of gastric microperfusion during laparoscopic sleeve gastrectomy. Obes Surg. 2017;27(926):9–32.
4. Varban OA, et al. Evaluating leaks after gastric bypass or technology? Surg Obes Relat Dis. 2016;12(2):264–72.
5. Varban OA, et al. The effect of operative technique on leaks after laparoscopic sleeve gastrectomy: a case-control study. Surg Obes Relat Dis. 2017;13(4):560–7.
6. Sepulveda, et al. Staple line reinforcement in laparoscopic sleeve gastrectomy: experience in 1023 consecutive cases. Obes Surg. 2017;27(6):1474–80.
7. Joo MK. Approach for major complications of bariatric surgery. Clin Endosc. 2017;50:31–41.
8. Aurora AR, Khaitan L, Saber AA. Sleeve gastrectomy and the risk of leak: a systematic analysis of 4,888 patients. Surg Endosc. 2012;26(6):1509–15.
9. Smith MD, Adeniji A, Wahed AS, Patterson E, Chapman W, Courcoulas AP, Dakin G, Flum D, McCloskey C, Mitchell JE, Pomp A, Staten M, Wolfe B. Technical factors associated with anastomotic leak after Roux-en-Y gastric bypass. Surg Obes Relat Dis. 2015;11(2):313–20.
10. Mbadiwe T, Prevatt E, Duerinckx A, Cornwell E 3rd, Fullum T, Davis B. Assessing the value of routine upper gastrointestinal contrast studies following bariatric surgery: a systematic review and meta-analysis. Am J Surg. 2015;209(4):616–22.
11. Rosenthal, et al. Sleeve gastrectomy expert panel consensus statement: best practice guidelines based on experience of >12,000 cases. Surg Obes Relat Dis. 2012;8(1):8–19.
12. Quezada N, Maiz C, Daroch D, Funke R, Sharp A, Boza C, Pimentel F. Effect of early use of covered self-expandable endoscopic stent on the treatment of postoperative stapler line leaks. Obes Surg. 2015;25(10):1816–21.
13. Mercky P, et al. Usefulness of over-the-scope clipping system for closing digestive fistulas. Dig Endosc. 2014;27:18–24.
14. Keren D, et al. Over-the-scope clip (OTSC) system for sleeve gastrectomy leaks. Obes Surg. 2015;25:1358–63.
15. Walsh C, Karmali S. Endoscopic management of bariatric complications: A review and update. World J Gastrointest Endosc. 2015;7(5):518–23. Moon RC, Shah N, Teixeira AF, Jawad MA. Management of staple line leaks following sleeve gastrectomy. Surg Obes Relat Dis. 2015;11(1):54–9.
16. Manta R, Caruso A, Cellini C, Sica M, Zullo A, Mirante VG, Bertani H, Frazzoni M, Mutignani M, Galloro G, Conigliaro R. Endoscopic management of patients with post-surgical leaks involving the gastrointestinal tract: a large case series. United European Gastroenterol J. 2016;4(6):770–7.
17. Joo MK. Endoscopy for post-bariatric complication. Clin Endosc. 2017;50:31–41.
18. Souto-Rodríguez R, et al. Endoluminal solutions to bariatric surgery complications. World J Gastrointest Endosc. 2017;9(3):105–26.

Chronic Leak and Fistulas

21

Luciano Antozzi, Priscilla Antozzi, and Mario Norberto Antozzi

Background

The worldwide acceptance of bariatric surgery is a result of its well-known results, but despite making our greatest efforts to achieve near-zero complications, some may appear. A new challenge starts when this happens, and the medical team must be prepared to manage them appropriately [1, 2].

A chronic complication means that during the acute phase, the problem could not be solved and this can be mentally exhausting and physically deteriorating for the patient, so a multidisciplinary approach with gastroenterology, interventional radiology, nutrition, and psychology is important to maintain good communication and attain good results.

Complication management, due to its low frequency, has a learning curve hard to overcome, and it could be beneficial to centralize it in high-volume centers. Endoscopic therapies require experienced physicians, but they are less invasive and usually don't interfere with surgical management, so, if the patient condition allows it, they should precede other major procedures like total gastrectomy, proximal gastrectomy with esophago-jejunal reconstruction, or fistulectomy with Roux-en-Y lateral anastomosis [3, 4].

Leaks appear when the integrity of the visceral lumen is not complete, and a communication is established with another organ or cavity. In some cases, a chronic tract conforms a fistula, an anastomotic or staple line defect that can be very morbid and possibly fatal. Gastric, enteric, gastro-bronchial, gastro-pleural, gastro-splenic, gastro-gastric, gastrocolic, gastro-cutaneous, and entero-cutaneous have been described, and when inflammation is significant, spontaneous closure is unusual [5–7].

A leak is defined as chronic when it persists more than 12 weeks and surpassed acute (<7 days), early (7–45 days), and late (45–90 days) stages. Predisposing and perpetuating factors related to the patient's characteristics are male sex and age older than 50 years, while demonstrated conditions like chronic heart failure, chronic renal failure, chronic lung disease, and diabetes significantly predispose to complications. To achieve the best possible results, nutritional and clinical management has to be optimal during treatment [8–10].

Sleeve gastrectomy leaks mostly occur at the lateral margin of the esophagogastric junction, the thinnest, least irrigated portion of the stomach that receives the highest pressure during gastric contraction. Continuous drain aspiration or negative pressure related to diaphragmatic

L. Antozzi (✉)
Department of Bariatric and Esophago-Gastric Surgery, Hospital Italiano Regional del Sur, Buenos Aires, Argentina

P. Antozzi · M. N. Antozzi
Department of General and Bariatric Surgery, Centro de Cirugías Especiales, Buenos Aires, Argentina

R. Lutfi et al. (eds.), *Global Bariatric Surgery*, https://doi.org/10.1007/978-3-319-93545-4_21

movement impacts negatively on resolution. The best described deleterious mechanisms are distal strictures; they can be anatomic when the gastric lumen narrows unevenly (frequently at the *incisura angularis*) or functional when asymmetry between posterior and anterior gastric walls alters normal motility [1, 11, 12].

In Roux-en-Y gastric bypass, a gastrojejunal anastomosis too small can perpetuate a pouch leak, but the most common acute location is in this anastomosis. Despite it rarely becomes chronic, an obstructed descending alimentary limb or small jejuno-jejunal anastomosis can difficult the healing process. The most common presentation of chronic fistulas is the gastro-gastric, normally detected after changes in the patient's eating capacity and weight regain [13, 14].

An infected cavity next to the leak and the presence of a drain inside its lumen are perpetuating factors that can be seen regardless of the surgical technique performed and have to be properly identified and treated (Figs. 21.1 and 21.2).

Before adopting therapeutic measures, evaluation with a computed tomography can indicate the presence of extravasation of liquid contrast and different fluid collection sites. A contrast swallow has interobserver variability, but it can assess gastric anatomy, leak location, size, strictures, kinking, and communication with other organs or cavities. Endoscopy can be safely performed and contributes with vital information about cavity characteristics, fistula size, stricture size, septum length, foreign bodies, and granulation process (Figs. 21.3 and 21.4). Utilization of caps at the tip of the endoscope can help evaluating leaks without the need of insufflation [15, 16].

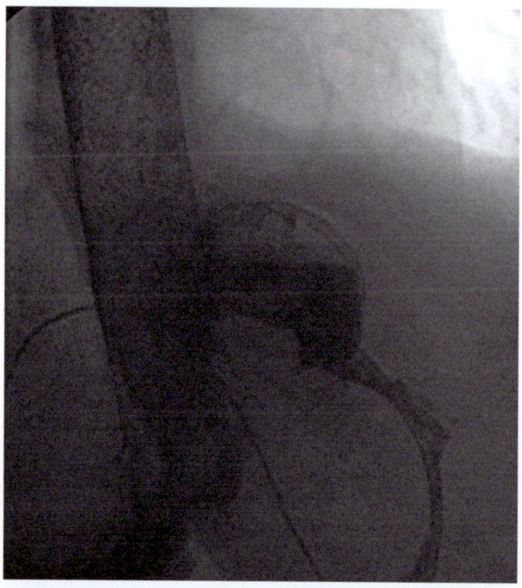

Fig. 21.1 Persistent sleeve gastrectomy leak with stent and percutaneous drain

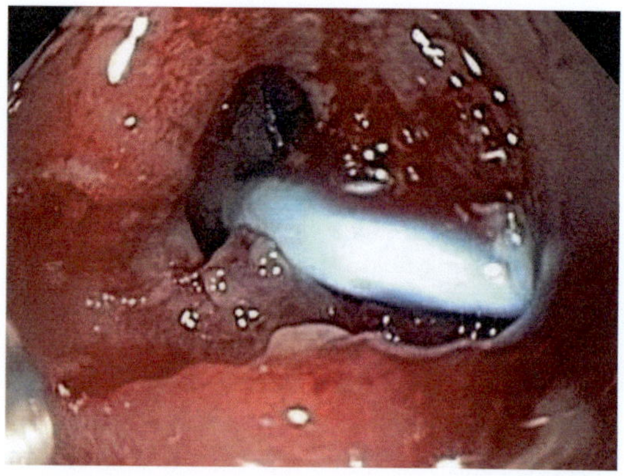

Fig. 21.2 After stent removal, it can be observed that the drain is inside the stomach

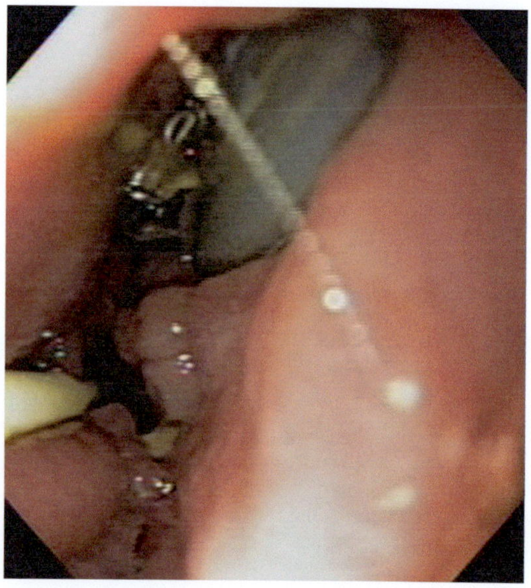

Fig. 21.3 Surgical drain inside gastric lumen

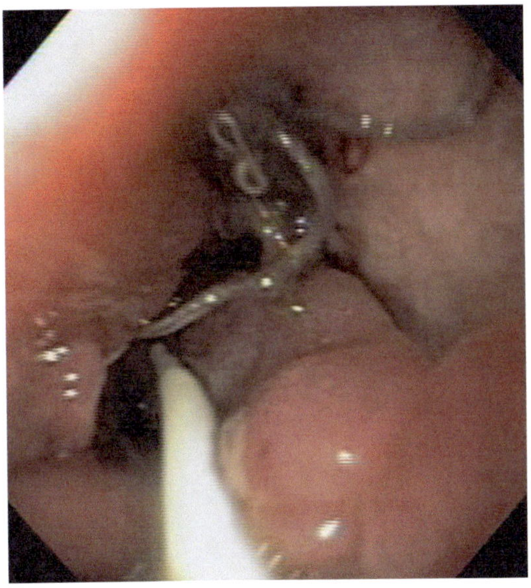

Fig. 21.4 After drain removal their staples and suture are observed

Treatment

Given the lack of established guidelines for early or acute leaks management, a patient with a chronic complication can present after varied and multiple failed treatment attempts. Decision-making must be focused on treating not only the leak but also perpetuating factors.

Endoscopic strategies aim to occlude a fistula, reduce its size, bypass it, or favor internal drainage while restoring normal progression of the alimentary bolus [17].

Stents

Unlike its use in early leaks, endoscopic stent placement in patients with chronic leaks and anastomotic strictures is discouraged due to unsatisfactory results on definitive healing. They can be placed to allow for oral nutrition and enteral resuscitation, but naso-enteric tubes despite being uncomfortable for the patients are more cost-efficient, are equally successful, and don't present the difficulties and risks of stent removal.

Internal Drainage

If a patient has a well-delimited collection next to the gastric wall that perpetuates sepsis and there is no access for percutaneous drainage, internal evacuation can be achieved with double pigtails. They are placed with a pusher through the staple line orifice leaving one end at the lumen and the other inside the cavity. The defect remains clean and granulation is stimulated due to the foreign body presence. This technique requires naso-enteric feeding, endoscopic control, and pigtail replacement every 4–6 weeks but reduces the chance of cutaneous fistulas.

EVT

When a cavity is large or multiple gastric wall orifices drain to a common cavity, endoscopic vacuum technique (EVT) has shown promising results reducing the defect size.

To assemble the system, a porous sponge is secured to a regular nasogastric tube with sutures, and an additional loop suture fixated to the tip facilitates traction. All the tube holes should be covered by the sponge so the vacuum acts only at this portion. After measuring the defect by endoscopy, the sponge shape and size are trimmed to the observed dimensions before insertion. The tube is progressed through a nostril, captured with an endoscopic grasping forceps at the pharynx, and then gently pushed from the loop into the defect. Care must be taken to avoid contact of the sponge with the mucosa or retrieval of the system when the endoscope is withdrawn. After insertion, the vacuum system is connected, and aspiration pressure of 125 mmHg has to be maintained. Oral food intake is not permitted during treatment, and the sponge has to be changed every 3–5 days. Success is considered when the cavity reduced the size up to the gastric wall edge. This modality should be avoided if vascular structures are close, because of hemorrhage risks [18, 19].

Septotomy and Dilation

When a large cavity is present with a gastric wall septum in between, infection perpetuates due to accumulation of detritus and bacteria that obstruct the healing process. Unification of the defect with the gastric lumen by sectioning the septum facilitates bolus progression and evacuation of contaminated material. Commonly a distal stricture coexist and if suspected it must also be treated.

Preferably argon plasma coagulation is used to cut the septum because it carries less risks of bleeding when compared to needle knife. The section is made toward the lateral edge of the stomach pointing to the cavity without exceeding its bottom. After completion of septotomy, sleeve gastrectomy strictures are aggressively dilated with a 30 mm achalasia balloon, with 15 PSI during 1–3 min under general anesthesia with fluoroscopic and endoscopic guidance (Figs. 21.5, 21.6, and 21.7). Smaller-sized balloons are used for RNYGB anastomosis (18–20 mm) (Figs. 21.8, 21.9, and 21.10) Multiple sessions are repeated as necessary.

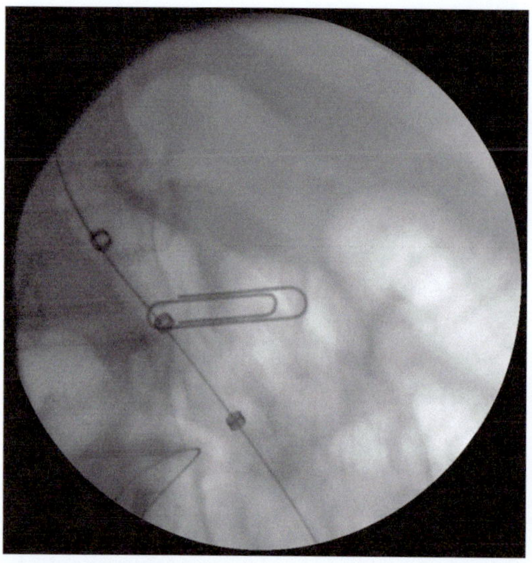

Fig. 21.5 External clip marking the stenotic site and 30 mm balloon positioned

Gastro-gastric Fistulas

It is proposed that this communication between the gastric pouch and remnant may appear after incomplete stapling during RNYGB or after undetected chronic leaks. Altered eating capacity

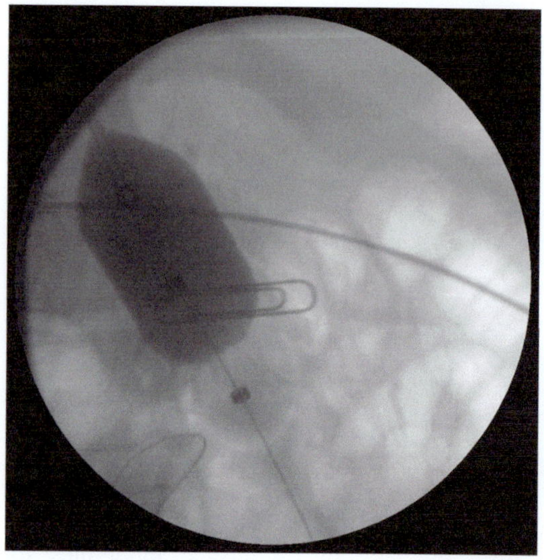

Fig. 21.6 The defect is recognized during balloon filling

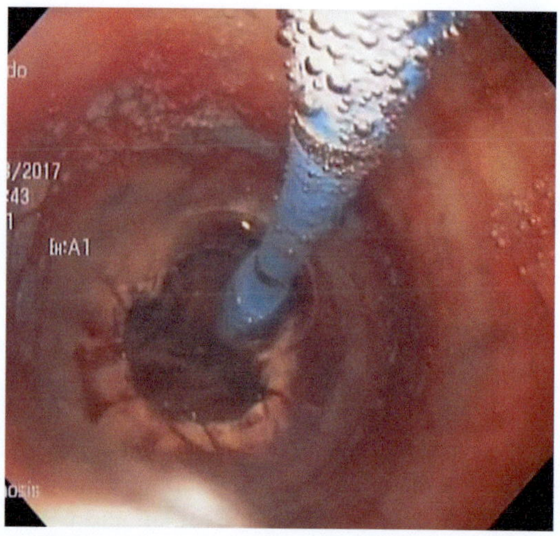

Fig. 21.7 Endoscopic control shows the *incisura angularis* stricture

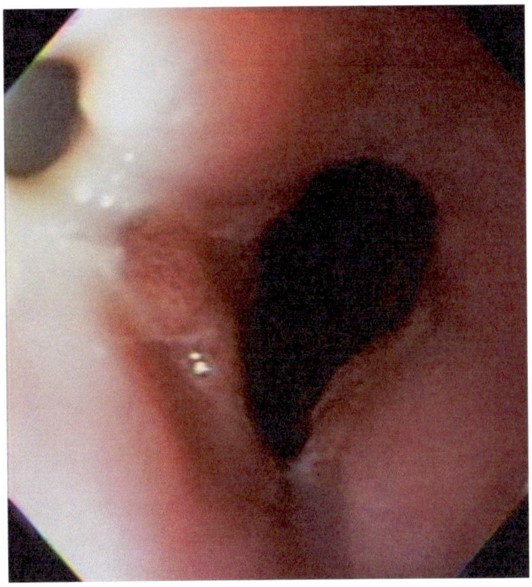

Fig. 21.8 Small fistula at EGJ after RNYGB

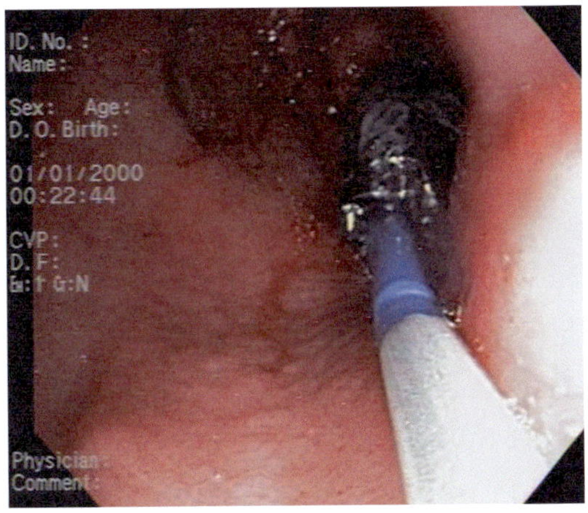

Fig. 21.10 Dilation with 18 mm balloon resolved the fistula without any further treatment

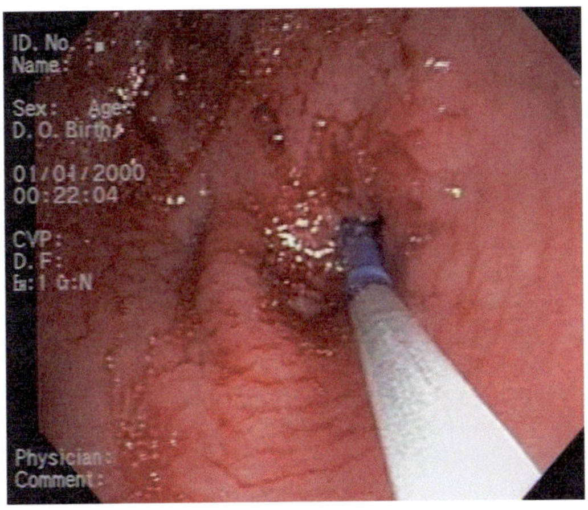

Fig. 21.9 Distal severe anastomotic stenosis

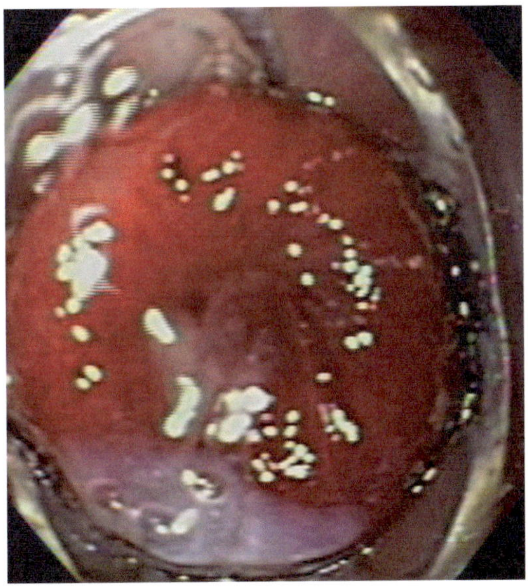

Fig. 21.11 OTSC clip with complete entry of the fistula wall

and weight regain in the absence of other causes are common symptoms, and it can be easily diagnosed with endoscopy or barium swallow.

Ideally a small fistula can be successfully closed with over-the-scope clips. During endoscopy, the fistula is positioned in front of the cap, the wall contacted and aspiration used to introduce the orifice completely into the cap, the clip released, and the result controlled by endoscopy (Figs. 21.11 and 21.12). A barium swallow confirms the result. If unsuccessful, surgery with intraoperative endoscopy is indicated to avoid closing the stapler over the previously deployed clip.

Gastro-bronchial Fistulas

A gastro-bronchial fistula is suspected when respiratory symptoms like productive cough and fever start in a patient with history of a chronic

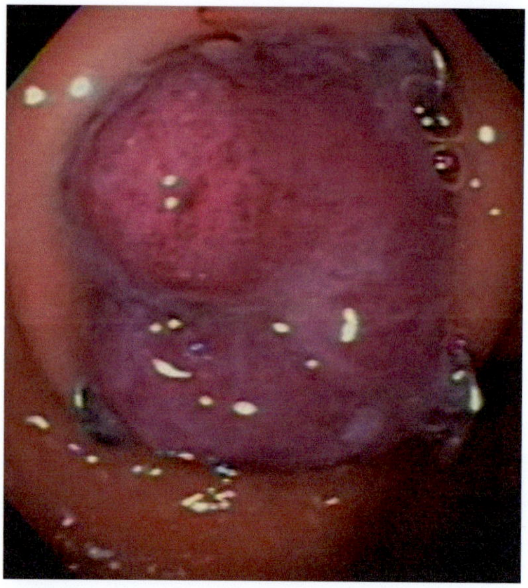

Fig. 21.12 OTSC clip deployed

leak. Frequency is higher in sleeve gastrectomy because of the usual association of distal stenosis and subphrenic abscess.

When it comes to management, there is no consensus, and reports of small series make it difficult to recommend any modality. Probably the one that the endoscopic team has more experience with would be best. Stent placement and septotomy with stricture dilation have been described as successful, and surgery is a last resort because it entails high morbidity.

References

1. Milone L, Strong V, Gagner M. Laparoscopic sleeve gastrectomy is superior to endoscopic intragastric balloon as a first stage procedure for super-obese patients (BMI > or =50). Obes Surg. 2005;15(5):612–7.
2. Imaz I, Martinez-Cervell C, Garcia-Alvarez EE, Sendra-Gutierrez JM, Gonzalez-Enriquez J. Safety and effectiveness of the intragastric balloon for obesity. A meta-analysis. Obes Surg. 2008;18(7):841–6.
3. Ubeda-Iglesias A, Irles-Rocamora JA, Povis-Lopez CD. Antral impaction and cardiorespiratory arrest. Complications of the intragastric balloon. Med Intensiva. 2012;36(4):315–7.
4. Deviere J, Ojeda Valdes G, Cuevas Herrera L, Closset J, Le Moine O, Eisendrath P, et al. Safety, feasibility and weight loss after transoral gastroplasty: first human multicenter study. Surg Endosc. 2008;22(3):589–98.
5. Moreno C, Closset J, Dugardeyn S, Barea M, Mehdi A, Collignon L, et al. Transoral gastroplasty is safe, feasible, and induces significant weight loss in morbidly obese patients: results of the second human pilot study. Endoscopy. 2008;40(5):406–13.
6. Familiari P, Costamagna G, Blero D, Le Moine O, Perri V, Boskoski I, et al. Transoral gastroplasty for morbid obesity: a multicenter trial with a 1-year outcome. Gastrointest Endosc. 2011;74(6):1248–58.
7. Fogel R, De Fogel J, Bonilla Y, De La Fuente R. Clinical experience of transoral suturing for an endoluminal vertical gastroplasty: 1-year follow-up in 64 patients. Gastrointest Endosc. 2008;68(1):51–8.
8. Brethauer SA, Chand B, Schauer PR, Thompson CC. Transoral gastric volume reduction as intervention for weight management: 12-month follow-up of TRIM trial. Surg Obes Relat Dis. 2011;8:296.
9. Schouten R, Rijs CS, Bouvy ND, Hameeteman W, Koek GH, Janssen IM, et al. A multicenter, randomized efficacy study of the EndoBarrier gastrointestinal liner for presurgical weight loss prior to bariatric surgery. Ann Surg. 2010;251(2):236–43.
10. Rodriguez-Grunert L, Galvao Neto MP, Alamo M, Ramos AC, Baez PB, Tarnoff M. First human experience with endoscopically delivered and retrieved duodenal-jejunal bypass sleeve. Surg Obes Relat Dis. 2008;4(1):55–9.
11. Gersin KS, Rothstein RI, Rosenthal RJ, Stefanidis D, Deal SE, Kuwada TS, et al. Open-label, sham-controlled trial of an endoscopic duodenojejunal bypass liner for preoperative weight loss in bariatric surgery candidates. Gastrointest Endosc. 2010;71(6):976–82.
12. de Moura EG, Martins BC, Lopes GS, Orso IR, de Oliveira SL, Galvao Neto MP, et al. Metabolic improvements in obese type 2 diabetes subjects implanted for 1 year with an endoscopically deployed duodenal-jejunal bypass liner. Diabetes Technol Ther. 2012;14(2):183–9.
13. Escalona A, Pimentel F, Sharp A, Becerra P, Slako M, Turiel D, et al. Weight loss and metabolic improvement in morbidly obese subjects implanted for 1 year with an endoscopic duodenal-jejunal bypass liner. Ann Surg. 2012;255(6):1080–5.
14. Sandler BJ, Rumbaut R, Swain CP, Torres G, Morales L, Gonzales L, et al. Human experience with an endoluminal, endoscopic, gastrojejunal bypass sleeve. Surg Endosc. 2011;25(9):3028–33.
15. Abu Dayyeh BK, Lautz DB, Thompson CC. Gastrojejunal stoma diameter predicts weight regain after Roux-en-Y gastric bypass. Clin Gastroenterol Hepatol. 2011;9(3):228–33.
16. Fernandez-Esparrach G, Lautz DB, Thompson CC. Peroral endoscopic anastomotic reduction improves intractable dumping syndrome in Roux-en-Y gastric bypass patients. Surg Obes Relat Dis. 2010;6(1):36–40.

17. Aly A. Argon plasma coagulation and gastric bypass – a novel solution to stomal dilation. Obes Surg. 2009;19(6):788–90.
18. Galvão Neto M, Rodriguez L, Zundel N, Ayala JC, Campos J, Ramos A. Endoscopic revision of Roux-en-Y gastric bypass Stomal dilation with a suturing device: preliminary results of a first out-of-United States series. Bariatric Times. 2011;8(6):32–4.
19. Abu Dayyeh BK, Jirapinyo P, Weitzner Z, Barker C, Flicker MS, Lautz DB, et al. Endoscopic sclerotherapy for the treatment of weight regain after Roux-en-Y gastric bypass: outcomes, complications, and predictors of response in 575 procedures. Gastrointest Endosc. 2012;76(2):275–82.

22 Intolerance to Oral Intake, Refractory Nausea, and Vomiting

Aaron Lee and Samuel Szomstein

Introduction

Obesity is not only an epidemic in the United States, but it has been observed beyond the western hemisphere as a pandemic phenomenon around the world. Obesity has become one of the leading healthcare problems today that carries potential socioeconomic burden to the society as a whole [1]. Many medical and surgical therapies have become available to the public with great success. Among all of the available therapies, weight loss surgery has become the gold standard treatment because of its durability and reproducible weight loss with resolution of comorbidities. Therefore, bariatric operations have become one of the fastest-growing operations performed [1]. As with all surgeries that are performed today, bariatric procedures, although safe and effective, are not free from potential complications.

Different procedures affect patients differently, but one of the most common complications or complaints that patients have after any bariatric operation is severe food intolerance, nausea, and/or vomiting secondary to stricture [2]. The incidence of poor PO tolerance after any bariatric procedure secondary to stricture can range from 2.3% to 16% [2]. Different procedures such as laparoscopic gastric band placement, sleeve gastrectomy, and gastric bypass, all have different incidences of stenosis or stricture. It has been shown that nausea/vomiting is the most common reason for hospital readmission after a bariatric surgery, exceeding the rates of abdominal pain and dehydration [3]. Healthcare providers should carefully consider the causes of nausea and vomiting because many physicians who are not familiar with bariatric patients may overlook the sentinel signs of what can be easily managed if the diagnosis was promptly made and treated (Table 22.1). Delayed diagnosis or improper treatment of PO intolerance can result in severe nutritional deficiencies, dehydration, early readmission, and prolonged hospital stay.

The goal of this chapter is to better understand some of the common causes of complications and their managements, especially for poor PO tolerance secondary to stricture.

Pathophysiology

Although PO intolerance is a relatively common problem after a bariatric procedure, the pathophysiology behind it is still poorly understood. The pathophysiology may vary depending on the etiology and the type of the procedure.

There is a psychosocial component to this particular problem. Few people understand that bar-

A. Lee
Department of General Surgery, Cleveland Clinic Florida – Weston, Weston, FL, USA

S. Szomstein (✉)
The Bariatric and Metabolic Institute, Cleveland Clinic Florida – Weston, Weston, FL, USA
e-mail: szomsts@ccf.org

R. Lutfi et al. (eds.), *Global Bariatric Surgery*, https://doi.org/10.1007/978-3-319-93545-4_22

Table 22.1 Causes of nausea/vomiting

Causes
Patient behavior
Non-compliant with the bariatric diet program
Bulky eating
Inadequate mastication
Physiologic
Gastric dysmotility
Gallstone
Dumping
Biliary dyskinesia
Dehydration
Vitamin deficiency
Medication
Infectious/inflammation
Esophagitis
Marginal ulcer
GERD
Mechanical
Gastrojejunostomy stricture
Sleeve narrowing/stricture
Twist of the sleeve
Band narrowing/stricture
Bezoar
Internal hernia
Adhesion causing the obstruction

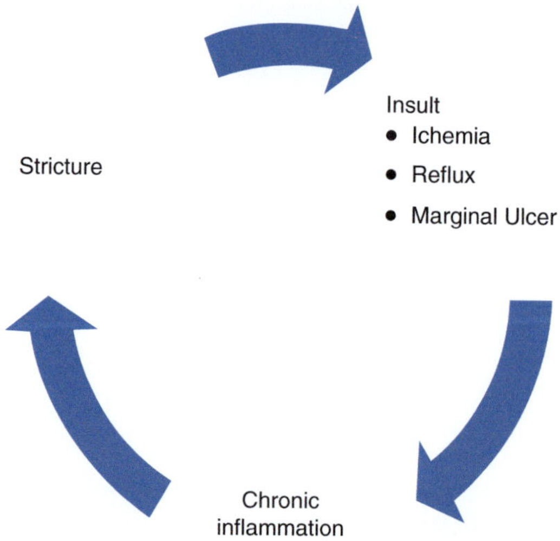

Fig. 22.1 Esophagitis and ulcer(s) can start a vicious cycle, which will cause chronic inflammation and fibrosis that can eventually lead to stricture

iatric surgery is a lifelong commitment and that people need to follow a strict bariatric diet for the rest of their lives. Bariatric Centers of Excellence are required to have a supervised diet and psychiatric/psychologic evaluation prior to any bariatric operation for this reason. Also, it has been shown that patients with anxiety or depression tend to have issues with dietary compliance after the surgery [4].

With rapid weight loss, the patients' body goes through significant physiologic changes that put them at a higher risk of developing biliary diseases up to 30% [5]. This occurs secondary to bile stasis, and up to 50% of bypass patients will develop gallstone(s)/sludge within 6 months of the index procedure. Nausea/vomiting and food intolerance are a few of the symptoms that can arise from any biliary disease.

Reflux or food regurgitation is one of the common complications that can occur after a sleeve gastrectomy, and it can occur in up to 25% of cases [6]. Post-sleeve gastrectomy reflux occurs because of the high-pressure system that is created. Experts agree that smaller bougies carry a higher risk of reflux secondary to an increased risk of stenosis [7]. Similarly, reflux is a common problem after gastric band placement, and the mechanism and pathophysiology are similar to the reflux after the sleeve. Reflux can have adverse effects on the patient's health and his/her quality of life by causing severe esophagitis or ulcer(s). The esophagitis and ulcer(s) can start a vicious cycle, which will cause chronic inflammation and fibrosis that can eventually lead to stricture (Fig. 22.1).

The mechanisms of weight loss from different procedures vary from purely restrictive to purely malabsorptive or a combination of both; therefore, even the same signs and symptoms may be derived by different pathways.

Gastric band and sleeve gastrectomy are restrictive procedures, and they can have both intrinsic and extrinsic causes of nausea and vomiting. The causes specific to sleeve gastrectomy are shown in Table 22.2. Gastric band can have similar phenomenon, but it is slightly different because the symptoms are caused mostly by the extrinsic compression secondary to the foreign body around the gastric cardia. Also, a foreign body causes chronic inflammation over time, which can lead to fibrosis and stricture. This type

Table 22.2 Causes specific to sleeve gastrectomy

Extrinsic	
	Edema
	Hematoma
	Oversewing
Intrinsic	
	Small bougie
	Gastric tube twisting
	Technical error

Table 22.3 Specific causes of sleeve gastrectomy

Procedure	Acute	Chronic
Band	Slippage	Fibrosis
	Hematoma	Erosion
Sleeve	Leak	Reflux
	Obstruction at the angle of incisura	Stricture at the angle of incisura
	Narrow gastric tube	Fistula
		Portal-SMV thrombosis
Bypass	Leak	Marginal ulcer
	Acute angulation of GJ	Stricture
	Small GJ anastomosis	
	Hematoma	

of stricture can be differentiated from an overly tightened band by emptying it completely and reevaluating the patient's symptoms.

After gastric bypass, research has shown that the anvil size is associated with postoperative stricture; therefore, it is recommended to use a 25 mm anvil if the circular EEA technique is utilized [8]. The stenosis still occurs with other techniques as well such as the completely hand-sewn anastomosis or the combination of posterior linear stapled and anterior hand-sewn anastomosis. Most surgeons hypothesize that this occurs because of chronic ischemia from the staple line or the suture. Also, a marginal ulcer is not an uncommon problem that occurs after gastric bypass that can potentially lead to symptomatic stenosis secondary to chronic inflammation and fibrosis.

As briefly discussed in the previous paragraph, the symptoms of nausea and vomiting or intolerance to PO intake can be summarized into two main categories, intrinsic and extrinsic in nature. Extrinsic causes are more common than the intrinsic ones because it is heavily dependent on the surgical technique such as the angle of stapling device at the incisura angularis, the bougie size, and the narrowing of the lumen with the oversewing of the staple line.

Clinical Presentation

The patient can either present with chronic symptoms to an outpatient facility or to an emergency room with more acute symptoms. The most common acute and chronic clinical presentations for different bariatric procedures are summarized in Table 22.3. The presentation will vary because of a variety of different pathologies. Although most patients will present with nausea and vomiting, it is prudent that the clinicians consider a wide variety of differential diagnoses when dealing with patients with poor PO tolerance.

Patients can develop PO intolerance as an acute symptom immediately after a procedure because of anesthesia, edema, hematoma, and narrowing of or tight gastric conduit. Most commonly, it is due to edema or a hematoma, which resolves over a short period of time as the swelling resolves. However, during the immediate postoperative period, intra-abdominal catastrophes such as a leak or perforation should be considered if the patient is having abdominal pain or early signs of sepsis along with nausea and vomiting.

One of the most common causes for a patient's poor PO tolerance after a bariatric procedure is non-compliance to the strict diet program postoperatively. These patients will present to the clinic or the ED with complaints of nausea and vomiting associated with food intake. The most common bariatric procedures that are performed in the United States are laparoscopic gastric band, laparoscopic sleeve, and laparoscopic Roux-en-Y gastric bypass. These procedures all share a common key component, which is to create a small gastric pouch. Because of the smaller neogastric pouch, patients will no longer be able to tolerate a big bulky meal. Non-compliant patients will complain of regurgitation of undigested food particles. Also, after gastric bypass, patients can develop dumping syndrome (DS) with high concentrated carbohydrate intake, which can present with poor PO tolerance along with other symptoms of DS including crampy abdominal pain, diarrhea, hypoglycemia, and fainting. It has been reported in the literature that patients can develop intolerance to certain foods, but the pathophysiology of this phenomenon is unknown [9].

Additionally, patients may have these symptoms because of either organic or functional causes such as gallbladder pathology and gastric or esophageal dysmotility. The incidence of cholecystectomy secondary to symptomatic cholelithiasis after bariatric surgery is about 3.4% within the first 12 months [10]. Those patients can present with nausea and vomiting along with other symptoms such as right upper quadrant abdominal pain associated with fatty meals and fever/chills. Also, it has been reported that bariatric surgery can have deleterious effects on esophageal motility, especially after sleeve gastrectomy or gastric band placement [11]. Patients with dysmotility will present with nausea and vomiting along with severe reflux and possibly retrosternal chest pain or food regurgitation.

Patients can develop symptoms because of uncorrected nutritional deficiencies especially vitamin B12, D, folate, iron, and zinc [12]. Different nutritional deficiencies will present with different signs and symptoms, which are summarized in Table 22.4. It is critical in severe cases of vomiting to rule out B1 (thiamine) deficiency. Severe deficiency can lead to Wernicke-Korsakoff syndrome, which could cause irreversible neurologic damage if left untreated.

Table 22.4 Nutritional deficiencies with clinical presentations

Nutritional deficiency	Complications
Vitamin B12	Anemia, neuropathy, neuropathy
Vitamin B1	Wernicke-Korsakoff syndrome
Vitamin D and calcium	Osteoporosis
Copper	CHF, neurologic and psychiatric disorders, unsteady ambulation
Folate	Megaloblastic anemia, neurologic and psychiatric conditions
Iron	Iron deficiency anemia
Zinc	Folate deficiency

Patients may present with poor PO tolerance after any bariatric surgery secondary to mechanical obstruction or stenosis. Patients can present with complete or partial obstruction depending on the degree of the stenosis. This can either occur during the acute or chronic phase. Acute phase is defined as within 2 weeks after the index procedure, and chronic phase is usually defined as time after the initial 2 weeks. Acute phase usually occurs because of poor surgical techniques, such as narrowing at the angle of incisura, usage of a small bougie or anvil, or narrowing with suturing; it can also occur because of intrinsic causes such as hematoma and/or edema. Most patients present with poor PO tolerance during the chronic phase. Because most of the stenosis or obstruction occurs secondary to chronic inflammation or fibrosis due to chronic ischemia, patients will complain of progressive dysphagia or reflux along with nausea/vomiting. If a patient has a combination of both stricture and poor compliance, patient may present with acute on chronic obstruction secondary to food bezoar.

When patients present with subtle signs of poor PO tolerance, physicians should have a high index of suspicion for common pathologies that can cause such symptoms; otherwise, patients may develop medical complications from malnutrition, dehydration, vitamin deficiency, etc.

Diagnosis

Most patients will have indolent and progressive symptoms for their poor PO tolerance. When a patient starts to develop signs and symptoms of nausea and vomiting, prompt work-up should be done to avoid complications. Physicians should tailor the work-up to cover a broad differential diagnosis. It is key to perform a thorough history and physical examinations to evaluate and rule out behavioral or psychosocial causes of his/her symptoms of PO intolerance. Also, basic laboratory tests along with vitamin levels need to be checked to rule out any nutrition and/or vitamin deficiencies.

A proposed algorithm is shown in Fig. 22.2. It is prudent to assess the acuity of the patient's

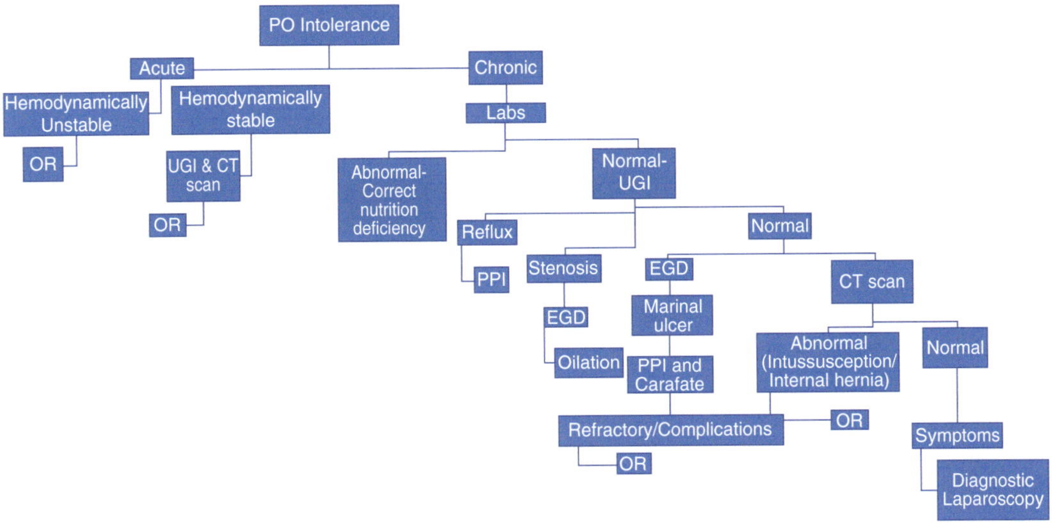

Fig. 22.2 PO intolerance algorithm

symptoms and the urgency of required therapeutic intervention. If a patient requires any emergent/urgent intervention, delayed diagnosis or intervention is associated with higher morbidity and mortality. Regardless of the procedure that the patient may have had in the past, it is important to rule out all potential causes that are acutely life-threatening. If the patient has a history of gastric band, a simple abdominal X-ray or an upper gastrointestinal series (UGI) can evaluate the position of the band and effectively rule out obstruction or band slippage. Either CXR or KUB can rule out free air, which is an important diagnosis to make when patient has a history of gastric bypass and/or marginal ulcer.

Also, after evaluating the stomach, which is the most common anatomic cause of poor PO intake, ultrasound of gallbladder and/or CT scan with PO contrast can assist in diagnosing other potential pathologies such as cholelithiasis, internal hernia, or intussusception. Although a CT scan lacks specificity or sensitivity in diagnosing either internal hernia or intussusception, it can be a valuable tool in conjunction with a surgeon's clinical suspicion [13]. A CT scan finding of target sign is highly suggestive of intussusception or mesenteric swirling for an internal hernia [14]. Patients who have lost a significant amount of weight are at higher risk of developing an intussusception. Also, these patients can develop internal hernia, especially after a gastric bypass procedure.

In the absence of other non-bariatric surgical causes of PO intolerance, UGI and EGD can diagnose and potentially be therapeutic in certain cases. The most common causes of poor PO tolerance after bariatric surgery are procedure specific. The most common cause after sleeve gastrectomy is narrowing of the conduit. Also, after a sleeve gastrectomy, the surgeon should carefully evaluate the degree of the reflux because it is reported that up to 25% of patients can suffer from symptomatic reflux after the procedure. A good-quality UGI can be utilized to evaluate both degree of the stricture and the reflux. After a gastric band placement, the patient can have poor PO tolerance secondary to tight extrinsic compression of the band or chronic fibrosis. For the banded patient, it is important to evaluate the degree of extrinsic compression before introducing any instrumentation because of the potential risk of perforation, especially if the patient has been having chronic symptoms. The patient may have developed esophageal dilation, which carries a higher complication rate than in the normal esophagus during the endoscopy [15]. It is recommended to deflate the balloon prior to planned EGD if the patient has a gastric band.

After a gastric bypass, patients can have obstructive symptoms because of marginal ulcer, stenosis, or food bezoar. Similar to other procedures, clinicians should start the evaluation with noninvasive UGI, and if clinically indicated, EGD can be performed. EGD can be both diagnostic and therapeutic at the same time.

If the above work-up is negative and the patient has clinical signs and symptoms of esophageal dysmotility disorder, further work-up should be taken with manometry. Also, if the patient's work-up failed to reveal any significant pathology but the chief complaint is reflux, it is advisable to perform an esophageal pH monitoring such as the Bravo test.

Management

Management for PO intolerance will vary depending on the underlying pathology that is causing the symptoms. If the proposed algorithm is followed, most of the common causes of obstructive symptoms should be addressed.

Patient's acuity of symptoms and urgency of potentially required intervention should be carefully assessed. During the immediate postoperative period, should the patient develop acute symptoms of PO intolerance, surgical or technical complications should be considered. If the patient presents with chronic symptoms, the patient should be assessed to determine whether or not he/she is physically fit to undergo any major operation. If the patient is severely dehydrated or malnourished (BMI <18), IV hydration and/or temporary parenteral nutrition with or without enteral feeding via remnant gastrostomy or jejunal feeding tube should be started.

Although the gastric band has fallen out of favor secondary to lack of efficacy and durability of weight loss, it was the most commonly performed bariatric procedure in the 1990s. It has its own set of complications that come with any intraperitoneally placed foreign body. The incidence of band slippage has been reported to be 1–22% [16, 17]. When it occurs, it could be a surgical emergency because it can cause stomach ischemia or necrosis which could lead to perforation. When band slippage is diagnosed, the first step is to deflate the band and immediately reassess the situation. If complete resolution of symptoms is not achieved or still there is any degree of intolerance to drinking, it is prudent to proceed to surgery and remove the band. When dealing with an emergent diagnosis, it is advisable to deal with the problem without any heroic measures. Sometimes, at the time of the surgery, a surgeon may encounter concomitant band erosion and perforation. When this occurs, an omentum or jejunal patch is recommended with adequate drainage and antibiotics. When a patient presents with more chronic symptoms, additional work-up can be done to diagnose the stenosis and fibrosis as described above. Once the diagnosis is made, the first thing to do is to make sure that the band is completely decompressed. However, if the patient has been having chronic symptoms associated with external compression of the stomach, band deflation alone may not be enough to control the symptoms. In those patients who are refractory to nonsurgical management, surgery should be considered with removal of the band. In the operating room, it is critical not only to remove the band with the scar tissue that is causing the external compression secondary to chronic inflammation and fibrosis.

Similar principles can be applied to patients who either had a sleeve gastrectomy or a gastric bypass. It is important to rule out any acute pathology with basic imaging and endoscopy, along with physical examinations. Leak, stenosis, or reflux can cause poor PO tolerance after sleeve gastrectomy. Any one of these diagnoses can present acutely or chronically. Management of each of these problems may vary depending on the patient's condition at the time of the presentation and the quality of the tissue found intraoperatively. For a leak that occurred acutely after the index operation, the patient should be returned to the OR promptly for repair and adequate drainage along with initiation of broad-spectrum antibiotics. In spite of adequate drainage, if the patient fails to heal (which can happen to sleeve patients because of the high-pressure system), a stent can be considered [18]. If the stent fails to control the leak, the patient will require a formal revision of the sleeve. For these patients, resection of the leaked portion of the stomach, which is usually located at the proximal part of the conduit, and reconstruction with esophagojejunostomy are a valid option.

Acute obstruction after a sleeve occurs due to narrowing at the incisura from technical reasons or more commonly because of postoperative edema or hematoma. The latter causes usually improve with observation only and rarely require surgery. However, narrowing at the incisura will most likely need surgical revision, often to a bypass.

Patients who had sleeve gastrectomy can present with chronic problems secondary to nonhealing fistula/leak, stenosis, or chronic reflux. Chronic stenosis can be managed with a stent [19]. Some surgeons believe that fistula and leaks do not heal after a sleeve because of the high-pressure system proximal to functional pylorus. Therefore, most of the problems can be safely and effectively addressed by converting to a low-pressure system such as gastric bypass. It is important to remove the diseased portion of the stomach with the site of the leak, fistula, and/or stenosis and send for pathology to evaluate for any underlying conditions. Although associated with high morbidity and complications, seromyotomy or segmental resection with gastro-gastrostomy can be considered for the patients who refuse revision to gastric bypass [20].

Gastric bypass has been proven to be the most effective and durable weight loss surgical option. However, patients can have complications in the immediate postoperative period or long after the surgery, and these complications can cause PO intolerance. As with all other surgical problems, early recognition is the key to decrease morbidity and mortality. For early acute pathologies with unstable patient, it is prudent to take the patient to the operating room for a second look with or without an intraoperative endoscopy especially if sepsis is present. If the patient is stable, most contained leaks can be effectively treated conservatively with a drain; however, if the patient is septic and not responding to nonsurgical management, the surgeon needs to evaluate the patient operatively [21, 22]. Endoscopy will be especially helpful in the setting in which an intragastric bleeding needs to be ruled out. When clinically indicated, endoscopy can be performed safely and effectively during the immediate postoperative period [23]. The patient's tissue quality and clinical factors will help determine further management intraoperatively. Primary repair, reinforcement with omentum, and re-doing the anastomosis are all viable options, but the most important part of the operation when returning to the OR for a leak is adequate drainage [21].

Gastric bypass patients can develop acute obstruction because of a hematoma or edema similar to sleeve patients. Conservative management is usually successful. Depending on the location and severity of the hematoma, the patient may need either an endoscopic or laparoscopic intervention to evacuate the source (gastrojejunal or jejuno-jejunal anastomosis). Acute obstruction can always arise from one of the trocars site in up to 1.6% of cases. In these cases, urgent exploration is required [24].

Another common problem that patients can develop after a gastric bypass is a marginal ulcer. Marginal ulcers can develop secondary to smoking, NSAID abuse, or high acid secretion from the retained antrum. It usually occurs at the jejunal side of the GJ anastomosis. Marginal ulcers can be diagnosed endoscopically, and usual treatment requires high-dose PPI with Carafate. If the patient is a smoker, it is absolutely critical to counsel the patient to cease smoking. Most marginal ulcers respond to medical therapy, but it can lead to stricture secondary to chronic fibrosis and inflammation. If stenosis occurs and the patient becomes symptomatic, UGI can help assess the degree of the stenosis. However, when a patient develops symptoms secondary to stricture that is confirmed with a radiographic study, the patient should undergo an EGD for both diagnostic and therapeutic purposes. During endoscopy, accurate assessment of the anastomosis can be made, and the performing physician can decide how aggressively he/she will dilate the stricture. It has been shown that the dilation can be performed safely without added risk of perforation or complication up to 16 mm [25]. When the balloon dilation is being considered as a therapeutic option, it can be dilated in increments. It has been shown that patients will require an average of two dilations or more. However, if the stenosis is a recurring problem and it is affecting the patient's quality of life or the marginal ulcer causes significant complications such as uncontrolled bleeding or perforation, surgical correction of the problem is warranted. Usually, the anastomosis and the ulcer need to be resected, and a new gastrojejunostomy should be reconstructed. Some surgeons advocate for completely removing the remnant stomach to decrease acid production for refractory marginal ulcers. There have been documented cases of concomitant vagotomy and remnant gastrectomy, but no level 1 data is available to support such procedures [26, 27].

Another chronic problem that can arise from a bypass surgery besides the stricture of the anastomosis and marginal ulcer is internal hernia. An internal hernia can occur approximately in 2.5% of the patients, and the most common sites are the transverse colon mesentery, Petersen's space, and at the enteroenterostomy site [28]. There are several proposed methods to prevent an internal hernia, but there is no consensus on which one is the most effective. The key is to recognize the problem since patients can present without any specific signs or symptoms and there is no gold standard diagnostic modality. When a patient presents with vague intermittent abdominal complaints with poor PO tolerance and there is no obvious pathology demonstrated during the work-up, diagnostic laparoscopy should be considered to rule out an internal hernia; if found, closure of the defect should be performed with nonabsorbable sutures [28].

Conclusion

Poor PO tolerance after a bariatric procedure can impact a patient's quality of life with significant medical consequences; therefore, it needs to be carefully addressed by the physician. There are broad differential diagnoses that need to be carefully worked up for these patients. Early recognition of the problem and appropriate treatment will decrease morbidity and mortality.

References

1. Elrazek AEMAA, et al. Medical management of patients after bariatric surgery. WJGS. 2014;6(11):220–8.
2. Ma IT, Madura JA. Gastrointestinal complications after bariatric surgery. Gastroenterol Hepatol. 2015;11(8):526–35.
3. Aman MW, et al. Early hospital readmission after bariatric surgery. Surg Endosc. 2016;30:2231–8.
4. Godoy CM, et al. Food tolerance in patients submitted to gastric bypass: the importance of using an integrated and interdisciplinary approach. Obes Surg. 2012;22:124–30.
5. Lopez PP, et al. Outpatient complications encountered following Roux-en-y gastric bypass. Med Clin N Am. 2007;91:471–83.
6. Brethauser SA. Sleeve gastrectomy. Surg Clin North Am. 2011;91:1265–79.
7. Rosenthal R, International Sleeve Gastrectomy Expert Panel. International sleeve gastrectomy expert panel consensus statement: best practice guidelines based on experience of > 12,000 cases. Surg Obes Relat Dis. 2012;8:8–19.
8. Dolce CJ, et al. Gastrojejunal strictures after roux-en-y gastric bypass with a 21-mm circular stapler. JSLS. 2009;13(3):306–11.
9. Graham L, et al. Taste, smell, and appetite change after Roux-en-Y gastric bypass surgery. Obes Surg. 2014;24(9):1463–8.
10. Pineda O et al. A prospective study of the conservative management of asymptomatic preoperative and postoperative gallbladder disease in bariatric surgery. Obes Surg. 2017;27(1):148-153. doi: 10.1007/s11695-016-2264-3.
11. Tolone S, Savarino E, Yates RB. The impact of bariatric surgery on esophageal function. Ann N Y Acad Sci. 2016;1381(1):98–103. doi: 10.1111/nyas.13107. Epub 2016 Jun 15.
12. Xanthakos SA. Nutritional deficiencies in obesity and after bariatric surgery. Pediatr Clin N Am. 2009;56(5):1105–21.
13. Daellenback K, Suter M. Jejunojejunal intussusception after Roux-en-Y gastric bypass: a review. Obes Surg. 2011;21(2):253–63.
14. Lockhart ME, et al. Internal hernia after gastric bypass: sensitivity and specificity of seven CT signs with surgical correlation and control. Am J Roentogenol. 2007;188(3):745–50.
15. Katzka DA, Castell DO. Review article: an analysis of the efficacy, perforation rates and methods used in pneumatic dilation for achalasia. Aliment Pharmacol Ther. 2011;34(8):832–9.
16. Suter M. Laparoscopic band repositioning for pouch dilatation/slippage after gastric banding: disappointing results. Obes Surg. 2001;11(4):507–12.
17. Eid I, et al. Complications associated with adjustable gastric banding for morbid obesity: a surgeon's guide. Can J Surg. 2011;54(1):61–6.
18. Nguyen NT, et al. The use of endoscopic stent in management of leaks after. Obes Surg. 2010;20(9):1289-92. doi: 10.1007/s11695-010-0186-z.

19. Ogra R, Kini GP. Evolving endoscopic management options for symptomatic stenosis post-laparoscopic sleeve gastrectomy for morbid obesity: experience at a large bariatric surgery unit in New Zealand. Obes Surg. 2015;2(2):242–8.
20. Vilallonga R, et al. Laparoscopic management of persistent strictures after laparoscopic sleeve gastrectomy. Obes Surg. 2013;23(1):1655–61.
21. Bekheit M, et al. Earliest signs and management of leakage after bariatric surgeries: single institute experience. Alex J Med. 2013;49(1):29–33.
22. Gonzalez R, et al. Diagnosis and contemporary management of anastomotic leaks after gastric bypass for obesity. J Am Coll Surg. 2007;204:47–55.
23. Walsh C, Karmali S. Endoscopic management of bariatric complications: a review and update. World J Gastrointest Endosc. 2015;7(5):518–23.
24. Pilone V, et al. Trocar site hernia after bariatric surgery: our experience without fascial closure. Int J Surg. 2014;12(1):83–6.
25. Go MR, et al. Endoscopic management of stomal stenosis after Roux-en-Y gastric bypass. Surg Endosc. 2004;18(1):56–9.
26. Patel RA, et al. Revisional operations for marginal ulcer after Roux-en-Y gastric bypass. SORD. 2009;5(3):317–22.
27. Steinemann DC, et al. Laparoscopic gastric pouch and remnant resection: a novel approach to refractory anastomotic ulcers after Roux-en-Y gastric bypass: case report. BMC Surg. 2011;11:33.
28. Iannelli A, et al. Internal hernia after laparoscopic Roux-en-Y gastric bypass for morbid obesity. Obes Srug. 2006;16(10):1265–71.

23 Postoperative Strictures

Mandi Joshi, Emanuele Lo Menzo,
Samuel Szomstein, and Raul J. Rosenthal

Bariatric Surgery Complications: GJ Stricture and Sleeve Stricture

Obesity is a global epidemic and has become a public health crisis in the United States. Multiple studies have shown the prevalence of this epidemic has been steadily increasing over the last three decades [1]. Reports published by the National Health and Nutrition Examination Survey (NHANES) from 2009 to 2010 showed one out of three American adults are obese and two out of three are overweight [2].

Bariatric surgery is considered the most effective way to achieve durable weight loss. Roux-en-Y gastric bypass (RYGB) and sleeve gastrectomy (SG) are two of the most commonly performed bariatric procedures and lead to excellent short-term and long-term outcomes. Due to the widespread adoption of these procedures, even the rare complications, such as gastrojejunal (GJ) anastomotic stricture and sleeve gastrectomy stricture, are now encountered more frequently.

M. Joshi
Department of Surgery, DaVita Medical Group, Albuquerque, NM, USA

E. L. Menzo · S. Szomstein
The Bariatric and Metabolic Institute, Cleveland Clinic Florida – Weston, Weston, FL, USA
e-mail: lomenze@ccf.org; szomsts@ccf.org

R. J. Rosenthal (✉)
Department of Surgery, Cleveland Clinic Florida, Weston, FL, USA
e-mail: rosentr@ccf.org

Gastrojejunal Anastomotic Stricture Following RYGB

Incidence

The incidence of GJ stricture varies from 3% to 30% in the literature (Table 23.1). The experience at our institution is about 6% [3]. The wide variation in the incidence is mostly dependent upon the surgical technique utilized. The data comparing open technique to laparoscopic technique is conflicting [4, 5]. Studies comparing the linear stapler technique to the circular stapler have shown an increased incidence of stricture with the latter. A retrospective study by Peterli et al. in 328 patients has shown the stricture to be 0% in the linear stapler group and 7% in the circular stapler group [6]. The diameter/size of the circular stapler used is another important factor. In fact, the 21 mm circular stapler causes significant stenosis (26.8%) compared to the 25 mm stapler (8.8%), as observed in a study by Nguyen et al. [7]. It is also important to note that the hand sewn anastomosis carries a similar incidence of stricture rate as compared to the linear staple [8]. Table 23.1 summarizes the incidence of GJ stricture in selected series of LRYGB.

R. Lutfi et al. (eds.), *Global Bariatric Surgery*, https://doi.org/10.1007/978-3-319-93545-4_23

Mechanism/Cause

Various mechanisms have been described in the literature for the formation of GJ stricture; however, none have strong evidence. Ischemia of the anastomosis with or without ulceration causing scarring and stricture is probably the most common mechanism. Other mechanisms include non-ischemic ulceration, probably due to high acid concentration in the gastric pouch, technical failure leading to acute angulation of the anastomosis, or too tight anastomosis creation [15, 16]. A large gastric pouch has also been postulated to play a role in GJ ulceration and stricture formation [17].

Table 23.1 Incidence of GJ stricture in selected series of LRYGB

Author/year	Number of patients	Incidence of strictures (%)	Mean BMI (kg/m^2)
Higa (2000) [9]	1040	4.9	50
Wittgrove (2000) [10]	500	1.6	45
Matheus (2000) [11]	48	27	52.3
Schwartz (2004) [12]	1000	3.2	45
McCarty (2005) [13]	2000	2.1	45
Rosenthal (2008) [3]	1012	6	45
Marmuse (2015) [14]	1500	3.4	

Presentation

The majority of patients present with symptoms of GJ stricture within the first 1–3 months of surgery. Presenting symptoms usually range from nausea, vomiting, intolerance to diet, dehydration, and abdominal pain to severe malnutrition and micronutrient/vitamin deficiency in longstanding cases.

Diagnosis

The diagnosis of GJ stricture is based on the clinical evaluation followed by radiographic evaluation and/or esophagogastroduodenoscopy (EGD). The upper gastrointestinal (UGI) study with oral contrast is still considered the radiographic study of choice [18]. A CT scan can also be performed if the UGI study is equivocal. However the CT scan only shows static signs of the stenosis, such as pouch enlargement, lack of passage of contrast in the Roux limb, and inflammatory changes at the anastomosis. The UGI instead will give a dynamic picture of the anatomy showing a dilated pouch, delayed emptying of pouch, visualization of stricture, and non-emptying of contrast in the jejunum (Fig. 23.1).

Flexible endoscopy is performed as both diagnostic and therapeutic modality in GJ stricture (Fig. 23.2). The inability to pass a standard adult upper endoscope with an external diameter of 10.5 mm easily through the anastomosis is con-

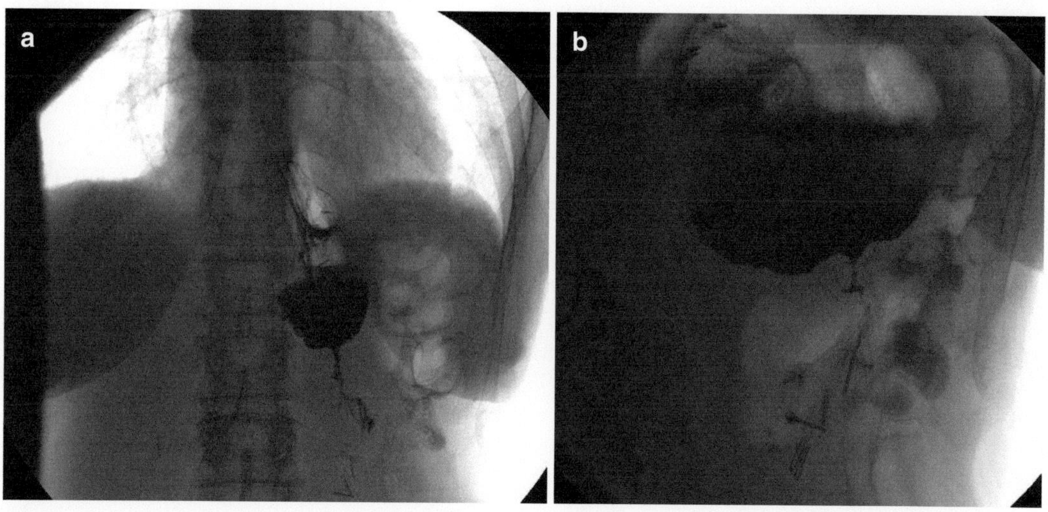

Fig. 23.1 (**a**, **b**) UGI contrast study depicting severe gastrojejunal anastomotic stricture and dilated gastric pouch

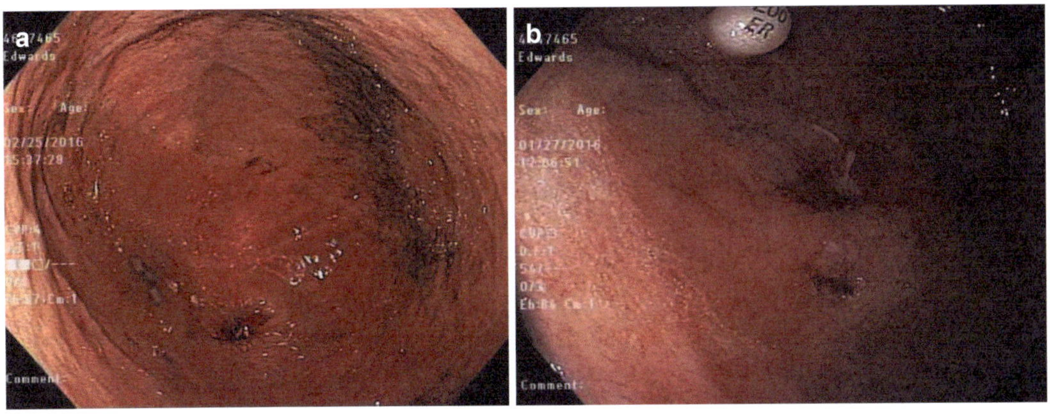

Fig. 23.2 (**a**, **b**) Flexible endoscopy showing dilated gastric pouch and stenotic gastrojejunal anastomosis

sidered diagnostic for stricture [16]. The EGD also allows for visualization of concomitant ulceration, if any is present. The GJ stricture can be endoscopically categorized into four grades (Table 23.2) [16].

Table 23.2 Grades of gastrojejunal anastomotic stricture

Grade I	Mild stenosis; 10.5 mm endoscope can be passed
Grade II	Moderate stenosis; 8.5 mm pediatric endoscope can be passed
Grade III	Severe stenosis; only guidewire can be passed
Grade IV	Complete or near-complete obstruction, pinhole/untraversable

Management

Nonsurgical Management

As mentioned above, flexible endoscopy can be used for both diagnostic and therapeutic purposes. Following the diagnosis of stricture, different dilatation techniques can be used. Commonly the through-the-scope (TTS) technique is utilized. In this technique, a balloon catheter (Fig. 23.3) of various sizes, depending upon the grade of stenosis, is passed via the working channel of the flexible endoscope and through the GJ stricture such that the midportion of the balloon lies at the stricture. The balloon is then inflated with water under direct vision to the specific pressure as per balloon sizes (Figs. 23.4 and 23.5) [15]. Repeated dilation up to three to four attempts is usually performed with intervals of 2–4 weeks between dilations in severe stenosis. Fluoroscopy-guided balloon dilation can be used in difficult stenosis, especially if only a guide wire can be advanced across the stenosis (Fig. 23.6). The most serious complication of balloon dilatation is perforation, which can occur in 4.9% of cases in our institutional experience [3].

Alternatively, a wire-guided dilatation with weighted bougies (Savary-Gilliard) can also be

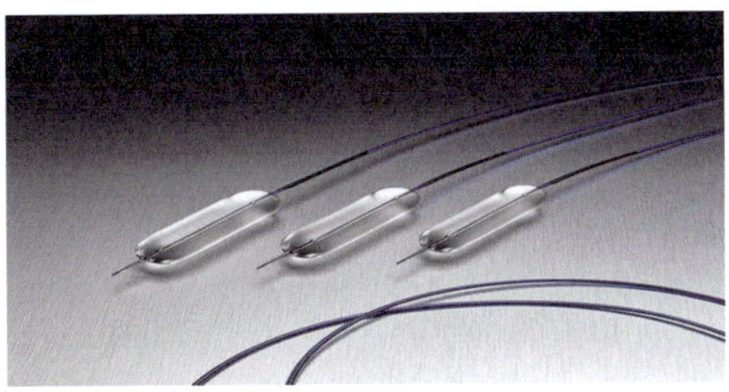

Fig. 23.3 Endoscopic balloon dilator available in various sizes

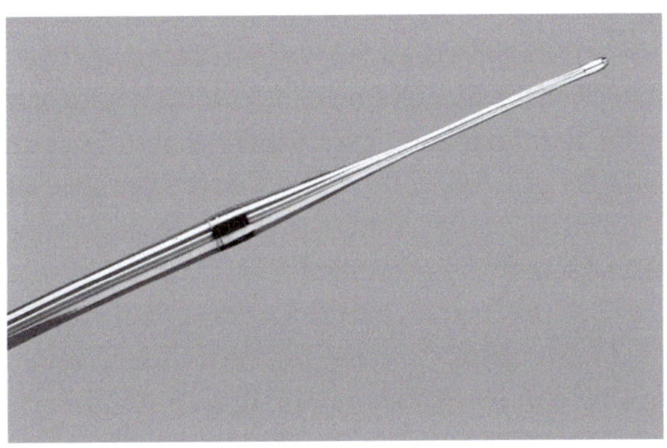

Fig. 23.4 Savary-Gilliard dilator

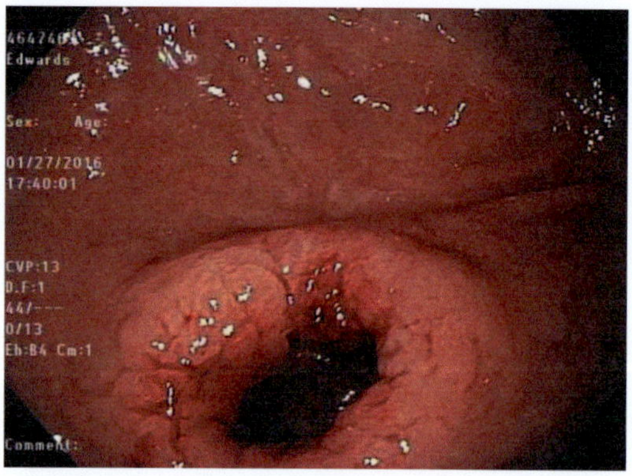

Fig. 23.5 Flexible endoscopy post-balloon dilation showing moderate dilation of gastrojejunal anastomotic stricture

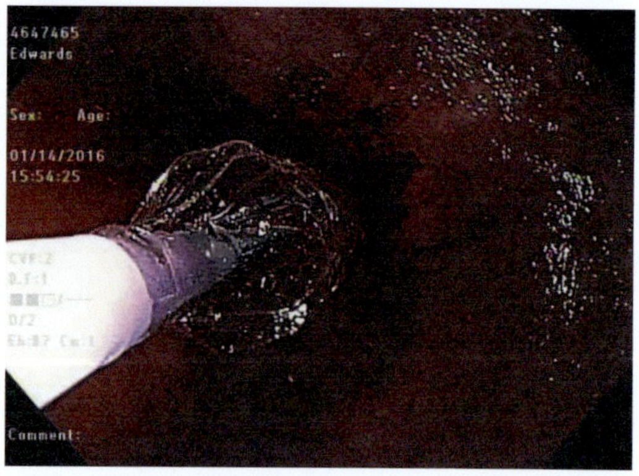

Fig. 23.7 Endoscopic balloon dilation of the stricture, balloon at inflated and deflated state

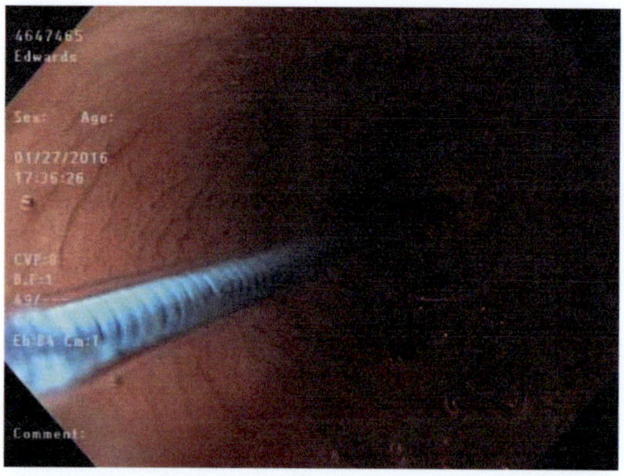

Fig. 23.6 Fluoroscopy-guided balloon dilation of gastrojejunal stricture and post dilation free passage of contrast

safely and effectively used for dilation of GJ stricture with good outcomes (Fig. 23.7); however, the data is limited [14]. The potential advantage of this technique is the ability of dilating by using shearing forces as opposed to just radial forces as in the TTS technique. In the case of refractory strictures, endoscopic stents have been used; however, stent migration and post placement pain have been frequently described [19].

Surgical Management

Surgical management is reserved for the strictures refractory to multiple attempts of endoscopic dilatation, complete occlusion of the anastomosis, or in case of perforation after dilatation [20]. Revisional bariatric surgery has good outcomes in experienced hands and high-volume centers. Meticulous dissection, with careful identification of anatomy and excision of the GJ anastomosis with partial gastric pouch resection and creation of new anastomosis, is the typical surgery for most of the cases of GJ stricture. Large populations and long-term studies are still lacking in the literature regarding the efficacy of revisional bariatric surgery for GJ stricture.

In summary, GJ anastomotic stricture is probably one of the most common complications seen after RYGB. If left untreated, it can lead to severe malnutrition, dehydration with multiple ER visits, and hospital admissions. The diagnosis is usually made clinically and with the aid of UGI radiographic study and flexible endoscopy. Most of the cases are successfully treated with serial dilation with endoscopy-guided balloon catheter, although it may require several attempts. Failed endoscopic management usually requires surgical revision of the GJ anastomosis. Revision surgery has good outcomes in experienced hands and high-volume bariatric centers.

Sleeve Stricture

Introduction

Sleeve gastrectomy is currently the most commonly performed bariatric procedure worldwide.

Table 23.3 Incidence of sleeve gastrectomy stricture in selected series

Author/year	Number of patients	Incidence of stricture (%)
Kini (2015) [21]	857	3.03
Braghetto (2013) [22]	717	0.69
Parikh (2012) [23]	230	3.5
Zundel (2010) [24]	1155	0.26
Rosenthal (2008) [25]	148	0.7
Cottam (2006) [26]	126	3.9

Consequently, with the increase in numbers of this procedure, rare but severe complications such as sleeve stricture are becoming more common. The incidence of sleeve stricture varies form 0.3% to 4% in various reports (Table 23.3). Various causes and mechanisms have been described in the literature. Among the potential different causes of stricture are the size of the bougie used, the technique of stapling the stomach, the proximity to the incisura angularis, the oversewing of the staple line, and the twisting of the sleeve.

Mechanism/Pathophysiology

The International Sleeve Gastrectomy Expert Panel has recommended using a bougie ranged between 32 and 38 Fr for sizing the sleeve [27]. Smaller bougie size has been associated with increased incidence of leak, but not strongly associated with sleeve stricture [28, 29]. However, currently there is significant variability in the size of the bougie, and some centers do not use a bougie at all. We routinely use a 38 Fr bougie at our center, and our stricture rate is in line with the literature (0.7%) [25]. The principal causes of sleeve stricture are technical or iatrogenic. Careful handling of the stapler and paying attention to stapling technique can prevent this complication most times. Overzealous attempts to make a narrow sleeve to achieve significant weight loss can definitely cause stricture and also sleeve leaks. Starting stapling too close to the pylorus or staying too close to the incisura can lead to sleeve stricture (Table 23.4).

Table 23.4 Prevention of stricture formation

Use of bougie while stapling the stomach
Avoiding stapling close to pylorus and incisura angularis
Suture reinforcement if done should be performed meticulously
Avoiding twisting of sleeve by maintaining symmetry of anterior and posterior wall of the stomach while stapling
Preservation of blood supply of the lesser curve
Careful attention to staple line hematoma
Use of intraoperative EGD if necessary [30]

Reinforcement of the staple line using continuous suturing is performed to prevent staple line bleeding and leaks. Although the data to demonstrate the association between staple line suturing and stricture is mixed, care needs to be taken not to take too much tissue, and not to include tissue too far apart, or too close to the lesser curvature. Also, twisting of the staple line secondary to malalignment of the stapler, or secondary to too much retraction of the anterior or posterior wall while stapling, can cause development of functional valve or angulation, thus causing stenosis. Other postoperative complications like hematoma and staple line leak can also eventually cause stenosis [24, 29].

Clinical Presentation and Diagnosis

Although the initial presentation of sleeve stricture can vary significantly depending upon the severity and the cause of it, most are symptomatic in the first 6 weeks after surgery. Similar to gastric bypass stricture, patients usually present with nausea, vomiting, and intolerance to diet. Dysphagia, sticking sensation of food, saliva and food regurgitation, and de novo GERD symptoms can also be seen in these patients [30]. Symptoms in the immediate postoperative period may be due to tissue edema, which usually resolves with conservative management. Persistent symptoms may warrant further investigations and management. The diagnosis is usually made with upper gastrointestinal (UGI) contrast study and flexible upper endoscopy.

The UGI contrast study can show any combinations of these findings: thin stenotic sleeve, kinking or tortuosity of the sleeve, lack of progression of the contrast column, or dilated fundus [24]. However, routine postoperative UGI study is not a good predictor of future symptomatic stenosis and/or leak and thus has been abandoned in many institutions.

Flexible endoscopy is the gold standard investigation for the diagnosis and evaluation of the stenosis. It helps in identifying the characteristics of the stenosis, such as location, length, angulation, and functional stenosis. Flexible endoscopy can be simultaneously diagnostic and therapeutic. Cautious intubation of the sleeve in early postoperative days should be done; however, it is a safe procedure in experienced hands. A narrow lumen with difficulty in passage of the adult flexible endoscope is considered a stricture.

Management

Nonsurgical Management

In the early postoperative period, a patient presenting with nausea and vomiting should be managed conservatively with nil per os, intravenous hydration, antiemetics, and protein pump inhibitors. Most of these early symptoms are due to tissue edema, causing stenosis, and they resolve spontaneously. Non-resolution of the symptoms would trigger further investigation, such as UGI contrast study and flexible endoscopy. Short-segment stenosis can be effectively managed with flexible endoscopy and balloon dilatation. At least two to five attempts of dilation are necessary for the resolution of symptoms and tolerance of diet. Endoscopic myotomy in four quadrants has been described in some centers for resolution of short-segment stenosis [24]. Endoscopic stenting has been used in cases of failed balloon dilation; however, the data still is not very convincing. Most often, the stents are removed within a week because of pain and stent migration [2].

Surgical Management

Surgical management of a sleeve stricture depends mainly on its location and length. Scarce data exists in the literature regarding standard surgical management of sleeve stricture. The possible techniques include stricturoplasty, wedge resection/segmental resection of the stricture, seromyotomy, and more radical technique such as conversion to RYGB and total gastrectomy with Roux-en-Y esophagojejunostomy. Immediate re-intervention for sleeve stricture in the early postoperative days includes evacuation of staple line hematoma if present, suture removal if used for staple line reinforcement, and untwisting and omentopexy of the sleeve.

Stricturoplasty

A Heineke-Mikulicz-type strictureplasty, as described initially for gastric outlet obstruction in peptic ulcer disease and also for small bowel stricture, can be performed for sleeve strictures as well. Sudan et al. described the technique in two patients with sleeve stricture with robotic assistance and satisfactory results [31]. The stricture was incised along the long axis the entire length and closed in the transverse axis, single layer, using permanent braided sutures.

Seromyotomy

Seromyotomy has been described by a few authors for long-sleeve strictures [32, 33]. The technique described involves the use of a monopolar hook or ultrasonic energy to perform the seromyotomy until the mucosa is visualized, along the entire length of the stricture and 1 cm beyond both proximally and distally (Figs. 23.8 and 23.9). Intraoperative esophagogastroscopy

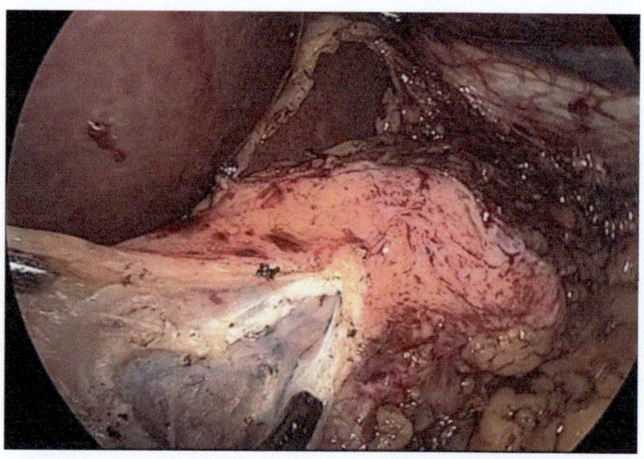

Fig. 23.8 Seromyotomy of the gastric musculature after LSG

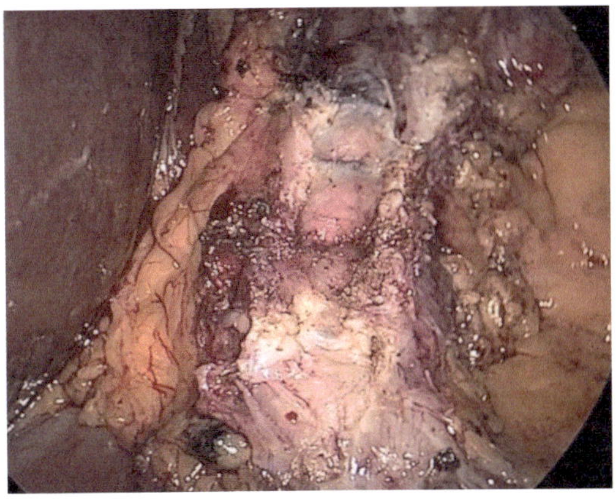

Fig. 23.9 Completed seromyotomy of the LSG

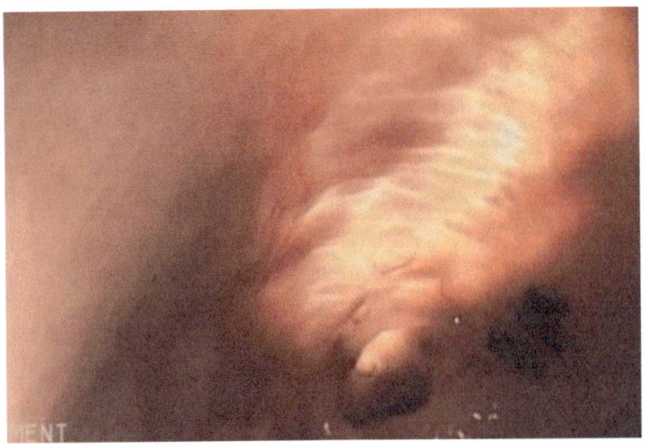

Fig. 23.10 Intraoperative esophagogastroscopy to assess completeness of the myotomy and patency of the sleeve

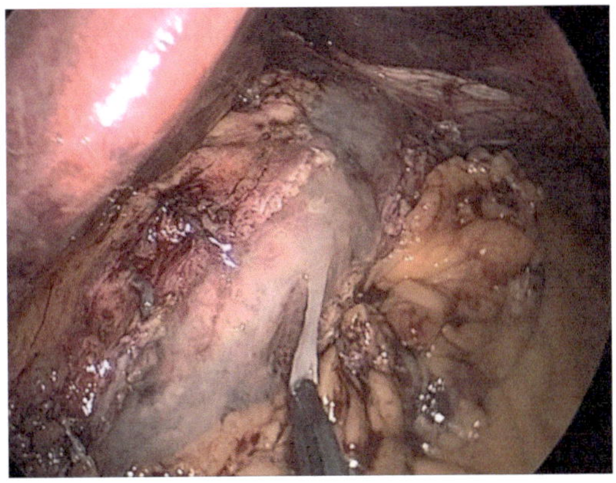

Fig. 23.11 Fibrin glue placed over the gastric myotomy

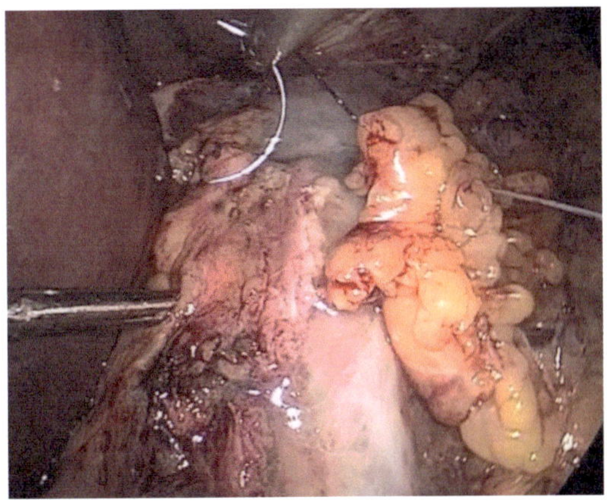

Fig. 23.12 The omentum is placed over the myotomy to provide reinforcement

can be used to assess the completeness of the seromyotomy intraoperatively (Fig. 23.10). Placement of fibrin glue and omentoplasty has also been described for reinforcement of the seromyotomy (Figs. 23.11 and 23.12). Despite satisfactory improvement of symptoms, high incidences of postoperative leak and reoperation have been seen following seromyotomy in some studies.

Wedge resection/segmental resection of the sleeve has also been proposed as a surgical technique for short-segment sleeve stricture [32]. Following resection of the segment with 1 cm margin, end-to-end anastomosis of the proximal and distal remaining stomach is done using a single-layer running suture. For patients with sleeve stricture not amenable to previously described techniques, RYGB or total gastrectomy with esophagojejunostomy should be performed [23]. The technique of RYGB in these patients is similar to revisional RYGB in patients with weight regain or failure of weight loss in sleeve gastrectomy. All patients undergoing surgery for sleeve stricture should begin with diagnostic laparoscopy and intraoperative flexible endoscopy to delineate the anatomy and the stricture. Revision surgery for sleeve stricture, similar to revision surgery in gastric bypass stricture, is a challenging operation and should be performed by experts in high-volume centers for better outcomes.

In summary, GJ anastomotic stricture and sleeve stricture are among the most common complications seen after bariatric surgery. If left untreated, they can lead to multiple ER visits and hospital admissions. The diagnosis is usually made clinically and with aid of UGI radiographic study and flexible endoscopy. Most cases are successfully treated with serial dilation with endoscopy-guided balloon catheter, usually after three to four attempts. Failed endoscopic management usually is treated with revisional surgery. Revisional surgery has good outcomes in experienced hands and in high-volume bariatric centers.

References

1. Wang Y, et al. Will all Americans become overweight or obese? Estimating the progression and cost of the US obesity epidemic. Obesity. 2008;16(10):2323–30.
2. Flegal KM, et al. Prevalence of obesity and trends in the distribution of body mass index among US adults, 1999–2010. JAMA. 2012;307(5):491–7.
3. Ukleja A, et al. Outcome of endoscopic balloon dilation of strictures after laparoscopic gastric bypass. Surg Endosc. 2008;22(8):1746–50.
4. Nguyen NT, et al. Laparoscopic versus open gastric bypass: a randomized study of outcomes, quality of life, and costs. Ann Surg. 2001;234(3):279–91.
5. Peifer KJ, et al. Successful endoscopic management of gastrojejunal anastomotic strictures after Roux-en-Y gastric bypass. Gastrointest Endosc. 2007;66(2):248–52.
6. Schneider R, et al. Linear compared to circular stapler anastomosis in laparoscopic Roux-en-Y gastric bypass leads to comparable weight loss with fewer complications: a matched pair study. Langenbeck's Arch Surg. 2016;401(3):307–13.
7. Nguyen NT, Melinda Stevens C, Wolfe BM. Incidence and outcome of anastomotic stricture after laparoscopic gastric bypass. J Gastrointest Surg. 2003;7(8):997–1003.
8. Kravetz AJ, et al. A comparative study of handsewn versus stapled gastrojejunal anastomosis in laparoscopic Roux-en-Y gastric bypass. Surg Endosc. 2011;25(4):1287–92.
9. Higa KD, Boone KB, Ho T. Complications of the laparoscopic Roux-en-Y gastric bypass: 1,040 patients-what have we learned? Obes Surg. 2000;10(6):509–13.
10. Wittgrove AC, Wesley Clark G. Laparoscopic gastric bypass, Roux en-Y-500 patients: technique and results, with 3–60 month follow-up. Obes Surg. 2000;10(3):233–9.
11. Matthews BD, et al. Initial results with a stapled gastrojejunostomy for the laparoscopic isolated Roux-en-Y gastric bypass. Am J Surg. 2000;179(6):476–81.
12. Schwartz ML, et al. Stenosis of the gastroenterostomy after laparoscopic gastric bypass. Obes Surg. 2004;14(4):484–91.
13. McCarty TM, et al. Optimizing outcomes in bariatric surgery: outpatient laparoscopic gastric bypass. Ann Surg. 2005;242(4):494–501.
14. Ribeiro-Parenti L, et al. Gastrojejunostomy stricture rate: comparison between antecolic and retrocolic laparoscopic Roux-en-Y gastric bypass. Surg Obes Relat Dis. 2015;11(5):1076–84.
15. Takata MC, et al. Predictors, treatment, and outcomes of gastrojejunostomy stricture after gastric bypass for morbid obesity. Obes Surg. 2007;17(7):878–84.
16. Goitein D, et al. Gastrojejunal strictures following laparoscopic Roux-en-Y gastric bypass for morbid obesity. Surg Endosc Other Interv Tech. 2005;19(5):628–32.
17. Mason EE, et al. Effect of gastric bypass on gastric secretion. Am J Surg. 1976;131(2):162–8.
18. Mathew A, et al. Gastrojejunal stricture after gastric bypass and efficacy of endoscopic intervention. Dig Dis Sci. 2009;54(9):1971–8.
19. Eubanks S, et al. Use of endoscopic stents to treat anastomotic complications after bariatric surgery. J Am Coll Surg. 2008;206(5):935–8.
20. Papasavas PK, et al. Laparoscopic management of complications following laparoscopic Roux-en-Y gastric bypass for morbid obesity. Surg Endosc Other Interv Tech. 2003;17(4):610–4.
21. Ogra R, Kini GP. Evolving endoscopic management options for symptomatic stenosis post-laparoscopic sleeve gastrectomy for morbid obesity: experience at a large bariatric surgery unit in New Zealand. Obes Surg. 2015;25(2):242–8.
22. Burgos AM, Csendes A, Braghetto I. Gastric stenosis after laparoscopic sleeve gastrectomy in morbidly obese patients. Obes Surg. 2013;23(9):1481–6.
23. Parikh A, et al. Management options for symptomatic stenosis after laparoscopic vertical sleeve gastrectomy in the morbidly obese. Surg Endosc. 2012;26(3):738–46.
24. Zundel N, et al. Strictures after laparoscopic sleeve gastrectomy. Surg Laparosc Endosc Percutan Tech. 2010;20(3):154–8.
25. Lalor PF, et al. Complications after laparoscopic sleeve gastrectomy. Surg Obes Relat Dis. 2008;4(1):33–8.
26. Cottam D, et al. Laparoscopic sleeve gastrectomy as an initial weight-loss procedure for high-risk patients with morbid obesity. Surg Endosc Other Interv Tech. 2006;20(6):859–63.
27. Rosenthal RJ, International Sleeve Gastrectomy Expert Panel. International Sleeve Gastrectomy Expert Panel Consensus Statement: best practice guidelines based on experience of > 12,000 cases. Surg Obes Relat Dis. 2012;8(1):8–19.
28. Parikh M, et al. Surgical strategies that may decrease leak after laparoscopic sleeve gastrectomy: a systematic review and meta-analysis of 9991 cases. Ann Surg. 2013;257(2):231–7.
29. Binda A, Jaworski P, Tarnowski W. Stenosis after sleeve gastrectomy–cause, diagnosis and management strategy. Pol J Surg. 2013;85(12):730–6.

30. Nimeri A, et al. The use of intraoperative endoscopy may decrease postoperative stenosis in laparoscopic sleeve gastrectomy. Obes Surg. 2016;26(7):1398–401.
31. Sudan R, et al. Sleeve gastrectomy strictures: technique for robotic-assisted strictureplasty. Surg Obes Relat Dis. 2010;6(4):434–6.
32. Vilallonga R, Himpens J, Van De Vrande S. Laparoscopic management of persistent strictures after laparoscopic sleeve gastrectomy. Obes Surg. 2013;23(10):1655–61.
33. Dapri G, Cadière GB, Himpens J. Laparoscopic seromyotomy for long stenosis after sleeve gastrectomy with or without duodenal switch. Obes Surg. 2009;19(4):495–9.

Postoperative Gastroesophageal Reflux Disease

24

Alexandra H. Leon Guerrero and Marina S. Kurian

Abbreviations

AGB	Adjustable gastric banding
GERD	Gastroesophageal reflux disease
LAGB	Laparoscopic adjustable gastric banding
LES	Lower esophageal sphincter
LSG	Laparoscopic sleeve gastrectomy
RYGB	Roux-en-Y gastric bypass
SG	Sleeve gastrectomy
TLESR	Transient lower esophageal sphincter relaxations

Introduction

Obesity is an epidemic in the United States and around the world [1]. As the number of individuals living with obesity and its associated comorbidities increases, so has the number of weight loss surgeries being performed. Over the last several decades, we have gained knowledge about the different comorbidities and complications that affect patients before and after bariatric surgery, gastroesophageal reflux disease among them. This chapter aims to discuss the medical and surgical strategies for the management of de novo or recurrent GERD after the three most commonly performed bariatric surgeries: adjustable gastric banding, Roux-en-Y gastric bypass, and sleeve gastrectomy.

A. H. Leon Guerrero (✉)
Department of Surgery, New York University Langone Medical Center, New York, NY, USA
e-mail: alex.leon.guerrero@gmail.com

M. S. Kurian
Department of Surgery, New York Minimally Invasive Surgery, PLLC, New York, NY, USA
e-mail: MARINA.KURIAN@NYUMC.ORG

Epidemiology of GERD

While some degree of gastroesophageal reflux is physiologic and characterized by postprandial, transient, and asymptomatic episodes, pathologic reflux is associated with bothersome symptoms or objective findings of mucosal injury not always correlated with symptoms. The most commonly reported symptoms associated with reflux include heartburn and regurgitation; however reflux has also been associated with symptoms of dysphagia, chest pain, globus sensation, cough, hoarseness, aspiration, and shortness of breath. Given the broad spectrum of conditions attributable to reflux and the lack of agreement on what constitutes typical reflux disease, a consensus statement known as the Montreal classification defines gastroesophageal reflux disease (GERD) as a condition that develops when gastric contents reflux abnormally into the esophagus causing "troublesome symptoms and/or complications" [2].

The pathophysiology by which GERD occurs is likely multifactorial but centers around lower esophageal sphincter (LES) dysfunction with

R. Lutfi et al. (eds.), *Global Bariatric Surgery*, https://doi.org/10.1007/978-3-319-93545-4_24

three dominant mechanisms: increased frequency of transient lower esophageal sphincter relaxations (TLESR), a hypotensive lower esophageal sphincter, and anatomic disruption of the gastroesophageal junction [3, 4]. Patients who experience GERD can manifest signs of mucosal inflammation on endoscopy, known as erosive esophagitis, or lack of mucosal damage, known as non-erosive reflux disease. Untreated and chronic GERD is associated with increasing frequency of esophagitis, the development of Barrett esophagus, and is a risk factor for adenocarcinoma of the esophagus [5].

GERD is a global problem with a significant impact on quality of life and considerable economic consequences. The prevalence of GERD has increased since 1995, with obesity, tobacco, and heredity the main risk factors. In a systematic review investigating the epidemiology of GERD, Dent and colleagues [6] reported a prevalence of 10–20% in Western populations and less than 5% in Asia. More recent studies, however, suggest an increasing prevalence of GERD in Asia over the last 10–20 years, with the most important factor being the increase in prevalence of obesity and metabolic syndrome in the region [7].

GERD and Obesity

Obesity is an independent risk factor for GERD. There is strong evidence demonstrating a higher prevalence of GERD in obese individuals compared to normal-weight individuals [8–12]. Jacobson and colleagues [13] used a supplemental GERD questionnaire added to the Nurses' Health Study to show that subjects who reported at least weekly symptoms had an increase in the adjusted odds ratio for reflux symptoms for each BMI stratum [13]. A systematic review by Corley and colleagues [14] further established the relationship between obesity and GERD by showing that, within the United States, there is a positive association between increasing BMI and the presence of GERD with odds ratios of 1.57 and 2.15 in overweight and obese individuals, respectively. Finally, obese patients have been shown to have an increased prevalence of complications of GERD, including Barrett's esophagus and esophageal adenocarcinoma [8, 11, 15, 16]. While the prevalence of obesity is lower outside the United States, several studies support the epidemiological relationship between obesity and GERD in both Europe and Asia [17–23].

The pathogenic link between obesity and GERD is likely multifactorial, but excessive abdominal fat, known as central obesity, is thought to be an important factor. Increased waist circumference has been associated with increases in intragastric pressure, frequency of tLESRs, and transdiaphragmatic pressure gradients, thereby increasing the potential for esophageal acid exposure [14, 24–26]. In a 24-h pH monitoring study, El-Serag and colleagues [26] showed obese patients had a mean percentage of time with pH <4 of 7.7%, 47% higher than normal-weight patients [26]. The altered transdiaphragmatic pressure gradients that promote this retrograde flow of gastric contents into the esophagus may also lead to disruption of the esophagogastric junction with widening of the angle of His and separation of the LES from the extrinsic crural diaphragm, also known as a hiatal hernia [27].

GERD Following Bariatric Surgery

Studies investigating the effect of bariatric surgery on GERD symptoms show an overall trend toward improvement of symptoms, yet until recently, there was insufficient data to reach a consensus. While it is broadly assumed that weight loss helps alleviate GERD symptoms, proof of this is difficult to derive. Bariatric surgery is the only reliable means of achieving significant and durable weight loss, so the procedures themselves become confounding variables.

Furthermore, there is significant variability in the efficacy of GERD improvement depending on the specific bariatric procedure performed. Pallati and colleagues [28] reviewed 116,136 patients in the Bariatric Outcomes Longitudinal Database, 36,938 of whom had preoperative evidence of GERD. They demonstrated that GERD scores improved by 56.5% after Roux-en-Y gastric bypass (RYGB), 46% after placement of an adjustable gastric band (AGB), and 41% after a sleeve gastrectomy (SG). Given the mixed pattern of outcomes, many studies have attempted to understand how each bariatric procedure independently affects both the subjective experience of GERD symptoms and objective markers of the disease process.

Roux-en-Y Gastric Bypass

Current evidence indicates there is clear improvement or resolution of GERD symptoms in the majority of patients following RYGB. Multiple studies have shown subjective improvement of GERD symptoms using patient questionnaires before and after RYGB [29–36]. Frezza and colleagues [32] surveyed 152 patients at a 12-month follow-up interval and found a significant reduction in reported GERD symptoms including heartburn (from 87% to 22%, $p < 0.001$), use of proton pump inhibitors (from 44% to 9%, $p < 0.001$), and use of H2 blockers (from 60% to 10%, $p < 0.01$). Similarly, Perry and colleagues [37] assessed 57 patients at a mean follow-up of 18 months with all patients reporting improvement or resolution of GERD symptoms. While patients had a mean weight loss of 40 kg, the authors point out that improvement of GERD symptoms was not always correlated with excess body weight lost.

Improvements in objective findings of GERD after RYGB measured by 24-h pH monitoring and endoscopic evaluation have also been reported [29, 30, 38–40]. Ortega and colleagues [39] performed esophageal manometry and 24-h pH monitoring in 40 patients both before and after RYGB at 3 months and 1 year postoperatively. The prevalence of GERD by pH metrics decreased from 80% preoperatively to 15% postoperatively, while there were no significant differences in all esophageal manometry parameters [39].

Mechanisms that explain the anti-reflux effect of RYGB go beyond just sustainable weight loss to include lowering acid production in the gastric pouch by decreasing the population of parietal cells, accelerated gastric pouch emptying, and the diversion of bile from the stomach [41, 42]. In a systematic review and meta-analysis comparing laparoscopic RYGB and SG to treat obesity-related comorbidities, Li and colleagues [43] determined that RYGB is a highly effective anti-reflux procedure with resolution of GERD seen in 70–80% of patients. As a result, the RYGB has become the gold standard treatment of morbidly obese patients with GERD who meet criteria for a bariatric operation [38, 44].

While traditional anti-reflux procedures have been shown to be safe in obese patients, the long-term functional outcomes remain a source of debate [45, 46]. Supporters of bariatric surgery argue that the prevalence of comorbid disease in the obese population make RYGB preferable to fundoplication due to the health benefits associated with durable weight loss. Also notable are several studies that have assessed the use of RYGB as a revision surgery for traditional anti-reflux procedures that have failed to alleviate GERD symptoms [47–50]. Using the Gastroesophageal Reflux Disease-Health-Related Quality of Life (GERD-HRQoL) scale, Raftopoulos and colleagues showed a significant reduction of GERD scores ($p = 0.006$) in seven patients with previous Nissen fundoplication undergoing revision to a RYGB [47].

Although the majority of patients experience improvement or resolution of GERD symptoms after RYGB, there remains a subset of patients who continue to be symptomatic after surgery, as well as patient who develop de novo reflux. The Early Results of the Swiss Multicentre Bypass or Sleeve Study trial reported a 4% rate of de novo GERD at a 1-year follow-up after RYGB [51]. DuPree and colleagues [52] performed a retrospective review of the Bariatric Outcomes Longitudinal Database which included 33,867 patients undergoing RYGB for morbid obesity and showed persistent and worsening GERD symptoms in 17.6% and 2.2% of patients, respectively. Madalosso and colleagues [30] performed a prospective study that showed pathologic esophageal acid exposure detected on pH monitoring 39 months after surgery in 9% of patients with normal preoperative pH monitoring. In addition, half of the patients who developed postoperative erosive esophagitis had normal 24-h pH monitoring [30].

Persistent or de novo reflux after RYGB has been attributed to either a large pouch resulting in remaining parietal cells and associated acid production or a short alimentary limb allowing for bile reflux [53]. However, several studies suggest that causes other than acid or bile reflux might also contribute to esophageal injury. In a recent study, Rebecchi and colleagues [54] prospectively assessed the long-term effects of RYGB on gastroesophageal function using both the GERD-HRQoL questionnaire and objective evaluations such as upper endoscopy, esophageal manometry, and 24-h impedance pH monitoring preoperatively at 12- and 60-month follow-up intervals. They showed that irrespective of the presence of symptoms, 75% of study participants presented with distal esophageal exposure to weakly acidic reflux with a high incidence of both microscopic and macroscopic esophagitis. They postulated that the high incidence of weakly acidic reflux after RYGB without clinical or endoscopic signs of gastric stasis may be related to functional dysmotility of the roux limb, independent of roux limb length [54].

Laparoscopic Adjustable Gastric Band

The laparoscopic adjustable gastric band (LAGB) has been reported to reduce or eliminate many obesity-related comorbidities; however the association with GERD and its effect on esophageal function is conflicting. Several studies have shown improvement of reflux symptoms either immediately after or within 6 weeks of band placement and before any major weight loss has occurred, suggesting an effect of the band itself, likely due to augmentation of the LES [55–58]. However, studies have also demonstrated worsened or newly developed GERD symptoms in patients postoperatively, particularly at longer-term follow-up intervals [56, 59–63].

In 2010, de Jong and colleagues [64] performed a systematic review assessing the influence of adjustable gastric banding on GERD and esophageal motility. They reported the prevalence of reflux symptoms decreased postoperatively from 32.9% to 7.7% and medication use from 27.5% to 9.5%. De novo reflux symptoms were found in 15% of patients, while newly developed esophagitis was observed in 22.9%. The authors concluded that AGB has anti-reflux properties resulting in resolution or improvement in reflux symptoms, normalized pH monitoring results, and a decrease of esophagitis in the short term but that worsening or newly developed reflux symptoms are found in a subset of patients at longer follow-up intervals [64].

In 2012, Woodman and colleagues [65] performed a 2-year interim analysis of patients in the 5-year prospective APEX study who reported GERD requiring daily medical therapy prior to the AGB procedure. Among 122 patients assess at a 2-year follow-up interval, complete resolution of GERD was reported in 80%, improvement in 11%, no change in 9%, and worsening in 2%. The data in this study, however, is limited due to an unrecorded number of hiatal hernia repairs that were conducted, as well as the unknown medical history among patients who reported worsening or de novo onset of GERD symptoms [65].

Possible reasons for worsening or de novo reflux after LAGB include reduced esophageal clearance, pouch formation, food stasis, and reversible esophageal dilation [55, 56, 59, 60, 66–69]. While a large pouch may be secondary to suboptimal technique at initial band placement, more often a correctly sized pouch may enlarge over time. Mechanisms of pouch enlargement include chronic over-tightening of the band or prolapse of the stomach through the band. This may explain why studies with shorter-term follow-up show anti-reflux properties of the band, while those with intermediate- to longer-term follow-up show increasing symptoms and findings of GERD. Further studies are needed to investigate the discrepancies between early and late effects of LAGB on reflux; however given that this bariatric procedure has since fallen out of favor for surgeons and patients, this is unlikely to occur.

Sleeve Gastrectomy

Initially introduced as the first step in a two-stage procedure to treat high-risk, super-obese patients, sleeve gastrectomy (SG) is now a stand-alone bariatric procedure [70]. Due to its technical simplicity and proven weight loss outcomes, SG is now the most commonly performed bariatric procedure [71, 72]. There have been many studies investigating the effect of SG on GERD. As with the LAGB, evidence has been controversial, with the majority of studies reporting worsening of GERD symptoms [73–80], while others have reported improvement [81–84].

In a retrospective review of the Bariatric Outcomes Longitudinal Database, Dupree and colleagues [52] demonstrated that among patients who had pre-existing GERD and underwent SG, 15.9% reported resolution after surgery, while 84.1% reported persistent symptoms. Of SG patients who did not demonstrate preoperative GERD, 8.6% developed de novo GERD postoperatively. In 2011, Chiu and colleagues [85] performed a systematic review assessing the effect of SG on GERD, but no clear consensus could be drawn due in part to the heterogeneity of studies [85]. In 2016, Oor and colleagues [86] reexamined the literature performing a meta-analysis of the pooled studies and reported a minimal trend toward an increased prevalence of GERD symptoms following SG, although without any statistical significance.

The relationship between GERD and SG is multifactorial. Anatomic factors and physiologic mechanisms that may explain the increased prevalence of GERD after LSG include hypotensive LES, disruption of the angle of His, resection of sling fibers, reduced gastric compliance with higher intragastric pressure, decreased gastric emptying, late dilatation of the sleeve, and occurrence of hiatal hernia. Factors associated with reduced GERD after LSG include weight loss, restoration of the angle of His, decreased acid production, and accelerated gastric emptying; however these are typically only seen after longer-term follow-up [85].

In 2014, Rebecchi and colleagues [87] performed a prospective clinical study evaluating gastroesophageal function in morbidly obese patient undergoing a LSG using a clinically validated questionnaire, upper endoscopy, esophageal manometry, and 24-h pH monitoring both before and 24 months after LSG. Patients with pathologic reflux were identified preoperatively using 24-h pH monitoring and after LSG were found to have statistically significant reductions in Gastroesophageal Reflux Disease Symptom Assessment Scale (GSAS) scores, DeMeester scores, and total acid exposure. In patients who did not have pathologic reflux preoperatively, the incidence of de novo GERD was 5.4%. Furthermore, no significant changes in lower esophageal sphincter pressures and esophageal peristalsis amplitudes were found. Of note, patients with large hiatal hernia were excluded, routine hiatal hernia repair was not performed for small hiatal hernias, and a 36-Fr bougie was used [87].

Beginning in 2007, there have been multiple international summits where expert surgeons gather to review all major aspects of SG. Best practice guidelines were developed in 2011 from a 2-day live expert consensus panel with a collective experience of >12,000 cases. There was 83% consensus that the presence of a hiatal hernia should always be assessed intraoperatively, including dissection of the phrenoesophageal membrane and inspection of the greater curvature side of the stomach. Accordingly, 82% of experts agreed that if a hernia is found, it should be repaired. For patients who developed GERD symptoms after LSG, 85% agreed that proton pump inhibitors should be the first line of treatment [88].

In 2016, results of an online anonymous survey of expert surgeons and general bariatric surgeon were compared with the aforementioned 2011 data. Based on the findings of Rebecchi and colleagues, the majority of expert surgeons now believe that GERD is overall improved after SG and it should not be a contraindication. Only one third of expert surgeons would recommend formal preoperative pH and manometry studies prior to SG, and not routinely but only very selectively. However, complications of GERD, including Barrett's esophagus, remain a contraindication to the LSG, necessitating preoperative gastroscopy. This is primarily because performing a sleeve gastrectomy precludes a gastric pull-through should severe dysplasia require a distal esophagectomy [71].

It is the author's opinion that Barrett's esophagus is a relative contraindication to SG. While the incidence of progression of Barrett's to dysplasia is fairly low, there is currently no data on progression of Barrett's with sleeve gastrectomy. It is the author's practice to offer a patient with Barrett's a laparoscopic RYGB, an anti-reflux procedure, because as previously discussed, there is clear data on the impact of anti-reflux procedures on Barrett's disease [89, 90]. It is important to describe the risks of SG compared with a RYGB in the patient with Barrett's. Furthermore, GERD-like symptoms may be an indication to perform a preoperative EGD to rule out Barrett's in all patients undergoing a LSG. A limitation in patients with asymptomatic disease will be missed.

Medical Management

Unlike GERD in the general population, evaluation of GERD-like symptoms after bariatric surgery should be approached with an expanded differential diagnosis. In the immediate postoperative period, there can be significant overlap between GERD and normal postoperative symptoms. Furthermore, surgery-specific postoperative complications can be masked by preexisting GERD or present as newly developed symptoms.

Once surgery-specific postoperative complications have been excluded, however, first-line therapy is like that of the general population with dietary modification and cessation of smoking and alcohol use. After bariatric surgery, dietary modifications in the form of changes to eating behaviors are important given the restrictive anatomy inherent in the AGB, SG, and RYGB. Eating too quickly or large quantities over a short period of time results in food stasis in the lower esophagus and consequently heartburn, dysphagia, and regurgitation. Paced swallowing, therefore, is a learned behavior that can ameliorate GERD symptoms.

Eating behaviors are especially important to elucidate in patients after AGB as GERD-like symptoms are frequently elicited by over-tightening of the band. It is common for patients who fail to achieve adequate weight loss to request tightening of their band. Oftentimes, the reason for weight loss failure is the consumption of inappropriate quantities or types of foods, such as liquid calories. A thorough knowledge of the patient's dietary history and counseling on eating behaviors can therefore prevent unnecessary and inappropriate over-tightening of the AGB system [91].

Second-line therapy for GERD after bariatric surgery is the use of acid-reducing medications. The use of acid-reducing medications has been shown to decrease from 37.7% to 29.6% at 1 year after bariatric procedures; however it was not uniform among the different operations, with 56.2% of patients who were previously on either a PPI or an H2-blocker discontinuing these medications after RYGB [92]. In a study with similar results, more patients after SG used acid-reducing medications as compared to RYGB (48.1% vs. 16.1%) [93].

In situations where acid-reducing medications are ineffective and weakly acidic reflux or food stasis due to either delayed gastric emptying or roux limb dysmotility has been established, promotility agents may be used as an adjunct to acid suppression and provide relief through improved esophageal clearance and gastric emptying [94]. Finally, while *H. Pylori* testing is typically performed as part of a patient's preoperative workup, testing may be warranted in a postoperative patient and treatment with triple therapy initiated if results are positive.

Surgical Management

Post-bariatric surgery GERD-like symptoms that are refractory to conservative management warrant further investigation to evaluate whether any surgical interventions are indicated for management. Surgery-specific complications should be identified and the history and clinical context in which symptoms occur need to be thoroughly understood.

After LAGB, the possible causes of GERD-like symptoms include over-tightening, a slipped band, gastric herniation, or a dilated pouch. Urgent surgical intervention may be indicated for a slipped band or gastric herniation given the risk for gastric ischemia. With a dilated pouch, the surgical options can be tailored based on the desired outcomes of the individual patients. Generally, the surgical options for patients with band complications or failure to lose weight include band removal, band repositioning, band replacement, or conversion to an alternate procedure. Band removal is associated with a high rate of weight regain and is an undesirable option for most patients [95].

Presentation of GERD after an LSG should prompt an assessment for a retained fundus, a kinking or stricturing of the sleeve, or a hiatal hernia. A radiological contrast study or endoscopy may help to make the diagnosis. In the case of a retained fundus, either a revision SG or conversion to a RYGB is a surgical option. While gastric strictures are more commonly associated with persistent nausea, emesis, and intolerance to solids, if this complication is diagnosed in the setting of GERD-like symptoms, treatment may lead to symptomatic improvement. Endoscopy is recommended to confirm the diagnosis of a stricture, with the possibility for therapeutic balloon dilation [96, 97]. Parikh and colleagues showed that symptomatic short-segment stenosis was more likely to be successfully treated with endoscopic balloon dilation, whereas patients with long stenoses or significant kinking are less likely to respond to endoscopic techniques and may ultimately require conversion to RYGB [97].

In patients with GERD after either a LAGB or LSG who have failed conservative management and in whom further work-up could not demonstrate any treatable causes, conversion to RYGB should be considered for its favorable outcomes as an anti-reflux procedure. The conversion rate of SG to RYGB due to GERD is reported as 2.9% [71]. Langer and colleagues demonstrated successful conversion of SG to RYGB in three patients, all of whom reported improvement in reflux symptoms and were able to discontinue acid-suppressive medications [98]. Abdemur and colleagues [99] similarly investigated reasons for and outcomes of conversions of LSG to RYGB. They reported nine patients who underwent conversion surgery for intractable GERD, six of whom reported complete resolution of their GERD symptoms, two who continued to report GERD symptoms and were maintained on PPI therapy, and one who was kept on a PPI for marginal ulcerations [99].

Given the significant alteration in anatomy that occurs with RYGB, it is paramount to understand the etiology of GERD after RYGB prior to performing any revision surgery. As previously discussed, persistent or de novo reflux after RYGB is most commonly due to either a large pouch resulting in remaining parietal cells and associated acid production or a short alimentary limb allowing for bile reflux [53]. Impedance studies can help to differentiate these and guide surgical management. A revision of the gastric pouch size may be indicated for a large pouch, whereas lengthening of the roux limb may be indicated if bile reflux is the offending etiology.

It is worth mentioning that while the RYGB is highly effective in controlling reflux symptoms, there are risks associated with this complex surgical procedure, and not all patients are candidates given unfavorable gastrointestinal anatomy or issues with malabsorption. Magnetic sphincter augmentation (MSA) is a new anti-reflux surgical technique for treating GERD. The LINX ® system is an MSA device that was approved by the FDA in 2012 for the treatment of reflux in the general public as an alternative therapy to the gold standard, a Nissen fundoplication. It controls reflux by physiologically reinforcing the lower esophageal sphincter (LES) with a ring of magnetic beads implanted around the gastroesophageal junction.

There are now short- and medium-term outcomes demonstrating the efficacy of the LINX for management of GERD [100]. Ganz and colleagues [101] studied the long-term outcomes of patients who received the LINX system and concluded that magnetic sphincter augmentation is capable of providing significant and sustained control of reflux with minimal side effects or complications. All study participants were using PPIs at baseline, and this decreased to only 15.3% at 5 years after device placement. Median GERD-HRQoL scores also decreased from 27 in patients not on PPIs, and 11 in patients taking PPIs, to 4 overall. The prevalence of bothersome gas bloat decreased from 57% at baseline to 1.2% at 5 years, with all study participants able to belch and vomit as needed. Dysphagia was the primary complaint in the postoperative period, but this seemed to be only a short-term complication as the prevalence of dysphagia symptoms returned to baseline by 5 years [101]. Laparoscopic removal of the LINX device can be safely performed, with the causes of removal being dysphagia, recurrent GERD, device-related pain, diagnosis of esophageal cancer, and device erosion [102, 103].

While the applications of MSA devices for management of reflux after bariatric surgery is still in its experimental stages, preliminary studies suggest similar outcomes in this specific population. Desar and colleagues [104] reported the LINX system is a safe and effective option for patients with reflux refractory to medical therapy after LSG despite adequate weight loss. The authors point to how the LINX is implanted in an area undisturbed with LSG, making it a relatively low-risk surgery compared with the alternative surgical option of conversion to a RYGB. Not to mention, implantation of the LINX does not preclude later conversion in the event of failure. Hawasli and colleagues [105] describe case demonstrating successful management of refractory reflux after a RYGB using the LINX system together with a hiatal hernia repair [105].

Endoscopic Management

For patients with refractory GERD after bariatric surgery who are either unwilling or not candidates for revision surgeries, endoluminal therapies are a reasonable option. There are multiple new and emerging techniques including the Stretta procedure (Mederi Therapeutics, Greenwich, Conn), the EsophyX® (EndoGastric Solutions, Redmond, Wash), and the MUSE™ system (Medigus Ultrasonic Surgical Endostapler, Medigus Ltd. Omer, Israel).

The Stretta procedure uses radio-frequency energy to treat GERD. It consists of a flexible catheter with a 30 F bougie tip and a balloon basket assembly consisting of radially placed electrodes that deliver radio-frequency energy to the gastroesophageal junction. The proposed mechanism by which the Stretta system works is twofold. First, the thermal injury causes scarring and collagen deposition at the gastroesophageal junction (GEJ) resulting in decreased compliance of the LES and a presumed reduction in transient LES relaxation. Second, the ablation of vagal afferent fibers may result in fewer transient LES relaxations. Mattar and colleagues [106] investigated the application of the Stretta procedure for patients with refractory GERD after RYGB. Of 369 patients, seven were identified who had refractory GERD and underwent the Stretta procedure. Five had complete resolution of their symptoms with normalization of pH studies, with one patient reporting persistent symptoms and one patient lost to follow-up evaluation [106].

The EsophyX® and MUSE™ system are both methods of transoral incisionless fundoplication. There is little to no data currently available for the application of these procedures for management of GERD after bariatric procedures. The device profiles are such that a large retained fundus or pouch would be needed to use the devices and may preclude their use for the treatment of GERD after LSG or RYGB.

Summary

GERD is a significant comorbidity in bariatric patients preoperatively and postoperatively. Management of GERD postoperatively can be challenging as the temporal presentation and underlying mechanisms for symptom occurrence may vary based on the specific bariatric procedure performed. Bariatric surgeons should be familiar with the appropriate evaluation, procedures choices, and management options. Revision surgery for reflux symptoms is often indicated; however the appropriate anatomy and outcomes should be considered when offering these interventions to patients.

References

1. Ogden CL, Carroll MD, Fryar CD, Flegal KM. Prevalence of obesity among adults and youth: United States, 2011–2014. NCHS Data Brief. 2015;219:1–8.
2. Vakil N, van Zanten SV, Kahrilas P, Dent J, Jones R, Global Consensus G. The Montreal definition and classification of gastroesophageal reflux disease: a global evidence-based consensus. Am J Gastroenterol. 2006;101(8):1900–20. quiz 1943
3. Festi D, Scaioli E, Baldi F, et al. Body weight, lifestyle, dietary habits and gastroesophageal reflux disease. World J Gastroenterol. 2009;15(14):1690–701.
4. Iovino P, Angrisani L, Galloro G, et al. Proximal stomach function in obesity with normal or abnormal oesophageal acid exposure. Neurogastroenterol Motil. 2006;18(6):425–32.
5. Shaheen N, Ransohoff DF. Gastroesophageal reflux, barrett esophagus, and esophageal cancer: scientific review. JAMA. 2002;287(15):1972–81.
6. Dent J, El-Serag HB, Wallander MA, Johansson S. Epidemiology of gastro-oesophageal reflux disease: a systematic review. Gut. 2005;54(5):710–7.
7. Goh KL. Gastroesophageal reflux disease in Asia: a historical perspective and present challenges. J Gastroenterol Hepatol. 2011;26(Suppl 1):2–10.
8. Hampel H, Abraham NS, El-Serag HB. Meta-analysis: obesity and the risk for gastroesophageal reflux disease and its complications. Ann Intern Med. 2005;143(3):199–211.
9. El-Serag HB, Graham DY, Satia JA, Rabeneck L. Obesity is an independent risk factor for GERD symptoms and erosive esophagitis. Am J Gastroenterol. 2005a;100(6):1243–50.
10. El-Serag HB. Obesity and disease of the esophagus and colon. Gastroenterol Clin N Am. 2005;34(1):63–82.
11. Friedenberg FK, Xanthopoulos M, Foster GD, Richter JE. The association between gastroesophageal reflux disease and obesity. Am J Gastroenterol. 2008;103(8):2111–22.
12. Chang P, Friedenberg F. Obesity and GERD. Gastroenterol Clin N Am. 2014;43(1):161–73.
13. Jacobson BC, Somers SC, Fuchs CS, Kelly CP, Camargo CA Jr. Body-mass index and symptoms of gastroesophageal reflux in women. N Engl J Med. 2006;354(22):2340–8.
14. Corley DA, Kubo A. Body mass index and gastroesophageal reflux disease: a systematic review and meta-analysis. Am J Gastroenterol. 2006;101(11):2619–28.
15. El-Serag HB, Hashmi A, Garcia J, et al. Visceral abdominal obesity measured by CT scan is associated with an increased risk of Barrett's oesophagus: a case-control study. Gut. 2014;63(2):220–9.
16. El-Serag HB, Kvapil P, Hacken-Bitar J, Kramer JR. Abdominal obesity and the risk of Barrett's esophagus. Am J Gastroenterol. 2005b;100(10):2151–6.
17. Nocon M, Labenz J, Willich SN. Lifestyle factors and symptoms of gastro-oesophageal reflux – a population-based study. Aliment Pharmacol Ther. 2006;23(1):169–74.
18. Murray L, Johnston B, Lane A, et al. Relationship between body mass and gastro-oesophageal reflux symptoms: the Bristol Helicobacter Project. Int J Epidemiol. 2003;32(4):645–50.
19. Diaz-Rubio M, Moreno-Elola-Olaso C, Rey E, Locke GR 3rd, Rodriguez-Artalejo F. Symptoms of gastro-oesophageal reflux: prevalence, severity, duration and associated factors in a Spanish population. Aliment Pharmacol Ther. 2004;19(1):95–105.
20. Rey E, Moreno-Elola-Olaso C, Artalejo FR, Locke GR 3rd, Diaz-Rubio M. Association between weight gain and symptoms of gastroesophageal reflux in the general population. Am J Gastroenterol. 2006;101(2):229–33.
21. Nilsson M, Johnsen R, Ye W, Hveem K, Lagergren J. Obesity and estrogen as risk factors for gastroesophageal reflux symptoms. JAMA. 2003;290(1):66–72.
22. Kang MS, Park DI, Oh SY, et al. Abdominal obesity is an independent risk factor for erosive esophagitis in a Korean population. J Gastroenterol Hepatol. 2007;22(10):1656–61.
23. Ma XQ, Cao Y, Wang R, et al. Prevalence of, and factors associated with, gastroesophageal reflux disease: a population-based study in Shanghai, China. Dis Esophagus. 2009;22(4):317–22.
24. Falk GW. Obesity and gastroesophageal reflux disease: another piece of the puzzle. Gastroenterology. 2008;134(5):1620–2.
25. Ayazi S, Hagen JA, Chan LS, et al. Obesity and gastroesophageal reflux: quantifying the association between body mass index, esophageal acid exposure, and lower esophageal sphincter status in a large series of patients with reflux symptoms. J Gastrointest Surg. 2009;13(8):1440–7.
26. El-Serag HB, Ergun GA, Pandolfino J, Fitzgerald S, Tran T, Kramer JR. Obesity increases oesophageal acid exposure. Gut. 2007;56(6):749–55.
27. Pandolfino JE, El-Serag HB, Zhang Q, Shah N, Ghosh SK, Kahrilas PJ. Obesity: a challenge to esophagogastric junction integrity. Gastroenterology. 2006;130(3):639–49.
28. Pallati PK, Shaligram A, Shostrom VK, Oleynikov D, McBride CL, Goede MR. Improvement in gastroesophageal reflux disease symptoms after various bariatric procedures: review of the Bariatric Outcomes Longitudinal Database. Surg Obes Relat Dis. 2014;10(3):502–7.
29. Mejia-Rivas MA, Herrera-Lopez A, Hernandez-Calleros J, Herrera MF, Valdovinos

MA. Gastroesophageal reflux disease in morbid obesity: the effect of Roux-en-Y gastric bypass. Obes Surg. 2008;18(10):1217–24.
30. Madalosso CA, Gurski RR, Callegari-Jacques SM, Navarini D, Mazzini G, Pereira Mda S. The impact of gastric bypass on gastroesophageal reflux disease in morbidly obese patients. Ann Surg. 2016;263(1):110–6.
31. Madalosso CA, Gurski RR, Callegari-Jacques SM, Navarini D, Thiesen V, Fornari F. The impact of gastric bypass on gastroesophageal reflux disease in patients with morbid obesity: a prospective study based on the Montreal Consensus. Ann Surg. 2010;251(2):244–8.
32. Frezza EE, Ikramuddin S, Gourash W, et al. Symptomatic improvement in gastroesophageal reflux disease (GERD) following laparoscopic Roux-en-Y gastric bypass. Surg Endosc. 2002;16(7):1027–31.
33. Clements RH, Gonzalez QH, Foster A, et al. Gastrointestinal symptoms are more intense in morbidly obese patients and are improved with laparoscopic Roux-en-Y gastric bypass. Obes Surg. 2003;13(4):610–4.
34. Foster A, Laws HL, Gonzalez QH, Clements RH. Gastrointestinal symptomatic outcome after laparoscopic Roux-en-Y gastric bypass. J Gastrointest Surg. 2003;7(6):750–3.
35. Smith SC, Edwards CB, Goodman GN. Symptomatic and clinical improvement in morbidly obese patients with gastroesophageal reflux disease following Roux-en-Y gastric bypass. Obes Surg. 1997;7(6):479–84.
36. Jones KB Jr. Roux-en-Y gastric bypass: an effective antireflux procedure in the less than morbidly obese. Obes Surg. 1998;8(1):35–8.
37. Perry Y, Courcoulas AP, Fernando HC, Buenaventura PO, McCaughan JS, Luketich JD. Laparoscopic Roux-en-Y gastric bypass for recalcitrant gastroesophageal reflux disease in morbidly obese patients. JSLS. 2004;8(1):19–23.
38. Patterson EJ, Davis DG, Khajanchee Y, Swanstrom LL. Comparison of objective outcomes following laparoscopic Nissen fundoplication versus laparoscopic gastric bypass in the morbidly obese with heartburn. Surg Endosc. 2003;17(10):1561–5.
39. Ortega J, Escudero MD, Mora F, et al. Outcome of esophageal function and 24-hour esophageal pH monitoring after vertical banded gastroplasty and Roux-en-Y gastric bypass. Obes Surg. 2004;14(8):1086–94.
40. Merrouche M, Sabate JM, Jouet P, et al. Gastroesophageal reflux and esophageal motility disorders in morbidly obese patients before and after bariatric surgery. Obes Surg. 2007;17(7):894–900.
41. Nadaleto BF, Herbella FA, Patti MG. Gastroesophageal reflux disease in the obese: pathophysiology and treatment. Surgery. 2016;159(2):475–86.
42. Khan A, Kim A, Sanossian C, Francois F. Impact of obesity treatment on gastroesophageal reflux disease. World J Gastroenterol. 2016;22(4):1627–38.
43. Li JF, Lai DD, Lin ZH, Jiang TY, Zhang AM, Dai JF. Comparison of the long-term results of Roux-en-Y gastric bypass and sleeve gastrectomy for morbid obesity: a systematic review and meta-analysis of randomized and nonrandomized trials. Surg Laparosc Endosc Percutan Tech. 2014;24(1):1–11.
44. Varela JE, Hinojosa MW, Nguyen NT. Laparoscopic fundoplication compared with laparoscopic gastric bypass in morbidly obese patients with gastroesophageal reflux disease. Surg Obes Relat Dis. 2009;5(2):139–43.
45. Telem DA, Altieri M, Gracia G, Pryor AD. Perioperative outcome of esophageal fundoplication for gastroesophageal reflux disease in obese and morbidly obese patients. Am J Surg. 2014;208(2):163–8.
46. Prachand VN, Alverdy JC. Gastroesophageal reflux disease and severe obesity: fundoplication or bariatric surgery? World J Gastroenterol. 2010;16(30):3757–61.
47. Raftopoulos I, Awais O, Courcoulas AP, Luketich JD. Laparoscopic gastric bypass after antireflux surgery for the treatment of gastroesophageal reflux in morbidly obese patients: initial experience. Obes Surg. 2004;14(10):1373–80.
48. Zainabadi K, Courcoulas AP, Awais O, Raftopoulos I. Laparoscopic revision of Nissen fundoplication to Roux-en-Y gastric bypass in morbidly obese patients. Surg Endosc. 2008;22(12):2737–40.
49. Stefanidis D, Navarro F, Augenstein VA, Gersin KS, Heniford BT. Laparoscopic fundoplication takedown with conversion to Roux-en-Y gastric bypass leads to excellent reflux control and quality of life after fundoplication failure. Surg Endosc. 2012;26(12):3521–7.
50. Kim M, Navarro F, Eruchalu CN, Augenstein VA, Heniford BT, Stefanidis D. Minimally invasive Roux-en-Y gastric bypass for fundoplication failure offers excellent gastroesophageal reflux control. Am Surg. 2014;80(7):696–703.
51. Peterli R, Borbely Y, Kern B, et al. Early results of the Swiss Multicentre Bypass or Sleeve Study (SM-BOSS): a prospective randomized trial comparing laparoscopic sleeve gastrectomy and Roux-en-Y gastric bypass. Ann Surg. 2013;258(5):690–4. discussion 695
52. DuPree CE, Blair K, Steele SR, Martin MJ. Laparoscopic sleeve gastrectomy in patients with preexisting gastroesophageal reflux disease: a national analysis. JAMA Surg. 2014;149(4):328–34.
53. Siilin H, Wanders A, Gustavsson S, Sundbom M. The proximal gastric pouch invariably contains acid-producing parietal cells in Roux-en-Y gastric bypass. Obes Surg. 2005;15(6):771–7.
54. Rebecchi F, Allaix ME, Ugliono E, Giaccone C, Toppino M, Morino M. Increased esophageal exposure to weakly acidic reflux 5 years after

laparoscopic Roux-en-Y gastric bypass. Ann Surg. 2016;264:871.
55. Dixon JB, O'Brien PE. Gastroesophageal reflux in obesity: the effect of lap-band placement. Obes Surg. 1999;9(6):527–31.
56. de Jong JR, van Ramshorst B, Timmer R, Gooszen HG, Smout AJ. The influence of laparoscopic adjustable gastric banding on gastroesophageal reflux. Obes Surg. 2004;14(3):399–406.
57. Spivak H, Hewitt MF, Onn A, Half EE. Weight loss and improvement of obesity-related illness in 500 U.S. patients following laparoscopic adjustable gastric banding procedure. Am J Surg. 2005;189(1):27–32.
58. Lew JI, Daud A, DiGorgi MF, Olivero-Rivera L, Davis DG, Bessler M. Preoperative esophageal manometry and outcome of laparoscopic adjustable silicone gastric banding. Surg Endosc. 2006;20(8):1242–7.
59. Gutschow CA, Collet P, Prenzel K, Holscher AH, Schneider PM. Long-term results and gastroesophageal reflux in a series of laparoscopic adjustable gastric banding. J Gastrointest Surg. 2005;9(7):941–8.
60. Suter M, Dorta G, Giusti V, Calmes JM. Gastric banding interferes with esophageal motility and gastroesophageal reflux. Arch Surg. 2005;140(7):639–43.
61. Korenkov M, Kohler L, Yucel N, et al. Esophageal motility and reflux symptoms before and after bariatric surgery. Obes Surg. 2002;12(1):72–6.
62. Klaus A, Gruber I, Wetscher G, et al. Prevalent esophageal body motility disorders underlie aggravation of GERD symptoms in morbidly obese patients following adjustable gastric banding. Arch Surg. 2006;141(3):247–51.
63. Frigg A, Peterli R, Peters T, Ackermann C, Tondelli P. Reduction in co-morbidities 4 years after laparoscopic adjustable gastric banding. Obes Surg. 2004;14(2):216–23.
64. de Jong JR, Besselink MG, van Ramshorst B, Gooszen HG, Smout AJ. Effects of adjustable gastric banding on gastroesophageal reflux and esophageal motility: a systematic review. Obes Rev. 2010;11(4):297–305.
65. Woodman G, Cywes R, Billy H, et al. Effect of adjustable gastric banding on changes in gastroesophageal reflux disease (GERD) and quality of life. Curr Med Res Opin. 2012;28(4):581–9.
66. Naef M, Mouton WG, Naef U, van der Weg B, Maddern GJ, Wagner HE. Esophageal dysmotility disorders after laparoscopic gastric banding – an underestimated complication. Ann Surg. 2011;253(2):285–90.
67. Gustavsson S, Westling A. Laparoscopic adjustable gastric banding: complications and side effects responsible for the poor long-term outcome. Semin Laparosc Surg. 2002;9(2):115–24.
68. Milone L, Daud A, Durak E, et al. Esophageal dilation after laparoscopic adjustable gastric banding. Surg Endosc. 2008;22(6):1482–6.
69. Victorzon M, Tolonen P. Mean fourteen-year, 100% follow-up of laparoscopic adjustable gastric banding for morbid obesity. Surg Obes Relat Dis. 2013;9(5):753–7.
70. Kueper MA, Kramer KM, Kirschniak A, Konigsrainer A, Pointner R, Granderath FA. Laparoscopic sleeve gastrectomy: standardized technique of a potential stand-alone bariatric procedure in morbidly obese patients. World J Surg. 2008;32(7):1462–5.
71. Gagner M, Hutchinson C, Rosenthal R. Fifth International Consensus Conference: current status of sleeve gastrectomy. Surg Obes Relat Dis. 2016;12(4):750–6.
72. Ponce J, DeMaria EJ, Nguyen NT, Hutter M, Sudan R, Morton JM. American Society for Metabolic and Bariatric Surgery estimation of bariatric surgery procedures in 2015 and surgeon workforce in the United States. Surg Obes Relat Dis. 2016;12(9):1637–9.
73. Nocca D, Krawczykowsky D, Bomans B, et al. A prospective multicenter study of 163 sleeve gastrectomies: results at 1 and 2 years. Obes Surg. 2008;18(5):560–5.
74. Arias E, Martinez PR, Ka Ming Li V, Szomstein S, Rosenthal RJ. Mid-term follow-up after sleeve gastrectomy as a final approach for morbid obesity. Obes Surg. 2009;19(5):544–8.
75. Himpens J, Dobbeleir J, Peeters G. Long-term results of laparoscopic sleeve gastrectomy for obesity. Ann Surg. 2010;252(2):319–24.
76. Lakdawala MA, Bhasker A, Mulchandani D, Goel S, Jain S. Comparison between the results of laparoscopic sleeve gastrectomy and laparoscopic Roux-en-Y gastric bypass in the Indian population: a retrospective 1 year study. Obes Surg. 2010;20(1):1–6.
77. Carter PR, LeBlanc KA, Hausmann MG, Kleinpeter KP, deBarros SN, Jones SM. Association between gastroesophageal reflux disease and laparoscopic sleeve gastrectomy. Surg Obes Relat Dis. 2011;7(5):569–72.
78. Howard DD, Caban AM, Cendan JC, Ben-David K. Gastroesophageal reflux after sleeve gastrectomy in morbidly obese patients. Surg Obes Relat Dis. 2011;7(6):709–13.
79. Braghetto I, Csendes A, Lanzarini E, Papapietro K, Carcamo C, Molina JC. Is laparoscopic sleeve gastrectomy an acceptable primary bariatric procedure in obese patients? Early and 5-year postoperative results. Surg Laparosc Endosc Percutan Tech. 2012;22(6):479–86.
80. Soricelli E, Iossa A, Casella G, Abbatini F, Cali B, Basso N. Sleeve gastrectomy and crural repair in obese patients with gastroesophageal reflux disease and/or hiatal hernia. Surg Obes Relat Dis. 2013;9(3):356–61.
81. Rawlins L, Rawlins MP, Brown CC, Schumacher DL. Sleeve gastrectomy: 5-year outcomes of a single institution. Surg Obes Relat Dis. 2013;9(1):21–5.

82. Melissas J, Koukouraki S, Askoxylakis J, et al. Sleeve gastrectomy: a restrictive procedure? Obes Surg. 2007;17(1):57–62.
83. Weiner RA, Weiner S, Pomhoff I, Jacobi C, Makarewicz W, Weigand G. Laparoscopic sleeve gastrectomy – influence of sleeve size and resected gastric volume. Obes Surg. 2007;17(10):1297–305.
84. Chopra A, Chao E, Etkin Y, Merklinger L, Lieb J, Delany H. Laparoscopic sleeve gastrectomy for obesity: can it be considered a definitive procedure? Surg Endosc. 2012;26(3):831–7.
85. Chiu S, Birch DW, Shi X, Sharma AM, Karmali S. Effect of sleeve gastrectomy on gastroesophageal reflux disease: a systematic review. Surg Obes Relat Dis. 2011;7(4):510–5.
86. Oor JE, Roks DJ, Unlu C, Hazebroek EJ. Laparoscopic sleeve gastrectomy and gastroesophageal reflux disease: a systematic review and meta-analysis. Am J Surg. 2016;211(1):250–67.
87. Rebecchi F, Allaix ME, Giaccone C, Ugliono E, Scozzari G, Morino M. Gastroesophageal reflux disease and laparoscopic sleeve gastrectomy: a physiopathologic evaluation. Ann Surg. 2014;260(5):909–14. discussion 914–905
88. Rosenthal RJ, International Sleeve Gastrectomy Expert P, Diaz AA, et al. International Sleeve Gastrectomy Expert Panel Consensus Statement: best practice guidelines based on experience of >12,000 cases. Surg Obes Relat Dis. 2012;8(1):8–19.
89. Braghetto I, Csendes A. Prevalence of Barrett's esophagus in bariatric patients undergoing sleeve gastrectomy. Obes Surg. 2016a;26(4):710–4.
90. Braghetto I, Csendes A. Patients having bariatric surgery: surgical options in morbidly obese patients with Barrett's esophagus. Obes Surg. 2016b;26(7):1622–6.
91. Flint RS, Coulter G, Roberts R. The pattern of adjustments after laparoscopic adjustable gastric band. Obes Surg. 2015;25(11):2061–5.
92. Varban OA, Hawasli AA, Carlin AM, et al. Variation in utilization of acid-reducing medication at 1 year following bariatric surgery: results from the Michigan Bariatric Surgery Collaborative. Surg Obes Relat Dis. 2015;11(1):222–8.
93. Barr AC, Frelich MJ, Bosler ME, Goldblatt MI, Gould JC. GERD and acid reduction medication use following gastric bypass and sleeve gastrectomy. Surg Endosc. 2017;31(1):410–5.
94. DeVault KR, Castell DO, American College of G. Updated guidelines for the diagnosis and treatment of gastroesophageal reflux disease. Am J Gastroenterol. 2005;100(1):190–200.
95. Lanthaler M, Strasser S, Aigner F, Margreiter R, Nehoda H. Weight loss and quality of life after gastric band removal or deflation. Obes Surg. 2009;19(10):1401–8.
96. Rebibo L, Hakim S, Dhahri A, Yzet T, Delcenserie R, Regimbeau JM. Gastric stenosis after laparoscopic sleeve gastrectomy: diagnosis and management. Obes Surg. 2016;26(5):995–1001.
97. Parikh A, Alley JB, Peterson RM, et al. Management options for symptomatic stenosis after laparoscopic vertical sleeve gastrectomy in the morbidly obese. Surg Endosc. 2012;26(3):738–46.
98. Langer FB, Bohdjalian A, Shakeri-Leidenmuhler S, Schoppmann SF, Zacherl J, Prager G. Conversion from sleeve gastrectomy to Roux-en-Y gastric bypass – indications and outcome. Obes Surg. 2010;20(7):835–40.
99. Abdemur A, Fendrich I, Rosenthal R. Laparoscopic conversion of laparoscopic sleeve gastrectomy to gastric bypass for intractable gastroesophageal reflux disease. Surg Obes Relat Dis. 2012;8(5):654.
100. Loh Y, McGlone ER, Reddy M, Khan OA. Is the LINX reflux management system an effective treatment for gastro-oesophageal reflux disease? Int J Surg. 2014;12(9):994–7.
101. Ganz RA, Edmundowicz SA, Taiganides PA, et al. Long-term outcomes of patients receiving a magnetic sphincter augmentation device for gastroesophageal reflux. Clin Gastroenterol Hepatol. 2016;14(5):671–7.
102. Harnsberger CR, Broderick RC, Fuchs HF, et al. Magnetic lower esophageal sphincter augmentation device removal. Surg Endosc. 2015;29(4):984–6.
103. Asti E, Siboni S, Lazzari V, Bonitta G, Sironi A, Bonavina L. Removal of the magnetic sphincter augmentation device: surgical technique and results of a single-center cohort study. Ann Surg. 2016.
104. Desart K, Rossidis G, Michel M, Lux T, Ben-David K. Gastroesophageal reflux management with the LINX(R) system for gastroesophageal reflux disease following laparoscopic sleeve gastrectomy. J Gastrointest Surg. 2015;19(10):1782–6.
105. Hawasli A, Phillips A, Tarboush M. Laparoscopic management of reflux after Roux-en-Y gastric bypass using the LINX system and repair of hiatal hernia: a case report. Surg Obes Relat Dis. 2016;12:e51-4.
106. Mattar SG, Qureshi F, Taylor D, Schauer PR. Treatment of refractory gastroesophageal reflux disease with radiofrequency energy (Stretta) in patients after Roux-en-Y gastric bypass. Surg Endosc. 2006;20(6):850–4.

Part VII

Endoscopy

25 Building Bariatric Endoscopy Practice for the Surgeon

Josemberg Campos,
Maíra Danielle Gomes de Souza,
Manoel Galvao Neto,
Milton Ignacio Carvalho Tube,
and Luiz Gustavo de Quadros

Introduction

The increasing number of patients undergoing bariatric surgery, the broad arsenal of surgical techniques available, and the growing number of complications that can be treated endoscopically have led to the emergence of bariatric endoscopy as an advanced diagnosis-treatment interface. There is therefore a need for endoscopists, gastroenterologists, and bariatric surgeons to acquire knowledge of specific endoscopic aspects and use them for diagnosis, thereby treating complications in a manner that is minimally invasive, safe, and effective [1].

Endoscopic bariatric treatment can be subdivided into three lines: primary treatment of obesity (patients who are not candidates for surgery, such as intragastric balloon placement), treatment of surgical complications, and secondary treatment of obesity after weight regain (revisional procedures, such as the use of argon plasma). When used as a primary approach, endoscopic treatment produces better results compared to clinical treatment, but it is still not as durable or effective as surgery [2–4].

Training in bariatric endoscopy has traditionally been carried out informally at an endoscopy unit in a manner similar to other areas of professional education [5, 6]. Bariatric endoscopy is currently evolving, using more sophisticated and more durable equipment, requiring the presence of a well-trained multidisciplinary team including surgeons, clinicians, endocrinologists, psychologists, nurses, physiotherapists, and nutritionists to reduce the likelihood of postoperative complications.

This chapter presents solutions to surgical challenges involving bariatric endoscopy and shows the importance of a team specialized in bariatric endoscopy for training of endoscopists/surgeons in diagnostic and therapeutic bariatric endoscopy.

Training in Bariatric Endoscopy for Surgeons

A multidisciplinary team is fundamental for ensuring good results and safety in bariatric endoscopy [4]. There is therefore an urgent need for training of new bariatric surgeons, as a way of

J. Campos (✉)
Department of Surgery, Federal University of Pernambuco, Recife, PE, Brazil

M. D. G. de Souza · M. I. C. Tube
Department of Surgery, University Federal of Pernambuco, Recife, PE, Brazil

M. G. Neto
Department of Surgery, Herbert Wertheim College of Medicine – Florida International University, Doral, FL, USA

L. G. de Quadros
Department of Surgery, ABC Medical School, Sao Jose Do Rio Preto, SP, Brazil

R. Lutfi et al. (eds.), *Global Bariatric Surgery*, https://doi.org/10.1007/978-3-319-93545-4_25

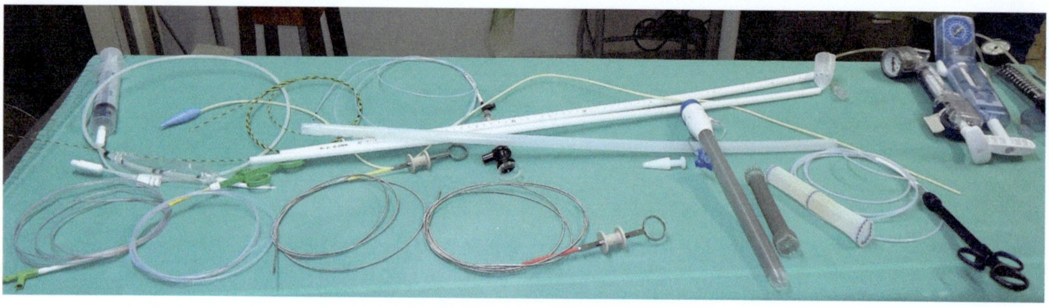

Fig. 25.1 Materials and equipment for bariatric endoscopy procedures

developing all-around understanding of obesity and achieving high success rates in both surgery and bariatric endoscopy. From the current pedagogical perspective, the need for knowledge and practical bariatric surgery skills requires the adoption of creative and innovative methodologies alongside traditional teaching.

Such a methodology requires a multidisciplinary team specialized in procedures such as fitting stents, dilation, septotomy, and removal of foreign bodies, among others. Implementation of a bariatric endoscopy training program certainly facilitates the teaching of novice bariatric surgeons [7].

The Federal University of Pernambuco's Postgraduate Program in Surgery has, since 2013, been conducting a study involving training of 50 physicians from 13 countries in Latin America and other parts of the world in bariatric endoscopy. These professionals were recruited by way of an internship program established by hospitals interested in training through direct contact with the researcher or on the recommendation of other interns who had already done the training. They included trainee bariatric surgeons and gastroenterological endoscopists interested in bariatric surgery.

The training took the form of 4–12-week academic internships divided into three stages:

First Stage

Teaching the fundamentals of endoscopy and general knowledge of equipment (assembling, manipulating, cleaning, and maintaining the endoscope and the endoscopy tower). Materials needed: intragastric balloon, partially covered esophageal stents, fully covered esophageal stents, needle knife, injector for control of bleeding, use of metal endoscopic clips, dilation balloon, Savary guide wire, and over tube (Fig. 25.1).

Second Stage

Training in bariatric endoscopy skills: anatomy and endoscopic approach under supervision of a teaching physician specialized in bariatric endoscopy; assemblage, placement, and removal; patient care; and handling of endoscopy materials presented in the first stage are the responsibility of the team's nursing monitor.

After instruction and training, the physicians are free to carry out procedures until they develop the level of skill required by the evaluation test. Training lasts on average 6 h, twice a week, varying according to the conditions of the inter-institutional agreement between the UFPE and the hospitals in the country of origin of each physician. Ex vivo pig models are used for all training procedures (airways, esophagus, stomach, and duodenum) [8] (Figs. 25.2 and 25.3).

Some techniques may be addressed and taught in this stage:

Balloon Dilatation

Gastrojejunal anastomosis stenosis or fistula may occur in isolation or concomitantly after bariatric surgery. Distal stenosis increases pressure in the gastric pouch, leading to development or exacerbation of fistula, which is unlikely to close spontaneously [9]. Endoscopic procedures, such as balloon dilation, have thus been used to effectively resolve complications.

When the stenosis has a diameter <10 mm, dilation treatment using a 20 and 30 mm balloon is effective and safe, enabling resolution of this serious complication [10]. The use of a stent for treatment of GJA fistula is indicated when the diameter of the fistula orifice is greater than 10 mm, especially in the early stages (less than 30 days after RYGB), when severe tissue fibrosis has not yet occurred [11] (Fig. 25.4).

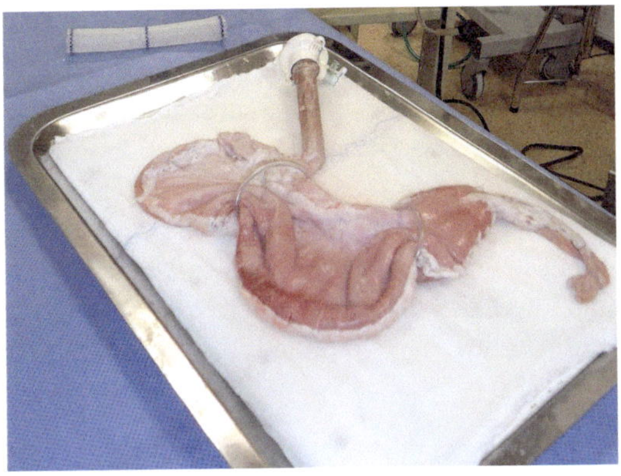

Fig. 25.2 Ex vivo pig stomach model used for endoscopy training

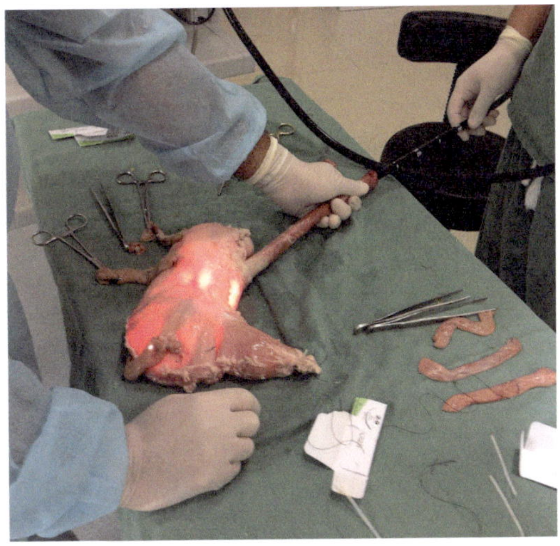

Fig. 25.3 Passage of endoscope into ex vivo pig stomach

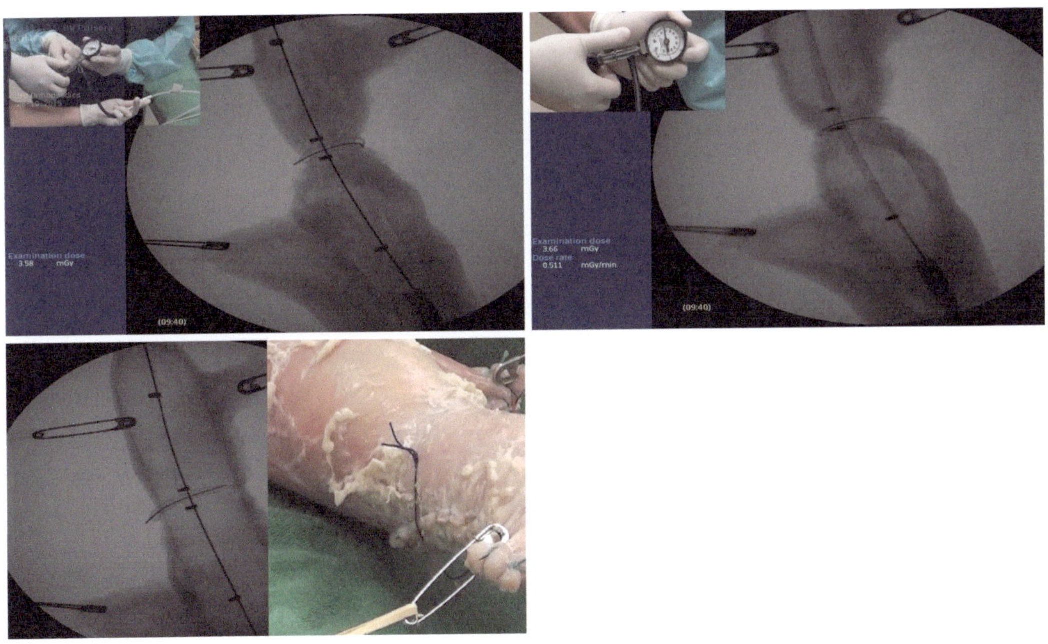

Fig. 25.4 Passage, positioning, and execution of procedure to break or widen contention ring using achalasia balloon in pig model

Performance of the Technique

- Procedure carried out in a hospital setting
- Patient in left lateral decubitus, under deep sedation, administered by an anesthesiologist
- Use of standard single-channel endoscope
- Identification of stenosis on the GJA and characteristics of the gastric pouch
- Passage of balloon with center positioned on the site of the GJA stenosis
- Balloon filled with liquid, using insufflator with manometer
- Gradual insufflation to avoid proximal or distal dislocation of the balloon, reducing the risk of laceration and perforation
- Endoscopic viewing of dilation
- Insufflation for around 1–3 min
- Desufflation and removal of balloon
- Endoscopic review to check for signs of bleeding or perforation
- Patient kept on a zero diet

Stent Placement

The self-expandable stent has been used for endoscopic treatment of fistulas [12, 13]. The aim is to reduce intragastric pressure, remodel the stomach, and isolate the fistula orifice. However, the stents traditionally available on the market were designed for apposition in the esophagus and do not adapt well to the sleeve gastrectomy format, as they are short and small caliber.

Owing to this difficulty and the large number of sleeve gastrectomies performed, some longer larger caliber stents have been developed specifically for the purpose of bariatric surgery. These stents have less potential for migration and are more efficient in reducing intragastric pressure, with the advantage of covering the whole stomach, providing better occlusion of the fistula and lower risk of migration. Increasingly consistent studies have reported good results [14] (Fig. 25.5).

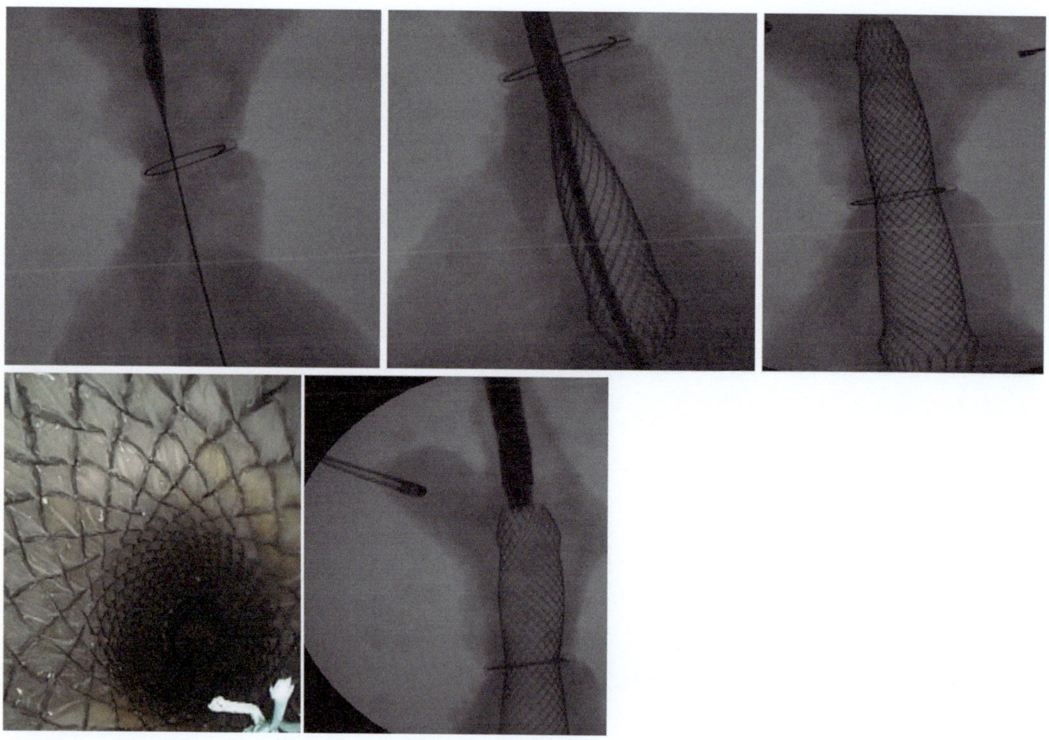

Fig. 25.5 Placement and removal of stent for treatment of ring slippage/fistula in pig model

Performance of the Technique

- Pneumatic dilation with 30 mm balloon and introduction of self-expandable stent
- Passage of guide wire into duodenum
- Passage of 30 mm pneumatic endoscopic dilation balloon over the ^^guide wire, positioned with the aid of radiology and endoscopic vision
- Dilation of the corpus-antrum axis, with balloon insufflated to 20 psi
- Insertion of double covered stent over the guide wire
- Endoscopic evaluation
- Proximal repositioning of stent, with foreign body forceps
- Radiological contrast test

Septotomy

Gastric fistula is one of the most serious complications of Roux-en-Y gastric bypass (RYGB), with a mean occurrence of 2.4%, and it is more common in the proximal segment, just below the gastroesophageal junction [15–17]. It is caused by local tension and tissue ischemia [18]. Septotomy is an innovative endoscopic treatment of gastrointestinal fistulas after gastroplasty. The procedure is based on treatment of Zenker's diverticulum, enabling internal drainage of the perigastric abscess, directing the flow of gastric secretion, reducing cavity contamination and intragastric pressure, and ensuring the gastric lumen is clear [19, 20]. It can be carried out with good results in cases where there is a fistula with perigastric cavity, with accumulation of secretions and debris and the presence of fibrous septum between the cavity and gastric pouch, whether in the angle of His, the gastric corpus, or the gastrojejunal anastomosis.

The procedure is carried out by cutting the septum, using electrocauterization or the application of argon plasma, with a view to guiding drainage of secretion into the pouch. It should ideally be combined with endoscopic dilation, which enables treatment of possible associated stenosis, facilitates the flow of secretions, and stimulates the formation of granulation tissue.

Performance of the Technique

- Patient in left lateral decubitus, under general anesthetic and orotracheal intubation
- Initial diagnostic endoscopy
- Pneumatic dilation of anastomosis with 14 mm balloon
- Irrigation and washing of perigastric cavity (abscess) debris
- Opening of septum between perigastric cavity and pouch
- Review of hemostasis

Third Stage

In this stage, the physicians are evaluated by the project coordinator, using the OSATS [21] scale modified for endoscopy, on a scale from 1 to 30, with a pass mark of 16.

As of the time of writing, 100% of physicians trained successfully developed bariatric endoscopy skills.

Discussion

The first challenge in endoscopy is to make an accurate diagnostic anatomo-endoscopic correlation in order, with the aid of associated exams and the patient's clinical history, to be able to arrive at a correct conclusion regarding the complication found. The study of the anatomy of the stomach, the general conditions of the patient, the presence of a team accustomed to working with the obese patient, and the environment are all crucial factors for adequate treatment.

The multidisciplinary focus on the field of bariatric surgery and endoscopy has become increasingly important in recent years. The positive results for integral management of bariatric patients have certainly led to improved treatments and lower incidence of complications.

The literature shows the importance of a multidisciplinary team, especially nurses, who can safely and effectively assist in endoscopy. Some reviews have explored the evidence supporting the performance of endoscopy by nonphysicians, the possible difficulties, and the requirements of a high-quality program to support training [7].

This dynamic and synchronized working methodology facilitates teaching of complex and difficult procedures, such as placement of partially covered esophageal stents for treatment of fistulas, placement of fully covered esophageal stents for ring removal, handling of septotomy materials (needle knife, injector to control bleeding, metal endoscopic clips), and materials for treatment of stenoses (dilation balloon, Savary guide wire, and over tube).

The concentration that the therapeutic procedure requires and the large quantity of materials that may be used in a single procedure mean that therapeutic endoscopy always performed by four, six, or eight hands. The assistant must have technical and anatomical knowledge and be familiar with the materials that may be needed during the procedure. Correct handling of endoscopic accessories and focus and concentration in performing tasks are of the utmost importance for the success of the procedure. During a "simple" gastrojejunal anastomosis dilation procedure, for example, the simple fact of the assistant having difficulty desufflating the balloon when the patient is agitated may lead to a deep laceration or even local perforation; correct handling of the guide wire during procedures may require it to be passed through repeatedly or even cause perforations; correct exposure of needles, scalpels, and so forth is essential for safe and effective endoscopy. In addition to the need for training of the team that works during the procedure, post-procedure care and correct nutritional guidelines are fundamental for ensuring a successful outcome. Therapeutic bariatric endoscopy ends with the resolution of the problem; during post-sleeve fistula treatment, for example, the endoscopist should be involved and accompany the patient throughout the process: diagnosis, choice of treatment, stent placement, follow-up and counseling while the stent is in place, removal of the stent, follow-up after removal of the stent, and so forth. It is a lengthy process, and adequate formal training and skilled referral services are essential for adequate management. Bariatric endoscopy is "a world apart," and most endoscopy or surgery schools do not provide adequate training in this field.

Final Considerations

- Endoscopy is now being widely used for minimally invasive, safe, and effective treatment of complications after bariatric surgery.
- Evaluation of the results of the study leads to the conclusion that a specialized multidisciplinary team improves the development of bariatric medicine skills.
- The introduction of training of professionals to attend patients with various types of postoperative complications is of crucial importance.
- Pre- and post-procedure management is as important as the procedures themselves, and a trained team is essential for this.

References

1. Campos JM, Neto MPG, Moura EGH, Silva CEJ. Endoscopia Pré e Peroperatoria. In: Campos et al. Endoscopia em Cirurgia da obcsidade.1nded. São Paulo: Santos; 2008. p. 49.
2. Cai JX, Schweitzer MA, Kumbhari V. Endoscopic management of bariatric surgery complications. Surg Laparosc Endosc Percutan Tech. 2016;26(2):93–101.
3. Sullivan S, Kumar N, Edmundowicz SA, Abu Dayyeh BK, Jonnalagadda SS, Larsen M, et al. ASGE position statement on endoscopic bariatric therapies in clinical practice. Gastrointest Endosc. 2015;82(5):767–72.
4. Maluf Filho F, Lima MS. The role of endoscopy in bariatric surgery. Einstein. 2006;Supl 1:S114–9. Disponivel em: http://apps.einstein.br/revista/arquivos/PDF/110-114-119.pdf.
5. Waschke KA, Anderson J, Macintosh D, Valori RM. Training the gastrointestinal endoscopy trainer. Best Pract Res Clin Gastroenterol. 2016;30(3):409–19.
6. Galvão-Neto MP, Zilberstein B, Guimarães P, Figueroa C, et al. Treinamento videocirurgico em animal de laboratório. Laparoscopic surgical training in laboratory animals. Res Gate. 2003;(2):38–42.
7. Ruco A, Walsh CM, Cooper MA, Rabeneck L. Training non-physicians to do endoscopy: feasibility,

effectiveness and cost-effectiveness. Best Pract Res Clin Gastroenterol. 2016;30(3):389–96.

8. Tube MIC, Netto FACS, Costa E, Lafayette DSA, Lima GAFCA, Menezes JIS, et al. Chest drainage teaching and training for medical students. Use of a surgical ex vivo pig model. Acta Cir Bras. 2016;31:353–63.
9. Campos JM, Pereira EF, Evangelista LF, Siqueira L, Neto MG, Dib V, et al. Gastrobronchial fistula after sleeve gastrectomy and gastric bypass: endoscopic management and prevention. Obes Surg. 2011;21(10):1520–9.
10. Campos JM, Mello FS, Ferraz AA, Brito JN, Nassif PA, Galvao-Neto Mdos P. Endoscopic dilation of gastrojejunal anastomosis after gastric bypass. Arq Bras Cir Dig: ABCD = Braz Arch Dig Surg. 2012;25(4):283–9.
11. Puli SR, Spofford IS, Thompson CC. Use of self-expandable stents in the treatment of bariatric surgery leaks: a systematic review and meta-analysis. Gastrointest Endosc. 2012;75(2):287–93.
12. Perisse LG, Perisse PC, Bernardo JC. Endoscopic treatment of the fistulas after laparoscopic sleeve gastrectomy and roux-en-Y gastric bypass. Revista do Colegio Brasileiro de Cirurgioes. 2015;42(3):159–64.
13. Murino A, Arvanitakis M, Le Moine O, Blero D, Deviere J, Eisendrath P. Effectiveness of endoscopic management using self-expandable metal stents in a large cohort of patients with post-bariatric leaks. Obes Surg. 2015;25(9):1569–76.
14. Leenders BJ, Stronkhorst A, Smulders FJ, Nieuwenhuijzen GA, Gilissen LP. Removable and repositionable covered metal self-expandable stents for leaks after upper gastrointestinal surgery: experiences in a tertiary referral hospital. Surg Endosc. 2013;27(8):2751–9.
15. Baker RS, Foote J, Kemmeter P, Brady R, Vroegop T, Serveld M. The science of stapling and leaks. Obes Surg. 2004;14(10):1290–8.
16. O'Rourke RW, Andrus J, Diggs BS, Scholz M, McConnell DB, Deveney CW. Perioperative morbidity associated with bariatric surgery: an academic center experience. Arch Surg (Chicago Ill: 1960). 2006;141(3):262–8.
17. Baretta G, Campos J, Correia S, Alhinho H, Marchesini JB, Lima JH, et al. Bariatric postoperative fistula: a life-saving endoscopic procedure. Surg Endosc. 2015;29(7):1714–20.
18. Podnos YD, Jimenez JC, Wilson SE, Stevens CM, Nguyen NT. Complications after laparoscopic gastric bypass: a review of 3464 cases. Arch Surg (Chicago Ill: 1960). 2003;138(9):957–61.
19. Adams J, Sheppard B, Andersen P, Myers B, Deveney C, Everts E, et al. Zenker's diverticulostomy with cricopharyngeal myotomy: the endoscopic approach. Surg Endosc. 2001;15(1):34–7.
20. Campos JM, Siqueira LT, Ferraz AA, Ferraz EM. Gastrobronchial fistula after obesity surgery. J Am Coll Surg. 2007;204(4):711.
21. Niitsu H, Hirabayashi N, Yoshimitsu M, Mimura T, Taomoto J, Sugiyama Y, et al. Using the objective structured assessment of technical skills (OSATS) global rating scale to evaluate the skills of surgical trainees in the operating room. Surg Today. 2013;43(3):271–5.

26 Endoscopic Bariatric Therapies

Anthony Choi and Reem Sharaiha

Gastric Endoscopic Bariatric Therapies

Traditional bariatric surgeries, whether Roux-en-Y gastric bypass surgery, gastric band, or sleeve gastrectomy, all share gastric volume reduction/restriction as a common component. Studies have shown that besides early satiety, such gastric manipulation may be affecting the neuroendocrine signaling in the body that may lead to weight loss [1]. In the endoscopic realm, several innovative therapies are offered to alter the stomach's capacity, including space-occupying devices, gastric remodeling methods, and aspiration therapy.

Intragastric Balloon

The Orbera intragastric balloon (Apollo Endosurgery, Austin, TX) is an FDA-approved, silicone-based balloon that is initially advanced along into the stomach in its deflated state. Once its position is confirmed via an endoscope, the balloon is inflated with fluids via an attached catheter, usually with saline. In the USA, a multicenter randomized non-blinded trial compared 125 patients receiving the Orbera balloon and lifestyle interventions to 130 patients receiving lifestyle interventions alone and noted a 10.7% total body weight loss for the former group and 4.7% in the latter group [2]. In terms of adverse events, no mortality was observed. Serious adverse events (4%) included gastric outlet obstruction with gastritis ($n = 1$), gastric perforation with sepsis ($n = 1$), mucosal esophageal tears ($n = 2$), and laryngospasm ($n = 1$). The most frequent adverse events were nausea, vomiting, and abdominal pain.

Because of its prolonged use outside of the USA, the data is the most robust for the Orbera intragastric balloon in comparison to other balloons. A meta-analysis of 17 studies including 1638 patients revealed a 25.44% mean excess body weight loss at 12 months [3]. Within those studies, three randomized control trials showed 26.9% difference in mean excess body weight loss between Orbera patients and controls. In terms of adverse events, pain and nausea were most frequent at 33.7%, and serious side effects included migration (1.4%) and gastric perforation (0.1%). Four deaths were reported in the literature.

The ReShape Duo (Reshape Medical, San Clemente, CA) derives its name from its dual-balloon system, which is filled with normal saline and methylene blue. The FDA-approved, dual-balloon implant is endoscopically placed and retrieved after 6 months. A prospective randomized trial evaluated 326 patients either to

A. Choi · R. Sharaiha (✉)
Division of Gastroenterology and Hepatology, New York Presbyterian-Weill Cornell Medical Center, New York, NY, USA
e-mail: ajc2006@nyp.org; rzs9001@med.cornell.edu

R. Lutfi et al. (eds.), *Global Bariatric Surgery*, https://doi.org/10.1007/978-3-319-93545-4_26

the dual balloon with lifestyle modifications group or the sham endoscopy with lifestyle modifications group. At 24 weeks, excess body weight loss was 27.9% in the dual-balloon group versus 12.3% in the sham group ($p = 0.0007$). Of note, ulcers occurred in 35% of dual-balloon patients, which led to a redesign of the distal device tip mid-trial that reduced ulcer frequency and size. Other most frequent adverse events were nausea, vomiting, and abdominal pain. Serious adverse events included esophageal mucosal tear ($n = 1$), ulcer-associated GI hemorrhage ($n = 1$), esophagus perforation ($n = 1$), and pneumonitis ($n = 1$).

The Obalon gastric balloon (Obalon Therapeutics, Inc., Carlsbad, CA) is another FDA-approved intragastric balloon. It is initially enclosed within a small disintegrating capsule that is connected to a long catheter. The pill is swallowed, disintegrates, and once its intragastric position is confirmed via fluoroscopy, is inflated with gas through the detachable catheter that protrudes out of the mouth. Up to three balloons can be swallowed in a patient, which are then removed between 12 and 26 weeks thereafter. A recent multicenter, randomized blinded clinical trial compared 185 patients with the Obalon balloon and 181 patients who underwent a sham procedure (both groups underwent lifestyle modifications). At 6 months, total body weight loss was 6.9% for the Obalon group versus 3.6% in the sham group [4].

The Spatz adjustable balloon system (Spatz Medical, Great Neck, NY) allows for adjustment of the volume of the balloon once inside the patient's stomach. The balloon is filled with saline solution and is equipped with an extractable inflation tube that allows the balloon to be adjusted depending on tolerance and desired effectiveness. A European trial showed that in 70 patients with a follow-up of up to 12 months, mean total body weight loss was 19% and excess body weight loss was 45.7%, with 38 of those patients losing additional 9.4 kg with adjustments [5]. Adverse events included intolerance, balloon deflations, and gastric ulcers. Currently, a multicenter trial is underway in the US [6].

Other Space-Occupying Devices

The TransPyloric Shuttle (BAROnova, Inc., Goleta, CA) is a silicone-based device that is comprised of a larger bulb connected to a smaller bulb by a flexible tether. The device is deployed endoscopically into the stomach, and while the larger bulb remains in the stomach, the size of the smaller bulb allows it to naturally migrate via peristalsis into the duodenum, thus assuming the transpyloric position. In this position, the larger bulb sits at the gastric antrum, creating an intermittent obstruction leading to delayed gastric emptying as well as early and prolonged satiety.

The first feasibility trial evaluated 20 patients, half who had the device for 3 months and half for 6 months [7]. The mean excess weight loss and total body weight loss were 25.1% and 8.9% in the 3-month group and 41.0% and 14.5% in the 6-month group. The most common adverse events were nausea, sore throat, and abdominal pain. There were two early device retrievals (at 2.5 and 5.5 months) due to epigastric pain, with immediate resolution of symptoms after device removal. A multicenter randomized trial is currently underway in the USA.

The Full Sense Device (Baker, Foote, Kemmeter, Walburn, LLC, Grand Rapids, MI) is another space-occupying endoscopic bariatric device that transpires between two parts of the GI tract: the lower esophagus and proximal stomach. The proximal portion of the device resembles an esophageal stent and connects via struts to a disk that resides in the cardia, inciting a feeling of satiety. There are currently no peer-reviewed data published.

Endoscopic Sleeve Gastroplasty

Endoscopic sleeve gastroplasty is an endoscopic procedure that imbricates the stomach to mimic a surgical sleeve gastrectomy. It differs from it slightly in that the fundus is not sutured down, and a small pouch is left behind. In the former, the Overstitch device (Apollo Endosurgery, Austin, TX) is introduced transorally to place a series of full-thickness triangular sutures endoluminally along the great curvature of the stomach. The stitches are positioned from the prepyloric antrum to the gastroesophageal junction and, when tightened, cause the greater curvature of the stomach to fold in on itself along its long axis, creating a smaller gastric sleeve/lumen. This procedure has been associated with early satiety and delayed gastric emptying [8].

After the initial feasibility study in 2013 [9], many groups have showed the safety and efficacy of this procedure [10–12]. A recent multicenter study was carried out with 248 patients at 3 centers over 24 months [13]. Total body weight loss was 15.17% at 6 months and 18.6% ($n = 92$, after accounting for loss to follow-up) at 24 months, with no significant variability between centers. Adverse events occurred in five cases and included perigastric inflammatory fluid collection ($n = 2$), hemorrhage from splenic laceration ($n = 1$), pulmonary embolism ($n = 1$), and pneumoperitoneum/pneumothorax ($n = 1$). One study also demonstrated improvement in A1C by 1% ($p = 0.03$), as well as improvement in systolic blood pressure and liver function tests [14].

Primary Obesity Surgery Endoluminal

Primary obesity surgery endoluminal (POSE) utilizes a peroral incisional operating platform (USGI Medical, San Clemente, CA, USA) to operate two graspers and one catheter with a needle tip. Using these tools to approximate and suture, the procedure involves placing transmural tissue anchor plications in the fundus and distal body of the stomach for reducing accommodation and delaying emptying. Following two single-arm studies, two multicenter randomized trials have been completed to date. In the MILEPOST study, 39 patients were analyzed in 3 centers, 30 in POSE with diet/exercise guidance group and 9 to the diet/exercise guidance-only control group [15]. At 12 months, statistical significance was seen in total body weight loss (13.0% vs 5.3%, $p < 0.01$) and excess body weight loss (45.0% vs 18.1%, $p < 0.01$) for the POSE groups vs the control group. No serious adverse events were reported, with only two patients experiencing minor postoperative bleeding.

In the ESSENTIAL study, besides 34 patients in an unblinded lead-in cohort, 221 patients were randomized to the POSE group and 111 patients to the sham surgery group [16]. At 12 months, the total body weight loss for the POSE group versus sham group was 4.95% versus 1.38% ($p < 0.0001$) and overall weight loss 4.81 kg versus 1.20 kg ($p < 0.0001$). In addition, statistical significance was seen in fasting glucose and HbA1c levels. The most common adverse events in the POSE group were pain (45.2%), sore throat (27.6%), and nausea (21.3%), and the most common device-related adverse events were gastric erosion (0.5%), pain (0.5%), and mouth trauma (0.9%). Serious adverse events occurred in 5% in the POSE group and included only procedure-related events: extra-gastric bleeding, nausea, and vomiting.

Aspiration Therapy

The AspireAssist system (Aspire Bariatrics, King of Prussia, PA) consists of interdependent devices used in aspiration therapy, in which a portion of the consumed food is removed directly from the stomach after one's meal. The A-tube is a removable, silicone-based tube that is inserted much like a standard percutaneous endoscopic gastrostomy tube, with a skin-port connection. One initiates aspiration about 20 min after a meal and lasts for about 10–15 min. For aspiration, the External Device and water reservoir, both of which are portable and detachable, are connected to the A-tube via the skin-port, and after subsequent rounds of aspiration and water flushes, about 30% of the food is removed from the stomach, decreasing the calories one's body absorbs.

The first studies were promising in terms of outcome, showing 14.8–20.1% total body weight loss and 40.8–54.6% excess body weight loss [17, 18], and exhibited adverse events similar to that of percutaneous endoscopic gastrostomy tubes. A 52-week, multicenter, randomized control trial compared the outcomes of 137 patients who were treated with the AspireAssist system and lifestyle counseling to 70 patients who received lifestyle counseling [19]. At 52 weeks, the AspireAssist group saw 31.5% mean reduction in excess body weight, while the lifestyle counseling-only group lost a mean of 9.8% ($p < 0.001$), and more participants in the AspireAssist group lost at least 25% excess weight loss than in the lifestyle counseling-only group (58.6% vs 15.3%, $p < 0.001$). The most common adverse events were peristomal granulation tissue (40.5%), abdominal pain within 4 weeks of A-tube placement (37.8%), nausea/vomiting (17.1%), and peristomal irritation (17.1%), while one patient each experienced a serious adverse event (severe abdominal pain, peritonitis, prepyloric ulcer, and A-tube replacement due to malfunction). About a quarter of the participants had intolerance/early removal of the device before 52 weeks [6].

Small Bowel Endoscopic Bariatric Therapies

In Roux-en-Y gastric bypass surgery, improvement in blood sugars and reduction or elimination of diabetic medication are often seen quickly after surgery, even before (and thus likely independent of) significant weight loss [20]. Furthermore, in duodenojejunal bypass surgery, HbA1c, glycemic control, and beta-cell response improve with minimal weight loss [21]. Though the exact mechanism is unknown, it is thought to be related to the bypass of the duodenum and the rapid delivery of nutrients to the mid to distal jejunum, causing a change in the gut endocrine environment. Hormones implicated include GLP-1 [22] (which enhances insulin secretion, inhibits glucagon release, causes delayed gastric emptying and decreased food intake, induces proliferation in islet beta cells, and inhibits beta-cell apoptosis), peptide YY [23] (which inhibits gastric motility and decreases appetite), and gastric inhibitory peptide [24], which has an insulinotropic effect.

Thus, by mimicking the effects and avoiding the invasiveness of classical bariatric surgery, increasing numbers of endoscopic therapies bypassing the proximal small bowel have been gaining traction in the bariatric therapy world to contribute to weight loss and diabetes management.

Duodenojejunal Bypass Liner

The EndoBarrier (GI Dynamics, Boston, MA) is a duodenojejunal bypass liner (DJBL). Via an endoscopic delivery system, this 80-cm-long fluoropolymer-based sleeve is anchored proximally with ten barbs and spans from the duodenal bulb just behind the pylorus to the proximal jejunum. Because of its impermeable nature, the length of the sleeve prevents any contact between the food and digestive juices in the duodenum and proximal jejunum, artificially causing malabsorption. In essence, the procedure mimics the excluded biliopancreatic limb of a Roux-en-Y gastric bypass.

There have been several trials that evaluated the safety and efficacy of the bypass liner. Of these, perhaps the most significant was a multicenter, randomized, sham-controlled trial that prior to early stoppage, enrolled 216 subjects in the DJBL arm to 109 in the sham arm. This study was stopped prior to completion of enrollment because of a 3.5% incidence of hepatic abscess; in addition, 11.7% of the subjects experienced serious adverse events that required early device removal [25]. In terms of efficacy, HbA1c decreased by 1% in the DJBL group and 0.3% in the sham group. A meta-analysis reviewed 271 implantations from 11 clinical trials, of which 9 reported adverse events and early removal rates [3]. It found that 18.37% implantations required early removal. Serious adverse events included migration (4.9%), GI bleeding (3.86%), sleeve obstruction (3.4%), liver abscess (0.126%), cholangitis (0.126%), acute cholecystitis (0.126%), and esophageal perforation (0.126%). As for efficacy, in three trials with at least 12-month follow-up and four randomized control trials with 12–14-week follow-up, the %EWL was 35.3% and 9.4%, respectively. Reductions in HbA1c of 0.7%, 1.7%, and 1.5% were also seen at 12, 24, and 52 weeks, respectively. Another analysis of 14 studies found that at time of explant of the DJBL, HbA1c decreased by 1.3 ($p < 0.0001$) [26]. More studies to gather data as well as improve on the design and safety of DJBLs are ongoing [27].

Gastroduodenojejunal Bypass Sleeve

The gastroduodenojejunal bypass sleeve (ValenTx endoluminal bypass; ValenTx Inc., Hopkins, MN) shares some similarities with the DJBL. It also mimics the anatomical changes of a Roux-en-Y gastric bypass with a fluoropolymer-based sleeve. However, as the name suggests, the stomach is also bypassed during this procedure, requiring a longer sleeve. Another difference is that this endoluminal implantation device is currently deployed endoscopically with laparoscopic assistance. The 120-cm sleeve is deployed through the pylorus and, after ensuring the distal end extends through the duodenum into the proximal jejunum, is anchored proximally at the GE junction with sutures.

The first-in-human prospective trial was published in 2011 [28]. After pre-procedural exclusion, 22 patients had attempted device implantation. All 22 patients had successful implantation and explantation without procedure-related complications. Five of these patients underwent explantation before the 12-week scheduled removal due to dysphagia, and symptoms resolved completely with explantation. In terms of the efficacy of the remaining 17 patients, the average excess weight loss was 39.7%, and average total weight loss was 16.8 kg. A subsequent trial was designed to follow patients who had the device implanted for 12 months [29]. Of the 12 patients, 2 had early explantation due to device intolerance. The remaining ten patients reached a 12-month follow-up. No periprocedural complications were noted, and all ten tolerated the sleeve device throughout the 12 months without bowel erosion, ulceration, bowel obstruction, or pancreatitis. At follow-up endoscopy, six patients had fully attached and functional devices, while four had partial cuff detachment. The former group had an average excess weight loss of 54%, while the average for all ten patients was 35.9%. Furthermore, five of the six patients who reached a year with a fully attached device were subsequently followed for an average of 14 months post-explant and maintained an average 30% excess weight loss. All of the studied patients who had diabetes, hypertension, or hypertriglyceridemia saw improvements of their disease (fasting glucose and HbA1c levels, blood pressure, triglyceride levels).

Duodenal Mucosal Resurfacing

The Revita duodenal mucosal resurfacing (DMR) (Fractyl, Lexington, MA) is another investigational, device-based, minimally invasive, transoral procedure. The theory behind the procedure stems from studies in type 2 diabetes rodent models, in which (1) their duodenal mucosa is characterized by abnormal hypertrophy and endocrine hyperplasia and (2) selective denudation of the duodenal mucosa via abrasion resulted in immediate lowering of glycemia during a glucose challenge [30]. In humans, the procedure involves injecting saline into the submucosal space of the duodenum to create a circumferential mucosal lift, followed by circumferential hydrothermal ablation. Following ablation of the "pathologic" mucosa, the duodenum re-epithelializes with normal mucosa, bringing along with it its associated benefits on glucose homeostasis.

The first-in-human clinical study on the safety, tolerability, and 6-month interim effectiveness was published in 2016 [30]. In terms of safety, there were no perioperative complications in all 40 treated patients. The most common adverse effect (8/40 patients) was postprocedural abdominal pain which self-resolved and duodenal stenosis (3/40 patients) that resolved after endoscopic balloon dilation. Gastrointestinal bleeding, perforation, pancreatitis, severe hypoglycemia, and evidence of malabsorption were not seen. All follow-up patients exhibited mucosal healing on endoscopy and biopsy. In terms of efficacy, HbA1c decreased by 1.2% at 6 months ($p < 0.001$) and that the predominant effect was on fasting hyperglycemia. Furthermore, the authors did not find a significant correlation between the amount of weight loss and level of HbA1c improvement.

Incisionless Magnetic Anastomosis System

The incisionless magnetic anastomosis system (GI Windows, Bridgewater, MA) is perhaps the most unique of the investigational, minimally invasive, endoscopic procedures. The technology relies on two self-assembling magnets that are designed to be deployed into adjacent hollow organs and couple. When the magnets come together, they cause necrosis of the tissue in between the coupled magnets, followed by a remodeling of the surrounding tissue and formation of an anastomosis. For the desired bariatric effect, one magnet is deployed via upper endoscopy to the jejunum and another via lower endoscopy to the ileum so that when a partial jejunal diversion is created, it allows for nutrients and digested fluids to circumvent part of the small bowel.

The first-in-human clinical study on the feasibility, safety, and 1-year interim effectiveness was very recently reported [31]. The study evaluated ten patients, of which four subjects had type 2 diabetes, three had prediabetes, and three did not have diabetes. All ten patients had successful patent anastomosis with no initial leak or perforation and no abnormal scarring, fibrosis, and significant change in size throughout the follow-up. All ten patients reported nausea, vomiting, and abdominal pain, all of which resolved with minimal intervention. In terms of efficacy, average total weight loss was 14.6%, and average excess weight loss was 40.2%. The diabetic patients saw an average of 1.9% reduction in HbA1c, and prediabetic patients saw an average of 1.0%.

Conclusion

Bariatric endoscopy is in its infancy. While mostly less effective than bariatric surgery, it does in most cases have a safer profile and surely would be more acceptable to many patients who fear an operation and permanent anatomical changes.

It could certainly fill the wide cap in obesity treatment, between diet and exercise, and invasive surgical solution.

More research and innovation are needed to better understand its value and improve its outcome, so it can serve well the millions of patients who would not present for a procedure otherwise.

References

1. Bazerbachi F, Vargas Valls EJ, Abu Dayyeh BK. Recent clinical results of endoscopic bariatric therapies as an obesity intervention. Clin Endosc. 2017;50(1):42–50.
2. Courcoulas A, Abu Dayyeh BK, Eaton L, et al. Intragastric balloon as an adjunct to lifestyle intervention: a randomized controlled trial. Int J Obes. 2017;41(3):427–33.
3. ASGE Bariatric Endoscopy Task Force and ASGE Technology Committee, Abu Dayyeh BK, Kumar N, et al. ASGE bariatric endoscopy task force systematic review and meta-analysis assessing the ASGE PIVI thresholds for adopting endoscopic bariatric therapies. Gastrointest Endosc. 2015;82(3):425–38.e5.
4. Sullivan S, Swain JM, Woodman G, et al. 812d The Obalon Swallowable 6-month balloon system is more effective than moderate intensity lifestyle therapy alone: results from a 6- month randomized sham controlled trial. Gastroenterology. 2016;150(4):S1267.
5. Brooks J, Srivastava ED, Mathus-Vliegen EMH. One-year adjustable intragastric balloons: results in 73 consecutive patients in the U.K. Obes Surg. 2014;24(5):813–9.
6. Abu Dayyeh BK, Edmundowicz S, Thompson CC. Clinical practice update: expert review on endoscopic bariatric therapies. Gastroenterology. 2017;152(4):716–29.
7. Marinos G, Eliades C, Raman Muthusamy V, Greenway F. Weight loss and improved quality of life with a nonsurgical endoscopic treatment for obesity: clinical results from a 3- and 6-month study. Surg Obes Relat Dis. 2014;10(5):929–34.
8. Abu Dayyeh BK, Acosta A, Camilleri M, et al. Endoscopic sleeve Gastroplasty alters gastric physiology and induces loss of body weight in obese individuals. Clin Gastroenterol Hepatol. 2017;15(1):37–43.e1.
9. Abu Dayyeh BK, Rajan E, Gostout CJ. Endoscopic sleeve gastroplasty: a potential endoscopic alternative to surgical sleeve gastrectomy for treatment of obesity. Gastrointest Endosc. 2013;78(3):530–5.

10. Sharaiha RZ, Kedia P, Kumta N, et al. Initial experience with endoscopic sleeve gastroplasty: technical success and reproducibility in the bariatric population. Endoscopy. 2015;47(2):164–6.
11. Lopez-Nava G, Galvão MP, da Bautista-Castaño I, Jimenez A, De Grado T, Fernandez-Corbelle JP. Endoscopic sleeve gastroplasty for the treatment of obesity. Endoscopy. 2015;47(5):449–52.
12. Galvão-Neto MDP, Grecco E, de Souza TF, de Quadros LG, Silva LB, Campos JM. Endoscopic sleeve gastroplasty – minimally invasive therapy for primary obesity treatment. Arq Bras Cir Dig. 2016;29(Suppl 1(Suppl 1)):95–7.
13. Lopez-Nava G, Sharaiha RZ, Vargas EJ, et al. Endoscopic sleeve gastroplasty for obesity: a multicenter study of 248 patients with 24 months follow-up. Obes Surg. 2017;27(10):2649–55.
14. Sharaiha RZ, Kumta NA, Saumoy M, et al. Endoscopic sleeve gastroplasty significantly reduces body mass index and metabolic complications in obese patients. Clin Gastroenterol Hepatol. 2017;15(4):504–10.
15. Miller K, Turró R, Greve JW, Bakker CM, Buchwald JN, Espinós JC. MILEPOST multicenter randomized controlled trial: 12-month weight loss and satiety outcomes after pose (SM) vs medical therapy. Obes Surg. 2017;27(2):310–22.
16. Sullivan S, Swain JM, Woodman G, et al. Randomized sham-controlled trial evaluating efficacy and safety of endoscopic gastric plication for primary obesity: the ESSENTIAL trial. Obesity (Silver Spring). 2017;25(2):294–301.
17. Sullivan S, Stein R, Jonnalagadda S, Mullady D, Edmundowicz S. Aspiration therapy leads to weight loss in obese subjects: a pilot study. Gastroenterology. 2013;145(6):1245–52.e1.
18. Forssell H, Norén E. A novel endoscopic weight loss therapy using gastric aspiration: results after 6 months. Endoscopy. 2015;47(1):68–71.
19. Thompson CC, Abu Dayyeh BK, Kushner R, et al. Percutaneous gastrostomy device for the treatment of class II and class III obesity: results of a randomized controlled trial. Am J Gastroenterol. 2017;112(3):447–57.
20. Rubino F. Is type 2 diabetes an operable intestinal disease? A provocative yet reasonable hypothesis. Diabetes Care. 2008;31(Suppl 2):S290–6.
21. Klein S, Fabbrini E, Patterson BW, et al. Moderate effect of duodenal-jejunal bypass surgery on glucose homeostasis in patients with type 2 diabetes. Obesity (Silver Spring). 2012;20(6):1266–72.
22. Rhee NA, Vilsbøll T, Knop FK. Current evidence for a role of GLP-1 in Roux-en-Y gastric bypass-induced remission of type 2 diabetes. Diabetes Obes Metab. 2012;14(4):291–8.
23. Vilarrasa N, de Gordejuela AGR, Casajoana A, et al. Endobarrier® in grade I obese patients with long-standing type 2 diabetes: role of gastrointestinal hormones in glucose metabolism. Obes Surg. 2017;27(3):569–77.
24. Knop FK. Resolution of type 2 diabetes following gastric bypass surgery: involvement of gut-derived glucagon and glucagonotropic signalling? Diabetologia. 2009;52(11):2270–6.
25. Quezada N, Muñoz R, Morelli C, et al. Safety and efficacy of the endoscopic duodenal-jejunal bypass liner prototype in severe or morbidly obese subjects implanted for up to 3 years. Surg Endosc. 2018;32(1):260–7.
26. Jirapinyo P, Haas AV, Thompson CC. 549 effect of the Duodenal-Jejunal bypass liner on glycemic control in type-2 diabetic patients with obesity: a meta-analysis with secondary analysis on weight loss and hormonal changes. Gastrointest Endosc. 2017;85(5):AB82–3.
27. Sullivan S, Edmundowicz SA, Thompson CC. Endoscopic bariatric and metabolic therapies: new and emerging technologies. Gastroenterology. 2017;152(7):1791–801.
28. Sandler BJ, Rumbaut R, Swain CP, et al. Human experience with an endoluminal, endoscopic, gastrojejunal bypass sleeve. Surg Endosc. 2011;25(9):3028–33.
29. Sandler BJ, Rumbaut R, Swain CP, et al. One-year human experience with a novel endoluminal, endoscopic gastric bypass sleeve for morbid obesity. Surg Endosc. 2015;29(11):3298–303.
30. Rajagopalan H, Cherrington AD, Thompson CC, et al. Endoscopic duodenal mucosal resurfacing for the treatment of type 2 diabetes: 6-month interim analysis from the first-in-human proof-of-concept study. Diabetes Care. 2016;39(12):2254–61.
31. Machytka E, Bužga M, Zonca P, et al. Partial jejunal diversion using an incisionless magnetic anastomosis system: 1-year interim results in subjects with obesity and diabetes. Gastrointest Endosc. 2017;86:904–12.

27 Endoscopic Management of Complications

Manoel Galvao Neto, Lyz Bezerra Silva, Luiz Gustavo de Quadros, and Josemberg Campos

Roux-en-Y Gastric Bypass (RYGB)

Anastomotic Stricture

Gastrojejunal anastomotic stricture is one of the most common complications of RYGB, defined when the diameter is <10 mm, and common endoscope (9.8 mm) passage is not possible [1]. Most common symptoms are food intolerance, vomiting, and epigastric pain, usually becoming symptomatic when solid diet is started [1, 2]. The treatment can be done through endoscopic hydrostatic balloon dilation, using TTS (through the scope) balloons, with diameters usually up to 15 mm. This approach reaches success in 98% of cases, in a mean of 1.7 sessions per patient, with a complication rate of 2.5%, mostly perforations and bleeding [3, 4]. Some reports also use the Savary-Gilliard bougie for dilation [5]. In cases of failure, endoscopic stenotomy can be performed, using an endoscopic cautery to make incisions on the stricture, followed by balloon dilation.

M. G. Neto (✉)
Department of Surgery, Herbert Wertheim College of Medicine – Florida International University, Doral, FL, USA

L. B. Silva · J. Campos
Department of Surgery, Federal University of Pernambuco, Recife, PE, Brazil

L. G. de Quadros
Department of Surgery, ABC Medical School, Sao Jose Do Rio Preto, SP, Brazil

Marginal Ulcers

Marginal ulcers after RYGB have a multifactorial etiology, including tobacco and alcohol consumption, nonsteroidal anti-inflammatory drug (NSAID) usage, gastrogastric fistulas, and foreign bodies. Ulcers are more common at the jejunal side of the anastomosis, with varying size and depth [6]. Main symptoms are epigastric pain, dysphagia, nausea, and vomiting, with some cases being asymptomatic [7]. Any foreign bodies, such as visible sutures and staples, should be endoscopically removed to improve ulcer healing, together with proton-pump inhibitor and sucralfate prescription [8]. Ulcers can cause strictures due to fibrotic scar formation, and these can be treated through stenotomy and balloon dilation [4] (Fig. 27.1).

Ring Complications: Intragastric Erosion

This complication has an incidence of 0,9 a 7%; most common symptoms of intragastric ring erosion are weight regain, nausea, vomiting, and bleeding [9]. Endoscopy may show the ring inside the gastric pouch, and in early stages, an ulcer at the erosion site can be the only visible sign. In this case, PPIs should be prescribed until complete ring erosion, with surveillance endoscopy performed. Once >30% of the ring circumference is visible inside the gastric pouch,

R. Lutfi et al. (eds.), *Global Bariatric Surgery*, https://doi.org/10.1007/978-3-319-93545-4_27

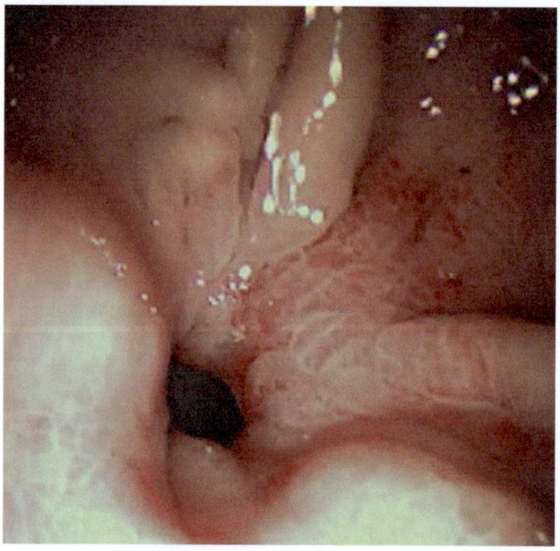

Fig. 27.1 Anastomotic stricture secondary to ulcer fibrotic scar tissue formation

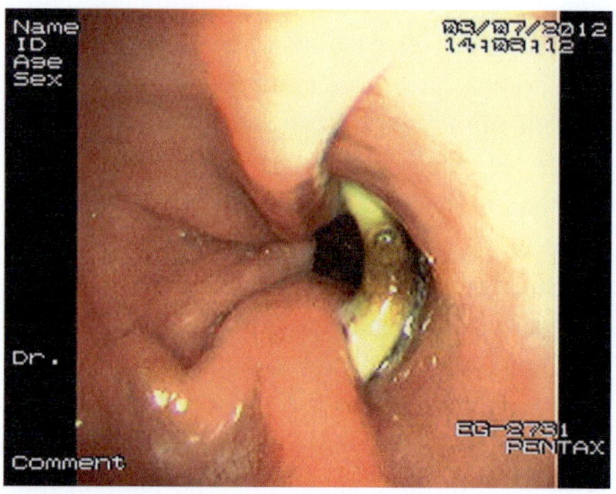

Fig. 27.2 Endoscopic view of eroded ring after RYGB, showing approximately 50% erosion; endoscopic removal with scissors

endoscopic removal is the gold standard. Removal is done using endoscopic scissors to section the ring. In cases of failure in cutting the ring, a gastric band cutter or lithotripter may be used. Treatment should be scheduled as soon as possible, due to the risk of gastric wall bleeding or food impaction [10] (Figs. 27.2 and 27.3).

Ring Slippage

Distal ring slippage promotes an angulation of the longitudinal axis of the gastric pouch, and

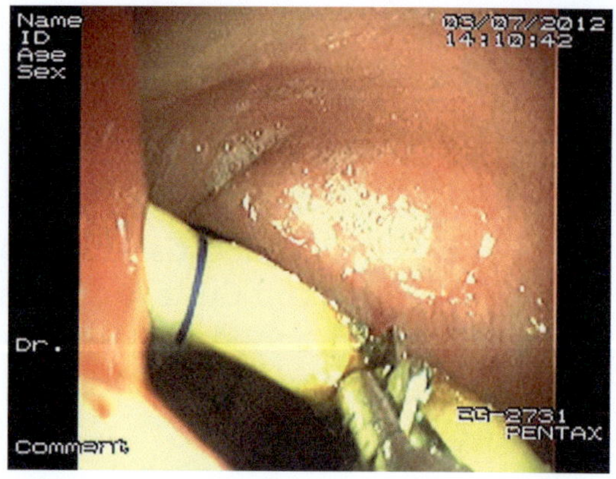

Fig. 27.3 Endoscopic view of eroded ring after RYGB, showing approximately 50% erosion; endoscopic removal with scissors

proximal gastric dilatation, leading to obstructive symptoms with an incidence lower than 1% [11]. Diagnosis can be made with contrast X-ray, showing an area of contrast retention, and endoscopy, which may show food stasis and convergence of the mucosal folds, caused by the jejunal obstruction just beneath the anastomosis [12].

Management can be done through endoscopic 30 mm achalasia balloon dilation that stretches or ruptures the thread running inside the ring, thus relieving symptoms with a low complication rate [11]. Stent placement can also be used for removal, causing an inflammatory/ischemic reaction around the ring, promoting intragastric erosion, with stent and ring removal possible after 10–15 days. A fibrotic scar tissue forms in the ring erosion area, restricting the pouch diameter, with better weight control when compared to dilation [13–15] (Figs. 27.4 and 27.5).

Food Intolerance

In some cases, vomiting episodes may occur after RYGB even when there is no ring slippage or gastric pouch/anastomotic stricture, which can be defined as ring-related food intolerance. This affects quality of life, with difficulties in food ingestion. Symptoms are similar to when there is a stricture: dysphagia, solid food intolerance, postprandial vomiting, and, in advanced stages, excessive weight loss, dehydration, and malnutrition.

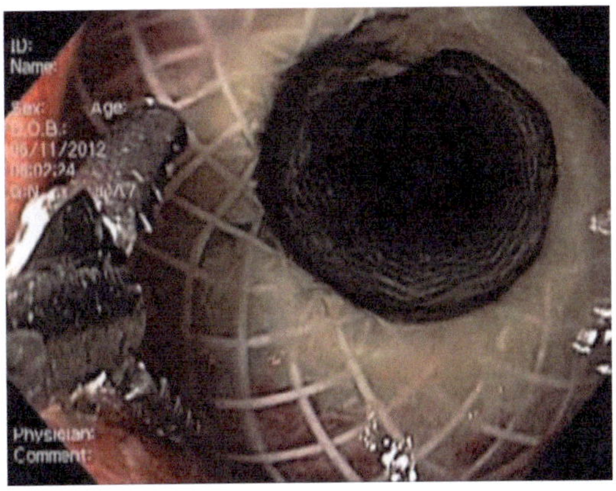

Fig. 27.4 Endoscopic view of plastic stent placed to induce ring erosion – possible to visualize ring compression on stent – and ring completely eroded after stent removal

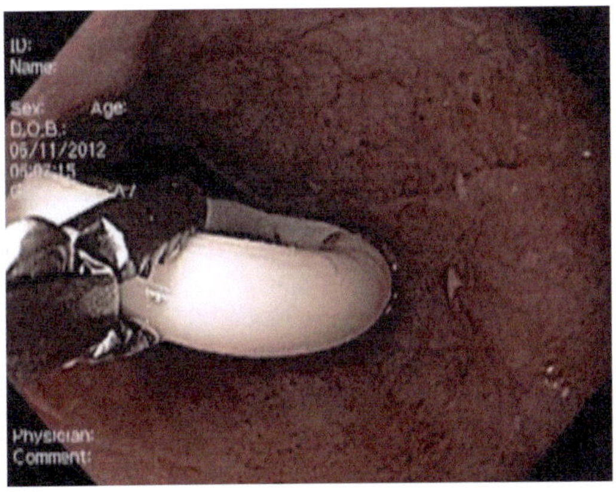

Fig. 27.5 Endoscopic view of plastic stent placed to induce ring erosion – possible to visualize ring compression on stent – and ring completely eroded after stent removal

These patients can also be treated by ring dilation or stenting, leading to improvement of symptoms in more than 96% of cases. The procedure has low cost and morbidity, with nonsignificant weight regain [16].

Sleeve Gastrectomy

Gastric Stricture

In post-sleeve gastric strictures, endoscopy can show a reduction in the gastric lumen, usually near the *incisura*, associated to a difficult endoscope progression or axis deviation. Typical symptoms include dysphagia, vomiting, and excessive weight loss. Treatment can be done with pneumatic 30 mm achalasia balloon dilation, associated to stenotomy when necessary [17, 18]. When endoscopic treatment fails, surgical management can be done through RYGB conversion, or, in some cases, total gastrectomy if surgical manipulation is too difficult [19] (Fig. 27.6).

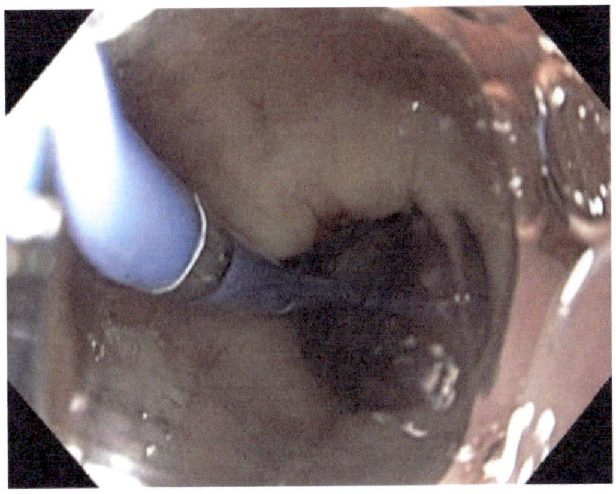

Fig. 27.6 Dilation of sleeve gastrectomy stricture with 30 mm achalasia balloon

RYGB and SG Leaks

Gastric leaks represent one of the most feared complications after RYGB and SG. Treatment modality is made according to patient status and local fistula conditions. Initial measures include drainage (surgical or percutaneous), antibiotics, and nutritional support [20, 21]. When there is contamination of the abdominal cavity – peritonitis/perigastric abscess –, surgical drainage can be an option. In a stable patient with a functioning and well-located peritoneal drain, conservative management may be suitable. Also, the perigastric abscess can be approached through percutaneous drainage, or, in selected cases, internal drainage through endoscopy [22].

Early diagnostic endoscopy allows evaluation of the leak internal orifice and identification of associated strictures and helps in correct positioning of abdominal drains and performance of internal abscess drainage. After initial leak control, specific surgical or endoscopic measures are taken. The endoscopic management is linked to decreased morbidity, involving internal drainage, septotomy, dilation, endoscopic suturing, clips, and in most cases, endoscopic stenting [23–29].

Endoscopic therapy has the aim of solving the three main issues perpetuating the leak: distal gastric stricture, increased intragastric pressure, and fistulous tract persistence. In SG, additionally, there can be an axis deviation with associated increased intragastric pressure [18].

Treatment choice is made according to time of onset, divided in four phases:

- Acute (<7 days): stent
- Early (1–6 weeks): stent + balloon dilation + septotomy (rare)
- Late (6–12 weeks): septotomy + balloon dilation + stent (rare)
- Chronic (>12 weeks): septotomy + balloon dilation [19]

In *acute and early leaks*, self-expandable metallic stents (SEMS) act by promoting occlusion of the leak orifice, correction of axis deviation, and distal strictures and also decreasing intragastric pressure, which leads to leak closure [19, 29].

Bariatric customized stents have been developed with a design customized for SG, with promising initial results and decreased complications [26, 30–33] (Fig. 27.7). Stents should not be left in place for 1–2 months, what is usually enough to correct strictures and deviations, with lower migration and easier removal [23]. After initial leak control, stent is removed even if complete orifice closure is not achieved. When needed, endoscopic treatment continues through septotomy, stenotomy, and balloon dilations, which will lead to complete fistula closure. In some early cases, internal drainage with pigtail drains has been described with success, especially in smaller leaks (<10 mm) with associated perigastric abscess [29, 34]. Other endoscopic approaches include usage of endoscopic clips, biologic glue, and tissue sealants, with controversial results [35, 36]. Endoscopic vacuum therapy has also been described [37, 38].

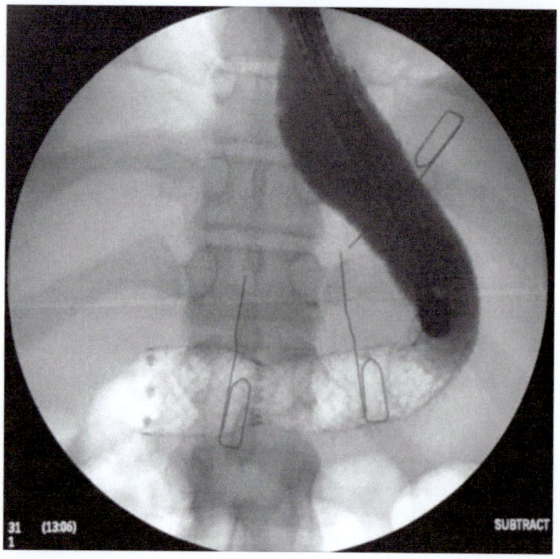

Fig. 27.7 Radioscopic view of long bariatric stent placed for sleeve gastrectomy leak treatment

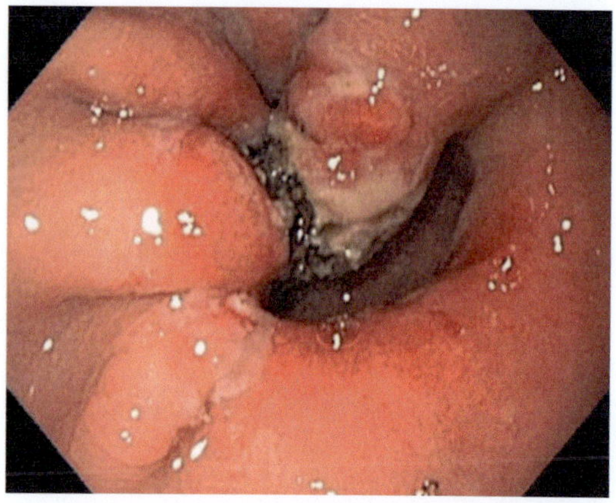

Fig. 27.8 Endoscopic view of septotomy: leak orifice on the left side, septum and gastric lumen on the right side

For *late and chronic leaks*, endoscopic multimodal treatment is usually done through multiple sessions using different techniques. When there is a septum adjacent to the fistulous orifice, septotomy is performed, decreasing flow of gastric contents through the fistula [39]. Septotomy is done with needle knife or argon plasma coagulation (associated to less bleeding), followed by balloon dilation (Fig. 27.8). When there is stenosis and fibrotic tissue associated, septotomy associated to balloon dilation may be used. This endoscopic therapy can be performed on an outpatient basis, with low morbidity and mortality and better quality of life.

The correction in digestive content flow will eventually lead to leak closure [18]. Stents can be used in selected cases, especially when there are anatomical defects.

Adjustable Gastric Band

Intragastric Band Erosion

This complication is one of the most common after this procedure, occurring in about 1.6% of patients, with nonspecific symptomatology [40]. The patient may present with weight regain, epigastric pain, portal infection, dysphagia, fever, hemorrhage, or obstruction. Endoscopy shows the presence of a segment of the gastric band in the gastric lumen, near the cardia, with better visualization under retroflection [4, 5].

In early stages of band erosion and asymptomatic patients, conservative approach is recommended, until intragastric erosion is greater than 50% of the circumference of the band. During this period, surveillance is essential, with use of proton-pump inhibitor, due to the risk of gastrointestinal bleeding or perigastric abscess [41, 42]. When there is enough intragastric migration (>50% of its circumference), endoscopic cutting and removal can be performed with high success and low complication rates, using endoscopic scissors or a gastric band cutter [41] (Fig. 27.9).

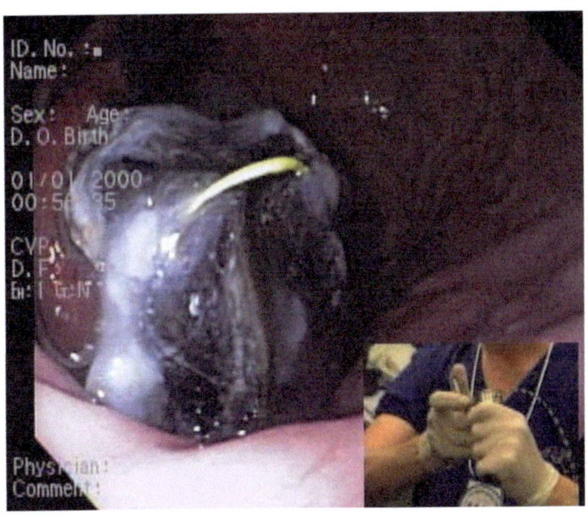

Fig. 27.9 Eroded adjustable gastric band, with removal using a gastric band cutter (similar to a lithotripter)

Band Slippage

Distal band slippage can cause proximal gastric reservoir dilation, with associated obstructive symptoms, like nausea, vomiting, dehydration, halitosis, excessive weight loss, heartburn, and abdominal pain [9]. Diagnosis can be confirmed with a contrast X-ray or endoscopy, which will show dilation in the gastric pouch with food stasis above the compression area of the band. Under retroflection, a retraction of the mucosa is seen in the slippage area, with exuberant and edematous folds, and difficult passage to the antrum [9].

For temporary symptom relief, an endoscopic maneuver can be done: hyperinflation of the gastric body, below the compression level, which can lead to band repositioning. The success of this maneuver does not modify the need for band removal [10].

Classical laparoscopic removal is the appropriate therapy, with attention to the risk of bronchial aspiration. To avoid this, and for temporary symptom relief, endoscopic approach under light sedation can be done, with aspiration of gastric contents. After passing of the endoscope past the band compression area, the stomach is hyperinflated, which will promote proximal slippage of the device, leading to a repositioning of the band to its usual site. This will relieve symptoms and decrease risks until definitive surgical removal is performed [43].

Endoscopic Treatment of Weight Regain

One of the potential causes of weight regain after RYGB is dilation of the gastrojejunal anastomosis and gastric pouch enlargement. In a study of 165 patients, it was found that the diameter of the anastomosis is a risk factor for weight regain after RYGB and that this variable should be included as a predictor of weight regain [44]. Recently, Ramos et al. published a study evaluating the size of the gastrojejunal anastomosis and its influence on weight loss. In a 2-year follow-up, a stoma diameter of 15 mm presented statistically better results than a 45 mm anastomosis [45]. The ideal anastomosis should have an approximate diameter of 10 mm, not exceeding 14 mm [44].

The most relevant aspects to indicate endoscopic treatment of weight regain after RYGB are a large gastric pouch and gastrojejunal anastomosis. However, there is a need to evaluate other alterations that may be leading the patient to gain weight, like gastrogastric fistula, ring slippage or stricture, and any type of stenosis [46]. A chronic stenosis causes food intolerance for which patients will, over the years, select food that most appeals to them, which are usually carbohydrates, sweets, and caloric liquids, which pass the stricture easily.

Development of endoluminal therapies for pouch and stoma revision can be a less invasive approach for failure or weight regain after bariatric surgery. Argon plasma coagulation leads to fusion of tissues and induces an inflammatory and fibrotic response. This fibrotic response is a side effect that is positive if used in order to reduce the anastomosis after RYGB [47]. Argon plasma coagulation can only be employed to narrow the anastomosis as it is not indicated in cases of enlarged pouches. The cost is low, is more accessible, and does not need a service of high complexity, with sedation being the means of anesthesia.

To produce the desired effect, the coagulation should be done in a circumferential way, involving the entire gastric side of the anastomosis, extending for 1–2 cm (Fig. 27.10).

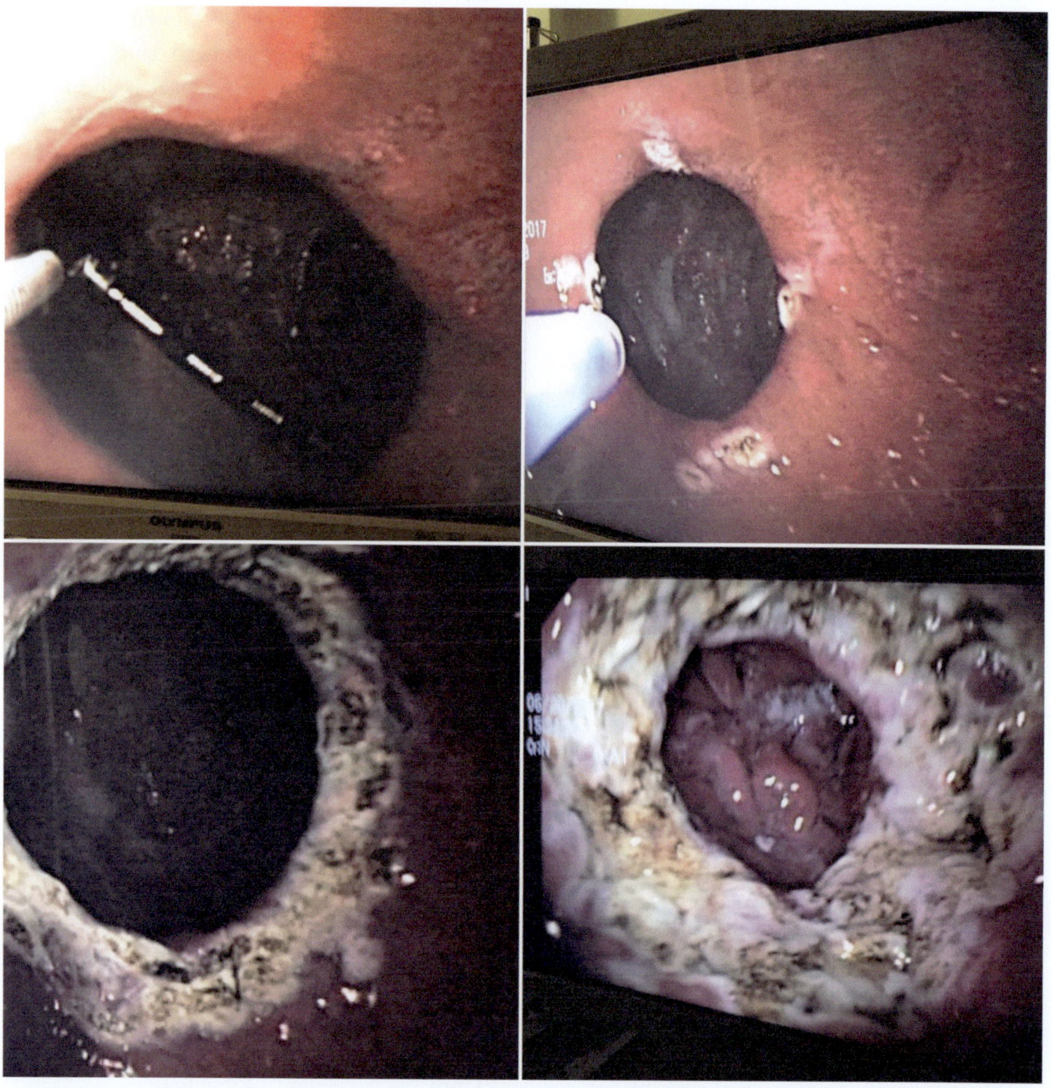

Fig. 27.10 Dilated RYGB gastrojejunal anastomosis, performance of argon plasma coagulation for stoma reduction

There is an initial edema and inflammatory response, causing immediate restriction. This effect decreases over time, and the edema is substituted by fibrosis. More than one session is usually necessary in order to achieve long-lasting effects [48]. Argon coagulation reduces the diameter of the anastomosis and consequently delays gastric emptying and early satiety and improves weight reduction [49]. One of the possible complications of argon plasma use is stricture of the coagulated anastomosis. This can be treated through endoscopic dilation with TTS balloons. In some cases, the obstructive symptoms will resolve by itself, hindering the need of intervention.

The use of sutures allows the concomitant treatment of a dilated anastomosis and a large pouch or the treatment of one or the other in isolation. A retrospective series of eight patients evaluated safety and short-term efficacy of the Overstitch™ in patients with weight regain and dilated gastrojejunostomy. Pre-procedure pouch size varied from 2 to 6 cm and stoma size from 20 to 40 mm. Procedure time ranged from 20 to 60 min (mean 38 min), all but one patient had three stitches applied, reducing stoma size to a 10 mm diameter. Post-procedure weight loss in a 90-day follow-up varied from 6 to 8 kg, with a mean % of regained weight loss of 28%. No postoperative complications were recorded [50].

References

1. Sullivan S, Kumar N, Edmundowicz SA, Abu Dayyeh BK, Jonnalagadda SS, Larsen M, et al. ASGE position statement on endoscopic bariatric therapies in clinical practice. Gastrointest Endosc. 2015;82(5):767–72.
2. Cai JX, Schweitzer MA, Kumbhari V. Endoscopic management of bariatric surgery complications. Surg Laparosc Endosc Percutan Tech. 2016;26(2):93–101.
3. Campos JM, Mello FS, Ferraz AA, Brito JN, Nassif PA, Galvao-Neto MP. Endoscopic dilation of gastrojejunal anastomosis after gastric bypass. Arq Bras Cir Dig. 2012;25(4):283–9.
4. de Moura EG, Orso IR, Aurelio EF, de Moura ET, de Moura DT, Santo MA. Factors associated with complications or failure of endoscopic balloon dilation of anastomotic stricture secondary to Roux-en-Y gastric bypass surgery. Surg Obes Relat Dis. 2016;12(3):582–6.
5. Escalona A, Devaud N, Boza C, Perez G, Fernandez J, Ibanez L, et al. Gastrojejunal anastomotic stricture after Roux-en-Y gastric bypass: ambulatory management with the Savary-Gilliard dilator. Surg Endosc. 2007;21(5):765–8.
6. Sapala JA, Wood MH, Sapala MA, Flake TM Jr. Marginal ulcer after gastric bypass: a prospective 3-year study of 173 patients. Obes Surg. 1998;8(5):505–16.
7. Huang CS, Forse RA, Jacobson BC, Farraye FA. Endoscopic findings and their clinical correlations in patients with symptoms after gastric bypass surgery. Gastrointest Endosc. 2003;58(6):859–66.
8. Garrido AB Jr, Rossi M, Lima SE Jr, Brenner AS, Gomes CAR Jr. Early marginal ulcer following Roux-en-Y gastric bypass under proton pump inhibitor treatment: prospective multicentric study. Arq Gastroenterol. 2010;47:130–4.
9. Huang CS, Farraye FA. Endoscopy in the bariatric surgical patient. Gastroenterol Clin N Am. 2005;34(1):151–66.
10. Fobi M, Lee H, Igwe D, Felahy B, James E, Stanczyk M, et al. Band erosion: incidence, etiology, management and outcome after banded vertical gastric bypass. Obes Surg. 2001;11(6):699–707.
11. Campos JM, Evangelista LF, Ferraz AA, Galvao Neto MP, De Moura EG, Sakai P, et al. Treatment of ring slippage after gastric bypass: long-term results after endoscopic dilation with an achalasia balloon (with videos). Gastrointest Endosc. 2010a;72(1):44–9.
12. Espinel J, Pinedo E. Stenosis in gastric bypass: endoscopic management. World J Gastrointest Endosc. 2012;4(7):290–5.
13. Marins Campos J, Moon RC, Magalhaes Neto GE, Teixeira AF, Jawad MA, Bezerra Silva L, et al. Endoscopic treatment of food intolerance after a banded gastric bypass: inducing band erosion for removal using a plastic stent. Endoscopy. 2016;48(6):516–20.
14. Blero D, Eisendrath P, Vandermeeren A, Closset J, Mehdi A, Le Moine O, et al. Endoscopic removal of dysfunctioning bands or rings after restrictive bariatric procedures. Gastrointest Endosc. 2010;71(3):468–74.
15. Wilson TD, Miller N, Brown N, Snyder BE, Wilson EB. Stent induced gastric wall erosion and endoscopic retrieval of nonadjustable gastric band: a new technique. Surg Endosc. 2013;27(5):1617–21.
16. Ferraz A, Campos J, Dib V, Silva LB, de Paula PS, Gordejuela A, et al. Food intolerance after banded gastric bypass without stenosis: aggressive endoscopic dilation avoids reoperation. Obes Surg. 2013;23(7):959–64.
17. Shnell M, Fishman S, Eldar S, Goitein D, Santo E. Balloon dilatation for symptomatic gastric sleeve stricture. Gastrointest Endosc. 2014;79(3):521–4.
18. Zundel N, Hernandez JD, Galvao Neto M, Campos J. Strictures after laparoscopic sleeve gastrectomy. Surg Laparosc Endosc Percutan Tech. 2010;20(3):154–8.
19. Rosenthal RJ, Diaz AA, Arvidsson D, Baker RS, Basso N, Bellanger D, et al. International sleeve gastrectomy expert panel consensus statement: best practice guidelines based on experience of >12,000 cases. Surg Obes Relat Dis. 2012;8(1):8–19.
20. Vix M, Diana M, Marx L, Callari C, Wu HS, Perretta S, et al. Management of staple line leaks

after sleeve gastrectomy in a consecutive series of 378 patients. Surg Laparosc Endosc Percutan Tech. 2015;25(1):89–93.
21. Bhayani NH, Swanstrom LL. Endoscopic therapies for leaks and fistulas after bariatric surgery. Surg Innov. 2014;21(1):90–7.
22. Baretta G, Campos J, Correia S, Alhinho H, Marchesini JB, Lima JH, et al. Bariatric postoperative fistula: a life-saving endoscopic procedure. Surg Endosc. 2015a;29(7):1714–20.
23. Campos JM, Pereira EF, Evangelista LF, Siqueira L, Neto MG, Dib V, et al. Gastrobronchial fistula after sleeve gastrectomy and gastric bypass: endoscopic management and prevention. Obes Surg. 2011;21(10):1520–9.
24. Silva LB, Moon RC, Teixeira AF, Jawad MA, Ferraz AA, Neto MG, et al. Gastrobronchial fistula in sleeve gastrectomy and Roux-en-Y gastric bypass-a systematic review. Obes Surg. 2015;25(10):1959–65.
25. Puli SR, Spofford IS, Thompson CC. Use of self-expandable stents in the treatment of bariatric surgery leaks: a systematic review and meta-analysis. Gastrointest Endosc. 2012;75(2):287–93.
26. Basha J, Appasani S, Sinha SK, Siddappa P, Dhaliwal HS, Verma GR, et al. Mega stents: a new option for management of leaks following laparoscopic sleeve gastrectomy. Endoscopy. 2014;46(Suppl 1 UCTN):E49–50.
27. Shehab HM, Hakky SM, Gawdat KA. An endoscopic strategy combining mega stents and over-the-scope clips for the management of post-bariatric surgery leaks and fistulas (with video). Obes Surg. 2015;2016:26–949.
28. Fischer A, Bausch D, Richter-Schrag HJ. Use of a specially designed partially covered self-expandable metal stent (PSEMS) with a 40-mm diameter for the treatment of upper gastrointestinal suture or staple line leaks in 11 cases. Surg Endosc. 2013;27(2):642–7.
29. Nedelcu M, Manos T, Cotirlet A, Noel P, Gagner M. Outcome of leaks after sleeve gastrectomy based on a new algorithm addressing leak size and gastric stenosis. Obes Surg. 2015;25(3):559–63.
30. van Wezenbeek MR, de Milliano MM, Nienhuijs SW, Friederich P, Gilissen LP. A specifically designed stent for anastomotic leaks after bariatric surgery: experiences in a tertiary referral hospital. Obes Surg. 2016;26(8):1875–80.
31. Fishman MB, Sedov VM, Lantsberg L. Laparoscopic adjustable gastric banding in treatment of patients with obesity. Vestn Khir Im I I Grek. 2008;167(1):29–32.
32. Galloro G, Magno L, Musella M, Manta R, Zullo A, Forestieri P. A novel dedicated endoscopic stent for staple-line leaks after laparoscopic sleeve gastrectomy: a case series. Surg Obes Relat Dis. 2014;10(4):607–11.
33. Bezerra Silva L, Galvao Neto M, Marchesini JC, SN Godoy E, Campos J. Sleeve gastrectomy leak: endoscopic management through a customized long bariatric stent. Gastrointest Endosc. 2017;85(4):865–6.
34. Pequignot A, Fuks D, Verhaeghe P, Dhahri A, Brehant O, Bartoli E, et al. Is there a place for pigtail drains in the management of gastric leaks after laparoscopic sleeve gastrectomy? Obes Surg. 2012;22(5):712–20.
35. Caballero Y, Lopez-Tomassetti E, Castellot A, Hernandez JR. Endoscopic management of a gastric leak after laparoscopic sleeve gastrectomy using the over-the-scope-clip (Ovesco(R)) system. Rev Esp Enferm Dig. 2016;108:746–50.
36. Keren D, Eyal O, Sroka G, Rainis T, Raziel A, Sakran N, et al. Over-the-scope clip (OTSC) system for sleeve gastrectomy leaks. Obes Surg. 2015;25(8):1358–63.
37. Seyfried F, Reimer S, Miras AD, Kenn W, Germer CT, Scheurlen M, et al. Successful treatment of a gastric leak after bariatric surgery using endoluminal vacuum therapy. Endoscopy. 2013;45(Suppl 2 UCTN):E267–8.
38. Hwang JJ, Jeong YS, Park YS, Yoon H, Shin CM, Kim N, et al. Comparison of endoscopic vacuum therapy and endoscopic stent implantation with self-expandable metal stent in treating postsurgical gastroesophageal leakage. Medicine (Baltimore). 2016;95(16):e3416.
39. Campos JM, Ferreira FC, Teixeira AF, Lima JS, Moon RC, D'Assuncao MA, et al. Septotomy and balloon dilation to treat chronic leak after sleeve gastrectomy: technical principles. Obes Surg. 2016;26:1992–3.
40. Nocca D, Frering V, Gallix B, de Seguin des Hons C, Noel P, Foulonge MA, et al. Migration of adjustable gastric banding from a cohort study of 4236 patients. Surg Endosc. 2005;19(7):947–50.
41. Neto MP, Ramos AC, Campos JM, Murakami AH, Falcao M, Moura EH, et al. Endoscopic removal of eroded adjustable gastric band: lessons learned after 5 years and 78 cases. Surg Obes Relat Dis. 2010;6(4):423–7.
42. Campos JM, Evangelista LF, Galvao Neto MP, Ramos AC, Martins JP, dos Santos MA Jr, et al. Small erosion of adjustable gastric band: endoscopic removal through incision in gastric wall. Surg Laparosc Endosc Percutan Tech. 2010b;20(6):e215–7.
43. Kang SH, Kim KC, Kim KH. Endoscopic treatment of gastric band prolapse. Obes Surg. 2014;24(6):954–7.
44. Abu Dayyeh BK, Lautz DB, Thompson CC. Gastrojejunal stoma diameter predicts weight regain after Roux-en-Y gastric bypass. Clin Gastroenterol Hepatol. 2011;9(3):228–33.
45. Ramos AC, Marchesini JC, de Souza Bastos EL, Ramos MG, de Souza MDG, Campos JM, et al. The role of gastrojejunostomy size on gastric bypass weight loss. Obes Surg. 2017;27:2317.
46. Yimcharoen P, Heneghan HM, Singh M, Brethauer S, Schauer P, Rogula T, et al. Endoscopic findings and outcomes of revisional procedures for patients with weight recidivism after gastric bypass. Surg Endosc. 2011;25(10):3345–52.
47. Fernandez-Esparrach G, Lautz DB, Thompson CC. Peroral endoscopic anastomotic reduction improves intractable dumping syndrome in Roux-

en-Y gastric bypass patients. Surg Obes Relat Dis. 2010;6(1):36–40.

48. Aly A. Argon plasma coagulation and gastric bypass – a novel solution to stomal dilation. Obes Surg. 2009;19(6):788–90.
49. Baretta GA, Alhinho HC, Matias JE, Marchesini JB, de Lima JH, Empinotti C, et al. Argon plasma coagulation of gastrojejunal anastomosis for weight regain after gastric bypass. Obes Surg. 2015b;25(1):72–9.
50. Galvão Neto M, Rodriguez L, Zundel N, Ayala JC, Campos J, Ramos A. Endoscopic revision of Roux-en-Y gastric bypass stomal dilation with a suturing device: preliminary results of a first out-of-United States series. Bariatric Times. 2011;8(6):32–4.

Part VIII

Special Surgical Situation and Consideration

Robotic Surgery

28

John Cole Cowling, Aarthy Kannappan, Erik B. Wilson, Keith C. Kim, and Shinil K. Shah

History of Robotics

For years, people have sought to advance technologies and processes to improve speed, efficiency, precision, safety, and reliability. These fundamentals seen in the automotive and airline industry and space exploration improved weapon systems in the military, computers, and electronics, as well as in the operating room to assist surgeons in safely performing increasingly complex procedures through less invasive approaches to improve patient outcomes.

The origins of robotics and applications to surgery started long before the introduction of platforms used today. While the term robot was first used in the early 1900s, derived from the word robota (Czech, definition – laborer or serf) [1], the first definition of the term "robot" was not established until 1979 by the Robotics Institute of America. The term robot is defined as a "reprogrammable, multifunctional manipulator designed to move material, parts, tools, or specialized devices through various programmed motions for the performance of a variety of tasks." [2]

In 1951, Raymond Goertz developed a teleoperated mechanical arm for radioactive materials [2]. In 1961, the first industrial robot (Unimate) was integrated into an assembly line at General Motors [1, 2]. In 1985, Kwoh described using the programmable universal machine for assembly (PUMA) robot to perform CT-guided brain tumor biopsies [3]. This same robot was used for a variety of urological procedures in 1988 in London, including transurethral resection of the prostate. This system eventually led to the development of surgeon-assistant robot for prostatectomy (SARP), prostate robot (PROBOT), and UROBOT [2, 4]. The first robotic system approved by the US Food and Drug Administration was ROBODOC (Integrated Surgical Supplies Ltd., Sacramento, CA), a system utilized in hip replacement [4].

After the advent of laparoscopic surgery, there was developing interest in developing robotic systems that could be applied to laparoscopy. Research into robotic systems and applications for surgical procedures were spearheaded by NASA and the US Department of Defense, which were interested in the possibility of surgeons remotely operating (without being physically present) on astronauts or soldiers [2].

Electronic Supplementary Material The online version of this chapter (doi:10.1007/978-3-319-93545-4_28) contains supplementary material, which is available to authorized users.

J. C. Cowling · E. B. Wilson · S. K. Shah (✉)
Department of Surgery, UT Health McGovern Medical School, Houston, TX, USA
e-mail: john.c.cowling@uth.tmc.edu; Shinil.k.shah@uth.tmc.edu

A. Kannappan
Department of Surgery, Loma Linda University, Loma Linda, CA, USA

K. C. Kim
Center for Metabolic and Obesity Surgery, Florida Hospital Celebration Health, Celebration, FL, USA

R. Lutfi et al. (eds.), *Global Bariatric Surgery*, https://doi.org/10.1007/978-3-319-93545-4_28

Initial robotic systems included the automated endoscopic system for optimal positioning (AESOP, Computer Motion, Inc., Goleta, CA, 1993), which allowed for control of a laparoendoscopic camera by voice commands. Intuitive Surgical Inc. (Mountain View, CA) developed the da Vinci surgical system, which was first used for a cholecystectomy in 1997 [1]. Computer Motion later developed the ZEUS system, which had a surgeon console with robotic arms. This was used first in 1998 for a fallopian tube anastomosis and was used for a variety of gastrointestinal, urologic, and cardiac operations [2]. In 2001, Dr. Marescaux, while in New York, used the ZEUS system to perform telesurgery on a patient that was located 4000 km away in Strasbourg [2, 5]. Computer Motion and Intuitive Surgical merged and the ZEUS system was taken off the market [1].

Current Status of Robotics in Weight Loss Surgery

Initial reports of minimally invasive weight loss surgery were published in the 1990s. The first known laparoscopic fixed gastric band placement was performed in 1992 [6]. In 1993, laparoscopic-adjustable gastric band placement, vertical banded gastroplasty, and Roux-en-Y gastric bypass were reported [7, 8]. Performing bariatric surgery using minimally invasive techniques has become the standard of care as it provides better patient outcomes, decreased rates of complications, faster recovery, and decreased overall costs.

Since the first report of robotic bariatric surgery in 1999 [9], surgeons have adopted this advanced technology into the practice of bariatric surgery at increasing rates. The robot offers several advantages to traditional laparoscopy, particularly when operating on the morbidly obese, where abdominal wall thickness, visceral fat, and patient body habitus can make the ergonomics of performing the operation difficult on the surgeon. Unfortunately, due to a lack of robust data comparing robotics to laparoscopy for these procedures, there is still much controversy when comparing the two approaches. In the following sections, we will review use of robotic platforms in the most common bariatric surgical procedures and the pros and cons associated with using the robot and examine potential learning curve and ergonomic benefits of robotic surgery.

Pros and Cons

Robotics and Adjustable Gastric Bands

Adjustable gastric band (AGB) placement is technically the simplest of all laparoscopic bariatric surgical procedures, requiring minimal dissection, tissue manipulation, and suturing. The procedure is often performed in the outpatient setting. However, its use has decreased substantially because of inferior excess weight loss and complications, including slips, erosions, and revision. The first robotic bariatric procedure performed was placement of a gastric band [9], but the literature has failed to note any significant benefits in performing this procedure robotically. Published series have demonstrated increased operative times and costs when compared to laparoscopy [10]. There may be a role in decreasing operative times in patients with very high body mass index (BMI), with one series demonstrating decreased times as compared to laparoscopy in patients with a BMI>50 [11]. From our personal experience, the robotic platform is probably most valuable in revising patients with previous laparoscopic AGB placement to other operations.

Robotics and Longitudinal Sleeve Gastrectomy

The increase in popularity in laparoscopic sleeve gastrectomy (SG) has been almost in parallel to the decreased number of patients choosing AGB placement. In experienced hands, this procedure offers low morbidity and better weight loss results than AGB and is perceived by most surgeons as technically straightforward.

Diamantis reported 19 patients undergoing robotic SG and found equivalent operative time in comparison to laparoscopy. They used two surgeons, one at the console and one bedside to operate the stapler [12]. Most other studies demonstrated longer operative times with the robotic approach. Ayloo et al. compared 30 robotic SG to 39 traditional laparoscopic SGs. They found longer robotic operative times by 21 min, which was attributable to the additional step of oversewing the staple line (not done in the laparoscopic group). There is no clear data that oversewing the staple line offers any outcome benefits, but this does provide trainees an opportunity to sew with the robotic platform, a skill that can be translated to more complex cases [13]. Romero et al. demonstrated similarly that robotic as compared to a systematic review of laparoscopic SG cases resulted in longer operative times. In this series, shorter hospital length of stay (approximately 1 day) was noted in the robotic group [14]. A series in adolescents (28 patients) also noted decreased hospital length of stay (median difference of approximately 6 h) with robotic SG, but longer median operative times and costs as compared to laparoscopic SG [15]. Other series have demonstrated longer operative times [16, 17] and/or costs [16, 18] with otherwise equivalent outcomes [19].

Increased operative times are a disadvantage, but some studies have demonstrated that this can be at least be partially addressed by repetition and training of the operating room staff. The learning curve to achieve decreases and normalization of the operative time for robotic SG is estimated to be about 20 cases [20]. Another potential advantage of this approach may occur with the continued development and refinement of robotic staplers, which may additionally eliminate the need for a bedside surgeon or assistant. Cost issues are prevalent in all discussions with robotic surgery; this is likely to become less of an issue with the introduction of multiple robotic platforms that may help to drive down costs.

In our experience, the robotic SG is a straightforward operation. SG may be a procedure that lends itself well to education of trainees in robotic surgery. A series of 411 patients demonstrated similar mean operative times as well as morbidity rates when compared to historical laparoscopic controls, albeit at increased costs [21].

Robotics and Roux-en-Y Gastric Bypass and Biliopancreatic Diversion/Duodenal Switch

Of the three most commonly performed bariatric operations in the current milieu (AGB, SG, and Roux-en-Y gastric bypass (RYGB)), the robot has arguably the most apparent benefits in the laparoscopic RYGB, especially with surgeons who use hand-sewn techniques. In patients with a higher BMI, the robot may afford better ergonomics as the surgeon does not feel the impact of the thickness of the abdominal wall in relation to torque on the instruments as compared to traditional laparoscopy.

While there is currently a paucity of controlled data comparing laparoscopic to robotic RYGB, the current data does suggest certain conclusions. It is important to note that most studies are retrospective or uncontrolled prospective studies, small, report a variety of techniques including partial or totally robotic operations, as well as may have issues with learning curve-related biases.

Series comparing robotic to laparoscopic RYGB have reported mostly uniformly increased operative times [22–28] and costs [29, 30], although several series describe decreased [31] or similar operative times [32]. Only one study demonstrated decreased costs with robotic RYGB [33], but most studies that report cost variables demonstrate, similar to other robotic operations, increased costs with the robotic approach [34].

Worrisome complications after RYGB include anastomotic leak as well as anastomotic strictures. A recent systematic review comparing laparoscopic to robotic RYGB demonstrated that the robotic approach was associated with decreased anastomotic stricture rates [35]. In addition, there have been smaller studies that have noted a reduction in leak rates [33, 36] as well as strictures [33] with the robotic approach. A series comparing 100 laparoscopic to 100 robotic RYGB demonstrated decreased length of stay and transfusions with the robotic approach [23]. Similarly, Buchs et al. demonstrated decreased conversion rates, leaks, early reoperations, and shorter hospital stay [24]. The most recent published systematic review and meta-analysis demonstrated decreased stricture rates, reoperations, and hospital length of stay with robotic as compared to laparoscopic RYGB [37].

In contrast, a series published by Benizri demonstrated increased 30-day complication rates and decreased operative times with the robotic as compared to the laparoscopic approach, with increased complication rates related primarily to leaks and post-op bleeding. It is important to note that the laparoscopic cases had a stapled gastrojejunal anastomosis as opposed to a sutured technique for the robotic cases [38]. A systematic review and meta-analysis demonstrated a higher conversion rate during robotic RYGB with otherwise equivalent outcomes [39]. Moon et al. reported higher leak rates and longer hospital stay in robotic RYGB as compared to laparoscopic RYGB in a single surgeon study comparing the first 64 robotic cases to 207 laparoscopic cases [40].

While there is still significant debate about the real advantage of the robotic approach in regard to outcomes, its real advantage may be in the learning curve. There have been a number of papers that have shown that the learning curve may be significantly shorter than with the traditional laparoscopic approach and that the rate of significant complications during the learning curve is not significantly increased [35, 41–43]. Most studies demonstrate significant decreases in operative times during the learning curve [44]. Given that the complications of RYGB, such as leaks, can be devastating for both the patient and the surgeon, the robotic platform may confer a significant advantage. In comparison, the rate of anastomotic leak during the learning curve for traditional laparoscopic Roux-en-Y bypass surgery can be as high as 10% [45].

In terms of biliopancreatic diversion (BPD) with duodenal switch (DS), there is little published data comparing the robotic to the traditional laparoscopic approach. The paucity of data is likely due to the small number of these operations performed. Sudan et al. published their initial case series of 47 patients demonstrating the feasibility and safety of the technique [45]. The authors have modified their technique to a single dock totally robotic operation with acceptable outcomes [46]. Others have reported series of robotic BPD/DS [47, 48]. We limit discussion on this topic given the relative absence of comparative data with the laparoscopic approach.

Robotics and Revisional Bariatric Surgery

As bariatric surgery continues to increase in popularity, there will be an increase in revisional operations, either to achieve improved weight loss or address complications related to other procedures.

Robotics may have advantages in revisional surgery. One such study compared robotic, laparoscopic, and open revisional weight loss surgery in 60 patients. Although the robotic operations required significantly longer operative times, the rate of conversion to an open procedure was 0% (versus 14.3% for the laparoscopic arm). Additionally, the robotic group had a lower complication rate and hospital length of stay [49]. Although series are small and mostly retrospective, series describing robotic revisional bariatric surgery report extremely low conversion rates with major complication rates approaching that of primary weight loss surgery operations [50–52].

While significantly more data is needed, it seems robotic platforms may offer an advantage in decreasing the rate of conversion to an open procedure with acceptable postoperative morbidity.

Robotics and Surgeon Ergonomics

The robot offers several ergonomic and visual advantages over traditional laparoscopy. The console offers a three-dimensional view of the surgical field, ability for the surgeon to control camera movement, additional degrees of freedom/motion of the instruments, motion scaling to translate surgeon movements precisely within a small operative field, as well as the ability to decrease translation of surgeon tremor to the operative field. It allows for decreased learning curve and improved dexterity in intracorporeal suturing as compared to laparoscopy, especially in novice surgeons [53–55]. One of the major current disadvantages of robotic platforms is the lack of haptic feedback.

The ability to sit at a console during surgery may decrease fatigue and strain in the upper extremities and back, especially during lengthy surgery. A survey of pediatric surgeons performing laparoscopic surgery found 78% complained of shoulder pain and 60% complained of other pain in their wrist and elbows, mostly related to length of surgery [56]. Other studies have demonstrated increased stress and fatigue associated with the ergonomics of laparoscopic surgery

[57]. There are limited studies evaluating the translation of the potential benefits of robotic surgery in actual perception of improved ergonomics. Although physical complaints seem to be lower in robotic surgery, Lee et al. demonstrated in a survey of over 400 surgeons that over half (56.1%) still report physical complaints/discomfort, most commonly in the fingers and neck [58]. Ergonomic training may help decrease physical complaints [59]. The ergonomic advantages of robotic surgery may be magnified in the bariatric population, where challenges such as abdominal wall thickness may provide increased difficulty with traditional laparoscopy.

Robotics and Training

With the introduction of any new technology, it is important that the surgeon and operating room staff are trained in its function and capability. The team must be able to efficiently set up, use, troubleshoot, and adjust to allow for safe and efficient implementation during surgery. This can be achieved in several fashions with respect to robotic surgery, including skill labs for introduction to the robotic platform, surgical simulators built into the robotic console that can be completed by a surgeon before performing any operations, fellowship or mini-fellowship training, and wet labs. Additionally there are standardized industry and nonindustry curriculums used for training of residents, fellows, and surgeons, including Fundamentals of Robotic Surgery (FRS) [60, 61].

It is also recommended to have a surgeon's initial experience be proctored by an experienced robotic surgeon and that they continue to use robotics on a regular basis to maintain their skill and efficiency. Lastly, robotics can be introduced in stages, with training and initial cases performed in less complex operations such as SG or by using the robot during portions of the RYGB.

Probably the major advantage in robotics in complex weight loss surgery (RYGB) is the decreased learning curve and, more importantly, the relatively lower complication rates during the learning curve [42, 62].

The learning curve for robotic bariatric surgery has been studied most in the RYGB. While the learning curve for performing laparoscopic RYGB has been reported to be about 100 cases, studies have demonstrated learning curves for performing this operation robotically to be less than 20–25 cases [31, 63, 64]. Yu et al. were able to demonstrate safe introduction of a robotic approach with performing a hand-sewn gastrojejunostomy reporting no leaks in over 100 cases of RYGB [42]. As discussed previously, nearly all series report significantly decreased operative times with increased experience.

Economics of Robotic Bariatric Surgery

Perhaps the largest criticism of robotic surgery has been cost. Inherent to introducing new technology is the cost of research and development. Nearly all studies demonstrated increased costs associated with using robotic platforms to perform bariatric surgery when compared to traditional laparoscopy. One such systematic review of ten studies reviewing 2557 patients compared robotic and laparoscopic RYGB. They found no differences in major or minor complications, but robotics was associated with nearly $3500 US dollars higher as compared to the laparoscopic group [34]. Similarly, a group in Brazil compared laparoscopic to robotic RYGB. While the outcomes were similar, they found the robotic costs to be twice as much, making it prohibitive for routine use in bariatric surgery there [18]. This finding has been reproduced in other studies [28, 30]. As mentioned earlier, there are only a few studies that demonstrate decreased costs of robotics [33].

Strategies to reduce cost include decreased operative time as surgeons progress along the learning curve, decreased major complication rates, length of stay, and readmission rates during the learning curve of new surgeons, using hand-sewn techniques to minimize or eliminate the use of endoscopic staplers, as well as continued development of competitive robotic platforms.

Insurance Issues and Challenge of Adding Cost to the Customer

There is a paucity of data to evaluate the reimbursements of hospitals and surgeons performing robotic bariatric surgery. In general, procedure codes do not differentiate robotic from laparoscopic cases, aside from prostatectomy. In general, the increased costs are absorbed by hospital systems. Indeed, in certain centers around the world, cost makes robotics for bariatric surgery not an economically feasible proposition [18]. Most hospital systems evaluate robotics in the broader sense of contribution margins. The increased costs are often justified when total hospital length of stay and/or complications are decreased, such as with the adoption of robotic hysterectomy as well as in colon/rectal surgery, which some studies demonstrate decreased conversion rates to open operations [19]. In other operations in which there have been no clear advantages to the robotic approach, such as in laparoscopic inguinal hernia, direct costs and contribution margins are nearly equivalent with robotic and laparoscopic procedures [65]. Most cost estimates do not take into account the initial investment made to purchase robotic and/or laparoscopic systems or service contracts to maintain the equipment, which is a drawback of most cost studies. This is an area ripe for future research to more clearly elucidate the cost issues associated with robotics, which is likely to become increasingly important in an environment of value-based healthcare.

Robotic Bariatric Surgery Internationally

Laparoscopic and robotic bariatric surgery has been pioneered in the United States, with Wittgrove reporting the first series of laparoscopic RYGB [8] and Mohr describing one of the first reports of totally robotic RYGB using the da Vinci robot platform in 2005 [31]. There is, however, a significant international experience with robotics and weight loss surgery.

From Brazil, Ramos et al. reported the first early Brazilian experience with robotic RYGB, with 5 surgeons operating on 68 patients, with a 30-day complication rate of 5.9% and no mortalities, leaks, or strictures [43]. Domene et al. reported on 100 patients undergoing robotic RYGB procedures with similar results [66]. Others have reported using the robotic platform in Brazil to perform AGB, SG, as well as RYGB [67]. Others in Brazil have reported their initial series, but cost precludes further use of the technology [18].

Vilallonga et al. (Spain) reported their initial experience with robotic SG, demonstrating a learning curve of about 20 cases [20]. This group has published on their large series of open, laparoscopic, as well as robotic weight loss surgery and has one of the larger series of robotic weight loss operations in Europe [17, 68, 69]. Bodner et al. reported on an initial robotic surgery experience in Austria, including ten robotic bariatric procedures. Given multiple factors including increased costs and times, it was not viewed by the authors as a feasible alternative [70]. Benizri et al. (France) reported a series of 100 robotic RYGB compared to 100 laparoscopic procedures, reporting shorter operative time but higher postoperative complication rates and hospital length of stay [38]. An additional series from Switzerland reported on 288 robotic RYGB, noting that in super obese patients (BMI>50) as compared to morbidly obese patients, there was increased conversion rates and length of stay among the patients with super obesity [71]. The published consensus statement from the European Association of Endoscopic Surgeons (EAES) on robotics in bariatric surgery states that robotics has comparable outcomes to laparoscopy [72]. Silverman et al. reported their initial series of ten robotic SG procedures, one of the initial published reports of robotic bariatric surgery in Australia [73].

Other groups globally have struggled to realize the technology. There have been reports of robotic RYGB [74] and SG [75] in India. In Japan currently, where the rates of morbid obesity are lower than in the West, the most common bariatric procedure is the laparoscopic SG, with placement of AGB or RYGB being uncommon. One reason of the decreased rates of RYGB is a fear of delayed diagnosis of gastric cancer in the gastric remnant after RYGB [76]. In Japan, robotic bariatric surgery has lagged behind other nations. Approval of the da Vinci platform occurred in 2009. Approval of new devices takes about 3–5 years, and most surgeons are using previous generations of the da Vinci robotic platform as newer versions await regulatory approval [77].

Robotic bariatric surgery is indeed developing at different paces and stages throughout the world. Cost is an important driver of surgical technology, especially in developing countries. It is also important that the published English literature does not reveal the full extent of application of robotic bariatric procedures, as groups may not publish their experience or publish in non-English language manuscripts.

Technical Pearls

Technical aspects of robotic-assisted SG and RYGB have been published extensively by our group [78] and others. Figure 28.1 demonstrates the typical docking with the da Vinci SI platform. A parallel side dock technique is utilized which allows for working space at the head of the bed for anesthesia as well as intraoperative endoscopy. With the da Vinci XI platform, the patient-side cart can be placed from any direction. Figures 28.2 and 28.3

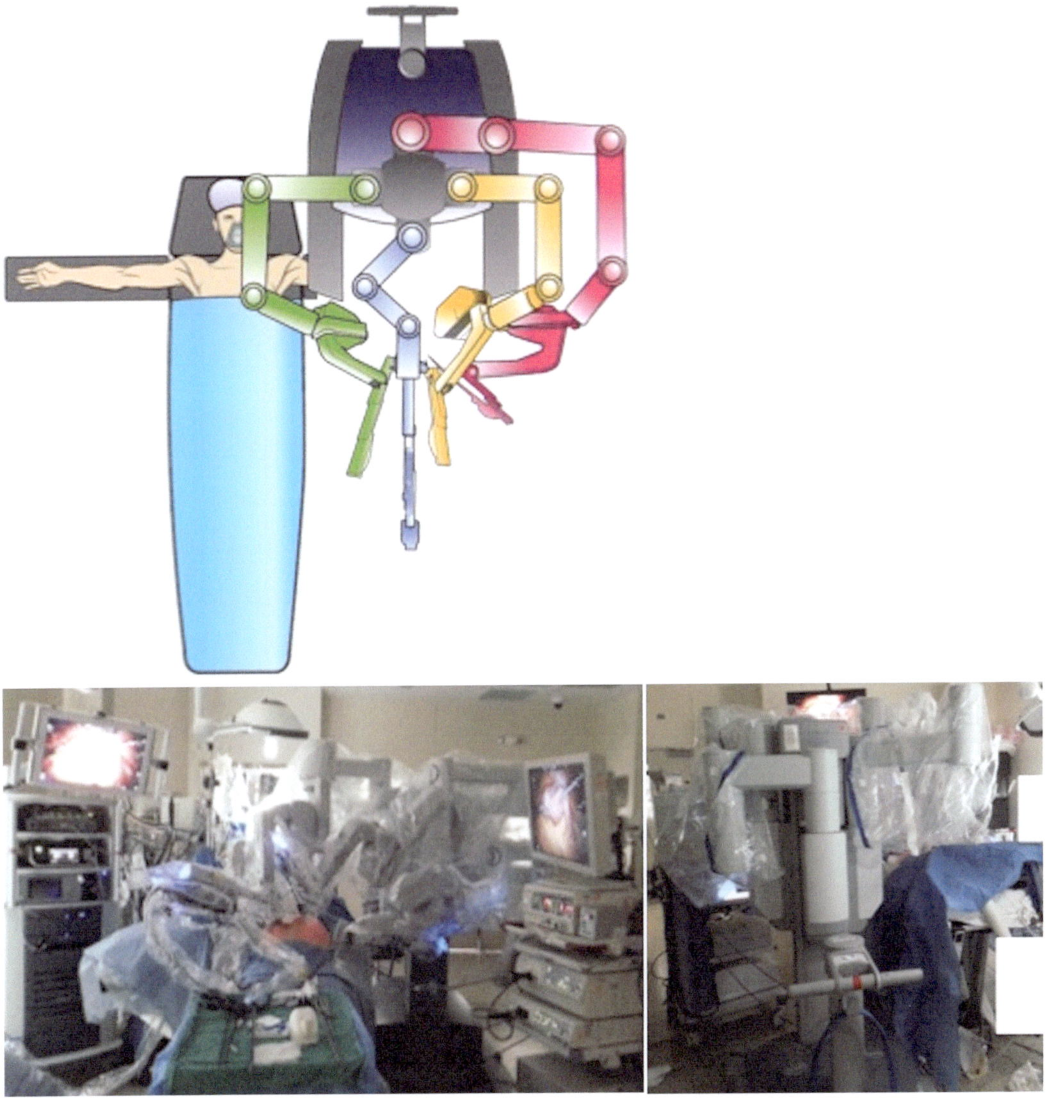

Fig. 28.1 Typical docking of the patient-side cart during robotic foregut and bariatric surgery. The parallel side dock technique allows for ease of access to the head for anesthesia as well as to aid in intraoperative endoscopy. (Reproduced with permission [78])

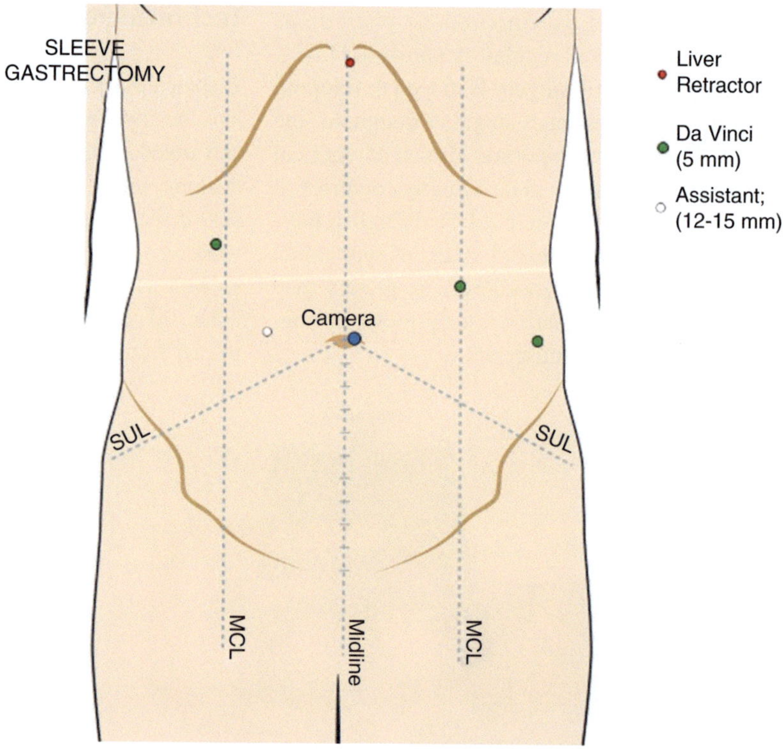

Fig. 28.2 Port placement for robotic sleeve gastrectomy. (Reproduced with permission [78])

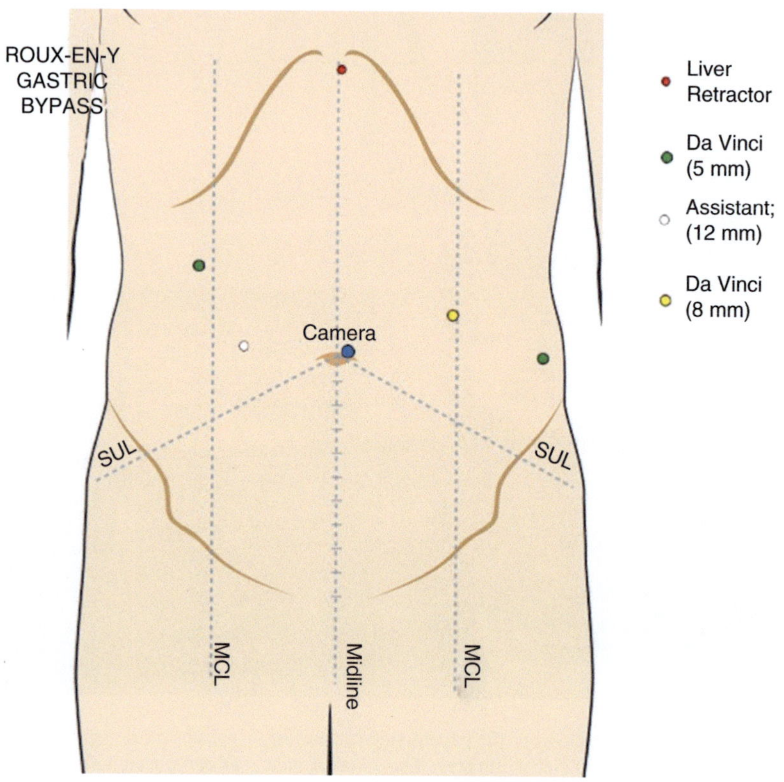

Fig. 28.3 Port placement for robotic Roux-en-Y gastric bypass. (Reproduced with permission [78])

demonstrate the port placement for robotic SG and RYGB, respectively. Port placement is similar, with the exception of an 8 mm port to allow for use of the robotic scissors. The left-sided ports are placed slightly lower for the totally robotic technique to allow for easier manipulation of the instruments to access the small intestine. Ports can be placed similarly for the da Vinci XI platform, although the ports are placed more in a horizontal line. The authors present an edited video of a robotic-assisted RYGB procedure (Video 28.1).

Available Commercial Robots for Gastrointestinal and Bariatric Surgery

While the most popular and widely used robotic platform is the da Vinci platform, over the next several years, multiple new platforms are expected to enter the sphere. There are several that deserve mention.

Titan Medical (Toronto, Ontario, Canada) is developing the SPORT™ Surgical System, which, while has many similar features to the da Vinci platform, uses a single-arm patient cart. Verb Surgical (Mountain View, CA), which started as a joint venture between Google Life Sciences and Ethicon, is currently developing a surgical robotic platform as is Medtronic (Minneapolis, MN). Medtronic has recently partnered with Mazor Robotics Ltd. (Israel), which has the Renaissance ® Guidance System utilized in spine and brain surgery. Transenterix (Morrisville, NC) developed the SurgiBot system, which represents a hybrid between conventional laparoscopy and robotic platforms, and is designed for use as a single-access surgical robotic. Recently, Transenterix acquired SOFAR S.p.A (Italy) which designed ALF-X surgical robot system, in which each robotic arm is on an individual patient cart and incorporates haptic feedback. Auris Surgical Robotics (San Carlos, CA), which recently acquired Hansen Medical, is developing surgical robotic technology and recently received US FDA approval for the ARES (Auris Robotic Endoscopy System) robot. It is believed that Auris is developing robotic platforms that may be utilized in endoluminal procedures, but little is known about this company. It may have similarities to the Flex ® Robotic System (Medrobotics, Raynham, MA), which recently received approval by the US FDA for applications in transoral robotic procedures in head/neck surgery.

Future Technology

Future advancements in robotics are likely to proceed along several avenues. New platforms will provide increased competition as well as potentially decreased costs and increased international adoption of the technology. Further development of single-port/single-access platforms, including flexible access platforms, may reopen applications in natural orifice or endoscopic (incisionless) surgery. Integration of haptic feedback may increase surgeon comfort and decrease learning curves further. Computer-aided navigation or creating no fly zones by integrating patient imaging with the surgical field may assist with reoperative surgery and decreasing complications.

References

1. Hockstein NG, et al. A history of robots: from science fiction to surgical robotics. J Robot Surg. 2007;1(2):113–8.
2. Leal Ghezzi T, Campos Corleta O. 30 years of robotic surgery. World J Surg. 2016;40:2550–7.
3. Kwoh YS, et al. A robot with improved absolute positioning accuracy for CT guided stereotactic brain surgery. IEEE Trans Biomed Eng. 1988;35(2):153–60.
4. Lanfranco AR, et al. Robotic surgery: a current perspective. Ann Surg. 2004;239(1):14–21.
5. Marescaux J, et al. Transatlantic robot-assisted telesurgery. Nature. 2001;413(6854):379–80.
6. Cadiere GB, et al. Laparoscopic gastroplasty for morbid obesity. Br J Surg. 1994;81(10):1524.
7. Batchelder AJ, et al. The evolution of minimally invasive bariatric surgery. J Surg Res. 2013;183(2):559–66.
8. Wittgrove AC, Clark GW, Tremblay LJ. Laparoscopic gastric bypass, Roux-en-Y: preliminary report of five cases. Obes Surg. 1994;4(4):353–7.
9. Cadiere GB, et al. The world's first obesity surgery performed by a surgeon at a distance. Obes Surg. 1999;9(2):206–9.

10. Muhlmann G, et al. Da Vinci robotic-assisted laparoscopic bariatric surgery: is it justified in a routine setting? Obes Surg. 2003;13(6):848–54.
11. Edelson PK, et al. Robotic vs. conventional laparoscopic gastric banding: a comparison of 407 cases. Surg Endosc. 2011;25(5):1402–8.
12. Diamantis T, et al. Initial experience with robotic sleeve gastrectomy for morbid obesity. Obes Surg. 2011;21(8):1172–9.
13. Ayloo S, et al. Robot-assisted sleeve gastrectomy for super-morbidly obese patients. J Laparoendosc Adv Surg Tech A. 2011;21(4):295–9.
14. Romero RJ, et al. Robotic sleeve gastrectomy: experience of 134 cases and comparison with a systematic review of the laparoscopic approach. Obes Surg. 2013;23(11):1743–52.
15. Pepper VK, et al. Robotic vs. laparoscopic sleeve gastrectomy in adolescents; reality or hype. Obes Surg. 2016;26(8):1912–7.
16. Elli E, et al. Laparoscopic and robotic sleeve gastrectomy: short- and long-term results. Obes Surg. 2015;25(6):967–74.
17. Vilallonga R, et al. Robotic sleeve gastrectomy versus laparoscopic sleeve gastrectomy: a comparative study with 200 patients. Obes Surg. 2013;23(10):1501–7.
18. Schraibman V, et al. Comparison of the morbidity, weight loss, and relative costs between robotic and laparoscopic sleeve gastrectomy for the treatment of obesity in Brazil. Obes Surg. 2014;24(9):1420–4.
19. Altieri MS, et al. Robotic approaches may offer benefit in colorectal procedures, more controversial in other areas: a review of 168,248 cases. Surg Endosc. 2016;30(3):925–33.
20. Vilallonga R, et al. The initial learning curve for robot-assisted sleeve gastrectomy: a Surgeon's experience while introducing the robotic Technology in a Bariatric Surgery Department. Minim Invasive Surg. 2012;2012:347131.
21. Ecker BL, et al. Resident education in robotic-assisted vertical sleeve gastrectomy: outcomes and cost-analysis of 411 consecutive cases. Surg Obes Relat Dis. 2016;12(2):313–20.
22. Park CW, et al. Robotic-assisted Roux-en-Y gastric bypass performed in a community hospital setting: the future of bariatric surgery? Surg Endosc. 2011;25(10):3312–21.
23. Myers SR, McGuirl J, Wang J. Robot-assisted versus laparoscopic gastric bypass: comparison of short-term outcomes. Obes Surg. 2013;23(4):467–73.
24. Buchs NC, et al. Laparoscopic versus robotic Roux-en-Y gastric bypass: lessons and long-term follow-up learned from a large prospective monocentric study. Obes Surg. 2014;24(12):2031–9.
25. Buchs NC, et al. Roux-en-Y gastric bypass for super obese patients: what approach? Int J Med Robot. 2016;12(2):276–82.
26. Smeenk RM, et al. The results of 100 robotic versus 100 laparoscopic gastric bypass procedures: a single high volume centre experience. Obes Surg. 2016;26(6):1266–73.
27. Ahmad A, et al. Laparoscopic versus robotic-assisted Roux-en-Y gastric bypass: a retrospective, single-center study of early perioperative outcomes at a community hospital. Surg Endosc. 2016;30(9):3792–6.
28. Lyn-Sue JR, et al. Laparoscopic gastric bypass to robotic gastric bypass: time and cost commitment involved in training and transitioning an academic surgical practice. J Robot Surg. 2016;10(2):111–5.
29. Artuso D, Wayne M, Grossi R. Use of robotics during laparoscopic gastric bypass for morbid obesity. JSLS. 2005;9(3):266–8.
30. Scozzari G, et al. Robot-assisted gastrojejunal anastomosis does not improve the results of the laparoscopic Roux-en-Y gastric bypass. Surg Endosc. 2011;25(2):597–603.
31. Mohr CJ, Nadzam GS, Curet MJ. Totally robotic Roux-en-Y gastric bypass. Arch Surg. 2005;140(8):779–86.
32. Ayloo SM, et al. Robot-assisted versus laparoscopic Roux-en-Y gastric bypass: is there a difference in outcomes? World J Surg. 2011;35(3):637–42.
33. Hagen ME, et al. Reducing cost of surgery by avoiding complications: the model of robotic Roux-en-Y gastric bypass. Obes Surg. 2012;22(1):52–61.
34. Bailey JG, et al. Robotic versus laparoscopic Roux-en-Y gastric bypass (RYGB) in obese adults ages 18 to 65 years: a systematic review and economic analysis. Surg Endosc. 2014;28(2):414–26.
35. Markar SR, et al. Robotic vs. laparoscopic Roux-en-Y gastric bypass in morbidly obese patients: systematic review and pooled analysis. Int J Med Robot. 2011;7(4):393–400.
36. Snyder BE, et al. Robotic-assisted Roux-en-Y gastric bypass: minimizing morbidity and mortality. Obes Surg. 2010;20(3):265–70.
37. Economopoulos KP, et al. Robotic vs. laparoscopic roux-En-Y gastric bypass: a systematic review and Meta-analysis. Obes Surg. 2015;25(11):2180–9.
38. Benizri EI, et al. Perioperative outcomes after totally robotic gastric bypass: a prospective nonrandomized controlled study. Am J Surg. 2013;206(2):145–51.
39. Maeso S, et al. Efficacy of the Da Vinci surgical system in abdominal surgery compared with that of laparoscopy: a systematic review and meta-analysis. Ann Surg. 2010;252(2):254–62.
40. Moon RC, et al. Robotic Roux-en-Y gastric bypass, is it safer than laparoscopic bypass? Obes Surg. 2016;26(5):1016–20.
41. Mohr CJ, et al. Totally robotic laparoscopic Roux-en-Y gastric bypass: results from 75 patients. Obes Surg. 2006;16(6):690–6.
42. Yu SC, et al. Robotic assistance provides excellent outcomes during the learning curve for laparoscopic Roux-en-Y gastric bypass: results from 100 robotic-assisted gastric bypasses. Am J Surg. 2006;192(6):746–9.
43. Ramos AC, et al. Early outcomes of the first Brazilian experience in totally robotic bariatric surgery. Arq Bras Cir Dig. 2013;26(Suppl 1):2–7.
44. Sanchez BR, et al. Comparison of totally robotic laparoscopic Roux-en-Y gastric bypass and traditional

laparoscopic Roux-en-Y gastric bypass. Surg Obes Relat Dis. 2005;1(6):549–54.
45. Sudan R, Puri V, Sudan D. Robotically assisted biliary pancreatic diversion with a duodenal switch: a new technique. Surg Endosc. 2007;21(5):729–33.
46. Sudan R, Podolsky E. Totally robot-assisted biliary pancreatic diversion with duodenal switch: single dock technique and technical outcomes. Surg Endosc. 2015;29(1):55–60.
47. Antanavicius G, Rezvani M, Sucandy I. One-stage robotically assisted laparoscopic biliopancreatic diversion with duodenal switch: analysis of 179 patients. Surg Obes Relat Dis. 2015;11(2):367–71.
48. Antanavicius G, Sucandy I. Robotically-assisted laparoscopic biliopancreatic diversion with duodenal switch: the utility of the robotic system in bariatric surgery. J Robot Surg. 2013;7(3):261–6.
49. Buchs NC, et al. Robotic revisional bariatric surgery: a comparative study with laparoscopic and open surgery. Int J Med Robot. 2014;10(2):213–7.
50. Snyder B, et al. Robotically assisted revision of bariatric surgeries is safe and effective to achieve further weight loss. World J Surg. 2013;37(11):2569–73.
51. Ayloo, S.M., N. Choudhury. Robotic revisional bariatric surgery: single-surgeon case series. Int J Med Robot. 2015;11(3):284–9.
52. Bindal V, Gonzalez-Heredia R, Elli EF. Outcomes of robot-assisted Roux-en-Y gastric bypass as a Reoperative bariatric procedure. Obes Surg. 2015;25(10):1810–5.
53. Jacobsen G, Berger R, Horgan S. The role of robotic surgery in morbid obesity. J Laparoendosc Adv Surg Tech A. 2003;13(4):279–83.
54. Stefanidis D, et al. Robotic assistance improves intracorporeal suturing performance and safety in the operating room while decreasing operator workload. Surg Endosc. 2010;24(2):377–82.
55. Chandra V, et al. A comparison of laparoscopic and robotic assisted suturing performance by experts and novices. Surgery. 2010;147(6):830–9.
56. Esposito C, et al. Work-related upper limb musculoskeletal disorders in paediatric laparoscopic surgery. A multicenter survey. J Pediatr Surg. 2013;48(8):1750–6.
57. Berguer R, et al. A comparison of surgeons' posture during laparoscopic and open surgical procedures. Surg Endosc. 1997;11(2):139–42.
58. Lee GI, et al. Surgeons' physical discomfort and symptoms during robotic surgery: a comprehensive ergonomic survey study. Surg Endosc. 2017;31(4):1697–706.
59. Franasiak, J et al. Feasibility and acceptance of a robotic surgery ergonomic training program. JSLS. 2014;18(4). pii: e2014.00166.
60. Foote JR, Valea FA. Robotic surgical training: where are we? Gynecol Oncol. 2016;143:179–83.
61. Smith R, Patel V, Satava R. Fundamentals of robotic surgery: a course of basic robotic surgery skills based upon a 14-society consensus template of outcomes measures and curriculum development. Int J Med Robot. 2014;10(3):379–84.
62. Starnes CC, et al. The economy of motion of the totally robotic gastric bypass: technique, learning curve, and outcomes of a fellowship-trained, robotic bariatric surgeon. J Laparoendosc Adv Surg Tech A. 2015;25(5):411–8.
63. Buchs NC, et al. Learning curve for robot-assisted Roux-en-Y gastric bypass. Surg Endosc. 2012;26(4):1116–21.
64. Ayloo S, Fernandes E, Choudhury N. Learning curve and robot set-up/operative times in singly docked totally robotic Roux-en-Y gastric bypass. Surg Endosc. 2014;28(5):1629–33.
65. Waite KE, Herman MA, Doyle PJ. Comparison of robotic versus laparoscopic transabdominal preperitoneal (TAPP) inguinal hernia repair. J Robot Surg. 2016;10(3):239–44.
66. Domene CE, Volpe P, Heitor FA. Robotic Roux-en-Y gastric bypass: operative results in 100 patients. Arq Bras Cir Dig. 2014;27(Suppl 1):9–12.
67. Abdalla RZ, et al. Brazilian experience in obesity surgery robot-assisted. Arq Bras Cir Dig. 2012;25(1):33–5.
68. Vilallonga R, et al. A bariatric surgery programme in adolescents. Preliminary results. Cir Esp. 2013;91(10):685–7.
69. Fort JM, et al. Bariatric surgery outcomes in a European Centre of Excellence (CoE). Obes Surg. 2013;23(8):1324–32.
70. Bodner J, et al. The da Vinci robotic system for general surgical applications: a critical interim appraisal. Swiss Med Wkly. 2005;135(45–46):674–8.
71. Buchs NC, et al. Robot-assisted Roux-en-Y gastric bypass for super obese patients: a comparative study. Obes Surg. 2013;23(3):353–7.
72. Szold A, et al. European Association of Endoscopic Surgeons (EAES) consensus statement on the use of robotics in general surgery. Surg Endosc. 2015;29(2):253–88.
73. Silverman CD, Ghusn MA. Early Australian experience in robotic sleeve gastrectomy: a single site series. ANZ J Surg. 2017;87(5):385–9.
74. Aggarwal S, et al. Totally robotic Roux-en-Y gastric bypass: technique. Indian J Surg. 2015;77(2):164–6.
75. Bhatia P, et al. Robot-assisted sleeve gastrectomy in morbidly obese versus super obese patients. JSLS. 2014;18(3). pii: e2014.00099.
76. Sasaki A, Wakabayashi G, Yonei Y. Current status of bariatric surgery in Japan and effectiveness in obesity and diabetes. J Gastroenterol. 2014;49(1):57–63.
77. Watanabe G. Medical care issues in Japan highlighted by the regulatory approval of the da Vinci surgical system. Surg Today. 2011;41(9):1182–3.
78. Shah SK, Walker PA, Snyder BE, Wilson EB. Essentials and future directions of robotic bariatric surgery. In: Kroh M, Chalikonda S, editors. Essentials of Robotic Surgery. Switzerland: Springer International Publishing; 2015. p. 73–80.

29 Bariatric Surgery in Adolescence

Marc Michalsky

Introduction

The increase in overall prevalence of childhood obesity in the U.S. and elsewhere appears to have continued to rise and, as a result, has been cited as a major threat to the health and well-being of millions of affected individuals [1]. Recent data estimate that approximately 17% of the US pediatric population is classified as being obese. Furthermore, it has been recently estimated that an additional 7% of the affected population in this country are further categorized as being "severely obese" (i.e., body mass index (BMI) ≥120% of the 95th percentile or BMI ≥35 kg/m^2) [1–5]. Although there have been some indications of a "leveling off" of obesity prevalence within specific subgroups of general pediatric population, obese adolescents and in particular, severely obese adolescents (age 12–19 years) have continued to show a steady rise in prevalence since the 1980s [1]. In addition to these alarming trends in the USA and other western countries, recent data also suggest that a correspondingly rapid increase in the rate childhood obesity has also been observed in the developing world and, as such, represents unique challenges to governments and populations that have traditionally struggled with significant problems associated with ongoing undernutrition [6–8]. In addition to a seemingly unabated rise in the prevalence of childhood obesity over the past several decades, an expanding body of corresponding literature highlighting the coexistence of many obesity-related comorbid disease states, including evidence of cardiovascular disease, dyslipidemia, impaired glucose metabolism, type 2 diabetes mellitus, hypertension, obstructive sleep apnea, polycystic ovarian disease, and fatty liver disease, has recently emerged [9–13]. The establishment of various related comorbid conditions, previously thought to primarily exist only within the severely obese adult population, coupled with evidence demonstrating poor outcomes related nonsurgical therapeutic interventions (i.e., exercise and diet and behavioral modification regimens) and evidence that severely obese youth have an extraordinarily high risk of becoming severely obese adults, has resulted in an increased interest in the application of weight loss surgery (i.e., bariatric surgery) during the adolescent time period [14–17].

The current chapter will focus on data regarding the development of several key comorbid conditions encountered in the severely obese adolescent population and review the current clinical indications for the use of surgical weight loss procedures among teens, including best practice guidelines and longitudinal outcomes related to the most commonly performed bariatric procedures. In addition, the chapter will review the use of bariatric surgery for pediatric

M. Michalsky
Department of Pediatric Surgery, Nationwide Children's Hospital, Columbus, OH, USA
e-mail: Marc.Michalsky@nationwidechildrens.org

R. Lutfi et al. (eds.), *Global Bariatric Surgery*, https://doi.org/10.1007/978-3-319-93545-4_29

patients with special considerations (i.e., the very young, individuals with syndromic or hypothalamic obesity, etc.). Lastly, the current consensus-driven guidelines for the development of a multidisciplinary care model designed to provide adolescent-specific treatment that is separate and distinct from the adult care as well as current challenges related to access to care for this underserved and vulnerable population will be presented.

Obesity-Related Comorbid Disease

As mentioned above, many of the recently observed obesity-related comorbid illnesses that have emerged within the affected pediatric population have previously been attributed only to populations of severely obese adults. Examples of these disorders include impaired glucose metabolism, obstructive sleep apnea, nonalcoholic fatty liver disease, various forms of cardiovascular disease, as well as evidence of increased cardiovascular risk factors, musculoskeletal disorders, pseudotumor cerebri, and psychological disorders to name a few [9, 12, 18–21]. In addition to the emerging picture of an obesity-related comorbid disease state in the affected pediatric population, it has been hypothesized that such related diseases, when developed during childhood, may result in a significantly different longitudinal impact compared to the development and progression of obesity-related diseases later in life. The potential for such a cumulative impact further supports the need for safe and effective therapeutic interventions including bariatric surgery.

Cardiovascular Disease

Although it has been well established that obesity is associated with the development of numerous cardiovascular risk factors as well as frank cardiovascular pathophysiology and related functional abnormalities, including atherosclerotic disease, heart failure, and stroke, and has been identified as the primary cause of premature mortality in the adult population, there is a relative paucity of investigations specifically focusing on the cardiovascular health among severely obese adolescents [12, 15]. In addition, very few contemporary studies have sought to directly address the potential changes in baseline cardiovascular health following surgically induced weight loss. As with other obesity-related comorbid illnesses that have been extensively documented in the adult population, a number of researchers have reported evidence of the pathologic impact of severe obesity on the adolescent population being considered for bariatric surgical intervention (i.e., hypertension, diastolic dysfunction, and elevated cardiac workload) [13, 19, 22]. In combination with the existence of numerous markers of generalized metabolic dysfunction (i.e., hypertension, dyslipidemia, and insulin resistance), an emerging body of literature serves to support the use of bariatric surgery earlier in life (i.e., during the adolescent time period) [10, 11, 23]. Recent examples include studies by Inge and Teeple, who've both reported a high prevalence of several markers of cardiovascular disease risk at baseline (i.e., before undergoing weight loss surgery) when compared to the lean pediatric population. Examples include elevated rates of hypertension, dyslipidemia, insulin resistance, and type 2 diabetes, among teenagers undergoing Roux-en-Y gastric bypass (RYGB). Longitudinal outcomes from both investigations showed significant improvements in nearly all variables by 2 years following bariatric surgery with marked improvement in most measured variable by 12 months. Corresponding data from both institutions highlight both the high baseline prevalence of impaired cardiovascular geometry and function as well as marked improvement in both biomarkers of cardiovascular risk and reversal of abnormal cardiac function (i.e., diastolic performance and cardiac workload) following bariatric surgical intervention [13, 19]. While such studies serve collectively to support the use of bariatric surgery as a safe and effective treatment algorithm, they are also fundamentally limited based on their relatively small sample sizes and the single institutional nature. In contrast, however, several ongoing studies including data from the Teen-Longitudinal Assessment of Bariatric Surgery (Teen-LABS) study, a prospective observational study of 242 adolescents undergoing bariatric surgery at five US centers, as well as the AMOS study (Swedish Nationwide Study), a prospective analysis of 81 adolescent bariatric surgery patients, offer more robust support of such early observations. In addition, these ongoing investigations are likely to continue to yield valuable insights with regard to cardiovascular health as well as several other important areas of study in this population [24, 25].

Impaired Glucose Metabolism

In conjunction with current reports citing the high prevalence of impaired glucose metabolism in the severely obese adult population, including a high prevalence of type 2 diabetes and evidence demonstrating significant clinical improvement following surgical weight loss [26–29], corresponding studies have shown a link between the increasing prevalence of childhood obesity and disruption of several aspects of normal glucose metabolism resulting in hyperinsulinemia (60–80%), impaired glucose tolerance (12–35%), and type 2 diabetes among individuals presenting for adolescent bariatric surgery. Recent studies charcterizing adolesent baratric patients show correspondingly high prevalences of hyperinsulinemia (71%), impaired fasting glucose (26%), and diabetes (14%) [9, 12, 23]. Not surprisingly, it is the adverse cumulative impact of diabetes and its association with the development of many other health-related problems that has prompted an ever-increasing level of interest in the development of aggressive therapeutic strategies to reverse the impact of severe obesity in the pediatric population [30]. This evolving consensus is supported by several recent studies that have demonstrated significant improvement in numerous biomarkers of metabolic performance [10, 11, 25]. Recent single center studies by Inge and Teeple have shown improvement in fasting serum glucose, insulin, hemoglobin A1c, and insulin resistance, as determined by homeostatic model assessment (HOMA-IR) among teens undergoing surgical weight loss procedures [10, 11]. More recently, the same group of investigators showed a 95% remission rate of type 2 diabetes by 3 years among a large cohort of teens undergoing bariatric surgery (sleeve gastrectomy or gastric bypass) [25].

Nonalcoholic Fatty Liver Disease

To date, there is a relative paucity of data regarding the overall prevalence of nonalcoholic liver disease (NAFLD) in the severely obese pediatric and/or adolescent population in general as well as the specific population undergoing metabolic and bariatric surgery. Furthermore, corresponding mechanistic data regarding the identification of specific risk factors for the development and longitudinal progression of NAFLD as well as the impact of surgical weight loss remain unclear [31]. From a pathophysiological standpoint, NAFLD is known to consist of a well-defined spectrum of histopathology ranging from simple and uncomplicated steatosis to a state of progressive hepatic inflammation resulting in the development of nonalcoholic steatohepatitis (NASH), cirrhosis, and eventual death [32, 33]. Although the prevalence of NASH among populations with severe adolescent obesity appear to be lower when compared to adult populations [34], evidence linking the development of NAFLD with obesity have shown that approximately 38% of obese children have excess fat deposition in the liver in which approximately 9% progress on to the frank development of NASH. Often considered a "hidden" disease with potentially devastating consequences, recent evidence demonstrating a decrease in the amount of hepatic steatosis and inflammation following surgical weight loss, the development of NASH is currently cited as an indication for bariatric surgery in adolescents (Table 29.1) [35–38]. Interestingly, the coexistence of certain cardio-metabolic risk factors (i.e., elevated alanine aminotransferase (ALT), hypertension, impaired fasting glucose, diabetes, etc.) rather than increasing BMI have been shown to be associated with increased severity of NAFLD [31].

Table 29.1 Current eligibility criteria for adolescent bariatric surgery

BMI (kg/m)	Comorbidities
≥35	Serious: type II diabetes mellitus, mod/severe OSA (AHI >15), pseudotumor cerebri, severe NASH
≥40	Other: mild OSA (AHI>5), insulin resistance, hypertension, impaired fasting glucose, dyslipidemia, impaired quality of life
Eligibility criteria	
Tanner stage	IV or V (unless severe comorbid disease warrants "early" WLS)
Skeletal maturity	≥95% estimated growth
Lifestyle changes	Demonstrate ability to understand dietary/physical changes (post-op)
Psychosocial	Evidence of mature decision-making
	Understands risk and benefits of surgery
	Evidence of family and social support
	Evidence that patient/family will be compliant with recommended pre- and postoperative care (dietary, medication, etc.)

Obstructive Sleep Apnea

Sleep-disordered breathing and obstructive sleep apnea (OSA), consisting of a spectrum of symptoms including apnea, hypopnea, and snoring, have become a source of growing concern among healthcare providers and has been shown to be highly prevalent within the obese pediatric population (46%) [9, 39, 40]. The clinical consequences of OSA, which is characterized by narrowing of the pharyngeal airway resulting in repeated episodes of airflow cessation, oxygen desaturation, and sleep disruption, result in various degrees of chronic fatigue, impaired scholastic performance and development, and progression of significant end-organ dysfunction such as hypertension, ventricular cardiac dysfunction, and heart failure. If left untreated, the end result is associated with an increased risk of early mortality [9, 41, 42]. In a recent series of adolescents presenting for bariatric surgery, Kalra et al. showed that 55% of study participants were noted to have a diagnosis of OSA. Repeat polysomnographic testing after bariatric surgery, however, showed significant improvement in all patients [42]. These results are similar to a number of published reports showing improvement in the severity of OSA following bariatric surgery in the adult population [43, 44] and, thereby, support the argument for surgical weight loss for adolescents who have documented moderate to severe OSA (e.g., of apnea-hypopnea index (AHI) >15 events/h) with a BMI ≥35 kg/m^2 or mild OSA (AHI ≥5 events/h) with a BMI ≥40 kg/m^2 (Table 29.1) [37, 38].

Pseudotumor Cerebri

Idiopathic intracranial hypertension, or pseudotumor cerebri, is characterized by raised intracranial pressure not attributed to mass lesions or focal structural abnormalities, resulting in pulsatile tinnitus, elevated cerebral spinal fluid pressure, severe headaches, and visual disturbances including blindness. Although considered a relatively uncommon disorder in the general population, with a reported incidence of 1 case per 100,000 per year, the corresponding incidence among the overweight population has been reported to be as high as 19 per 100,000 per year. Widely considered to be a complication of severe obesity, the exact pathophysiological event(s) leading to its development and progression are poorly understood. Despite the relative paucity of literature related to *pseudotumor cerebri* within the bariatric surgical population, which consists mostly of case reports demonstrating improved symptomatology in affected adults following surgical weight loss, recent data demonstrating a higher than expected prevalence among bariatric surgery patients highlights the importance of screening for this often asymptomatic disorder [45]. The establishment of this diagnosis is considered a strong indication for bariatric surgery in both adults and adolescents [37, 46–49].

Musculoskeletal Pain and Impaired Functional Mobility

The adverse consequences of obesity on functional mobility and associated musculoskeletal pain, potentially leading to impairment in overall quality of life and even early morbidity, have been previously described in the adult population. Corresponding data in the pediatric and adolescent populations, however, are extremely limited. Current data suggest that like obese adults, obese youth are not immune from the cumulative effects of being overweight or obese and demonstrate a high prevalence of musculoskeletal pain (12–44%) and impairment in functional mobility when compared to lean counterparts [20, 21, 50]. Similar to other disappointing outcomes related to lifestyle interventions, documented improvements in cardiovascular fitness and walking distance may only be of temporary benefit secondary to the poor adherence to structured physical activity programs in the pediatric age group [51–53]. Bout-Tabaku et al. recently showed that 49% of subjects had poor functional status while 76% reported associated musculoskeletal pain prior to undergoing weight loss surgery [20]. Lower back pain was the most prevalent (63%) followed by ankle/foot, knee (49%), and hip (31%) pain. In additional analysis of function (i.e., walking) and physiological measures (i.e., heart rate), Ryder et al. showed durable improvement in time to completion of the 400 m walk test as well as improvement in resting heart rate 2 years after undergoing an adolescent bariatric procure [21].

Psychological Disorders

A large and consistent body of evidence reporting high rates of psychosocial comorbidity related to severe obesity in adults exists. Based on estimated epidemiological trends showing that a significant proportion of the affected adult population report the onset of various symptoms during their preceding childhood years (i.e., depression, anxiety disorder, binge eating disorder, etc.), it is reasonable to assume that baseline rates of obesity-related psychosocial disorder are high among the pediatric population presenting for weight loss surgery [54]. Despite this, however, there continues to be a relative knowledge gap related to our overall understanding of the psychosocial comorbidities that exist in addition to the numerous medical and/or physiological consequences of obesity and severe obesity during youth. In addition, there have been few studies that specifically address these issues among the pediatric population seeking out bariatric surgical intervention. Recent reports have emerged that highlight potential links between obesity and interference with normal psychological development during childhood. The consequences of such impaired behavioral development may result in a negative impact affecting the normal transition from childhood into early adulthood [55]. Preliminary studies (mostly consisting of small single institutional cohorts) suggest the presence of at-risk subgroups of psychiatric comorbidity including individuals with depressive symptoms (14–38%) and eating disorders [56–58]. In a recent study by Zeller et al., investigators report significant improvement in health-related quality of life (HR-QOL) measures and depressive symptomology in the 1st year following bariatric surgery (RYGB) among 31 subjects at a single institution [56]. More recently, the same group of investigators examined 141 surgical subjects from multiple sites in comparison to a nonsurgical obese control group ($n = 83$) in an effort to correlate self-reported data characterizing psychopathology. Results showed that while both groups were at greater risk for psychopathology compared to national adolescent base prevalence rates, the nonsurgical cohort appeared to be at higher risk for pathological behavior. Therefore, the investigators suggest that individuals that achieve candidacy for weight loss surgery may represent a section bias and represent lower overall psychosocial risk when compared to counterparts seeking nonsurgical methods of weight reduction (i.e., behavior modification, diet, and exercise) [54]. Additional longitudinal studies, including anticipated long-term analysis from the Teen-LABS research consortium, should offer additional insight on the potential impact of surgical weight loss on psychosocial health.

Best Practice Guidelines

Although the use of bariatric surgery in the treatment of severe obesity in the adult population has been described as early as the 1960s and has had formalized clinical guidelines since the early 1990s with release of the heavily cited National Institutes of Health (NIH) consensus guidelines statement [59], a corresponding framework for clinical eligibility in the pediatric population has only developed within the last decade. Originally proposed by Inge et al. in 2004, the first published recommendations and guidelines for the use of bariatric surgery in adolescents were predicated on the previously established adult clinical guidelines and, similarly, relied heavily on anthropomorphic criteria (i.e., minimal BMI) in combination with concurrent identification of specific obesity-related comorbid diseases. Despite general similarities to the adult inclusion criteria, the authors of the initial adolescent recommendations supported a somewhat more conservative approach compared to adults. Adolescent-specific guidelines at that time called for a BMI $\geq$40 kg/m^2 in the presence of severe obesity-related comorbidities or BMI $\geq$50 kg/m^2 with less severe comorbidities. As shown in Table 29.1, the more recently updated recommendations while not identical to the original adult criteria have adopted a somewhat less conservative approach [37, 38]. As an example, more than a decade after publication of the original set of recommendations by Inge and colleagues, and in the context of a mounting body of evidence supporting the safe and efficacious use of bariatric surgery in adolescents, the paradigm has shifted toward lower preoperative BMI thresholds. Although the use of BMI as a critical benchmark for bariatric surgery eligibility has been recently brought into question, as evidence by the increased acceptance of bariatric surgery for the treatment of uncontrolled diabetes among adults with BMI $\leq$35 kg/m^2 [60], recent data demonstrating a potential "ceiling effect" in association with preoperative BMI and postoperative improvement in cardio-metabolic health suggest that efforts should be made to refer adolescent for bariatric surgery earlier in the spectrum of BMI progression [61]. Taken together, these factors have led to the establishment of specific recommendations for the adolescent population. Furthermore, current consensus supports the development of adolescent-centered bariatric treatment facilities based on a multidisciplinary model designed to address the specific needs of the pediatric population in order to optimize outcomes. In 2011 the Children's Hospital Association (CHA) published the proceedings of a multidisciplinary collaborative (FOCUS on a Fitter Future) which was convened in order to develop expert recommendations pertaining to all aspects of childhood obesity prevention and treatment strategies. Recommendations brought forth by the panel included the use of surgical weight reduction for the treatment of severe adolescent obesity [62]. Furthermore, the authors presented a consensus-driven road map for institutional development of age-appropriate bariatric surgery programs and highlighted the importance of the multidisciplinary care model using pediatric and adolescent-specific healthcare resources. Several additional reports highlight the need for behavioral screening by a qualified pediatric provider as well as the need to screen for common micronutrient and vitamin deficiencies (i.e., ferritin, vitamin A, and vitamin D) both before and following adolescent bariatric surgery [25].

In a series of steps designed to assign consensus-driven guidelines to the development of pediatric-specific bariatric surgical care that are both separate and distinct from the adult care model, the American Society for Metabolic and Bariatric Surgery (ASMBS) published a position statement and best practice guidelines in 2012 for the use of bariatric surgery in the adolescent population. The purpose of this important publication was to raise professional awareness regarding the need for safe and effective treatment strategies in order to counter the serious nature of obesity-related comorbid disease(s), widely believed to have profound immediate and future health implications [37]. Also in 2012, ASMBS and the American College of Surgeons (ACS) announced a decision to combine their respective national bariatric surgery accreditation programs by forming the Metabolic and Bariatric Surgery Quality Improvement Program (MBSAQIP). This national registry (https://asmbs.org/about/mbsaqip) currently collects prospective data designed to assess clinical effectiveness and safety and current accounts for more than 90% of bariatric procedures performed in the USA and Canada, representing 722 accredited clinical centers as of August 2016 [63]. Building on an emerging body of favorable outcomes related to bariatric surgery in the adolescent population as well as the previously published ASMBS best practice guidelines, it was determined that MBSAQIP would also define accreditation standards for centers that provide care to the pediatric population. Center awarded separate pediatric designations are required to demonstrate access to pediatric and adolescent-specific clinical resources designed to deliver optimal care. Such resources include incorporation of pediatric healthcare providers with expertise in general pediatric medicine, nutrition, and behavioral disciplines.

Patients with Special Considerations

Several subgroups within the pediatric population, including the very young (i.e., preteens) and individuals with hypothalamic, monogenic, and/or syndromic forms of obesity, warrant special consideration. While the majority of current literature regarding the use of bariatric surgery in the pediatric population is focused on the adolescent age group (i.e. 12–19 years), a small number of studies have emerged that aim to address the use of surgical weight loss procedures in the very young. Current data relating to this controversial topic have mostly emerged from single center retrospective experiences consisting for the most part of case reports comprised of one or two patients [64–66]. In contrast to such studies, which raise a number of concerns regarding the patient selection process and long-term follow-up, Alqahtani et al., recently presented a comprehensive analysis of 116 children younger than 14 years of age following sleeve gastrectomy (mean age 11.2 ± 2.5 years) [67]. This important analysis serves to refute some of the concerns regarding the potential for bariatric surgery in the very young to interfere with vertical growth and physiological maturation; however, additional factors, including the long-term impact on nutritional status (micro- and macronutrient deficiencies), longitudinal neurocognitive development, and cardio-metabolic health, remain unanswered.

Obesity related to disruption of normal hypothalamic-pituitary pathways, also referred to as hypothalamic obesity (HyOb), can be attributed to several conditions. HyOb has been reported to develop in more than 50% of individuals following surgical resection of an underlying craniopharyngioma, a benign and slow-growing epithelial neoplasm generally located in the area of the pituitary and hypothalamus [68]. Weight gain related to hypothalamic damage, from direct tumor infiltration and/or surgical resection, is often severe and refractory to medical management. The consequences of this pathological process and its treatment lead to serious negative impact on quality of life and the consideration for the use of bariatric surgical intervention [68, 69]. In a recent meta-analysis examining the use of bariatric surgery in this extremely challenging population, investigators identified a total of 21 cases and reported that the maximal mean weight loss after 6 and 12 months was observed in subjects undergoing RGYB. In addition to HyOb related to craniopharyngioma, several monogenic forms of obesity including Prader-Willi syndrome (PWS), Bardet-Biedl syndrome (BBS), and individuals with hypothalamic melanocortin signaling defects have also been the subject of investigation in the context of bariatric surgical intervention. Alqahtani et al. recently reported effective weight reduction and comorbid disease resolution in a comparative analysis of 24 adolescent subjects with PWS versus a matched control group of non-PWS adolescents undergoing weight loss surgery. While initial reports such as these are encouraging, the role of bariatric surgery, including specific procedural recommendations in this subpopulation, remains uncertain and will require additional prospective analysis [70]. In addition to the use of bariatric surgery in special forms of obesity briefly touched on above, the implications and outcomes of its use in the cognitively impaired population also remain largely unexplored [71]. Although detailed reports highlighting this population are lacking in both the adolescent and adult literature, it would seem reasonable to pursue consideration of surgical weight reduction on a case-by-case basis and taking into account the need for robust family, behavioral, and social support resources.

Types of Bariatric Procedures

Although there is no lack of anecdotal opinion regarding which operation(s) offer optimal intervention for adolescents considering surgical weight reduction, no clear evidence-based consensus has yet to emerge based on contemporary data. In light of the corresponding lack of definitive data regarding “the best” bariatric procedure in the adult population, until rigorously designed prospective comparative data become available, the debate will no doubt continue for the foreseeable future. Currently, the vast majority of adolescent bariatric operations being carried out in both the USA and elsewhere are identical to the most common procedures being performed for adult patients and include RYGB, adjustable gastric band (AGB), and the vertical sleeve gastrectomy (VSG). In addition, similar to the “adult” experience, recent evidence has shown that there has been a shift in procedural prevalence during the past decade such that RYGB and AGB appear to have been surpassed by VSG [23]. Finally, while strictly malabsorptive procedures such as the biliopancreatic diversion (BPD) or duodenal switch (DS) have been performed in adolescents, these types of operations are generally considered inappropriate in children over concerns for the potential of severe malabsorption during the postoperative time period [72].

A recent meta-analysis of studies involving RYGB in adolescents by Treadwell et al., consisting of 6 studies with a total 131 adolescent patients, showed significant as well as sustained weight loss as well as improvement in comorbid diseases including type 2 diabetes mellitus and hypertension [15]. In one of the largest series of adolescent patients undergoing RYGB, the ongoing Teen-LABS study has also demonstrated significant improvement in nearly all measured variables including anthropomorphic measurements, cardio-metabolic risk markers, musculoskeletal and physical function disorders, and quality of life [21, 25]. These results, along with others, show generally favorable outcomes that are similar to the large body of literature pertaining to the adult population [10, 11, 42, 61, 73, 74]. Postoperative complication rates, including anastomotic leaks/strictures, wound infections, postoperative bleeding, bowel obstructions, deep venous thrombosis, the need for reoperation, and/or 30-day hospital readmission rate, appear to be similar if not better when compared to corresponding adult studies on adults [23–25, 55].

The adjustable gastric band (AGB), which was approved by the US Food and Drug Administration (FDA) in 2001 for adults (age ≥18 years), experienced a rapid increase in use in both the USA and Europe following its initial introduction. Since that time, however, the procedural prevalence has declined significantly for a multitude of reasons including higher than expected complication and reoperation rates as well as evidence of disappointing weight loss durability. Secondary to current age restrictions (i.e., the AGB is currently not approved for use in patients <18 years of age in the USA), data in relation to the adolescent population remains limited to a series of small and mostly retrospective single institutional reports. In a recent meta-analysis of adolescent bariatric surgery outcomes, investigators showed that adolescents undergoing AGB demonstrated results similar to numerous adult studies in terms of weight loss and comorbidity resolution. The majority of postoperative complications were related to device malfunction [15]. A randomized control trial involving adolescents undergoing (AGB) versus lifestyle modification offers some of the most compelling evidence for the advantageous use of bariatric surgery as compared to nonsurgical means of weight reduction. These investigators demonstrated a 28% decrease in BMI over 2 years as compared to 3% in the lifestyle intervention group [55]. Taken together, mixed reports related to outcomes in both the adolescent and adult population as well as decreasing procedural prevalence leave a number of unanswered questions regarding the overall appropriateness of AGB use in the pediatric population.

A number of recent studies of adolescents undergoing sleeve gastrectomy demonstrate safety and efficacy profiles that are similar to reports in the adult literature. Although there is a limited number of studies evaluating its use in this population, recent evidence from both the Teen-LABS research consortium and others have been able to show significant reduction in BMI as well as reversal on many comorbid disease states related severe adolescent obesity [23, 25, 75–77]. Ongoing analysis by Teen-LABS investigators is expected to yield more comprehensive data specifically designed to assess comparative longitudinal outcomes for adolescents undergoing RYGB versus VSG.

Access to Care

Despite current literature in support of weight loss surgery for adolescents, the number of operations being performed on an annual basis is only a fraction of the number of the potentially eligible individuals based on anthropomorphic criteria alone [17, 78]. In addition, while the number of publications related to adolescent bariatric surgery continues to increase, recent data from the USA suggests that procedural prevalence has plateaued during the past decade [17]. While there are numerous factors that may impact these observations, attitudes among primary care providers as well as limitations in obtaining healthcare cost coverage appear to be prominent factors [79, 80]. Recent data from both the USA and UK suggest that attitudes toward adolescent bariatric surgery among medical versus surgical providers differ between countries and may result in major differences in procedural prevalence [80, 81]. The hesitation to refer severely obese pediatric patients to multidisciplinary bariatric centers may lead to a delay in intervention. Furthermore, recent data from a multi-institutional retrospective review examining insurance coverage for adolescent bariatric surgery demonstrates an apparent disparity in coverage availability compared to adults. In comparison to the relatively high success rate for procedural insurance authorization among adults seeking bariatric surgery, investigators showed that less than half of adolescents who met requirement for weight loss surgeries were initially approved. This is in stark contrast to 80–85% of adults who meet criteria for bariatric surgery and then gain approval on the initial request. Insurance approval was ultimately obtained (80%) when patients engaged in the complex insurance appeal process; however, approval in some cases was withheld despite numerous separate appeals for some (as many as five) [79]. The implications of such healthcare disparity resulting in limited access become even more compelling when considering the previously discussed evidence demonstrating the potential for differential response rates based on the relative severity of preoperative BMI [61]. Further advocacy efforts on behalf of this vulnerable population in combination with the results of ongoing studies will hopefully result in greater access to care in the future.

Conclusion

The increasing prevalence of obesity and in particular severe forms of obesity among the pediatric and adolescent population is especially concerning when considering the concurrent rise in prevalence of numerous related comorbid diseases. Increasing evidence supports the use of bariatric surgery in adolescent population and has been shown to be associated with significant and long-lasting improvements in various related disease states. Despite encouraging outcomes, the pediatric population faces ongoing barriers including age-related disparity in access to available procedures that must be challenged with strong advocacy from the medical community.

References

1. Ogden CL, Carroll MD, Lawman HG, et al. Trends in obesity prevalence among children and adolescents in the United States, 1988–1994 through 2013–2014. JAMA. 2016;315(21):2292–9.
2. Skinner AC, Skelton JA. Prevalence and trends in obesity and severe obesity among children in the United States, 1999–2012. JAMA Pediatr. 2014;168(6):561–6.

3. Kimm SY, Obarzanek E. Childhood obesity: a new pandemic of the new millennium. Pediatrics. 2002;110(5):1003–7.
4. Ogden CL, Carroll MD, Curtin LR, McDowell MA, Tabak CJ, Flegal KM. Prevalence of overweight and obesity in the United States, 1999–2004. JAMA. 2006;295(13):1549–55.
5. Daniels SR, Kelly AS. Pediatric severe obesity: time to establish serious treatments for a serious disease. Child Obes. 2014;10(4):283–4.
6. Lasserre AM, Chiolero A, Paccaud F, Bovet P. Worldwide trends in childhood obesity. Swiss Med Wkly. 2007;137(9–10):157–8.
7. Wang Y, Lobstein T. Worldwide trends in childhood overweight and obesity. Int J Pediatr Obes. 2006;1(1):11–25.
8. de Onis M, Blossner M, Borghi E. Global prevalence and trends of overweight and obesity among preschool children. Am J Clin Nutr. 2010;92(5):1257–64.
9. Brandt ML, Harmon CM, Helmrath MA, Inge TH, McKay SV, Michalsky MP. Morbid obesity in pediatric diabetes mellitus: surgical options and outcomes. Nat Rev Endocrinol. 2010;6(11):637–45.
10. Inge TH, Miyano G, Bean J, et al. Reversal of type 2 diabetes mellitus and improvements in cardiovascular risk factors after surgical weight loss in adolescents. Pediatrics. 2009;123(1):214–22.
11. Teeple EA, Teich S, Schuster DP, Michalsky MP. Early metabolic improvement following bariatric surgery in morbidly obese adolescents. Pediatr Blood Cancer. 2012;58(1):112–6.
12. Michalsky MP, Inge TH, Simmons M, et al. Cardiovascular risk factors in severely obese adolescents: the Teen Longitudinal Assessment of Bariatric Surgery (Teen-LABS) study. JAMA Pediatr. 2015;169(5):438–44.
13. Michalsky MP, Raman SV, Teich S, Schuster DP, Bauer JA. Cardiovascular recovery following bariatric surgery in extremely obese adolescents: preliminary results using Cardiac Magnetic Resonance (CMR) imaging. J Pediatr Surg. 2013;48(1):170–7.
14. O'Brien PE, Sawyer SM, Laurie C, et al. Laparoscopic adjustable gastric banding in severely obese adolescents: a randomized trial. JAMA. 2010;303(6):519–26.
15. Treadwell JR, Sun F, Schoelles K. Systematic review and meta-analysis of bariatric surgery for pediatric obesity. Ann Surg. 2008;248(5):763–76.
16. Freedman DS, Mei Z, Srinivasan SR, Berenson GS, Dietz WH. Cardiovascular risk factors and excess adiposity among overweight children and adolescents: the Bogalusa Heart Study. J Pediatr. 2007;150(1):12–17 e12.
17. Kelleher DC, Merrill CT, Cottrell LT, Nadler EP, Burd RS. Recent national trends in the use of adolescent inpatient bariatric surgery: 2000 through 2009. Arch Pediatr Adolesc Med. 2012:1–7.
18. Freedman DS, Dietz WH, Srinivasan SR, Berenson GS. The relation of overweight to cardiovascular risk factors among children and adolescents: the Bogalusa Heart Study. Pediatrics. 1999;103(6 Pt 1):1175–82.
19. Ippisch HM, Inge TH, Daniels SR, et al. Reversibility of cardiac abnormalities in morbidly obese adolescents. J Am Coll Cardiol. 2008;51(14):1342–8.
20. Bout-Tabaku S, Michalsky MP, Jenkins TM, et al. Musculoskeletal pain, self-reported physical function, and quality of life in the Teen-Longitudinal Assessment of Bariatric Surgery (Teen-LABS) cohort. JAMA Pediatr. 2015;169(6):552–9.
21. Ryder JR, Edwards NM, Gupta R, et al. Changes in functional mobility and musculoskeletal pain after bariatric surgery in teens with severe obesity: Teen-Longitudinal Assessment of Bariatric Surgery (LABS) study. JAMA Pediatr. 2016;170:871–7.
22. Cuspidi C, Rescaldani M, Tadic M, Sala C, Grassi G. Effects of bariatric surgery on cardiac structure and function: a systematic review and meta-analysis. Am J Hypertens. 2014;27(2):146–56.
23. Inge TH, Zeller MH, Jenkins TM, et al. Perioperative outcomes of adolescents undergoing bariatric surgery: the Teen-Longitudinal Assessment of Bariatric Surgery (Teen-LABS) study. JAMA Pediatr. 2014;168(1):47–53.
24. Olbers T, Gronowitz E, Werling M, et al. Two-year outcome of laparoscopic Roux-en-Y gastric bypass in adolescents with severe obesity: results from a Swedish Nationwide Study (AMOS). Int J Obes. 2012;36(11):1388–95.
25. Inge TH, Courcoulas AP, Jenkins TM, et al. Weight loss and health status 3 years after bariatric surgery in adolescents. N Engl J Med. 2016;374(2):113–23.
26. Dixon JB, le Roux CW, Rubino F, Zimmet P. Bariatric surgery for type 2 diabetes. Lancet. 2012;379(9833):2300–11.
27. Mokdad AH, Ford ES, Bowman BA, et al. Prevalence of obesity, diabetes, and obesity-related health risk factors, 2001. JAMA. 2003;289(1):76–9.
28. Schauer PR, Mingrone G, Ikramuddin S, Wolfe B. Clinical outcomes of metabolic surgery: efficacy of glycemic control, weight loss, and remission of diabetes. Diabetes Care. 2016;39(6):902–11.
29. Purnell JQ, Selzer F, Wahed AS, et al. Type 2 diabetes remission rates after laparoscopic gastric bypass and gastric banding: results of the longitudinal assessment of bariatric surgery study. Diabetes Care. 2016;39(7):1101–7.
30. Pinhas-Hamiel O, Zeitler P. The global spread of type 2 diabetes mellitus in children and adolescents. J Pediatr. 2005;146(5):693–700.
31. Xanthakos SA, Jenkins TM, Kleiner DE, et al. High prevalence of nonalcoholic fatty liver disease in adolescents undergoing bariatric surgery. Gastroenterology. 2015;149(3):623–34. e628
32. Schwimmer JB, Deutsch R, Kahen T, Lavine JE, Stanley C, Behling C. Prevalence of fatty liver in children and adolescents. Pediatrics. 2006;118(4):1388–93.
33. Matteoni CA, Younossi ZM, Gramlich T, Boparai N, Liu YC, McCullough AJ. Nonalcoholic fatty liver disease: a spectrum of clinical and pathological severity. Gastroenterology. 1999;116(6):1413–9.

34. Xanthakos S, Miles L, Bucuvalas J, Daniels S, Garcia V, Inge T. Histologic spectrum of nonalcoholic fatty liver disease in morbidly obese adolescents. Clin Gastroenterol Hepatol. 2006;4(2):226–32.
35. Mathurin P, Gonzalez F, Kerdraon O, et al. The evolution of severe steatosis after bariatric surgery is related to insulin resistance. Gastroenterology. 2006;130(6):1617–24.
36. Kral JG, Thung SN, Biron S, et al. Effects of surgical treatment of the metabolic syndrome on liver fibrosis and cirrhosis. Surgery. 2004;135(1):48–58.
37. Michalsky M, Reichard K, Inge T, et al. ASMBS pediatric committee best practice guidelines. Surg Obes Relat Dis (Official Journal of the American Society for Bariatric Surgery). 2012;8(1):1–7.
38. Pratt JS, Lenders CM, Dionne EA, et al. Best practice updates for pediatric/adolescent weight loss surgery. Obesity (Silver Spring). 2009;17(5):901–10.
39. Styne DM. Childhood and adolescent obesity. Prevalence and significance. Pediatr Clin N Am. 2001;48(4):823–54. vii
40. Kalra M, Inge T. Effect of bariatric surgery on obstructive sleep apnoea in adolescents. Paediatr Respir Rev. 2006;7(4):260–7.
41. Young T, Shahar E, Nieto FJ, et al. Predictors of sleep-disordered breathing in community-dwelling adults: the Sleep Heart Health Study. Arch Intern Med. 2002;162(8):893–900.
42. Kalra M, Inge T, Garcia V, et al. Obstructive sleep apnea in extremely overweight adolescents undergoing bariatric surgery. Obes Res. 2005;13(7):1175–9.
43. Guardiano SA, Scott JA, Ware JC, Schechner SA. The long-term results of gastric bypass on indexes of sleep apnea. Chest. 2003;124(4):1615–9.
44. Rasheid S, Banasiak M, Gallagher SF, et al. Gastric bypass is an effective treatment for obstructive sleep apnea in patients with clinically significant obesity. Obes Surg. 2003;13(1):58–61.
45. Hamdallah IN, Shamseddeen HN, Getty JL, Smith W, Ali MR. Greater than expected prevalence of pseudotumor cerebri: a prospective study. Surg Obes Relat Dis (Official Journal of the American Society for Bariatric Surgery). 2013;9(1):77–82.
46. Jamal MK, DeMaria EJ, Johnson JM, et al. Impact of major co-morbidities on mortality and complications after gastric bypass. Surg Obes Relat Dis (Official Journal of the American Society for Bariatric Surgery). 2005;1(6):511–6.
47. Sugerman HJ, Felton WL 3rd, Sismanis A, Kellum JM, DeMaria EJ, Sugerman EL. Gastric surgery for pseudotumor cerebri associated with severe obesity. Ann Surg. 1999;229(5):634–40. discussion 640–2
48. Sugerman HJ. Multiple benefits of bariatric surgery. Manag Care. 2005;14(10 Suppl):16–21.
49. Chandra V, Dutta S, Albanese CT, Shepard E, Farrales-Nguyen S, Morton J. Clinical resolution of severely symptomatic pseudotumor cerebri after gastric bypass in an adolescent. Surg Obes Relat Dis (Official Journal of the American Society for Bariatric Surgery). 2007;3(2):198–200.
50. Tsiros MD, Coates AM, Howe PR, Grimshaw PN, Buckley JD. Obesity: the new childhood disability? Obes Rev (An Official Journal of the International Association for the Study of Obesity). 2011;12(1):26–36.
51. Mendelson M, Michallet AS, Perrin C, Levy P, Wuyam B, Flore P. Exercise training improves breathing strategy and performance during the six-minute walk test in obese adolescents. Respir Physiol Neurobiol. 2014;200:18–24.
52. Danielsson P, Kowalski J, Ekblom O, Marcus C. Response of severely obese children and adolescents to behavioral treatment. Arch Pediatr Adolesc Med. 2012;166(12):1103–8.
53. Knop C, Singer V, Uysal Y, Schaefer A, Wolters B, Reinehr T. Extremely obese children respond better than extremely obese adolescents to lifestyle interventions. Pediatr Obes. 2015;10(1):7–14.
54. Rofey DL, Zeller MH, Brode C, et al. A multi-site view of psychosocial risks in patients presenting for bariatric surgery. Obesity (Silver Spring). 2015;23(6):1218–25.
55. Thakkar RK, Michalsky MP. Update on bariatric surgery in adolescence. Curr Opin Pediatr. 2015;27(3):370–6.
56. Zeller MH, Modi AC, Noll JG, Long JD, Inge TH. Psychosocial functioning improves following adolescent bariatric surgery. Obesity (Silver Spring). 2009;17(5):985–90.
57. Kim RJ, Langer JM, Baker AW, Filter DE, Williams NN, Sarwer DB. Psychosocial status in adolescents undergoing bariatric surgery. Obes Surg. 2008;18(1):27–33.
58. Messiah SE, Lopez-Mitnik G, Winegar D, et al. Changes in weight and co-morbidities among adolescents undergoing bariatric surgery: 1-year results from the Bariatric Outcomes Longitudinal Database. Surg Obes Relat Dis (Official Journal of the American Society for Bariatric Surgery). 2013;9(4):503–13.
59. Gastrointestinal surgery for severe obesity. Proceedings of a National Institutes of Health Consensus Development Conference. March 25–27, 1991, Bethesda, MD. Am J Clin Nutr 1992;55(2 Suppl):487S–619S.
60. Sjoholm K, Anveden A, Peltonen M, et al. Evaluation of current eligibility criteria for bariatric surgery: diabetes prevention and risk factor changes in the Swedish obese subjects (SOS) study. Diabetes Care. 2013;36(5):1335–40.
61. Inge TH, Jenkins TM, Zeller M, et al. Baseline BMI is a strong predictor of nadir BMI after adolescent gastric bypass. J Pediatr. 2010;156(1):103–108 e101.
62. Michalsky M, Kramer RE, Fullmer MA, et al. Developing criteria for pediatric/adolescent bariatric surgery programs. Pediatrics. 2011;128(Suppl 2):S65–70.
63. Blackstone R, Dimick JB, Nguyen NT. Accreditation in metabolic and bariatric surgery: pro versus con. Surg Obes Relat Dis (Official Journal of the American Society for Bariatric Surgery). 2014;10(2):198–202.

64. Baltasar A, Serra C, Bou R, Bengochea M, Andreo L. Sleeve gastrectomy in a 10-year-old child. Obes Surg. 2008;18(6):733–6.
65. Dan D, Harnanan D, Seetahal S, Naraynsingh V, Teelucksingh S. Bariatric surgery in the management of childhood obesity: should there be an age limit? Obes Surg. 2010;20(1):114–7.
66. Mohaidly MA, Suliman A, Malawi H. Laparoscopic sleeve gastrectomy for a two-and half year old morbidly obese child. Int J Surg Case Rep. 2013;4(11):1057–60.
67. Alqahtani A, Elahmedi M, Qahtani AR. Laparoscopic sleeve gastrectomy in children younger than 14 years: refuting the concerns. Ann Surg. 2016;263(2):312–9.
68. Bingham NC, Rose SR, Inge TH. Bariatric surgery in hypothalamic obesity. Front Endocrinol (Lausanne). 2012;3:23.
69. Inge TH, Pfluger P, Zeller M, et al. Gastric bypass surgery for treatment of hypothalamic obesity after craniopharyngioma therapy. Nat Clin Pract Endocrinol Metab. 2007;3(8):606–9.
70. Alqahtani AR, Elahmedi MO, Al Qahtani AR, Lee J, Butler MG. Laparoscopic sleeve gastrectomy in children and adolescents with Prader-Willi syndrome: a matched-control study. Surg Obes Relat Dis (Official Journal of the American Society for Bariatric Surgery). 2016;12(1):100–10.
71. Daigle CR, Schauer PR, Heinberg LJ. Bariatric surgery in the cognitively impaired. Surg Obes Relat Dis (Official Journal of the American Society for Bariatric Surgery). 2015;11(3):711–4.
72. Marceau P, Marceau S, Biron S, et al. Long-term experience with duodenal switch in adolescents. Obes Surg. 2010;20(12):1609–16.
73. Zeller MH, Reiter-Purtill J, Ratcliff MB, Inge TH, Noll JG. Two-year trends in psychosocial functioning after adolescent Roux-en-Y gastric bypass. Surg Obes Relat Dis (Official Journal of the American Society for Bariatric Surgery). 2011;7(6):727–32.
74. Sugerman HJ, Sugerman EL, DeMaria EJ, et al. Bariatric surgery for severely obese adolescents. J Gastrointest Surg (Official Journal of the Society for Surgery of the Alimentary Tract). 2003;7(1):102–7. discussion 107–8
75. Boza C, Viscido G, Salinas J, Crovari F, Funke R, Perez G. Laparoscopic sleeve gastrectomy in obese adolescents: results in 51 patients. J Gastrointest Surg (Official Journal of the American Society for Bariatric Surgery). 2012;8(2):133–7. discussion 137–9
76. Alqahtani AR, Antonisamy B, Alamri H, Elahmedi M, Zimmerman VA. Laparoscopic sleeve gastrectomy in 108 obese children and adolescents aged 5 to 21 years. Ann Surg. 2012;256(2):266–73.
77. Pepper VK, Rager TM, Diefenbach KA, Raval MV, Teich S, Michalsky MP. Robotic vs. laparoscopic sleeve gastrectomy in adolescents; reality or hype. Obes Surg. 2016;26:1912–7.
78. Gortmaker SL, Wang YC, Long MW, et al. Three interventions that reduce childhood obesity are projected to save more than they cost to implement. Health Aff. 2015;34(11):1932–9.
79. Inge TH, Boyce TW, Lee M, et al. Access to care for adolescents seeking weight loss surgery. Obesity (Silver Spring). 2014;22(12):2593–7.
80. Woolford SJ, Clark SJ, Gebremariam A, Davis MM, Freed GL. To cut or not to cut: physicians' perspectives on referring adolescents for bariatric surgery. Obes Surg. 2010;20(7):937–42.
81. Michalsky MP. Adolescent bariatric surgery in the United Kingdom; a call for continued study and open dialogue. Arch Dis Child. 2014;99(10):885–6.

Large Ventral Hernias

30

Luciano G. Tastaldi, David M. Krpata, and Michael J. Rosen

Scope of the Problem

Obesity has become endemic in the last 50 years, with 30–50% of the population considered overweight or obese. This epidemic has increased throughout America with approximately 36% of US citizens being considered obese (BMI>30). From a global perspective, 5% of the world population is morbidly obese (BMI>40), with rates increasing yearly [1–3]. Rising prevalence of obesity carries significant implications to our healthcare system, as it has led to increasing costs [2] and defining new patterns of care to manage this specific population and the multiple comorbidities associated with it.

Approximately four to five million major abdominal operations are performed each year, and about 20% of patients will develop incisional hernias despite refinements on abdominal wall closure techniques, technology implementation, and all measures taken by the surgeon to prevent hernia formation. As a result, ventral hernia repair remains one of the most common procedures performed by general surgeons [4]. Consequently, general, bariatric, and hernia surgeons are facing more complex scenarios and surgical management dilemmas while taking care of this increasingly more common population. The presence of a ventral hernia in the morbidly obese patient represents a frequent example of those challenging situations. Even though it has been largely studied, the subject still creates controversies among specialists and lacks sufficient data to recommend specific and uncontestable guidelines.

Pathophysiology of Hernias in the Morbidly Obese Population

Obesity is a well-known and largely documented risk factor for the development of incisional hernias, and the incidence of herniation is positively correlated with the progressive increase in body mass index (BMI). Incisional hernia formation after midline laparotomies in this population reaches 50%, thus illustrating the magnitude of the problem and the need for hernia formation and recurrence prevention initiatives.

Incisional hernia formation is a complex and multifactorial event, and many theories have been proposed to explain the higher prevalence in this subgroup [5–9]. When BMI increases, fat deposition in the mesentery, guts, and retroperitoneal space creates visceral adiposity that subsequently increases intra-abdominal pressure. Visceral adiposity, thicker subcutaneous layers, and increased intra-abdominal pressure create a tense closure of the abdomen that results in poor tissue approximation. Thicker subcutaneous layers often demand large flaps dissection,

L. G. Tastaldi (✉) · D. M. Krpata · M. J. Rosen
Digestive Disease And Surgery Institute, Cleveland Clinic Foundation, Cleveland, OH, USA
e-mail: TASTALL@CCF.ORG; KRPATAD@CCF.ORG; ROSENM@CCF.ORG

R. Lutfi et al. (eds.), *Global Bariatric Surgery*, https://doi.org/10.1007/978-3-319-93545-4_30

increasing rates of wound complications and infection, predisposing to hernia formation [6]. Additionally, excess fat deposition in the wound causes defects in tissue structure and decreases healing capacity. Lastly, comorbidities associated with morbid obesity act synergistically to impair healing capacity contributing to the higher rates of incisional hernias.

The burden of obesity is not only related to hernia formation. It is notable that obesity also makes hernia repair more difficult. Ventral hernia repair in the obese population has been marked by high recurrence rates, reported to be as high as 40% [10–15]. Great advances have been accomplished with large application of mesh, tension-free fascial closures and implementation of minimally invasive techniques. However, recurrence rates in this population remain high, implying that factors other than suboptimal tissue approximation and healing capacity might contribute to hernia formation and recurrence in this subset [6].

For example, increases in BMI are associated with concurrent increases in intra-abdominal pressure (IAP) [16, 17], creating an environment of chronic intra-abdominal hypertension. This may explain the contribution of obesity to hernia formation and recurrence, as this environment contributes to other *pressure-related comorbidities*, including hypertension, stress incontinence, venous insufficiency, gastroesophageal reflux disease (GERD), and obstructive sleep apnea [6, 17].

Further complicating factor is that obesity is also correlated with the development of medical and wound complications following hernia repair. Several studies associate obesity with increased rates of adverse events after hernia repair, including wound complications, infection, readmissions, and prolonged length of stay [18–23]. Surgical complications directly correlated to obesity include nosocomial infections, surgical site infections and abscess formation, pulmonary and thromboembolic events, and higher readmission rates. The aforementioned factors that contribute to hernia formation and hernia recurrence highlight the need for preoperative optimization in order to improve outcomes.

Special Consideration in Approaching Hernias in the Morbidly Obese Population

Preoperative Weight Loss/ Preoperative Optimization

Recent guidelines associate obesity with poor outcomes after elective ventral hernia repair and recommend that no elective ventral hernia repair should be undertaken without preoperative weight loss in morbidly obese patients. While dealing with a large ventral hernia in a morbidly obese patient, it is imperative to recognize that the postoperative outcomes will be closely affected by the quality of a well-guided preoperative optimization program. Operating on this specific population without preoperatively taking care of modifiable risk factors for complications will most certainly result in higher morbidity, recurrence rates, and cost of care. Therefore, patient counseling, patient selection, and a rational and evidence-based use of the hernia surgery armamentarium are critical in order to provide safe and durable repairs. Importantly, a multidisciplinary approach with medical weight loss specialists, bariatric surgeons, and a comprehensive team of caregivers is needed to provide adequate care for these patients.

Morbidly obese patients with large and recurrent abdominal defects are frequently referred to bariatric and hernia surgeons in a search for a miraculous resolution of their problems. Surgically treating morbid obesity and concurrently providing a functional and durable hernia repair is desirable; however, not always realistic or wise in practice. Preoperative weight loss is the cornerstone of adequate and successful surgical planning. Defining the patients that are suitable candidates for bariatric surgery and those who aren't is the first step in deciding the weight loss approach to employ for an individual patient. As important as the weight loss approach are providing education and motivating the patient to take part in the process, allowing them to consider themselves part of the solution rather than part of the problem. A well-educated and motivated patient is more likely to achieve preoperative weight loss and comorbidity control, improving their chances of a successful outcome after hernia surgery. We follow a specific preoperative optimization algorithm when dealing with comorbid patients which include preoperative weight loss (surgical or not), smoke cessation, and comorbidities control, such as glucose control in diabetic patients. Only when all preoperative goals are achieved, patients will be offered hernia repair. Table 30.1 summarizes the components of a suggested preoperative optimization protocol for obese patients undergoing ventral hernia repair.

No standardized or evidence-based approach to perioperative weight loss for hernia patients currently exists. Despite the potential benefits of preoperative weight loss in hernia patients, there remains a paucity of literature about medically supervised weight loss programs achieving better outcomes after ventral hernia repair. Several small studies report suboptimal results with medical weight loss and have cast doubt on the feasibility of preoperative, nonsurgical weight loss in morbidly obese patients [2].

It is undeniable that bariatric procedures offer rapid and long-term weight loss [24] and could be the salvation to obese patients with ventral hernias. Nevertheless, several factors might make bariatric surgery unviable in this population. Loss of domain, fistulas, and current infection from previous meshes usually make bariatric surgery not feasible. Lastly, a proportion of obese patients with hernias simply does not desire bariatric surgery. Such factors leave a significant amount of morbidly obese patients with large and/or complex abdominal wall defects that require preoperative optimization with a nonsurgical weight loss approach.

Table 30.1 Suggested preoperative optimization protocol for obese patients undergoing ventral hernia repair

Preoperative weight loss	Medically supervised weight loss with PSMF diet or surgical weight loss
	Target BMI<30 kg/m^2
	In some instances a BMI<40 kg/m2 might be acceptable
Smoke cessation	Minimum 6 weeks before the operation
	Cotinine urine testing is encouraged prior VHR
Glucose control	Referral for endocrinology for diabetes control
	Target: HbA1C <6.5%

Surgery should be postponed when:
HBA1C>8,0%
BMI>40 kg/m^2
Active smoking

Nonsurgical Weight Loss

Our group, in collaboration with medical weight loss specialists, has taken an aggressive approach with regard to preoperative weight loss [2]. A collaborative effort among surgical and medical weight loss specialists that delivers a clear and unified message to all patients is the main objective. Patients are educated about how important it is that they take an active role in their care if they want to have a good outcome after their hernia repair. A clear understanding of how obesity results in recurrent hernias and increased infectious and wound complication rates with unacceptable perioperative morbidity is presented to the patient. The crucial and imperative weight loss in the preoperative optimization period is largely discussed with the patient to demonstrate that a positive outcome is a result of not only medical or health professionals but, importantly, patient efforts. Surgical repair is not offered to patients until they achieve the desired weight loss. Our group advocates that patients achieve a BMI of less than 40 prior to undertaking a complex hernia repair.

Dietary Approach

Our medical weight loss specialists employ a protein-sparing modified fast (PSMF) diet in order to achieve a reasonable weight loss in a fast and safe manner. This dietary approach consists of a protein ingestion of 1.2–1.4/kg/day, calculated according to the patient's ideal body weight (BMI 25). A maximum daily carbohydrate ingestion of 40 g is permitted and the maximum caloric intake is 800 kcal/daily. All patients receive multivitamin and mineral supplementation during the weight loss treatment. Patients are encouraged to follow this program until they reach an ideal body weight with a BMI ranging from 25 to 27 or they plateau. Often, when patients are operated prior to achieving their ideal body weight, they are reintroduced to the PSMF during the postoperative period and continue until they achieve the desired goal.

After this initial weight loss period, and particularly after the surgery, maintaining the weight loss can be a challenge; however, this is essential to maintaining good long-term outcomes. Patients are encouraged to maintain a healthy, balanced, and individualized long-term maintenance diet for at least 5 years. Physical activity is encouraged according to the individuals' physical capacity, with a goal of at least 30 min a day, four times a week. Psychological counseling is provided according to the patient's needs and inclination.

The time it takes patients to achieve the necessary preoperative weight loss varies, ranging from 6 to 36 months. Using this approach, an expected body weight reduction of 18–20% can be achieved, and according to our experience, approximately 80% of the patients will lose and maintain the weight loss during long-term follow-up.

Like any other nonsurgical weight loss method, this approach is only feasible and successful for a motivated patient, who is willing to take part in their treatment.

Surgical Weight Loss

Bariatric procedures should be offered to the patients that desire surgery and are determined appropriate candidates after meticulous clinical, nutritional, and psychological evaluation. Included in this is documentation of a failed nonsurgical weight loss programs despite evidence of adequate involvement. We typically offer upfront bariatric consultation for super morbidly obese (BMI>50) and super-super morbidly obese (BMI>60) patients, in which nonsurgical weight loss would demand an excessive amount of time and would delay hernia repair. The initial weight loss is imperative to achieve adequate comorbidities control thus reducing intraoperative and postoperative complications. Bringing a super morbidly obese patient or a super-super morbidly obese patient to a BMI around 40 also enhances patient's capacity for physical activity, positively contributing to subsequent weight loss and comorbidities control, further improving outcomes and reducing surgical risk.

The specific bariatric procedure should be decided among a multidisciplinary evaluation and at the discretion of the bariatric and hernia surgeons. A laparoscopic sleeve gastrectomy is a good option for patients with large and complex ventral hernia patients, as it offers good weight loss results and avoids intestinal mobilization. Also, it can subsequently be converted to a Roux-en-Y gastric bypass at a future time if necessary. Additionally, leaving the hernia undisturbed during the bariatric procedure may decrease complications and reduce the chance of incarceration after surgery. Another option is going straight to the gastric bypass. However, this can be challenging as there is typically a large portion of small bowel involved in the hernia. For smaller and less complex hernias without intestinal involvement in the hernia sac, the laparoscopic gastric bypass is a safe option. Lastly, the intragastric balloon has arisen as an option for preoperative weight loss, but there is little data to support its efficacy in patients with ventral hernias.

Optimal Time to Intervene

After weight loss surgery, we recommend waiting a minimum of 6 months and assessing for weight stabilization prior to attempting a hernia repair in minimally symptomatic hernias. When symptoms cause quality of life impairment and/or predispose to incarceration, the abdominal wall operation should be scheduled as is clinically indicated.

Management of Ventral Hernias Found Intraoperatively During Bariatric Procedures

Hernias found intraoperatively are seldom encountered, and different strategies to address these defects have been proposed [4, 25, 26]. Surgeons should keep in mind that during the bariatric procedure, the ultimate goal is to perform the bariatric surgery safely, and the hernia repair should be only made in order to avoid postoperative complications and not in an attempt to provide a definitive repair. Leaving smaller hernias untouched raises concerns related to the risk of bowel incarceration and obstruction in the rapid weight loss period following the surgery. This risk has been reported as high as 37% in some series [25]. Repairing large and complex hernias concurrently, as already stated before, carries significant recurrence and complication rates and should not be undertaken at the same time as the bariatric operation. Nevertheless, even for smaller hernias that were repaired at the time of the bariatric procedure, recurrence rates of up to 100% [10] have been documented.

In smaller hernias with only omentum in the hernia sac, the repair can be delayed, as the incarcerated omentum prevents intestinal incarceration during the weight loss period. When an empty hernia sac is found or when small bowel is the hernia sac content, considering the risk of bowel obstruction and incarceration, the best option is to reduce its contents and close the defect primarily with transfascial sutures. It's easy and feasible and limits any additional operative time. Although recurrence rates are expected to be high, the risk to benefit ratio tends to be for this approach. Another option for smaller hernias is bridging the defect with bioresorbable or biologic mesh. The utility of this repair is limited, as biologic scaffolds are costly and recurrences for bridging repairs are high, making this a low-value approach. Nonetheless, it can be used in difficult situations to limit the risk of hernia-related postoperative complications. Definitive repair can then be undertaken later when there is no gastrointestinal violation with a concomitant procedure.

In larger and complex hernias, the staged hernia repair is the preferred approach. The risk of incarceration is small and repairing large hernias concurrently has not proven beneficial. When possible, the contents of large hernias should be left intact during the bariatric procedure, which will decrease the risk of complications in the postoperative period. When reduction of the hernia and adhesiolysis are essential so that a gastric bypass can be performed, we recommend bridging the defect with bioresorbable or biologic mesh, reducing the risk of incarceration and making definitive hernia repair in the future easier.

Surgical Management of Ventral Hernias in Obese Patients: Tips and Tricks

Tips for Abdomen Closure in Obese Patients with Large Defects

Despite the fact that many systematic reviews have been published in recent years comparing types of sutures and different techniques for abdominal closure [27–29], there remains a lack of strong data to recommend a universal technique for abdominal wall closure. Mainly, the group's heterogeneity and the lack of adequate comparison between elective and emergency laparotomies in the studies limit the ability to make definitive recommendations [29]. As it's a faster method for closing the abdomen, current recommendation is to utilize a running suture for closure. Peritoneal closures have not proven beneficial in short or long-term data and may increase surgery duration. Thus, peritoneal closure can be avoided [28].

Following current recommendations [29], we suggest performing a running suture for fascial closure. For running closures, the small bites technique (stitches with a 5 mm separation and 5–8 mm fascial bites) has shown a significant reduction in surgical site infections and incisional hernia formation [30, 31]. With respect to suture materials, slowly absorbable sutures are recommended, leading to decreased hernia formation when compared to rapidly absorbable sutures [31]. There has also been some implication that slowly absorbable sutures lead to less chronic wound pain and sinus formation when compared to nonabsorbable sutures [27].

Optimal Operation in the Morbidly Obese Patient with Large Ventral Hernias

More often than not, morbidly obese patients have large abdominal wall defects. Weight gain, multiples attempts of hernia repair, and subsequent recurrences contribute to increased hernia size and complexity. The surgeon's main objective when managing large abdominal wall defects is to employ a technique that will provide a tension-free medialization of the rectus muscles with reconstitution of the linea alba, resulting in a functional repair. Multiple factors have to be taken into account during surgical decision-making, but in general, for defects larger than 8 cm, an open approach is required for formal reconstruction.

For years, open hernia repair consisted of primary repair, with or without onlay mesh reinforcement, leading to high recurrence rates due to tension applied to tissue structures in the postoperative period. The increased rate of wound complications in the obese population makes onlay mesh less desirable in morbidly obese patients. Significant reduction in surgical site complications and hernia recurrence were seen with the retro-rectus dissection and sublay mesh placement, the Rives-Stoppa repair. Nevertheless, it is still difficult to achieve a tension-free fascial closure on larger defects with this approach. The advent of components separation technique introduced by Ramirez in 1990 [32] created the opportunity to achieve fascial closure in larger defects. Nevertheless, this approach as originally described was associated with high wound morbidity rates related to extensive raising of skin flaps. As previously stated, the creation of large skin flaps with wide subcutaneous tissue dissection leads to soft tissue devascularization by injuring perforators that arise from the rectus muscle and result in increased rates of wound complications.

The ideal technique should be one that provides tension-free fascial closure with wide overlap mesh reinforcement while avoiding subcutaneous flaps. One technique that meets these criteria is the posterior component separation with transversus abdominis release. This approach allows for wide mesh overlap in sublay position, while avoiding the need for large skin flaps but also resulting in equivalent myofascial advancement when compared to the anterior components separation. The retromuscular sublay position, unlike onlay or intraperitoneal mesh placements, also has the advantage of maintaining the mesh in a well-vascularized position which benefits tissue integration. Adhesions to the mesh, fistula formation, and fixation-related complications are also avoided by not placing the mesh intraperitoneally.

Open Retromuscular Ventral Hernia Repair with Posterior Component Separation and Transversus Abdominis Release

Surgical Planning Considerations

Preoperative imaging is routinely obtained with a non-contrast CT scan to provide adequate surgical planning, assessing the integrity of the abdominal wall musculature, measuring the defect dimensions, and detecting previous meshes or occult infections. With respect to mesh choice, a permanent synthetic mesh can safely be utilized in clean cases. A medium- or heavy-weight polypropylene mesh can be used for most repairs. However, the authors tend to utilize an uncoated, medium-weight, macroporous polypropylene mesh due to its improved capacity of bacterial clearance in case of infection. In a contaminated surgical field, bioresorbable or biologic meshes can be used but are related to increased cost and higher rates of eventration.

Operative Steps [33]

1. Patient Preparation and Positioning

   The patient should be maintained in dorsal decubitus position, under general anesthesia. Prophylactic antibiotics are administered according to institutional protocols. Special attention should be given to prophylaxis of venous thromboembolic events, as patients with large ventral hernias are at high risk for such complications.

2. Incision, Adhesiolysis, and Prior Mesh Removal

   A generous midline laparotomy should be performed with excision of the previous scar. The electrocautery for subcutaneous dissection should be minimized, in order to decrease seroma formation due to lipolysis. Manual traction is the best way to fracture a thick subcutaneous tissue. The abdominal cavity is entered sharply, taking caution that underlying abdominal wall adhesions may be present. A complete adhesiolysis is performed, taking down all adhesions between the visceral contents and the abdominal wall. Sharp dissection should be used exclusively, avoiding the use of cautery in order to prevent bowel thermal injuries. For recurrent hernia repairs, the presence of prior mesh may impact healing and tissue integration of the new mesh. As such, we suggest complete mesh removal at this time. After all adhesiolysis is completed, attention is then turned to the abdominal wall.

3. Retro-rectus Dissection

   Figures 30.1 and 30.2 illustrate operative steps of posterior rectus sheath incision and retromuscular dissection. The retro-rectus space is accessed by incising the posterior rectus sheath just lateral to the linea alba. The incision is performed 0.5–1.0 cm below linea alba and should be extended the full extent of the abdominal wall. The posterior rectus sheath should be grasped with Kocher clamps and retracted medially. The linea alba can be grasped with Kocher clamps by the assistant and retracted straight up. Using electrocautery, the retromuscular space is dissected laterally until the linea semilunaris is identified; blunt finger or gauze dissection often leads to bleeding and should be avoided. The neurovascular bundles that penetrate the rectus muscle should be carefully preserved. Transecting neurovascular bundles leads to rectus muscle denervation, causing weakness, laxity, and impaired abdominal

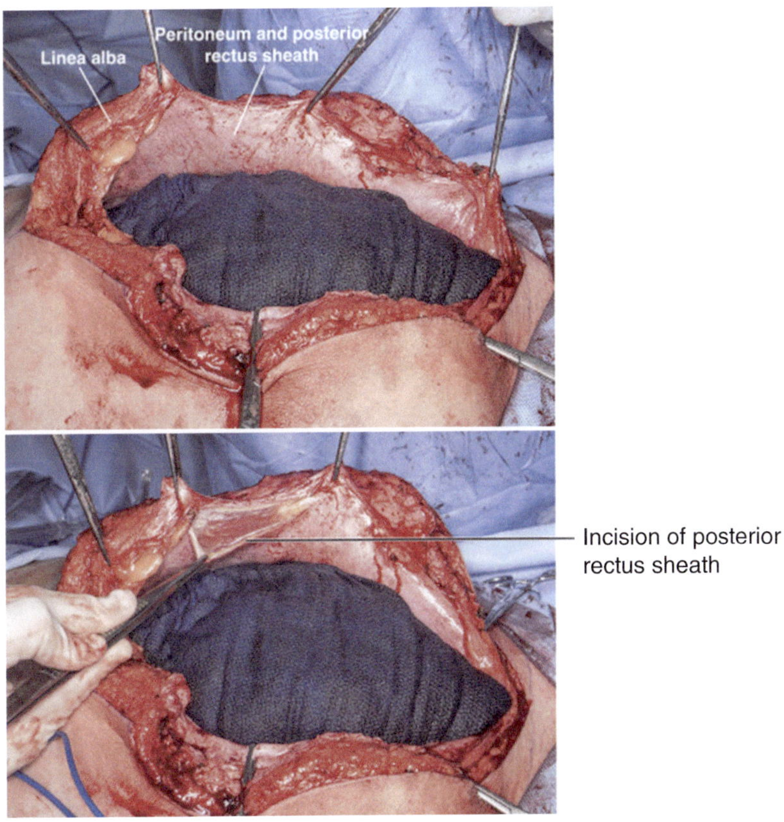

Fig. 30.1 Posterior rectus sheath incision. (Reprinted from [33], Chapter 5, Page 87, Copyright (2017), with permission from Elsevier)

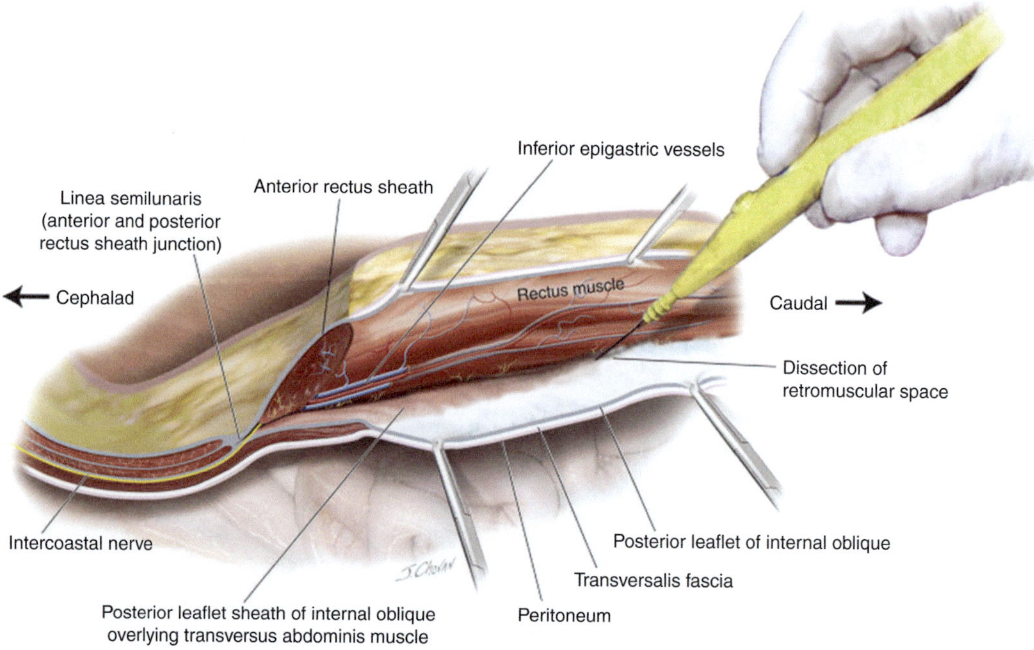

Fig. 30.2 Retromuscular dissection. (Reprinted from [33], Chapter 5, Page 89, Copyright (2017), with permission from Elsevier)

wall functionality. Additionally, the deep epigastric vessels which will be running anteriorly on the posterolateral surface of rectus muscles should be identified and preserved. Upon completing the retromuscular dissection, assessment of tension when bringing the fascia to midline is performed in order to determine if a posterior component separation with transversus abdominis release will be needed to achieve tension-free fascial closure.

4. The Posterior Component Separation

Figures 30.3 and 30.4 illustrate operative steps of posterior component separation. The posterior rectus sheath should be incised just medial to the entry of the neurovascular bundles. The incision can begin in the most cranial or caudal position depending on the exposure. The initial layer released is the posterior lamella of the internal oblique. Release of the posterior lamella of the internal oblique exposes the transversus abdominis muscle. With the aid of a right-angle clamp, tranversus abdominis fibers are dissected from the underlying peritoneum and transected with cautery. The correct plane consists of fatty areolar tissue and peritoneum. By transecting tranversus abdominis fibers, lateral forces are released allowing medial advancement of the posterior structures. A preperitoneal plane in the lateral abdominal wall is entered and developed using blunt dissection. This dissection is extended to the retroperitoneum in order to gain adequate space for wide mesh overlap. The medial border of the Psoas muscle marks the end of your lateral dissection. Dissection is carried out in the same manner on the contralateral side.

5. Pelvic Dissection

Preperitoneal dissection is extended to the pelvis entering the space of Retzius. Dissection should be performed using the epigastric vessels as guides to prevent disorientation and vascular injuries. Anatomic landmarks are pubic bone and Cooper's ligaments medially and both iliac crests laterally. Medially, Cooper's ligaments are exposed, and the bladder is swept down. The lateral aspect of the pelvis is exposed, and cord structures skeletonized. In females, the round ligaments are divided to facilitate advancement of the peritoneum.

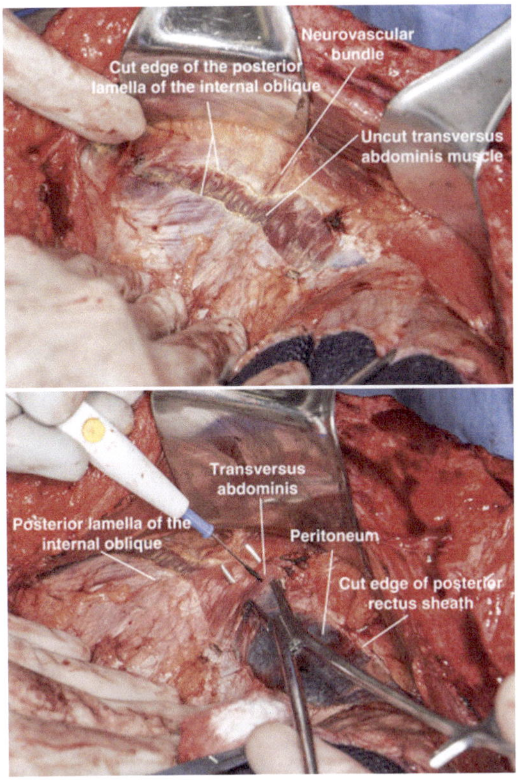

Fig. 30.3 Identification and transection of transversus abdominis muscle fibers. (Reprinted from [33], Chapter 5, Page 87, Copyright (2017), with permission from Elsevier)

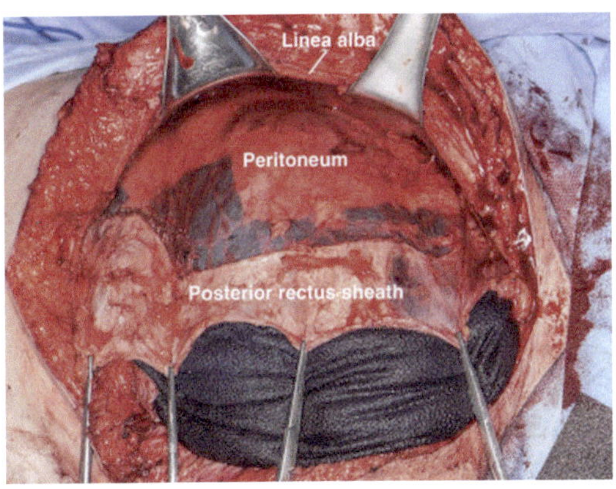

Fig. 30.4 Completed posterior component separation with transversus abdominis release (TAR). (Reprinted from [33], Chapter 5, Page 99, Copyright (2017), with permission from Elsevier)

6. Subxyphoid Dissection

   For hernias located in the mid-abdomen, cranial dissection 5–7 cm above the defect is typically adequate for repair. If the defect extends to the subcostal region or the xyphoid process, subxiphoid dissection is imperative to achieve adequate mesh overlap. Each leaflet of the posterior sheath is incised to its insertion on the xyphoid process. The peritoneum can be cleared off the diaphragms and taken all the way down to the central tendon of the diaphragm. This creates a large pocket to accommodate mesh, ensuring that mesh overlap is extended above the costal margins. Figure 30.5 illustrates final aspect of pelvic and subxiphoid dissections, respectively.

7. Posterior Rectus Sheath Closure: Recreation of the Visceral Sac

   Figure 30.6 illustrates posterior rectus sheath closure and mesh placement and fixation. After bilateral releases are complete, eventual peritoneal defects should be closed with absorbable sutures. The posterior rectus sheath is then reapproximated in the midline with running absorbable suture. This layer does not provide structural support to the abdominal wall, and its intent is to exclude the mesh from the visceral sac and prevent bowel herniation below the mesh. Uncoated permanent synthetic mesh should not be placed if the entire posterior rectus sheath and peritoneum are not intact. In those cases, a rapidly absorbable mesh or omental patch can be used to reconstruct the posterior sheath and exclude the mesh from the viscera prior to mesh placement.

8. Mesh Placement and Fixation

   An appropriately sized mesh is brought to the operative field and placed in a diamond configuration. In the pelvis, the mesh is fixated to both Cooper's ligaments with interrupted slowly absorbable sutures. Superiorly, the mesh is placed beyond the costal margin. This overlap can be extended beyond the xiphoid process and down to the central tendon of the diaphragm when necessary. Interrupted absorbable sutures are used for fixation at the xiphoid.

   Circumferentially, full-thickness transfascial sutures using #1 slowly absorbable material are used to fixate the mesh with the aid of a Carter-Thomason (CooperSurgical, Trumbull, CT) suture passer. For such, a small

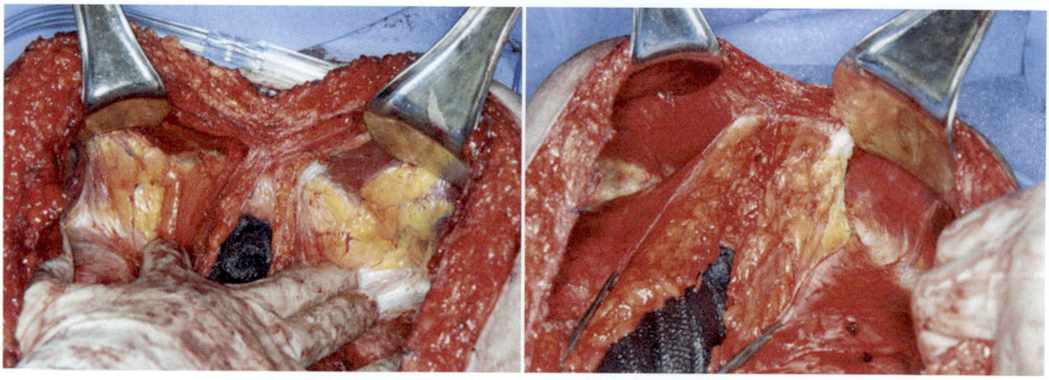

Fig. 30.5 Final aspect of pelvic and subxyphoid dissections. (Reprinted from [33], Chapter 5, Pages 91 and 93, Copyright (2017), with permission from Elsevier)

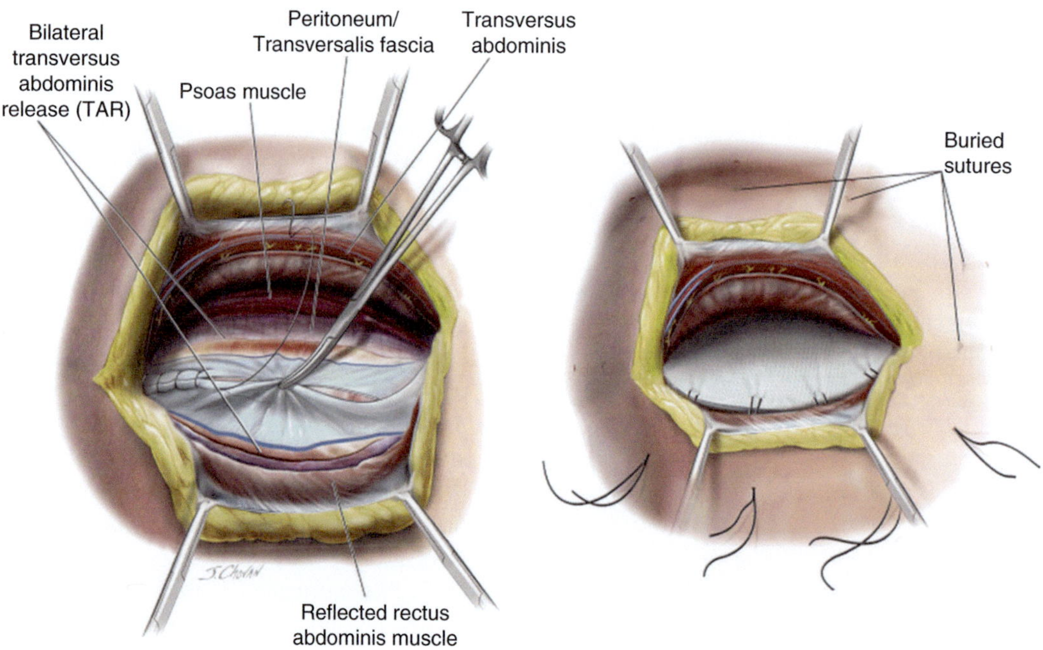

Fig. 30.6 Posterior rectus sheath closure and mesh fixation. (Reprinted from [33], Chapter 5, Pages 101 and 103, Copyright (2017), with permission from Elsevier)

stab incision is made in the skin with a #11 blade; the suture passer is introduced through the skin incision and abdominal musculature to retrieve a suture which has already been placed through the mesh. The suture passer is introduced again through the same incision and catches the opposite end of the suture. Three sutures are typically placed on each side of the abdomen. Once all transfascial sutures are placed, they are then tied.

9. Linea Alba Closure/Drainage/Skin Closure

Two large closed suction drains are placed in the retromuscular space (above the mesh) and exteriorized through the lateral abdominal wall on separate skin incisions. The anterior rectus sheath is reapproximated in the midline with a running or figure-of-eight suture of #1 slowly absorbable suture. The subcutaneous tissue and skin are closed in layers.

Laparoscopic Ventral Hernia Repair

Role of Laparoscopy

The laparoscopic approach to ventral hernia surgery has been widely adopted. Its safety and feasibility and a significant reduction in wound morbidity have been proven in multiple studies. Additionally, less postoperative pain, shorter length of stay, and faster return to normal activities are just a few examples of the numerous advantages provided by the laparoscopic approach [34–38].

The main benefits of laparoscopy are directly related to less tissue trauma and a blunted inflammatory response which may reduce general complications seen in obese patients during long hospital stays. Laparoscopy also reduces wound morbidity by avoiding the large, deep surgical wounds seen with open surgery. All these elements make a laparoscopic hernia repair a formidable approach to the obese hernia patient. However, not all hernias are amenable to laparoscopic repair. Patients with multiple prior abdominal surgeries, previous intra-abdominal meshes, adhesions, and large defect sizes increase the complexity and can make the laparoscopic repair difficult and sometimes impossible.

Initially, laparoscopic hernia repairs consisted of bridging the defect with intraperitoneal mesh placement. Intraperitoneal mesh placement with anti-adhesive barriers, which avoid intestinal adhesions to the prosthetic material, is fast and easy and provides reasonable long-term recurrence-free results. When amenable, defect closure can be achieved with transfascial sutures. For larger defects, frequently seen in obese and morbidly obese patients, tension-free defect closure cannot be achieved without employing myofascial release techniques. In these cases, the open approach is preferable. There is no well-defined cutoff for defect size for laparoscopy. In general, we reserve laparoscopy for defects with less than 8 cm.

Laparoscopic Ventral Hernia Repair

In this section, we will describe step-by-step the standard laparoscopic ventral hernia repair with intraperitoneal mesh placement [38]. Preoperative optimization, as mentioned before, remains as important and shouldn't be deferred.

Surgical Planning Considerations

The surgeon has to keep in mind some contraindications for laparoscopy when making the decision to perform laparoscopic ventral hernia repair. Contraindications include loss of domain, skin alterations (ulcerations, skin grafts), active infection, hypercoagulability, and patient expectations (i.e., scar revision). Surgeons should reasonably consider their laparoscopic skills prior to undertaking laparoscopic ventral hernia repairs, since adhesiolysis will demand ability and patience, and outcomes will dramatically change if not correctly performed. Abdominal imaging should be obtained preoperatively, especially in the morbidly obese, helping to define defect size, hernia sac contents, previous intra-abdominal meshes, and loss of domain.

Operative Steps

1. Patient Preparation and Positioning

   Prophylactic antibiotics and thromboprophylaxis should be administered according to institutional protocols. Patients are placed supine with arms tucked to maximize intra-abdominal accessibility. In the morbidly obese, arm sleds are often required due to patient and surgical bed dimensions. For off-midline defects, a bump should be placed under the hip on the same side as the hernia. Bladder and gastric decompression should be obtained after induction of anesthesia.
2. First Port Placement and Pneumoperitoneum

   Figure 30.7 illustrates suggested port placement. Initial port placement should take into consideration previous surgeries and hernia location. Palmer's point (below left costal margin) is a safe area to gain abdominal access. We suggest using the cutdown technique, since adhesions from previous surgeries may lead to unrecognized bowel injuries during abdominal punction and first trocar placement. Once the abdominal cavity is accessed, two additional 5 mm trocars can be

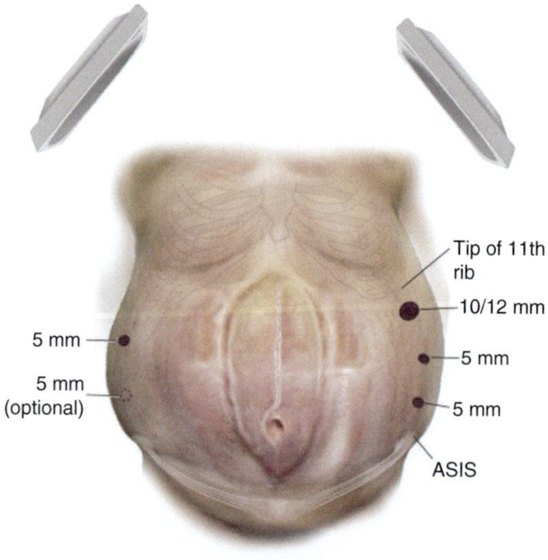

Fig. 30.7 Port placement. (Reprinted from: Atlas of Abdominal Wall Reconstruction, 2nd Edition, Michael J. Rosen, Laparoscopic Repair of Ventral Hernias: Standard, Chapter 2, Page 27, Copyright (2017), with permission from Elsevier)

placed laterally on the same side of the first trocar, under direct vision. Auxiliary 5 mm trocars can be positioned on the contralateral side and help visualization and traction during adhesiolysis.

3. Laparoscopic Adhesiolysis

   After all trocars are placed, all adhesions between visceral contents and the abdominal wall should be undertaken using exclusively cold, sharp dissection. It is critical to avoid using energy devices at this point, which could lead to thermal injuries. The primary tool during adhesiolysis will be endoscopic scissors, sharply dissecting and cutting adhesions while they are under traction with bowel graspers.

4. Sizing the Defect

   After all adhesions are taken down, measuring the defect is a critical step and shouldn't be neglected. We suggest measuring the defect inside the abdominal cavity and with the abdomen insufflated with the help of paper or plastic ruler. Spinal needles can be inserted into the defect edges to assist in measurement, but aren't mandatory. Hernia width and length should be measured in order to plan adequate mesh overlap. A minimum overlap of 4 cm is adequate for most hernias.

5. Defect Closure

   Transfascial sutures using permanent monofilament sutures are a fast way to achieve defect closure before mesh placement. Defect closure during laparoscopic ventral hernia repair has become routine since it's been associated with fewer seroma formation. This measure still lacks high-quality data to become a formal recommendation, but its benefits have already been addressed in case series and suggested by experienced laparoscopic hernia surgeons. Utilizing a Carter-Thomason suture passer, the defect can be closed with simple or figure-of-eight sutures. Starting at one of the defect's edges, a stab incision is made in the skin at the center of the defect. Under direct visualization, the suture passer device passes the permanent suture through the abdomen in one edge of the defect. Using the same stab incision, the device is passed on the contralateral edge of the defect and grasps the suture, pulling it out through the incision (Fig. 30.8).

   This process is repeated every 2–3 cm until the full length of the defect is approximated. After all sutures are passed, they can be tied down sequentially, with the abdomen deflated. After tying and cutting the sutures, a Kelly clamp is placed into the skin incision to allow the knot to fall below the skin. For smaller defects, surgeons skilled in laparoscopic suturing can close the defect intraperitoneally with the aid of barbed sutures in a running fashion.

6. Mesh Placement and Fixation

   Figure 30.9 illustrates mesh placement and fixation. The edges of the closed defect are marked on the skin with a surgical pen. Placing the mesh on the abdomen will help plan the adequate mesh overlap. Remember that meshes for laparoscopic ventral hernia repair must be coated with an antiadhesive barrier, preventing prosthetic material adhesions to intraperitoneal contents. After the size of the mesh is defined, sutures can be placed on its edges to allow pulling the mesh through the abdominal wall. We suggest using four nonabsorbable monofilament sutures, each placed on cardinal points. The tails of mesh sutures are tucked in, and the mesh is rolled and inserted through a 10–12 mm port. After mesh introduction, the mesh is unrolled and placed in the proper orientation. The sutures on cardinal edges of the mesh will help to achieve the correct orientation. The first suture to be pulled out is at the cranial edge of the mesh. A small stab incision is made in the appropriate location, and the suture is pulled out using the suture passer device. The same process is done with all cardinal sutures, leaving sutures untied and taut to the skin with hemostatic clamps. After all cardinal sutures are pulled out of the abdomen, they can be tied.

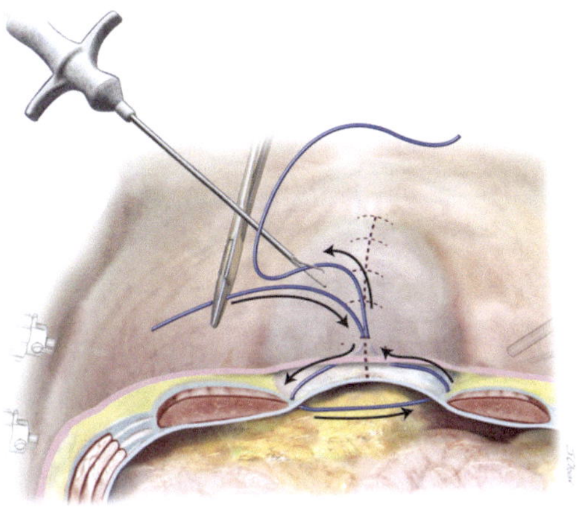

Fig. 30.8 Defect closure with transfascial sutures. (Reprinted from: Atlas of Abdominal Wall Reconstruction, 2nd Edition, Michael J. Rosen, Laparoscopic Repair of Ventral Hernias: Standard, Chapter 2, Page 32, Copyright (2017), with permission from Elsevier)

Tacks are then placed every 1 cm along the edge of the mesh circumferentially. A double-crown technique with an inner circle of tacks is placed in the periphery of the mesh. The inner row of tacks can be spaced out every 2–4 cm. If needed, additional transfascial sutures can be placed at this moment.

A careful review of the entire abdominal cavity is performed prior to removing the ports under direct visualization. If a 10 mm port was required, the fascia at the port site should be closed prior to terminating the operation.

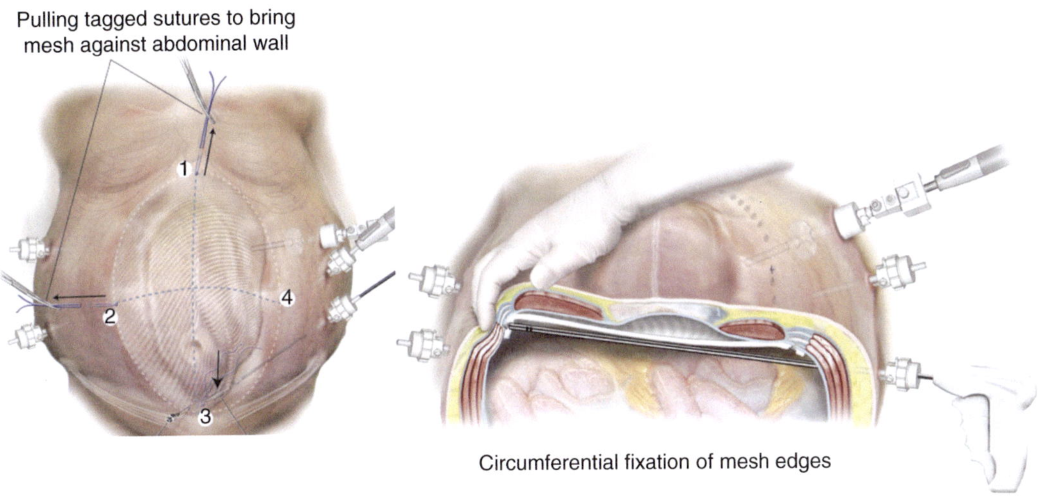

Fig. 30.9 Mesh placement and fixation. (Reprinted from: Atlas of Abdominal Wall Reconstruction, 2nd Edition, Michael J. Rosen, Laparoscopic Repair of Ventral Hernias: Standard, Chapter 2, Page 41, Copyright (2017), with permission from Elsevier)

Conclusion

Large ventral hernias in morbidly obese patients are a frequent and challenging clinical scenario that surgeons will be facing with increasing frequency on clinical practice. We have included three suggested algorithms according to our current practices to aid in surgeon decision-making (Figs. 30.10, 30.11, and 30.12), when dealing with morbidly obese patients with ventral hernias. Clinical judgment remains necessary to tailor the options of the surgical armamentarium according to patient's needs and expectations.

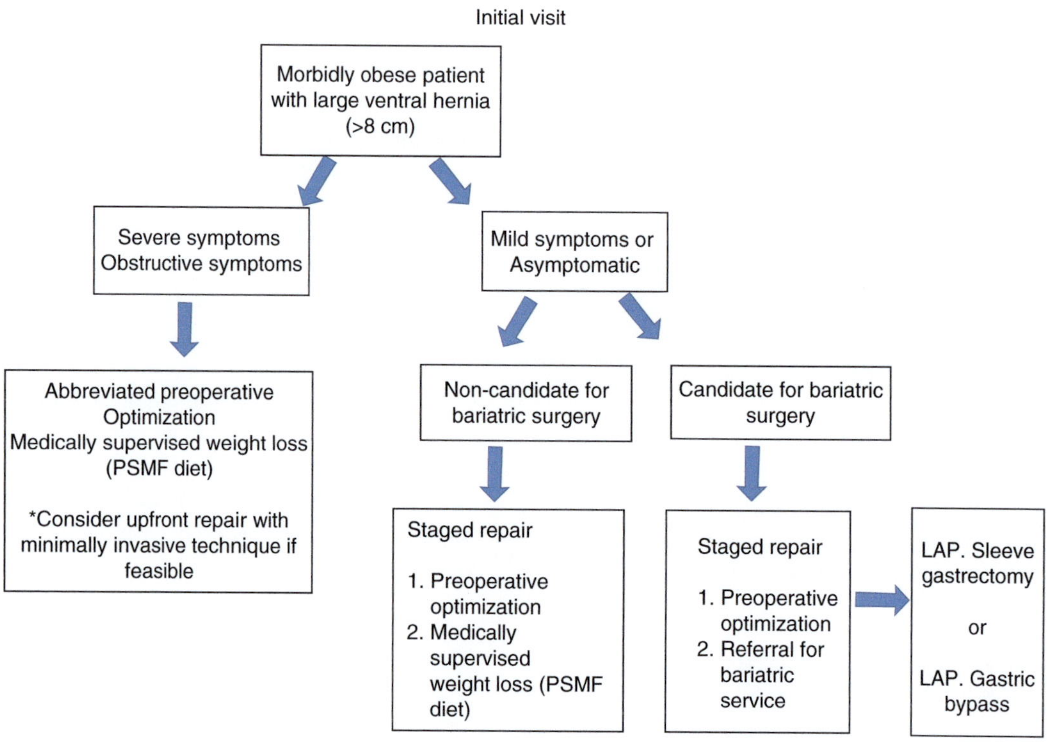

Fig. 30.10 Algorithm 1 – suggested management of morbidly obese patients with large ventral hernias

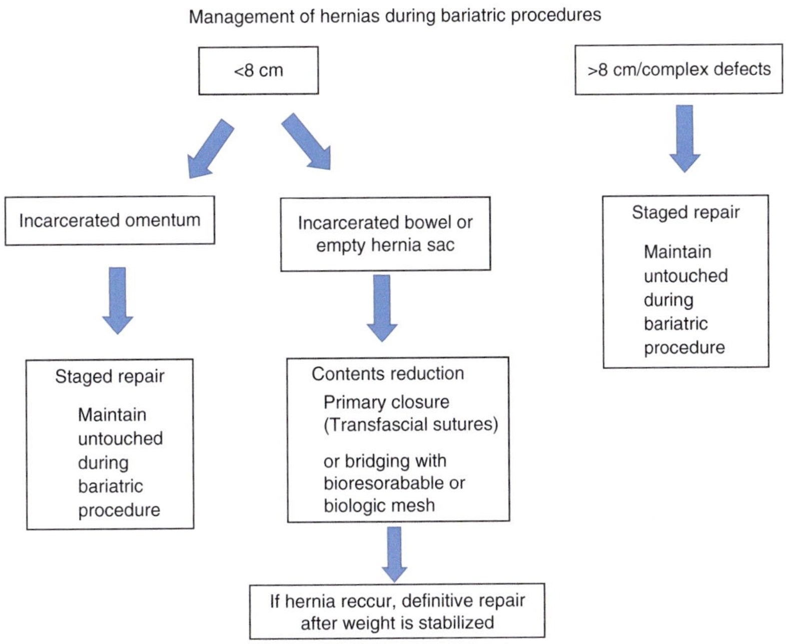

Fig. 30.11 Algorithm 2 – suggested management of hernias during bariatric procedures

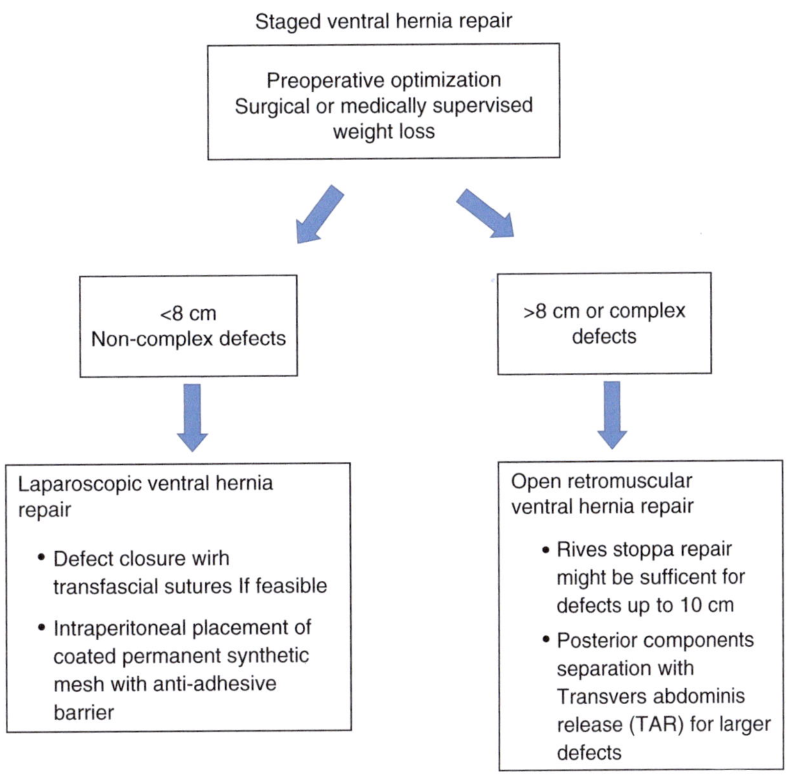

Fig. 30.12 Algorithm 3 – suggested operative strategy after preoperative optimization and weight loss

References

1. Ogden CL, Carroll MD, et al. Prevalence of obesity among adults and youth: United States, 2011–2014. NCHS Data Brief. 2015;219:1–8.
2. Rosen MJ, Aydogdu K, Grafmiller K, Petro CC, Faiman GH, Prabhu A. A multidisciplinary approach to medical weight loss prior to abdominal wall reconstruction: is it feasible? J Gastrointest Surg. 2015;19:1399–406.
3. Krpata DM, Criss CN, Gao Y, Sadava EE, Anderson JM, Novitsky YW, Rosen MJ. Effects of weight reduction surgery on the abdominal wall fascial wound healing process. J Surg Res. 2013:78–83.
4. Eid GM, Wikiel KJ, Entabi F, Saleem M. Ventral hernias in morbidly obese patients: a suggested algorithm for operative repair. Obes Surg. 2013;23: 703–9.
5. Sugerman HJ, Kellum JM Jr, Reines HD, et al. Greater risk of incisional hernia with morbidly obese than steroid-dependent patients and low recurrence with prefascial polypropylene mesh. Am J Surg. 1996;171(1):80–4.
6. Praveenraj P, Gomes RM, Kumar S, et al. Concomitant bariatric surgery with laparoscopic intra-peritoneal onlay mesh repair for recurrent ventral hernias in morbidly obese patients: an evolving standard of care. Obes Surg. 2016;26(6):1191–4.
7. Szczesny W, Bodnar M, Dabrowiecki S, et al. Histologic and immunohistochemical studies of rectus sheath in obese patients. J Surg Res. 2013;180(2): 260–5.
8. Klinge U, Si ZY, Zheng H, et al. Collagen I/III and matrix of metalloproteinases (MMP) 1 and 13 in the fascia of patients with incisional hernias. J Investig Surg. 2001;14(1):47–54.
9. Veljkovic R, Protic M, Gluhovic A, et al. Prospective clinical trial of factors predicting the early development of incisional hernia after midline laparotomy. J Am Coll Surg. 2010;210(2):210–9.
10. Newcomb WL, Polhill JL, Chen AY, et al. Staged hernia repair preceded by gastric bypass for the treatment of morbidly obese patients with complex ventral hernias. Hernia. 2008;12(5):465–9.
11. Tsereteli Z, Pryor BA, Heniford BT, Park A, Voeller G, Ramshaw BJ. Laparoscopic ventral hernia repair (LVHR) in morbidly obese patients. Hernia. 2008;12:233–8.
12. Hesselink VJ, Luijendijk RW, de Wilt JH, et al. An evaluation of risk factors in incisional hernia recurrence. Surg Gynecol Obstet. 1993;176(3):228–34.
13. Pitkin RM. Abdominal hysterectomy in obese women. Surg Gynecol Obstet. 1976;142(4):532–6.
14. Regnard JF, Hay JM, Rea S, Fingerhut A, Flamant Y, Maillard JN. Ventral incisional hernias: incidence, date of recurrence, localization and risk factors. Ital J Surg Sci. 18(3):259–65.
15. Rath AM, Chevrel JP. The healing of laparotomies: a bibliographic study. Hernia. 4:41–8.
16. Frezza EE, Shebani KO, Robertson J, Watchel MS. Morbid obesity causes chronic increase of intraabdominal pressure. Dig Dis Sci. 2007;52(4):1038–41.
17. Varela JE, Hinojosa M, Nguyen N. Correlations between intra-abdominal pressure and obesity-related co-morbidities. Surg Obes Relat Dis. 5(5): 524–8.
18. Kaoutzanis C, Leichtle SW, Mouawad NJ, et al. Risk factors for postoperative wound infections and prolonged hospitalization after ventral/incisional hernia repair. Hernia. 2015;19(1):113–23.
19. Fekkes JF, Velanovich V. Amelioration of the effects of obesity on short-term postoperative complications of laparoscopic and open ventral hernia repair. Surg Laparosc Endosc Percutan Tech. 2015;25(2): 151–7.
20. Le D, Deveney CW, Reaven NL, et al. Mesh choice in ventral hernia repair: so many choices, so little time. Am J Surg. 2013;205(5):602–7.
21. Fischer JP, Basta MN, Wink JD, et al. Optimizing patient selection in ventral hernia repair with concurrent panniculectomy: an analysis of 1974 patients from the ACS-NSQIP datasets. J Plast Reconstr Aesthet Surg. 2014;67(11):1532–40.
22. Berger RL, Li LT, Hicks SC, et al. Development and validation of a risk stratification score for surgical site occurrence and surgical site infection after open ventral hernia repair. J Am Coll Surg. 2013;217(6):974–82.
23. Goodenough CJ, Ko TC, Kao LS, et al. Development and validation of a risk stratification score for ventral incisional hernia after abdominal surgery: hernia expectation rates in intra-abdominal surgery (the HERNIA Project). J Am Coll Surg. 2015;220(4):405–13.
24. Buchwald H, Avidor Y, Braunwald E, et al. Bariatric surgery: a systematic review and meta-analysis. JAMA. 2004;292(14):1724–37.
25. Eid GM, Mattar SG, Hamad G, et al. Repair of ventral hernias in morbidly obese patients undergoing laparoscopic gastric bypass should not be deferred. Surg Endosc. 2004;18(2):207–10.
26. Rao RS, Gentileschi P, Kini SU. Management of ventral hernias in bariatric surgery. Surg Obes Relat Dis. 2011;7(1):110–6.
27. van't Riet M, Steyerberg EW, Nellensteyn J, et al. Meta-analysis of techniques for closure of midline abdominal incisions. Br J Surg. 89(11):1350–6.
28. Gurusamy KS, Cassar Delia E, Davidson BR. Peritoneal closure versus no peritoneal closure for patients undergoing non-obstetric abdominal operations. Cochrane Database Syst Rev. 2013;(7):CD010424. https://doi.org/10.1002/14651858.CD010424.pub2.
29. Muysoms FE, et al. European Hernia Society guidelines on the closure of abdominal wall incisions. Hernia. 2015;19(1):1–24.
30. Millbourn D, Cengiz Y, Israelsson LA. Effect of stitch length on wound complications after closure of midline incisions: a randomized controlled trial. Arch Surg. 2009;144(11):1056–9.

31. Diener MK, Voss S, Jensen K, Buchler MW, Seiler CM. Elective midline laparotomy closure: the INLINE systematic review and meta-analysis. Ann Surg. 2010;251(5):843–56.
32. Ramirez OM, Ruas E, Dellon AL. "Components separation" method for closure of abdominal wall defects: method for closure of abdominal wall defects: an anatomic and clinical study. Plast Reconstr Surg. 1990;86(3):519–26.
33. Rosen MJ. Posterior component separation with transversus abdominis release. In: Rosen MJ, editor. Atlas of abdominal wall reconstruction. 2nd ed. Philadelphia: Elsevier; 2017.
34. Novitsky YW, Cobb WS, Kercher KW, Matthews BD, Sing RD, Heniford BT. Laparoscopic ventral hernia repair in obese patients – a new standard of care. Arch Surg. 2006;141(1):57–61.
35. Park A, Birch DW, Lovrics P. Laparoscopic and open incisional hernia repair: a comparison study. Surgery. 1998;124(4):816–21.
36. Ramshaw BJ, Esartia P, Schwab J, et al. Comparison of laparoscopic and open ventral herniorrhaphy. Am Surg. 1999;65(9):827–31.
37. Heniford BT, Park A, Ramshaw BJ, Voeller G. Laparoscopic repair of ventral hernias: nine year's experience with 850 consecutive hernias. Ann Surg. 2003;238:391–9.
38. Orenstein SB, Cobb WS. Laparoscopic repair of ventral hernias: standard. Rosen MJ. Atlas of abdominal wall reconstruction. 2nd. Philadelphia: Elsevier; 2017.

31 Post-Bariatric Body Contouring

Ramsen Azizi

Introduction

Along with the increase of obesity in the general population has come an increase in bariatric surgery for its control. Patients who successfully undergo massive weight loss and attain their ideal weight are often left with a new body that brings its own challenges. These patients have developed a moderate to severe amount of skin excess and laxity and are enthusiastic to begin the reconstructive process. They should be congratulated on their weight loss and taking steps to ensure their own health as well as counseled pre- and postoperatively through the process. Although the rate of minor wound complications can be frequent, the vast majority of patients are very happy and satisfied with their newly contoured bodies.

Abdominoplasty

Introduction

One of the most commonly performed aesthetic procedures, and often the first procedure that massive weight loss patients undergo is abdominoplasty. It can make the most dramatic difference in the patient's body contour as well as helping to reshape an area that has been a lifetime concern. Patients who have been fortunate enough to lose a great amount of weight from bariatric surgery can have difficulty accepting their new body with the skin excess that has resulted [1]. Abdominoplasty can help to return the patient's self-confidence and renew their resolve in their new healthy lifestyle.

Several different abdominoplasty type excisions and resections have been developed since the procedure was first described in the late 1800s [2]. The classic and proven procedure as well as common modifications will be reviewed. Mastering the basic technique prior to adding modifications can help to decrease complications in the beginning learning curve.

History and Physical Exam

As with any procedure, a thorough history is essential. The goal is to identify patient's areas of concern and to rule out any habits which may lead to wound complications, nonadherence to recovery instructions, and suboptimal results. Interview should begin with noting patient's BMI, weight loss history and fluctuations, possibility of further weight loss, smoking history, and plans for further pregnancy. Ideal patients are those with excess of abdominal skin and with BMI scores of 30 or less. Slightly higher BMI patients can be selected if it is felt that the majority of their weight does not affect the abdominal region. However, careful attention must be paid to

R. Azizi
R.A.M. Plastic Surgery, Chicago, IL, USA
e-mail: DrAzizi@RAMPlasticSurgery.com

R. Lutfi et al. (eds.), *Global Bariatric Surgery*, https://doi.org/10.1007/978-3-319-93545-4_31

decreasing wound tension and limiting perforator dissection in order to decrease complications. Patients who are current or casual smokers are contraindicated to undergo abdominoplasty and procedure should be postponed until they are able to stop smoking. Studies have shown that patients should stop smoking at least 4 weeks prior to surgery [3]. If there is skepticism of the patient's nonadherence to smoking cessation protocol, it is prudent to have a urine nicotine test done on the day of surgery or to delay indefinitely.

Patients that are actively losing weight stand to have better postoperative results if surgery is performed after weight has been stable for 3–6 months. Excellent surgical results can often turn into average results if the patient loses or gains significant weight after the procedure. History and lab values should also investigate any nutritional deficiencies the patient may have. The vast majority of bariatric patients presenting for abdominoplasty have stable weight and are taking multivitamins. However, many over-the-counter multivitamins can contain ingredients that increase bleeding and therefore should be stopped along with aspirin, 2 weeks prior to surgery [4]. For optimal results, patients who are still planning on becoming pregnant are counseled to delay surgery until they have completed having children. However, pregnancies after abdominal contouring have still been shown to have enduring results [5].

Physical examination should carefully include the entire abdominal wall and flanks. Special concerns are paid to any previous surgical scars that may have affected blood supply to the abdominal wall. Lower abdominal appendectomy, cesarean section, and hysterectomy scars generally do not affect abdominoplasty results and can be included in the excision pattern for an improved result. Laparoscopic access scars do not significantly affect blood flow. However, open cholecystectomy, transverse upper abdominal, or laparotomy scars can leave reverse abdominoplasty as the patient's only option. The majority of patients have lower abdominal striae indicating a degree of irreversible skin damage. It should be noted to patients that striae above the umbilicus will unlikely be removed.

Examination should note the extent of rectus diastasis and abdominal wall laxity. If there is concern of ventral hernia, it is prudent to have CT imaging to help with surgical planning. Small- or medium-sized umbilical hernias can easily be repaired during the procedure. A large amount of patients have increased fat and fullness in the upper midline abdomen. These areas of fullness should be noted to patients preoperatively as regions that will have limited improvement after the procedure. Patients with BMI levels higher than 30 should also be counseled of a significantly increased thromboembolic risk. Caprini scores should be calculated in all patients in order to identify those that need preoperative prophylactic heparin and early ambulation [6]. It is much easier to treat mildly increased bleeding than a DVT or pulmonary embolism in an elective procedure.

Special attention should also be paid to the distance between the umbilicus and the proposed lower abdominal scar. This is the area that the umbilicus excision site needs to traverse in order to not result in a vertical scar at the lower abdomen. Patients with a large excess of lower abdominal skin on "pinch" test can be identified as having a more straightforward excision with minimal undermining. In patients with less lower abdominal laxity and a large umbilical to scar distance, "floating" of the umbilicus should be considered. In this modification, the umbilicus is left connected to the surrounding skin and the lower stalk is transected. It is allowed to move downward a conservative distance and does not need to be inset back into the flap as with traditional abdominoplasty.

Abdominoplasty Procedure

The procedure begins with preoperative markings while the patient is standing. It is helpful to have the patient wear their typical bathing suit or underwear in order to mark an inferior excision that is lower. The midline of the patient is first marked from the xyphoid down to the midline mons or penis. The midline, inferior scar is marked in a range of 6–8 cm above the vaginal introitus. Placing it at the 6 cm mark can increase tension on the wound and also create a temporary change in the urethral angle. However, placing it at the 8 cm mark can cause a high-riding scar with which patients are not satisfied. For the beginning surgeon, placing the scar at unstretched skin 7 cm above the introitus allows an acceptable compromise that can be changed with more experience.

The elliptical excision pattern markings are drawn out with a gradual line that moves laterally from this first midline mark. The classic teaching is to mark to the laterality level of the anterior superior iliac spine (although not as high). However, if the patient has significant flank fullness, they are often happy to have this removed in exchange for a longer scar. It is helpful to mark the superior aspect of the proposed elliptical excision pattern. It can help as a guide during surgery if the upper abdominal flap is either more or less difficult to mobilize as expected. The upper markings are begun with placing a transverse line about 1 cm above the umbilicus and gradually curving the line down to both lower corner markings.

The procedure is performed with the patient supine, routine preoperative antibiotics, and sequential compression devices on the lower legs. The lower transverse incision is made and dissection is taken down to the level of the anterior rectus fascia. Medium to large vessels such as the inferior superficial epigastrics can be ligated with hemoclips. Dissection is then taken superiorly toward the umbilicus. Dissection is relatively easily done in the loose areolar plane above the rectus, but some surgeons find that leaving a "carpet" of fat or areolar tissue on the fascia decreases postoperative serous drainage. Once the level of the umbilicus is attained, attention is turned to the overlying skin. The umbilicus is marked in a circle around its margins and the skin is incised. Metzenbaum scissors can be used to dissect around the umbilicus down to the anterior rectus fascia. Careful attention must be paid to saving a rim of periumbilical fat as this is where the vascular supply comes from. About 1 cm of periumbilical fat can be left in place to protect these perforators. Once the umbilicus has been dissected away from the abdominal wall skin and flap, it can be helpful to incise the inferior abdominal flap vertically, from the umbilical defect down to the lower abdominal transverse incision. This is done in full thickness through the flap and leaves two triangular portions of tissue that will eventually become the final excision.

Dissection is continued past the umbilicus, upward toward the costal margins. Medium to large perforators are often encountered and it is helpful to ligate these to limit postoperative hematoma. The traditional teaching is to undermine to the level of the xiphoid in the midline and the costal margins laterally. It should be noted that the more undermining this is done laterally, the more that vital perforators will be coagulated. A good technique for the new abdominoplasty surgeon is to create a narrow tunnel of dissection in the midline above the umbilicus. The margins of this tunnel can be the linea semilunaris. If there is increased tension of the closure or dimpling of the upper abdominal skin, more lateral resection can be done as needed.

Once the upper flap has been elevated, the markings for rectus plication can be made. The medial edge of the rectus muscle is identified either by visual inspection or using the electrocautery to cause muscle contraction. The medial edge is marked from the xiphoid down to the pubic tubercle. Both edges can be grasped with an Allis clamp and brought together to test the tension. The plication can be done with either permanent or long duration absorbable suture and with either interrupted or running fashion. The author uses a tensile strength 0 barbed 6-month-long duration absorbable suture to run from the xiphoid down to the level of the inferior rectus attachment. Careful attention is paid to only pass the needle through the medial edge of the fascia and not the muscle itself. A long umbilical stalk will often retract downward by plicating the rectus around it. However, it is important not to constrict the stalk and the aforementioned periumbilical perforators. After the initial running suture, the author reinforces the repair with several, interrupted permanent 0 sutures over the previous suture.

After the rectus plication is done, the operating table is reflexed so the hips are bent at about a 20–30° angle. This allows the upper flap to come down to the lower incision and decreases tension on the closure. If undue tension is encountered at this stage, more lateral dissection up to the costal margins can be done. In the rare patient, it may be necessary to leave a small vertical element of the scar in the midline to facilitate closure. As the superior flap is brought inferiorly, progressive tension sutures can be used to decrease the dead space and relieve tension off the closure. This has been shown to decrease seroma risk, as well [7]. For this technique, absorbable 2-0 Vicryl suture is used to suture the underside of the flap to the anterior rectus fascia. This is done symmetrically from a superior to inferior fashion.

Two 10 mm drains are typically placed in the dissection space. It is important to mark the location on the umbilicus on the anterior abdominal wall for later inset prior to closing the incision. The Scarpa's fascia layer is then approximated with interrupted sutures from the midline to approximately 15 cm laterally. The author prefers to use 2-0 Vicryl suture for this portion. It is helpful to place a few of the sutures through the anterior rectus fascia to prevent upward scar migration due to tension. Finally, the skin is closed with multiple interrupted, buried dermal sutures and a running subcuticular with a 3-0 Monocryl. The final part of the procedure is the umbilicus inset. Various incision types have been reported for inset (gentle "V" shape, vertical "cross" shape, inverted "V"). These eventually become a personal decision of the surgeon as to which aesthetic is desired. After the incision has been made in the aforementioned marked location, dissection is done with electrocautery to ensure hemostasis of the tunnel. The umbilicus is delivered anteriorly and sutured into place with interrupted dermal and running subcuticular sutures.

Steristrips and gauze sterile dressings are placed over all incisions. It can be beneficial to place a small wad of Xeroform in the umbilicus to aid in keeping its shape until the first postoperative appointment.

Recovery

The patient is allowed to shower after 48 h but no bathing or soaking for 2 weeks. Patients are kept in an abdominal binder for a minimum of 3 weeks after surgery. This is done to decrease edema through compression as well as to serve as a gentle reminder to limit abdominal activity. The patients are instructed to sleep in a semi-fowler "beach chair" position to take tension off of the incision. Drains are removed when they capture less than 30 mL of fluid per 24 h period, which typically takes 1–2 weeks. A small portion of patients may feel more tired than normal for the 1st month after surgery, but it is important to have a low threshold for dyspnea and pulmonary embolism workup. Small dehiscence of wounds is treated with daily bacitracin and gauze dressing. The vast majority of dehiscence closes without surgical intervention. The majority of edema in the anterior abdomen resolves in 3 weeks, but patients are instructed that it may last as long as 2–3 months. They are allowed to begin light exercise at 6 weeks and to gradually increase as tolerated.

Breast Contouring

Introduction

Breast lift surgery has grown 97% from 2000 to 2016 according to American Society of Plastic Surgeons statistics [8]. Following massive weight loss (MWL), the breasts will often undergo dramatic changes. Women who have become used to larger breasts are now faced with both ptosis as well as volume loss. However, the changes seen with MWL are often more severe than with natural aging.

Several characteristic changes are seen in the MWL breast. Most significant is upper pole deflation and volume loss. The skin has typically been stretched beyond its limits and presents with severe stretch damage. The nipples become more medialized and grade 3 ptosis is very common. Asymmetry in the MWL breast is often the rule rather than the exception. Lack of definition in the lateral breast happens as it begins to blend with the lateral chest rolls from the back [9].

History and Physical Exam

History begins with evaluating for occult breast pathology. History of breast lumps, abnormal discharge, pain, or suspicious mammograms is ruled out. Family history of breast cancer must be investigated prior to any breast surgery. Patients are expected to have a stable weight for at least 3–6 months and have no realistic plans for further weight loss. In the event of active weight loss, patients are encouraged to delay surgery until they have stabilized. Not only does this optimize the results of surgery, but it decreases the chances of future revisional surgery. Patients 50 years and older require a mammogram, and most surgeons will get one for 40-year-old patients, prior to surgery. Women who are younger than 40 with suspicious findings on exam or family history of breast cancer should undergo preoperative imaging [10]. Smoking is an absolute contraindication and should be eliminated at least 4 weeks prior to surgery. Active smokers are counseled about the vastly increased risk of wound healing problems and overall complication risk.

Physical exam begins with inspection for masses and clinically positive lymph nodes. Routine measurements are taken of the suprasternal notch to nipple distance, breast width, and nipple to inframammary fold (IMF) distance. It is helpful to document nipple to midline distance with asymmetrical breasts. The quality of the breast soft tissue envelope is examined. Severe skin damage evidence often will predispose patients to soft tissue envelopes that will stretch after surgery [11]. It may be necessary to do more parenchymal shaping in these patients than to rely on a “skin-only” mastopexy technique for increased longevity of results. Raising the deflated breast to the appropriate position and simulating the mastopexy result help in determining if patients need volume augmentation. Those patients who are unhappy with the size of their breasts while wearing a bra often will need a breast implant to increase volume and upper pole fullness.

The Pittsburgh Rating Scale was developed by Song et al. to describe post-bariatric body shapes and give relative recommendations for treatment. Patients with grade 1 breasts (ptosis grade 1/2 or severe macromastia) are benefitted by traditional vertical or Wise pattern mastopexy, reduction, or augmentation techniques. Those with grade 2 breasts (ptosis grade 3 or moderate volume loss) can be treated with traditional mastopexy with or without augmentation. Patients with grade 3 breasts (severe lateral rolls or volume loss with loose skin) are treated with auto-augmentation using parenchymal flaps and dermal suspension to the pectoralis [12]. The overall goals of MWL breast shaping is to raise the nipple to the appropriate position, tighten the overall skin envelope, and reshape the parenchyma into a more pleasing shape.

Mastopexy Procedure with Auto-augmentation

In MWL patients, it is helpful to recruit as much of their native breast parenchyma as possible during the lifting procedure. Despite appearing very deflated and ptotic, the breasts can have a surprisingly high amount of volume in the parenchyma once it becomes lifted to the appropriate position. The patient is marked in the standing position with the full weight of gravity. Vertical lines are drawn from the clavicle down the breast and onto the abdomen to mark the breast meridian. This confirms the future midline of the breast. Next, the inframammary fold (IMF) is transposed onto the anterior breast and marked at the meridian line. This will become the future nipple position. A keyhole marking pattern can be done at this point which predetermines the excision pattern for the future nipple-areola complex. However, for the beginning surgeon, it can be advantageous to mark the excision pattern without committing to the areola and do an inset/marking intraoperatively. In this case, the previous nipple marking is used as a guideline for an equilateral triangle with 8 cm arms. The apex of the triangle is placed 1 cm above the nipple marking and the bottom line is not drawn. The traditional Wise pattern markings are then done, with gentle curving line from the inferior aspect of the vertical 8 cm limps both medially and laterally to meet the IMF. The IMF is marked from the medial fold of the breast to the lateral extension of the breast. Often, the lateral marking is longer due to increased breast fullness in this region. An 8–10-cm-wide inferior pedicle is marked from the IMF up to the level of the current nipple. The lateral pedicle markings are curved above the current nipple, leaving at least 2 cm above in all directions.

The procedure is performed in the supine position, ensuring the bed can be raised to 90° to check for symmetry intraoperatively. Routine preoperative antibiotic and sequential compression device prophylaxis is used. A 42 mm cookie cutter is used to mark out the margins of the areola. The inferior pedicle is sharply de-epithelialized with a scalpel from the previously mentioned 2 cm semicircular rim down to the IMF. Electrocautery can be used to remove the medial pole and lateral pole skin overlying the triangular breast parenchyma tissue in the excision pattern. The medial, superior, and lateral breast skin flap is dissected using electrocautery. This is done with at least a 2 cm width of skin and fat (about twice the thickness of a thick mastectomy flap. The primary goal here is not to skeletonize the skin flaps, but to allow a robust blood supply to course through the fat down to the distal edges of the flap. There are significant perforators at the medial T2 intercostal level as well as from the superior, lateral thoracoacromial region which should be avoided during dissection. The superior flap is dissected up to the level of the clavicle. This aids in allowing room for the inferior pedicle to lie within the new soft tissue envelope.

When dissecting the posterior and lateral margins of the inferior pedicle, care must be taken to bevel the electrocautery away from pedicle tissue in order to not undermine it accidentally. Dissection is taken down to the pectoralis fascia. Leaving a "carpet" of 1 cm of parenchyma on the pectoralis muscle decreases postoperative pain and minimizes pectoralis trauma. Once the superior breast flaps and inferior pedicle have been dissected and the excess tissue eliminated, breast shaping can begin. The medial and lateral triangular extensions of the inferior pedicle are rotated upward 90° and sutured with absorbable 2-0 braided suture to the inferior pedicle. This allows both medial and lateral fullness to remain and maximizes the use of remaining parenchyma following massive weight loss. A temporary 3-0 silk suture is used to bring together the superior flap corners to the "triple point" at the midline of the lower inferior pedicle. The vertical and transverse incisions are then tailor tacked with staples, and the bed is adjusted to bring the patient to a sitting position to evaluate for symmetry.

At this point, the breasts are evaluated for symmetry and areas of excess fullness can be marked for excision. If volume is satisfactorily symmetrical, the previous cookie cutter is used to mark the nipple-areola inset. The ideal inset is at the most projected portion of the breast and typically lies at the superior aspect of the vertical scar. Ideal nipple position is 5–7 cm above the IMF. It is beneficial to use a loose silk tie suture to compare the sternal notch to nipple distance from the left to right breast for symmetry. Care must be taken to not place the nipple position too high. As the lower breast skin settles and expands in the postoperative position, the nipple can come to migrate too high or point upward. A high-riding nipple is difficult for the patient to mask while wearing swimwear or revealing blouses.

The patient is laid back down flat, and the vertical and horizontal skin is closed with 3-0 Monocryl absorbable suture and a running 3-0 Monocryl subcuticular suture. The marked areola position is sharply incised and removed full thickness with its parenchyma with electrocautery. It is helpful to bevel outward slightly so as not to create a tight "tunnel" for the nipple-areola complex to be pulled through. Once the complex is carefully brought through the new inset position, it is sutured into place circumferentially with 3-0 Monocryl interrupted dermal sutures and a running 4-0 Monocryl subcuticular suture. Sterile dressings are applied as well as a surgical bra.

Recovery

The patient is allowed to shower in 48 h, but it is helpful to avoid direct water to the incisions on the chest. It is recommended to wear the surgical bra as much as possible during the first 2–3 weeks. This helps the patient's comfort and support, as well as decreasing edema. Ecchymosis generally resolves in 1–2 weeks. Edema can last for up to 2 months, but the majority resolves in 4 weeks. Patients are allowed to wear a bra that is more comfortable to them at the 4 week point. However, they must avoid an underwire bra in order to not add pressure to the transverse incision. If wound dehiscence occurs, it is most commonly at the inferior "triple point." Typically this happens in a minor fashion with less than 1 cm of separation or epidermolysis. It is treated with bacitracin daily dressings and generally heals very well in this hidden area. Patients are asked to follow up at 1 week, 2 weeks, 1 month, 3 months, 6 months, and 1 year postoperatively to observe healing and "settling" of the breast shape.

Upper Extremity Contouring

Introduction

One of the greatest complaints of patients with massive weight loss is the resultant excess skin and tissue at the proximal upper extremity. Brachioplasty is often the next procedure patients undergo after breast and trunk reshaping. The scar in the upper extremity is not as easily hidden as the abdomen. Therefore, patients must be counseled that brachioplasty is a "trade-off" between the hanging skin they dislike and a scar that can often become hypertrophic due to the mobility of the region. Despite this concern, the vast majority of patients are very much satisfied with the new contour and ability to more easily shop for clothing [13].

History and Physical Exam

History should include the amount of weight loss and ability to remain stable at their new lower weight. If patients are still losing significant weight, the excision procedure should be delayed until they are stable for a period of at least 3 months. Patients should be asked to describe any history of localized rashes, lymphedema, nerve sensation changes, areas of particular concern, and goals of surgery.

When examining the arm in the MWL patient, it can be helpful to assess the skin and fat separately. Skin exam should include noting which areas from proximal to distal have the majority of excess. This helps to guide the extent to which an incision must be made [14]. Next, one should note which areas of localized adiposity remain. Patients often have localized adiposity on the posterior upper extremity, and the excess skin lies medial and anterior. Deflation of the skin comes with descent of the posterior axillary fold when the patient abducts the arm. The region of the mid-humerus will often have the greatest degree of descent, followed by the proximal arm. Care should be taken to determine if the skin excess extends onto the upper lateral chest wall.

Surgical Decision-Making

Both liposuction and skin excision are tools to reshape the proximal upper extremity. The choice of modality is dictated by degree of skin excess and presence of skin damage in the form of stretch marks. It is rare to find a MWL patient with a mild to moderate amount of localized adiposity and good skin quality. However, these patients are best served with conservative liposuction. Good skin quality will often benefit the patient by properly retracting following liposuction. Patients who have a moderate to high amount of skin excess will require a skin excisional procedure with or without the use of liposuction. The upper extremity is not as forgiving as the trunk when treated with liposuction. Therefore, it is prudent to have a low threshold for skin excision procedures.

The majority of patients have a combination of moderate to severe skin excess as well as localized adiposity on the posterior arm. These patients can be treated with either a combination liposuction and brachioplasty procedure or a staged excision. Patients who have mild to moderate posterior arm adiposity are able to be treated with liposuction at the beginning of procedure then an excision of the resultant skin excess as it is drawn up medially. Those who still have a large amount of fat on the posterior arm and a severe skin excess should be offered a staged procedure. In these cases, more fat is able to be removed in the initial liposuction procedure, and the skin is allowed to retract. A second procedure in 3 months' time can then be performed to excise the resultant skin excess.

Brachioplasty Procedure

The patient is seen in the preoperative area and marked in the standing position with arms abducted 90° at the axilla. Markings are done in order to have the final scar lie just posterior to the bicipital groove. This allows the scar to be hidden while the arms are in a relaxed position, as well as from anterior and posterior views. While the patient holds their arms in the "victory" position, an initial line is drawn from the axilla, across the bicipital groove, to just medial to the elbow. The distal aspect of the line corresponds with the distal excess of skin. Next, the previously drawn line is pulled downward with the left hand to simulate tension and the right hand marks where it previously lay as the anterior/upper aspect of the excision. The medial apex of the ellipse in the axilla is then drawn downward, curving slightly. This is taken down to the inferior extent of skin excess on the lateral chest wall, if present. It is often no more than 6 cm. A pinch test of the inferior/posterior aspect of skin is done to determine the posterior extent of the excision. It is pulled upward toward the superior anchor line and the skin is marked. This creates the lower/posterior line of the ellipse of excision. This is taken from the distal elbow mark to the proximal axilla mark. It is then curved downward toward the inferior apex of the previously marked 6 cm vertical axilla line. The inferior line is only a guide. Vertical hash marks are drawn across the arm to help with alignment intraoperatively.

The patient is laid in the supine position with the arms abducted to 90°. Standard sterile prep is used. One percent lidocaine with epinephrine is infiltrated into the incision lines to help with hemostasis. The vertical axillary line is incised along with the superior anchor line. Dissection is taken down through the subcutaneous fat into a level just above the brachial fascia. Care must be taken to leave a small "carpet" of tissue on the brachial fascia to preserve the medial antebrachial cutaneous nerve. It is often seen in the middle of the dissection. A uniform flap thickness is carried posteriorly at the level of the brachial fascia toward the previously marked "pinch test" line. Once the tissues have been fully undermined, the flap is brought upward toward the anchor line. The previous vertical hash marks act as guides for the segmental resection.

The lower flap is held with penetrating towel clamps at its edge and brought up and over the superior anchor line. The resection level is double checked at this point. Starting at the distal most hash mark, a knife is used to incise vertically downward until the lower flap meets the superior anchor line. A staple holds this temporarily together. The other two proximal hash marks are incised vertically in the same fashion. This segmental type resection ensures that too much skin is never removed and is a safe way to eliminate difficulties in closure. The final excess skin is drawn into the axilla, and the incision is drawn downward to meet the inferior axilla vertical marking. This leaves a 90° final scar at the axilla which prevents scar contracture mobility issues. Using a 2-0 permanent suture, the superficial fascial system of the inferior flap is sutured to the clavipectoral fascia at the axilla. This prevents scar migration and hypertrophy in the final result. The incision is closed with 2-0 Vicryl suture for the superficial fascial system approximation. Following, 3-0 Monocryl interrupted dermal sutures and a running 3-0 Monocryl subcuticular suture are used for the skin closure. Drains are typically not needed in the author's opinion, although may be used. Adhesive sterile tape strips are applied to the incisions, and an ACE elastic wrap is placed from the elbows to the axilla. In lieu of wrapping the arms from wrist to axilla, the patient is told that they will have distal arm swelling secondary to the upper arm wraps.

Recovery

The ACE wraps are removed on the 1st week postoperative visit, and more comfortable shirts with compressive sleeves are encouraged for the first 3 weeks. Patients are encouraged to begin range of motion movement at 1 week but to continue to avoid heavy lifting for 3 weeks. If the medial antebrachial cutaneous nerve was not transected, distal parasthesias are generally temporary and return to normal in a couple months. Scar reduction techniques such as scar massage and silicone strip therapy are begun at the 3-week point to attempt to prevent hypertrophy. It is not uncommon to have small areas of dehiscence, and these are treated with bacitracin daily dressings in the traditional fashion. Patients are instructed preoperatively and reminded at the 3 week point that scars will continue to improve over the course of the year.

Thigh Contouring

Introduction

One of the greatest areas of concern for MWL patients is the medial thigh excess tissue that develops. Complaints include persistent rashes, difficulty with clothing, and a general dissatisfaction with the appearance of the excess skin. The thighs are a complex area to reconstruct. The medial thigh tissues have less adherent skin and fat than laterally which leads to significant descent. Lateral and medial aspects of the thigh are treated separately and each side influences the other to a very limited degree. For the scope of this chapter, focus will be on medial thigh contouring as this area is most often symptomatic in MWL patients.

History and Physical Exam

As with all MWL patients, a stable weight for at least 3 months is the initial requirement. Patients should attempt to achieve their goal weight before undergoing thigh resection procedures because laxity after further weight loss is difficult to correct. History of lymphedema, lower extremity surgery, rashes, and areas of concern should be noted. On physical exam, one should note the distal extent of skin excess. The area around the knee will occasionally have increased adiposity which requires an element of liposuction rather than skin excision. Performing a "pinch test" of the medial thigh tissues aids in showing the patient the extent of improvement as well as indicating that lateral thigh will be relatively unaffected. In patients who have significant adiposity still, one can consider doing a two-stage procedure. The first stage is a relatively aggressive debulking liposuction of the stubborn areas. This is followed by the actual skin excision medial thigh lift procedure. In the initial consultation, patients are also instructed that there is a relatively high rate of minor wound healing complications, but the procedure has been found to improve the quality of life overall.

Medial Thigh Lift Procedure

The patient is marked while lying in bed with the legs abducted in a "frog leg" position. A curvilinear vertical line is marked lateral to the mons, along the perineal crease into the posterior part of the mid-thigh. The medial thigh skin is pulled anteriorly to simulate tension and the perineal line is extended longitudinally downward toward the knee. It ends just proximal to the medial knee, where the skin excess dissipates. Using a "pinch test" of the medial thigh skin, the anterior aspect of the excision is marked from superior to inferior. A gentle line joins these pinch test markings from the superior aspect of the perineal marking down toward the previously marked distal incision. The anterior marked line serves as an estimate of how much skin will be resected, whereas the posterior line is generally the scar anchor line. A final pinch test of the entire elliptical-shaped segment ensures adequate skin has been marked for removal. Transverse hash marks made every 6 cm are helpful in alignment at the end of surgery.

The patient is brought into the operating room and placed in a "frog leg" position. The leg skin is prepped in the standard sterile fashion circumferentially. The incisions are infiltrated with 1% lidocaine with epinephrine to help with hemostasis. The anterior incision is made first from the perineum down to the knee. Dissection is kept at just deep to the subcutaneous fat level, ensuring that the saphenous system is not injured. Using electrocautery, dissection is taken posteriorly, toward the previously marked posterior suture anchor line. Once this is reached, the skin flap is held with penetrating towel clamps and pulled up and over the anterior incision. A pinch test is once again done to ensure that the posterior line reaches the anterior one [15].

Starting distally, the first hash mark is incised from the flap edge until the anterior incision is reached. A temporary towel clamp or staple is placed here to hold the posterior flap to the anterior incision. Then, moving sequentially through the hash marks from distal to proximal, the resection is segmentally done and temporarily stapled in place. The final amount of excess skin is drawn up into the perineal region and incised to prevent a "dog ear." At this point, each segment is incised where it meets the anterior incision. Tension is avoided especially in the female perineal area in order to prevent labial spreading, postoperatively. Ten millimeter drains are placed from the perineum and into the distal aspect of the dissection in order to collect the gravity-dependent drainage. The incisions are closed with 2-0 braided absorbable suture for the superficial fascial system. This is followed by 3-0 absorbable monofilament interrupted dermal sutures and a running 3-0 absorbable monofilament subcuticular suture. Sterile dressing adhesive tape is used to offload more tension from the wound. The legs are wrapped with an ACE bandage for compression.

Recovery

The patient is seen 1 week postoperatively. The drains are removed when they reach less than 30 cc of fluid in a 24 h period. ACE wraps are kept for 4 weeks postoperatively, but patients are allowed to switch into compressive legwear if that is more tolerable. Patients are instructed to avoid strenuous activity for 3 weeks postoperatively. It is relatively common to have small areas of delayed wound healing. These are treated with daily bacitracin dressing changes and allowed to close spontaneously. Scar improvement techniques such as massage and silicone therapy are instituted at the 3 week mark. Lower extremity edema is very common in the first few weeks after surgery and patients are instructed to use elevation to decrease this.

Conclusion

Although the rate of minor wound healing complications is common in post-bariatric body contouring, the ultimate result is very satisfactory. Patients are ready to transition into their newly contoured bodies as a reward for having lost all their excess weight. Staging procedures help with decreasing operative times and improving recovery when there is only a single surgeon available for the operation. Proper patient selection, discussion of realistic expectations, conservative and safe operative technique, and management of minor complications make way for a very happy patient population.

References

1. Song AY, Rubin JP, Thomas V, Dudas JR, Marra KG, Fernstrom MH. Body image and quality of life in post massive weight loss body contouring patients. Obesity. 2006;14(9):1626–36.
2. Moufarrege R. The moufarrège horseshoe abdominoplasty. Aesthet Surg J. 1997;17(2):91–6.
3. Mustoe TA, Rohrich R. Clearing the smoke: the scientific rationale for tobacco abstention with plastic surgery by Jeffery K. Krueger, M.D. Rodney J. Rohrich, M.D. Plast Reconstr Surg. 2001;108(4):1074–5.
4. Wang C-Z, Moss J, Yuan C-S. Commonly used dietary supplements on coagulation function during surgery. Medicines. 2015;2(4):157–85.
5. Nahas F. Pregnancy after abdominoplasty. Aesthet Plast Surg. 2002;26(4):284–6.
6. Gutowski KA. Evidence based medicine. Plast Reconstr Surg. 2018;141:286e–99e.

7. Janis JE, Khansa L, Khansa I. Strategies for postoperative seroma prevention. Plast Reconstr Surg. 2016;138(1):240–52.
8. Plastic Surgery Statistics. American Society of Plastic Surgeons. https://www.plasticsurgery.org/news/plastic-surgery-statistics. Accessed 8 Feb 2018.
9. Rubin JP, Gusenoff JA, Coon D. Dermal suspension and parenchymal reshaping mastopexy after massive weight loss: statistical analysis with concomitant procedures from a prospective registry. Plast Reconstr Surg. 2009;123(3):782–9.
10. Greco R, Noone B. Evidence-based medicine. Plast Reconstr Surg. 2017;139(1):204e–29e.
11. Coombs DM, Srivastava U, Amar D, Rubin JP, Gusenoff JA. The challenges of augmentation mastopexy in the massive weight loss patient. Plast Reconstr Surg. 2017;139(5):1090–9.
12. Pang JH, Coombs DM, James I, Fishman J, Rubin JP, Gusenoff JA. Characterizing breast deformities after massive weight loss. Ann Plast Surg. 2018:1. https://doi.org/10.1097/sap.0000000000001338.
13. De Runz A, et al. Liposuction-assisted medial brachioplasty after massive weight loss. Plast Reconstr Surg. 2015;135(1):74e–84e.
14. Nguyen AT, Rohrich RJ. Liposuction-assisted posterior brachioplasty: technical refinements in upper arm contouring. Plast Reconstr Surg. 2010;126(4):1365–9.
15. Armijo BS, et al. Four-step medial thighplasty. Plast Reconstr Surg. 2014;5:134.

The Super Super-Obese

32

Kelvin D. Higa and Alan C. Wittgrove

Super-obesity as defined as BMI (body mass index) > 50 Kg/m^2 appears to be increasing at a faster rate than BMI < 50 kg/m^2. This is relevant as individuals with higher BMIs are more likely to have more complex health issues such as obstructive sleep apnea, metabolic syndrome, and hepatic steatosis which are associated with higher surgical risk, readmission rates, and long-term complications [1]. Also, higher BMIs have been shown to be more resilient to treatment, with less absolute weight loss and comorbidity resolution [2]. See Figs. 32.1 and 32.2.

The higher surgical risk and the trend to offer more complex operations, such as the duodenal switch, have prompted recommendations for the super-obese individuals to have surgery only at accredited centers. However, with the emphasis on performance, length of stay, readmission rates, and overall complications, there is a rising trend to avoid these patients for financial and access issues; some insurance plans will unilaterally eliminate centers that are above arbitrary complication rates regardless of risk stratification. Ironically, the patients who have the most urgent need for surgical intervention may be eliminated from consideration by virtue of the quality improvement programs originally conceived to ensure their safety.

As we continue to recognize the need to eliminate BMI as criteria for metabolic intervention, the availability of qualified surgeons and programs will be strained; our fear is that those individuals with the highest risk will be abandoned for the reasons already stated. This chapter will deal with the special consideration for treatment of the super-obese from a practical and philosophical perspective.

Preoperative Workup and Evaluation

The super-obese individual presents many challenges to the health-care system. At the extreme, gurneys, hospital beds, wheelchairs, and facilities must be able to accommodate extremes of weight. Personnel must be trained on moving such individuals, and lifts must be available for transport or simply to assist a patient who has fallen back into bed. Every piece of equipment has a weight limit or size capacity. Specialists often show their frustration and lack of empathy knowing the extra effort needed to care for persons of size. The super-obese have more comorbidities and are more often neglected by the medical community; therefore they will require a more extensive workup and preparation than the lower BMI patients.

K. D. Higa, MD, FASMBS, FACS (✉)
Minimally Invasive and Bariatric Surgery, Fresno Heart and Surgical Hospital, Fresno, CA, USA

A. C. Wittgrove, MD, FASMBS, FACS
Wittgrove Bariatric Center, Del Mar, CA, USA
e-mail: ACWMD@lapbypass.com

R. Lutfi et al. (eds.), *Global Bariatric Surgery*, https://doi.org/10.1007/978-3-319-93545-4_32

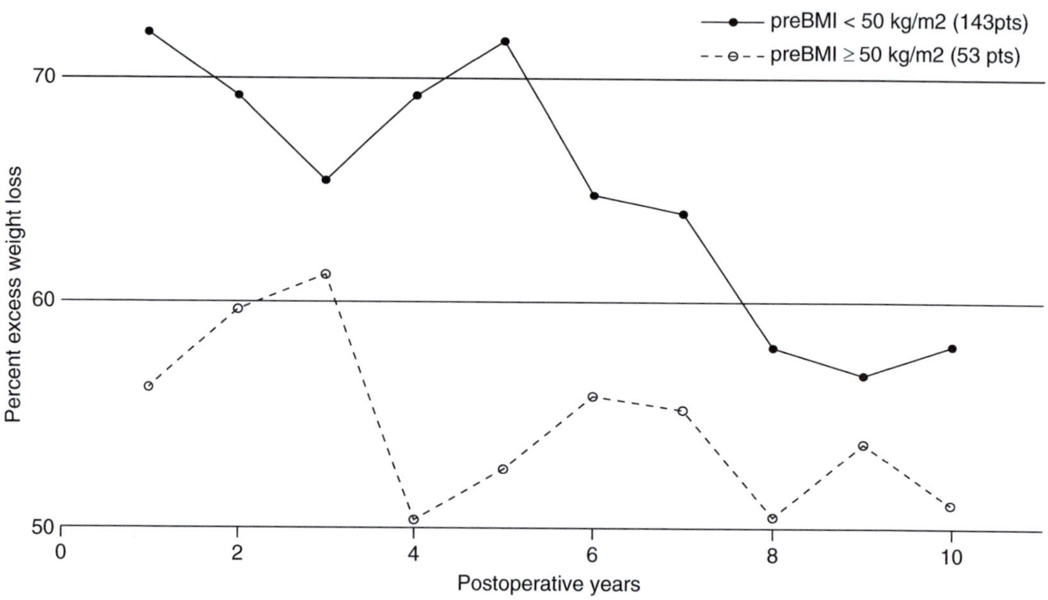

Fig. 32.1 Higher BMIs have been shown to be more resilient to treatment, with less absolute weight loss and comorbidity resolution

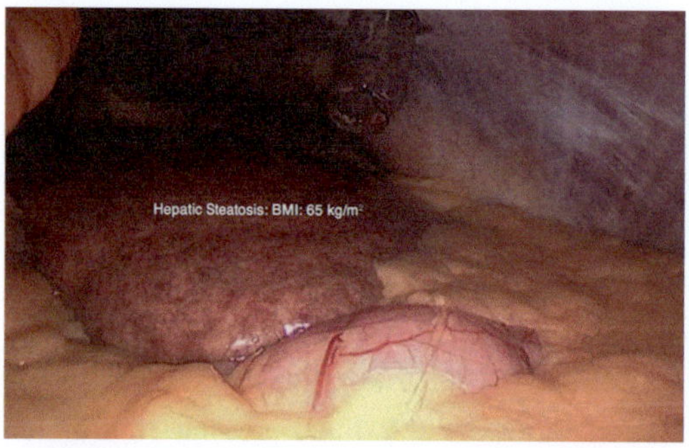

Fig. 32.2 Individuals with higher BMIs are more likely to have more complex health issues such as obstructive sleep apnea, metabolic syndrome, and hepatic steatosis which are associated with higher surgical risk, readmission rates, and long-term complications

Apart from the health-care maintenance items, the super-obese will require sleep studies and cardiopulmonary evaluation. Psychological and nutritional optimization is imperative. An objective risk assessment and multidisciplinary discussion is often helpful in advising a treatment program but also in deciding which surgical procedure to offer. Anecdotally, in our practices, these patients appear to have more psychosocial issues and are on more psychotropic medications than BMI < 50 kg/m^2 patients.

Preoperative Weight Loss

Preoperative weight loss has been shown to decrease surgical risk and operative time purportedly by decreasing liver volume and fat adiposity [3]. However, preoperative weight loss has not been shown to increase postoperative weight loss in at least two randomized controlled studies. Therefore, it is reasonable to advise preoperative weight loss for all patients, especially the super-obese, through lifestyle modification and pharmaceuticals for those patients who seem to be a higher risk by virtue of their central obesity. Contrarily, failure to achieve weight loss should not be a sign of non-compliance and eliminate an individual from surgical consideration.

As the intragastric balloon (IGB) is now available in the United States, it has been recommended as a bridge therapy to decrease surgical risk by immediate weight loss and improvement of medical comorbidities prior to bariatric/metabolic surgery. In a case controlled study, Busetto et al. demonstrated reduced risk of conversion and intraoperative complications in patients undergoing adjustable gastric banding [4]. However, in a multicenter, randomized trial, Coffin et al. found that IGB increased complications in patients undergoing gastric bypass despite superior weight loss to the control group [5]. Out of 55 patients randomized to IGB, 5 patients experienced significant complications of hemorrhage, abscesses, fistula, peritonitis, and occlusions ($p = 0.02$). In addition 35% of patients experienced significant complications at the time of explant. In addition, there was not improvement in surgical time, hospitalization stay, or postoperative weight loss at 6 months. It was conjectured the reason for increased complications had to do with the changes to the gastric wall, innervation, and blood distribution.

Operative Considerations

Larger patients require additional considerations during the operative procedure. Patient positioning with attention to pressure points and fixation are important as these cases often are more difficult and take longer to complete. Video-assisted intubation devices should be standard, as well as the capability for proper monitoring. Mechanical and chemo VTE prophylaxis is advised. Unfractionated heparin can have unpredictable pharmacokinetics; so low-molecular-weight heparin is advised. Continuing prophylaxis for several weeks after discharge may be indicated, especially in the sleeve patients for prevention of portal and deep vein thromboembolism. Longer instrumentation, trocars, and staplers are often necessary as well as sturdy liver retraction devices.

Postoperative Considerations

In our centers, most patients do not require ICU post-op. However, we do have 24-h oxygen saturation monitoring and capnography available on the surgical floor. Having patients bring their own CPAP machines is critical in some cases because the patient already is familiar with the machine type, the pressure, and the mask fit. Because more individuals in this category suffer with obstructive sleep apnea (and narcotic and anesthetics aggravate sleep apnea) and there may be a more difficult intubation, they present a more challenging re-intubation. To offset this risk, the anesthetist may delay extubation until the patient has shown they are well able to protect their airway. In the preoperative educational process, the patient should be informed that they may awaken in the recovery room still intubated and they will not be able to talk, but a nurse will be right there, and it does not mean anything went wrong with the operation; it is designed for their safety! Physical therapy and ambulatory protocols are necessary. Increasing BMI has been shown to influence the postoperative course and anesthetic outcomes after surgery. However, with aggressive preparation and clinical pathways, it is possible to limit the BMI influence [6]. See Fig. 32.3.

The use of drains and G-tubes should not be routine, but use in certain circumstances should be considered. For example, if an operation is particularly difficult because of the challenging anatomy and there is increased risk for fistula, then placement of drains prophylactically and a G-tube for potential enteral feedings might avoid a reoperation, especially when the patient exceeds the weight limit for CT drainage. Gastric distension and early leaks are often difficult to diagnose in the super-obese patient, yet early detection and treatment is critical to their survival.

Routine use of urinary catheters is becoming less frequent as operative times are reduced. However, fluid status is important in the metabolically challenged patient with multiple system involvement, and accurate measurement of urine output may be impossible depending on the mobility of the individual patient.

Choice of Procedure

At the time of this publication, there are four procedures that encompass more than 99% of all operations: the adjustable gastric band, the gastric bypass (including single anastomosis and banded forms), the sleeve gastrectomy, and the duodenal switch. The algorithm for recommending a particular operation is not as controversial as it is inconsistent among different surgeons, even within a single practice. Add to this, the lack

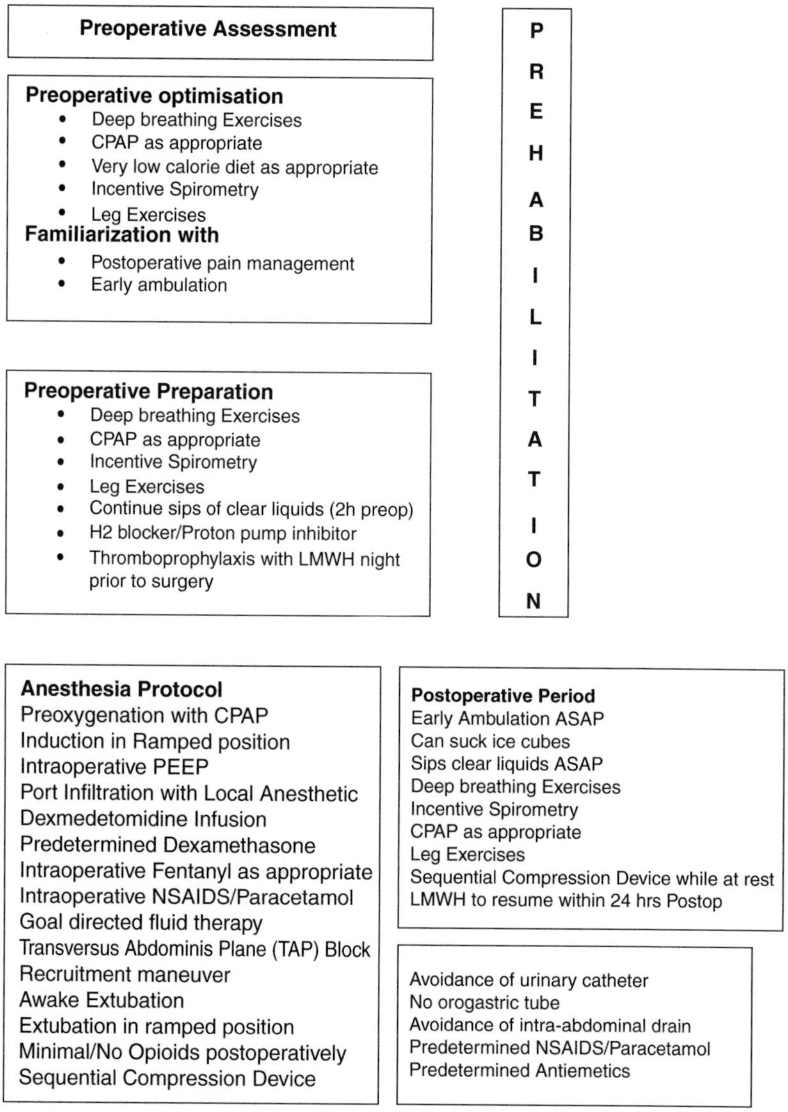

Fig. 32.3 Increasing BMI has been shown to influence the postoperative course and anesthetic outcomes after surgery. However, with aggressive preparation and clinical pathways, it is possible to limit the BMI influence

of standardization, outcomes interpretation is nearly impossible given the paucity of high-level studies that exist today. Systemic reviews only seem to amplify the uncertainty and add little to the process. Given the lack of consensus, one must and should rely upon his or her personal experience, assuming diligent data collection and analysis.

In a rapid evidence review of bariatric surgery in the super-obese, Peterson, et al. summarize (2) systematic reviews, (2) RCT, and (19) retrospective cohort studies. The only comparison that has over 5-year follow-up is between the gastric bypass and duodenal switch. The DS achieves better weight loss (p = 0.001), and higher risk of readmissions (p = 0.02), but comparable diabetes remission and mortality [7]. Using the Bariatric Outcomes Longitudinal Database (BOLD) from 2007 to 2012 (Celio et al.), although GBP had higher reoperation and readmission rates compared to SG ($p < 0.001$), percent total weight loss (%TWL) ($p < 0.001$), diabetes ($p < 0.001$), hypertension ($p < 0.001$), hyperlipidemia ($p < 0.001$), GERD ($p < 0.001$), and obstructive sleep apnea (p = 0.058) were higher at 1 year compared with SG [8].

It is generally agreed that the adjustable gastric band is a poor choice for most patients whose BMI > 50 kg/m^2.

As conversion from gastric bypass to duodenal switch is one of the more complex procedures and with consideration that the sleeve gastrectomy can give similar metabolic response in the less than 50 kg/m^2 patient, it has been advised to use the sleeve gastrectomy as a staging operation toward the duodenal switch. Response to the sleeve gastrectomy, as well as ongoing evaluation as to the compliance of the patient, gives additional information prior to committing to this procedure. For these reasons, sleeve gastrectomy may be the better option initially for many super-obese patients. As the patient and the surgeon are determining the proper operation for that specific patient, the surgeon needs to be clear about their own feelings about following patients who have undergone a malabsorptive operation, and they need to be sure the patient fully understands the potential medical and social issues, even to the amount and type of supplements required. Not every program is designed to care for patients who have undergone a malabsorptive operation.

Although more aggressive operations such as the duodenal switch are associated with greater weight loss and metabolic syndrome resolution or control, trade-offs include a higher propensity for vitamin, mineral, and protein-calorie malnutrition. The breakpoint for safety and performance is still to be determined; recommendations for each patient must be individualized.

The super morbidly obese patient presents many challenges for the health-care system. Access to care is often limited because of the disability preventing employment and insurability. These patients often do not participate in health-care maintenance of preventative measures and are often ostracized by the medical community. Surgical programs are inadvertently encouraged not to operate on these higher-risk patients or provide the care they deserve. Surgical procedures are more difficult, time-consuming, and less rewarding by virtue of a disease that is more difficult to control. Yet, these are the patients for whom the system should prioritize: those individuals whose higher risk makes therapy more urgent.

References

1. Sturm R, Hattori A. Morbid obesity rates continue to rise rapidly in the United States. Int J Obes. 2013;37(6):889–91.
2. Higa K, Ho T, Tercero F, Yunus T, Boone K. Laparoscopic Roux-en-Y gastric bypass: 10 year follow-up. Surg Obes Relat Dis. 2011;7:516–25.
3. Edholm D, Kullberg J, Haenni A, et al. Preoperative 4-week low calorie diet reduces liver volume and intrahepatic fat, and facilitates laparoscopic gastric bypass in morbidly obese. Obes Surg. 2011;21:345–50.
4. Busetto L, Segato G, De Luca M, et al. Preoperative weight loss by intragastric balloon in super-obese patients treated with laparoscopic gastric banding: a case-control study. Obes Surg. 2004;14:671–6.
5. Coffin B, Maunoury V, Pattou F, et al. Impact of intragastric balloon before laparoscopic gastric bypass on patients with super obesity: a randomized multicenter study. Obes Surg. 2017;27:902–9.
6. Sinha A, Jayaraman L, Punhani D, Chowbey P. Enhanced recovery after bariatric surgery in the severely obese, morbidly obese, super-morbidly obese and super-super morbidly obese using evidence-based clinical pathways: a comparative study. Obes Surg. 2017;27:560–8.
7. Peterson K, Anderson J, Boundy E, Ferguson L, Erickson K. Rapid evidence review of bariatric surgery in super obesity (BMI ≥ 50 kg/m^2). J Gen Intern Med. 2017;32(Suppl 1):56–64.
8. Celio A, Wu Q, Kasten K, Manwaring M, Pories W, Spaniolas K. Comparative effectiveness of Roux-en-Y gastric bypass and sleeve gastrectomy in super obese patients. Surg Endosc. 2017;31:317–23.

Optimizing the Staple Line

33

Edgardo Serra and Carlos Eduardo Jacob†

Background

> The idea stemmed from the need that the surgeon has to open the digestive tract with its highly contaminated lumen, thereby, risking consequent peritonitis with its associated increase in mortality. Simple manual suturing of the infected lumen of the intestine is time consuming, thus prolonging surgery and increasing the risk of mortality for patients under anaesthesia. Written by Aladár Petz (Oláh 2002) [1, 2]

To optimize means to make something as good as possible. This is the aim of a surgeon when performing any surgical procedure, including all bariatric techniques. Gastrointestinal surgeries are performed either openly or through minimally invasive techniques using regular sutures or mechanical staplers. Mechanical staplers are a mainstay of laparoscopic gastrointestinal surgery, in particular bariatric surgery.

Stapling devices can create transections and anastomoses quickly, safely, and with minimal, if any, bleeding or spillage. Staple-line failure, although uncommon, can result in significant morbidity and mortality [3].

Despite the routine nature of intestinal anastomosis procedures, the rate of complications, such as anastomotic leakage and strictures, is between 1% and 19% and remains unchanged in spite of the introduction of newer techniques and technologies. Postoperative leak can occur in 1–3% of patients submitted to sleeve gastrectomy and 0.1–5.6 after a laparoscopic Roux-en-Y bypass [4].

The long staple line in sleeve gastrectomy is a potential risk for disruption, especially near the esophagogastric junction, and sometimes this leakage is difficult to heal probably due to high gastric pressure and the presence of biliary and gastric contents [5, 6].

After a gastric bypass, surgeons care about gastrojejunal anastomosis because a leakage can mean reoperation and risk of death.

Staple-line failure is the most common cause of postoperative gastrointestinal hemorrhage after sleeve gastrectomy and Roux-en-Y gastric bypass and occurs in 1–3% and 1.9–4.4%, respectively (Aurora et al., Committee et al.). Possible factors that affect the risk of bleeding can be related to the device (staple height, type of device), to the tissue (anatomical location, tissue viscosity), and also to the surgeon's experience [7].

Although several papers discuss postoperative leaks and bleeding, few discuss intraoperative events. It seems that intraoperative bleeding and staple failure are not frequent, but it is clearly

Electronic Supplementary Material The online version of this chapter (doi:10.1007/978-3-319-93545-4_33) contains supplementary material, which is available to authorized users.

E. Serra (✉)
Bariatric Surgery, Centro CIEN, Corrientes, Argentina

†C. E. Jacob
Division of Gastrointestinal Surgery and Coloproctology – Hospital das Clínicas, University of Sao Paulo School of Medicine, Sao Paulo, Brazil

R. Lutfi et al. (eds.), *Global Bariatric Surgery*, https://doi.org/10.1007/978-3-319-93545-4_33

affected by surgeons' experience and methods used to prevent these events. Staple-line reinforcement with sutures, tissue sealants, glues, or buttressing materials can address these problems. In this chapter we will discuss the role of staple-line reinforcement [8].

World Staple History

There were several changes and improvements in the digestive surgery field. As wrote Dietz, "within the past 200 years, gastrointestinal anastomosis has been transformed from a life-threatening adventure to a safe and routinely performed procedure."

Difficult to evaluate its impact, the stapler, like laparoscopic approach, is one of the most useful inventions and has advanced surgery. Its applications were adopted worldwide from 100 years ago and help surgeons in many fields.

It was Hümer Hültl, a Hungarian surgeon, who started with the idea of a mechanical suture machine in 1907. He met with Victor Fischer, a surgical instruments manufacturer, and designed the first stapler. In May of 1908, this stapler was used clinically by its designer.

Another Hungarian surgeon, Aladár von Petz, worked on the disadvantages of the Hültl machine and designed a modern version of the stapler that was lightweight, easy to clean, and easy to refill and had better structure. This new instrument was first used clinically in 1920 and became a landmark in the history of surgery and surgical instruments. Later, Mark Ravitch introduced this technology in United States in 1959 [9].

Through time, mechanical stapling changed gastrointestinal surgery, reducing operating time and complications; this simultaneously decreased the cost of procedures and improved outcomes for the individual patients.

From the clamp, scissors, and suture, to the actual devices with two lines of three rows of staples, and the simultaneous transection and the simplicity and security in use, we can say, thanks to this machine, we have the possibility of bariatric surgery.

Thought Behind Enforcing

All surgeons' aim is to decrease the risk of complications. Therefore, many use various materials to provide hemostasis and reinforce the staple line. According to the report from the Fourth International Consensus Summit on Sleeve Gastrectomy, 75% of surgeons choose to perform staple-line reinforcement, and among them, 57% use buttressing materials and 43% oversew the staple line [11, 12].

Twenty-five years ago, gastric leak and fistula were the most significant complications of gastrointestinal surgical procedures like duodenal switch. Today, gastric leak still persists as a complication of the long suture of sleeve gastrectomy [9, 11]. Ischemic factors and intraluminal pressure could be the explanation of the disruption of the staple line. Other technical factors are considered causes as well.

The current generation of surgical staplers has remarkable reliability. However, staple-line complications do still occur and can result in significant morbidity and mortality. Because of this, gastrointestinal surgeons, especially bariatric surgeons, seek out techniques and devices that can reduce this risk [10].

One point to be stressed is the use of intraoperative testing as a recommendation for leak prevention during a sleeve gastrectomy and gastric bypass. Three papers reviewed the role of this kind of test after a sleeve gastrectomy. Aurora et al. reviewed 29 publications with 4888 patients and found that the test was performed in 15 studies (52%). Parikh et al. published a systematic review of 112 studies with 9991 patients submitted to sleeve gastrectomy and noticed that leak testing was used in 6717 patients (67%) and 62 studies (55%). Some measures were suggested by Abu Rached et al. to decrease the incidence of staple-line failure: staple-line reinforcement, larger bougie size, and routine use of dye intraoperative test.

Three other retrospective publications considered the value of intraoperative leak testing after sleeve gastrectomy [12]. These studies recognized the importance of the test allowing to detect and fix intraoperative leaks due to staple-line disruption, avoiding postoperative complications.

Four papers studied intraoperative leaks and bleeding after gastric bypass. Studied upper GI hemorrhage and found that gastrojejunal anastomosis was the site of bleeding in 90% of the patients [14].

Found 8.26% of the patients had staple-line dehiscence or evidence of gastric pouch/gastrojejunal anastomosis leak [15]. They proposed the selective use of fibrin glue and omental reinforcement.

Investigated the use of intraoperative endoscopy in managing leaks [16]. Air leak test detected problems in 11 patients (3.79%) and prompted repair with oversewing [3].

The Longitudinal Assessment of Bariatric Surgery study, published by [17], is a prospective multicenter research of intraoperative events in 2973 patients. They found a 0.98% incidence of equipment failure including stapler misfiring.

There are several controversies regarding staple-line reinforcement's role in the prevention of complications, especially preventing leaks. Wang tell us "staple line reinforcement did not significantly influence the frequency of staple line leakage overall" [4].

In fact, staple-line integrity is important to achieve good results, either to gastric bypass or sleeve gastrectomy, and has been the focus of continuing innovation by medical companies.

The potential physiologic effect of reinforcement is to improve the durability of staple line, increase the burst pressure of the intestinal or anastomotic mechanic suture, distribute the compressive force of the staples, improve the technical failures of the staple line, and decrease hemorrhage, among others. Buttressing materials add thickness and potentially strength [6].

We need to take into account other factors that reduce complications, like the correct use of laparoscopic instruments and devices, gentle handling of tissue with specific intestinal grasper, and correct use of energy devices to reduce ischemia, perforations, and lacerations. The correct use of stapler devices, such as the appropriate stapler election for tissue thickness, sustaining compression to the device over the tissues before firing to wash out the fluids, and the soft handling of the staple line are other necessary recommendations. And of course, the general condition of the patients and patient's preparations before the surgery, as in bariatric surgery, improve the general results over complications rates [8].

There are reasons for non-reinforcement of the staple line in laparoscopic surgery in bariatric surgery. The author's opinion is that reduction on operative time is one of the most important explanations from surgeons who do not reinforce. Other situations like cost reduction or lack of technical skills in laparoscopic suture and buttressing handle are at the top of our considerations as causes of non-reinforcement from the surgical community. The above situations win to the controversial results of some papers as the cause of non-reinforcement use.

Available Technology

Surgeons choose between multiple surgical options including no reinforcement, staple-line reinforcement with suture oversewing, nonabsorbable bovine pericardial strips, polymer membrane, or biological sealant [11]. All of these methods have been used to try to reduce the incidence of complications.

Without Reinforcement

What are the fundamentals for non-reinforcement of staple line in laparoscopic bariatric surgery? We think that reduction of operative time is one of the most important explanations from surgeons who do not reinforce. Others like cost reductions, lack of technical skills in laparoscopic suture, and buttressing handle are in the top of our consideration as a cause of non-reinforcement for the surgical community [2].

We believe that the above situations win to the controversial results of some papers as the cause of non-reinforcement use.

Oversewing

In bariatric surgery the most chosen method of reinforcement of the staple line is oversewing as reported by Rosenthal et al. during the International Sleeve Gastrectomy Expert Panel Consensus Statement. This is the cheaper method of reinforcement, but it increases surgical time. There are several techniques for oversewing the staple line: baseball stitch, simple oversewing, locking, imbricating, and more. It is possible to choose nonabsorbable or absorbable suture material. The surgeon could reinforce the cross-section between the staple line or, as we prefer, reinforce all the staple line. In our protocol, we reinforce all the staple line with a simple oversewing with absorbable material (Video 33.1).

Oversewing has same disadvantages like possible ischemia and increased blood loss. Despite that, it seems to reduce the general rate of hemorrhage and leak compared to non-reinforcement. In our experience, over 1055 sleeve gastrectomies, we had 0.47% of leak, without any reoperations because of hemorrhage and only 0,1% of blood transfusions.

However, for those who suture oversews, there is no consensus as to which suture material (absorbable vs. nonabsorbable) or type of sewing technique (baseball stitch, simple oversewing, locking, imbricating, etc.) is best. In addition, while some surgeons oversew the entire staple line, others only selected regions of the staple line. Oversewing a staple line has not unanimously been shown to be beneficial and might, in fact, lead to a greater.

In our technical protocol of sleeve gastrectomy, we reinforce the entire staple line with a simple oversewing with absorbable material. We prefer simple oversewing close to the staple rows because it has less sleeve gastric lumen reduction that imbricate suture (Fig. 33.1).

As reported by Shikora et al. (1), oversewing is better than no reinforcement in sleeve gastrectomy, but not as good as buttressing with bovine pericardium. But, Baxter, the company owner of the buttressing bovine pericardium material, supported the article.

Buttressing Material

Several publications show staple-line buttressing to decrease bleeding and to possibly reduce leak rates. It is well known that it increases staple-line burst pressure.

The hemostatic action of the roofing material is possibly related to the compression of the gastrointestinal wall transected and the hemostatic effect of the materials. Others explain that buttressing materials add thickness on the tissue stapled and distribute the tension of each individual staple over the length of the buttress material as a hemostatic effect. These factors are related to decrease the general rates of leaks, too. But there is no statistic significance, especially compared with other reinforcement techniques like oversewing suture [11].

On the other hand, there are controversies in the operative time when comparing buttressing reinforcement use versus not using. Dapri showed us extra procedures timed longer with the

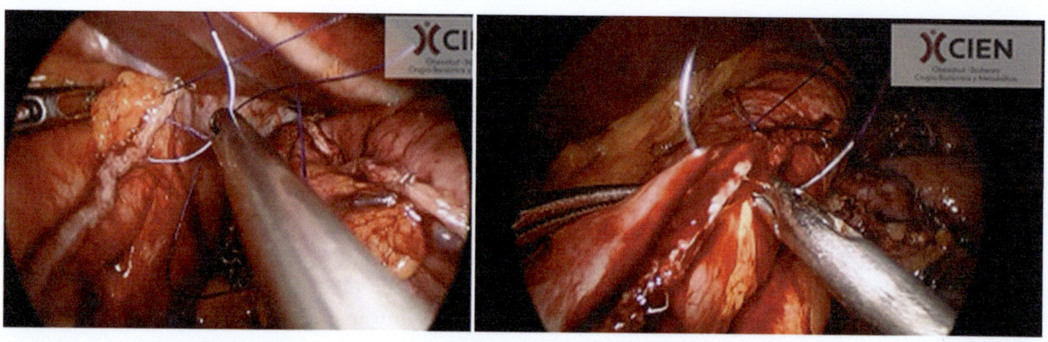

Fig. 33.1 Oversewing reinforcement of all the staple line of sleeve gastrectomy

application of buttressing/roofing material. Although others gave different results, they didn't find statistical significance in his series [11].

Buttressing material must be preloaded onto the stapler device and delivered at the moment of stapler firing. The buttressing strip should be flexible and thin because it needs to be easily cut by the blade of stapler device, leaving the buttress incorporated into the staple line. However, the cost of the product is only one factor when determining total cost. To better assess the total financial cost, one must also take into account other factors such as operating room time and improvements in outcome (i.e., reduction of complications, the need for other resources, reduction of hospital length of stay).

Bovine Pericardium

It is a biologic collagen matrix developed from bovine pericardium (Peristrips Dry and PSD Veritas; Synovis Surgical Innovations, St Paul, MN). The strip adds 1 mm. of thickness when this material is stapled onto the tissue when the device is fired. Two dehydrated BPS are secured on each side of a foam spacer by a plastic mounting unit. BPS (PSD) hydrogel creates a temporary bond between the strips and the forks of the stapler, promoting rehydration of the strips. Application of BPS requires some training and experience. Increased care is necessary to choose the correct cartridge size to fit the tissue thickness; if the staple height is too small to accommodate the tissue and the BPS, or if BPS is improperly loaded, the stapler may misfire [12].

In one of the largest meta-analyses, it was demonstrated that reinforcement of staple line reduces leakage and bleeding and bovine pericardium was superior in complication preventions versus suture reinforcement and biocompatible glycolide copolymer buttress. Others studies show different results [11].

It seems collagen matrix biologic buttress has more hemostatic power than synthetic buttress.

Biocompatible Glycoside Copolymer

This material synthesized from polyglycolic acid and trimethylene carbonate (Gore Seamguard®; W.L. Gore & Associates, Inc., Flagstaff, AZ) is bioabsorbable and developed with a 0,5 mm thickness. The strength effect into the staple line is maintained 4–5 weeks and it is completely absorbed within 6 months. The use of this buttress material requires extra operative time and a well-trained team in the surgery room.

In term of blood loss reduction, the effect can be related to the compression of the reinforcement material on the transected tissue.

Fibrin Sealant

This agent has two components, thrombin and fibrinogen, and provides hemostasis, sealing, and adhesion [1]. It is a biological tissue adhesive that, in contact of small amounts of factor XIII and calcium, initiates the last step of the coagulations and forms fibrin polymer and then precipitates as fibrin fibrils in the tissue. This fibrin sealant is expected to be completely resorbed in 10–14 days.

Technically, after the methylene blue test, two boxes (8 ml) of human fibrin sealant are sprayed along the suture line and posterior to the sleeved stomach through a delicate laparoscopic set.

Comparative Studies

Eight prospective comparative studies are always cited as the source of evidence when we discuss staple-line reinforcement after sleeve gastrectomy.

Published a prospective analysis of 75 patients comparing no reinforcement with staple-line reinforcement using Seamguard (WL Gore Inc., Flagstaff, AZ) and staple-line suturing. The use of buttress material reduced blood loss during stomach sectioning and overall blood loss. No difference was evidenced concerning postoperative leaks. Of course, the first group was associated with lower operative time.

Aggarwal et al. (2013) analyzed 60 patients; half of them submitted to staple-line reinforcement with continuing suture, and for the others, no reinforcement was used. There was no statistical difference between the two groups although two leaks were observed in the no-reinforcement group. No bleeding was observed in both groups. On the other hand, found that oversewing the staple line reduced the chance of bleeding. Albanopoulos also suggested oversewing the staple line to improve strength.

Studies by Shah and Musella et al.'s suggested that use of buttress or roof material reduces intraoperative events and, in this way, reduces the overall surgical time.

Two meta-analyses were published about staple-line reinforcement over the last years since this subject became a trending topic in bariatric surgery.

Analyzed 1345 patients from two randomized control trials and six cohort studies. They found that staple-line reinforcement decreased postoperative leaks and overall complications. A subgroup analysis showed that reinforcement of the suture line with buttress material may decrease the risk of staple-line hemorrhage and overall complications.

Reviewed 8 randomized controlled trials with 791 patients comparing no reinforcement and suture-line reinforcement. The last group was associated with a lower risk of staple-line hemorrhage and overall complications and longer operative time. No difference was observed regarding postoperative leakage. The subgroup analysis showed that hemorrhage is lower after application of buttressing materials, but not with oversewing when compared with no reinforcement.

It is also important to cite the meta-analysis published by Shikora and Mahoney that analyzed 253 studies about staple-line reinforcement in gastrointestinal surgery, most of them concerning bariatric surgery. Forty percent of the patients had no reinforcement with higher leak (2.75%) and bleed (3.45%) rates. Any type of staple-line reinforcement was better than no reinforcement concerning bleeding and leak rates (Tables 33.1, 33.2, and 33.3).

Since the basal leak rate is rather low, powering a study sufficiently to result in statistically significant differences would require large numbers of patients and is likely impossible to perform. Yet despite the relatively low incidence, leaks are often highly clinically significant and can result in prolonged hospitalization, critical illness, sepsis, debilitation, and even death.

Table 33.1 Leak rate by reinforcement type (sleeve and gastric bypass)

Buttress material	N of study arms	Event rate (%)	Number of patients
None	116	2.75	26,023
Glycolide copolymer	52	2.61	3693
Oversuture	92	2.45	19,755
Bovine pericardium	41	1.28	6838

Modified from Shikora and Mahoney [13]
Bovine pericardium versus none, $p < 0.001$; bovine pericardium versus oversuture, $p < 0.001$; bovine pericardium versus glycolide copolymer, $p < 0.01$

Table 33.2 Bleed rate by reinforcement type (sleeve and gastric bypass)

Buttress material	N of study arms	Event rate (%)	Number of patients
None	83	3.45	17,808
Oversuture	58	2.69	14,368
Glycolide copolymer	44	2.48	2929
Bovine pericardium	30	1.23	6759

Modified from Shikora and Mahoney [13]
Bovine pericardium versus none, $p < 0.001$; bovine pericardium versus glycolide copolymer, $p < 0.01$; bovine pericardium versus oversuture, $p \leq 0.05$; glycolide copolymer versus none, $p < 0.01$

Table 33.3 Bleed rate by reinforcement type for sleeve gastrectomy

Buttress material	N of study arms	Event rate (%)	Number of patients
None	25	4.94	2865
Oversuture	33	2.41	4682
Glycolide copolymer	28	2.09	1997
Bovine pericardium	14	1.16	1632

Modified from Shikora and Mahoney [13]
Bovine pericardium versus none, $p < 0.001$; oversuture versus none, $p < 0.001$; glycolide copolymer versus none, $p < 0.001$; bovine pericardium versus oversuture, $p < 0.05$; bovine pericardium versus glycolide copolymer, $p < 0.05$.

More high-quality randomized controlled studies with large sample sizes should be undertaken to better evaluate the effects of different methods of staple-line reinforcement.

Costs

Ghosh referred that published studies were insufficient to address the economic impact of bleeds and leaks or interventions, but development of improved stapler designs that obviate the need for SLR may reduce costs and improve outcomes.

The experience of the surgeon and the interaction with devices are one of the most important points in the creations of anastomosis and intestinal sutures with sufficient staple-line integrity, reducing leak and healing complications.

Shah and Musella et al.'s studies suggested that using buttressing or roof material is associated with decreased operative time because B/R material reduced intraoperative complications and thus saved time, while Dapri and Sroka et al. showed that application of B/R materials required extra procedures and it took longer time. The pooled data suggested that using B/R materials didn't significantly affect the operative time.

Staple-line buttressing has been shown in several publications to decrease bleeding, increase staple-line burst pressure, and possibly even reduce leak rates. However, as stated above, its use is not widespread. This may be due in part to the concern of added cost. However, the cost of the product is only one factor when determining total cost [11]. To better assess the financial cost, one must also take into account other factors, such as operating room time and improvements in outcome (i.e., reduction of complications, the need for other resources, and reduction of hospital length of stay). For example, while several studies have confirmed that buttressing materials reduce intraoperative bleeding, the difference in estimated blood loss was clinically insignificant [3]. However, in some studies, with the use of buttressing materials, the reduction in costly operating room time was greater than 30 min per case and the length of hospitalization was reduced almost a full day.

References

1. Abou Rached A, Basile M, El Masri H. Gastric leaks post sleeve gastrectomy: review of its prevention and management. World J Gastroenterol. 2014;20:13904–10.
2. Aggarwal S, Sharma AP, Ramaswamy N. Outcome of laparoscopic sleeve gastrectomy with and without staple line oversewing in morbidly obese patients: a randomized study. J Laparoendosc Adv Surg Tech A. 2013;23:895–9.
3. Al Hajj GN, Haddad J. Preventing staple-line leak in sleeve gastrectomy: reinforcement with bovine pericardium vs oversewing. Obes Surg. 2013;23:1915–21.
4. Alasfar F, Chand B. Intraoperative endoscopy for laparoscopic Roux-en-Y gastric bypass: leak test and beyond. Surg Laparosc Endosc Percutan Tech. 2010;20:424–7.
5. Albanopoulos K, Alevizos L, Flessas J, Menenakos E, Stamou KM, Papailiou J, Natoudi M, Zografos G, Leandros E. Reinforcing the staple line during laparoscopic sleeve gastrectomy: prospective randomized clinical study comparing two different techniques. Preliminary results. Obes Surg. 2012;22:42–6.
6. Aurora AR, Khaitan L, Saber AA. Sleeve gastrectomy and the risk of leak: a systematic analysis of 4,888 patients. Surg Endosc. 2012;26:1509–15.
7. Aydin MT, Aras O, Karip B, Memisoglu K. Staple line reinforcement methods in laparoscopic sleeve gastrectomy: comparison of burst pressures and leaks. JSLS. 2015;19.
8. Bulbuller N, Aslaner A, Oner OZ, et al. Comparison of four different methods in staple line reinforcement during laparoscopic sleeve gastrectomy. Int J Clin Exp Med. 2013;6:985–90.
9. Casella G, Soricelli E, Genco A, Ferrazza G, Basso N, Redler A. Use of platelet-rich plasma to reinforce the staple line during laparoscopic sleeve gastrectomy: feasibility study and preliminary outcome. J Laparoendosc Adv Surg Tech. 2015;3.
10. Cha J, Shademan A, Le HND, Decker R, Kim PCW, Kang JU, Krieger A. Multispectral tissue characterization for intestinal anastomosis optimization. J Biomed Opt. 2015;20(10):106001.
11. Gagner M, Buchwald JN. Comparison of laparoscopic sleeve gastrectomy leak rates in four staple-line reinforcement options: a systematic review. Surg Obes Relat Dis. 2014;10:713–23.
12. Gagner M, Deitel M, Erickson AL, et al. Survey on laparoscopic sleeve gastrectomy (LSG) at the Fourth International Consensus summit on sleeve gastrectomy. Obes Surg. 2013;23:2013–7.
13. Shikora SA, Mahoney CB. Clinical benefit of gastric staple line reinforcement (SLR) in gastrointestinal surgery: a meta-analysis. Obes Surg. 2015;25:1133–41.

14. Jamil KM, Rahman AS, Bardhan PK, Khan AI, Chowdhury F, Sarker SA, Khan AM, Ahmed T. Micronutrients and anaemia. J Health Popul Nutr. 2008;26(3):340–55. Review
15. Madan AK, Martinez JM, Lo Menzo E, Khan KA, Tichansky DS. Omental reinforcement for intraoperative leak repairs during laparoscopic Roux-en-Y gastric bypass. Am Surg. 2009;75(9):839–42.
16. Alasfar F, Chand B. Intraoperative endoscopy for laparoscopic Roux-en-Y gastric bypass: leak test and beyond. Surg Laparosc Endosc Percutan Tech. 2010;20(6):424–7.
17. Greenstein AS. New targets and opportunities at the level of the endothelium. Hypertension. 2012;60(4):896–7. https://doi.org/10.1161/HYPERTENSIONAHA.112.198325. Epub 2012 Aug 20

Part IX

Medical Management and Special Disorders

Preoperative Preparation and Workup

34

Paul R. Kemmeter and Eric J. Krebill

Introducation

Obesity rates continue to increase worldwide with an estimated 400 million adults being classified as obese and an estimated 300,000 yearly deaths attributable to complications of obesity such as heart disease, diabetes, and hypertension [1, 2]. Bariatric surgery remains the most efficacious treatment for obesity and its comorbidities. Over the past 15 years, surgery-associated morbidity and mortality rates have decreased substantially secondary to the development of dedicated minimally invasive bariatric surgery fellowships, centers of excellence, defined protocols and procedures, databases, and ongoing research. Attention to appropriate patient selection, preoperative workup, and preparation are essential to continue these trends. The purpose of this chapter is to share our group's experience and knowledge combined with that of the published literature in the preoperative process. Although we are aware that this process can seem lengthy and may result in a delay to surgery, our aim is to fulfill the essence of the Hippocratic Oath: first do no harm. Additionally, at least within the USA, bariatric surgery continues to be quite litigious, and proper attention to the development of a thorough preoperative process can prove "an ounce of prevention is worth a pound of cure."

P. R. Kemmeter (✉)
Department of Surgery, Grand Health Partners, Mercy Health Saint Mary's, Grand Rapids, MI, USA
e-mail: pkemmeter@grandhealthpartners.com

E. J. Krebill
Department of Surgery, Grand Health Partners, North Ottawa Community Health System, Grand Rapids, MI, USA
e-mail: ekrebill@grandhealthpartners.com

Patient Selection and Preparation

In 1991, the National Institute of Health (NIH) developed a consensus statement for bariatric surgery candidacy with the accepted criteria including (1) BMI ≥40 kg/m^2 or BMI = 35–40 kg/m^2 with associated comorbidities (Table 34.1), (2) patients who are motivated and well-informed about the benefits and risks of bariatric procedures, (3) failure of nonsurgical weight loss, (4) psychiatric stability without current alcohol dependence or illicit drug use, and (5) no medical problems that would preclude surgery [3]. Over the past two and a half decades, our understanding of obesity and its metabolic detriments has increased substantially, and it is now recognized that bariatric surgery has a significant metabolic component. Worldwide, the criteria for surgery vary based on regional/ethnic differences in metabolic derangements, with the most notable being type II diabetes mellitus (T2D). In various parts of Asia and the Middle East, where T2D is more prevalent, the BMI criterion has essentially been eliminated.

Within the USA, the NIH criteria continue to be the basis for eligibility for bariatric surgery;

R. Lutfi et al. (eds.), *Global Bariatric Surgery*, https://doi.org/10.1007/978-3-319-93545-4_34

Table 34.1 Obesity-related comorbidities (partial list)

Metabolic
Type II diabetes mellitus, dyslipidemia, hypercholesterolemia
Cardiovascular
Hypertension, coronary artery disease, pulmonary hypertension, venous stasis, arrhythmias, stroke
Pulmonary
Obstructive sleep apnea, asthma, hypoventilation syndrome
Gastrointestinal
Gastroesophageal reflux disease, nonalcoholic fatty liver disease, cholelithiasis
Psychiatric
Depression, anxiety, binge eating disorder, history of physical/sexual abuse
Decreased quality of life
Musculoskeletal
Degenerative joint disease, back pain, immobility, gout, fibromyalgia
Oncologic
Cancers of breast, ovary, endometrial, colon and rectum, pancreas, esophagus, kidney, prostate, liver, gallbladder

Table 34.2 Our preoperative office check list

Prior to initial office visit
Referral from primary care provider (if required)
Initial education with an informational seminar (online or in-person) with review of office processes, surgical procedural choices and mechanisms of action, and potential complications
Provide complete health history questionnaire (including diet attempts)
Office consultations
Bariatrician consult with complete history and physical with appropriate behavioral counseling (dietary, physical exercise) and preparatory surgical education (including brochures). Additional testing ordered as needed, including referrals to specialists. Psychiatric questionnaire provided
Behaviorist consult with review of questionnaire and 1 h interview. Referral to outside psychologist/psychiatrist as needed
Bariatric surgeon consult with focused history and physical, further education on bariatric procedures (brochures provided), and selection of bariatric procedure. Additional testing ordered as needed
Subsequent visits
Dietitian visit with education on food choices, nutrition label comprehension, and vitamin supplementation
Exercise physiologist visit with in-office exercise demonstration and recommendations
Screening upper endoscopy
2-week preoperative visit
Group visit led by physician assistant educating on very low-calorie diet, hospital processes including in-hospital expectations, and review of potential surgical complications
Dietitian-led group visit detailing very low-calorie diet (VLCD)
Individual physician assistant visit for adjusting medications and signing of operative consents
1-week preoperative visit
Final history and physical with evaluation for weight loss and possible side effects of VLCD (i.e., dehydration), review of labs, and final education prior to surgery

however, these criteria are just the starting points in the selection process. The overall goal with bariatric surgery is to safely provide lifelong treatment for obesity and its metabolic and life-altering sequelae. Unfortunately, bariatric surgery can be associated with weight recidivism and concomitant relapse in comorbidities, along with psychological alterations such as alcoholism and suicide. To our knowledge, there are currently no data demonstrating how to identify patients who will have "success" versus those who will have "failure," with neither of these terms being defined uniformly. Therefore, a goal in picking the "right" patient is impossible. However, our group's experience with over 13,000 patients has provided us some insight on patient selection and preoperative preparation. We employ a multidisciplinary approach in patient selection utilizing our entire staff including surgeons, bariatricians, advanced practice providers, dietitians, behaviorists, exercise physiologists, receptionists, coordinators, and office administration. When appropriate, we also seek input from our colleagues in pulmonology, endocrinology, cardiology, and psychiatry. Every member of the team has the responsibility of identifying patients who may require additional screening, as we have found that patients can behave very differently depending on which team member they interact with (Table 34.2). Additionally, the American College of Surgeons (ACS) has utilized the National Surgical Quality Improvement Program (NSQIP) database to develop a Bariatric Surgery Risk Calculator (http://glyconverter.altervista.org/basscore/index.html) attempting to improve patient and physician decisions about bariatric surgery [4]. Identifying patients at increased risk for a post-surgical complication and, when possible, modifying these risks preoperatively should be the goal of preoperative preparation. Identification of unmodifiable risk factors should heighten the bariatric surgery team's awareness for any possible postoperative complications.

Age

The influence of increasing age on postoperative morbidity and mortality has been evaluated in numerous studies with some suggesting no relationship and others demonstrating increased rates. Secondary to smaller sample size, most studies have divided patients into age groups. However a study utilizing the ACS-NSQIP data of over 20,000 patients demonstrated that with each increased year of age, there was a 1% increase in odds of complications [5]. Additionally, an analysis of the German Bariatric Surgery Registry showed a 1.13-fold increase in complication rate with every 10 years increase in age [6]. Although many centers will limit surgery to patients under a certain age, the NIH criteria do not indicate an upper age limit. Our group has identified that "chronologic age" does not predict "physiologic age," and we have performed bariatric surgery in patients up to 78 years of age with acceptable outcomes [7].

Although the NIH criteria do limit bariatric surgery to patients ≥18 years of age, surgery has been successfully performed on adolescents for well over the past decade, with acceptable morbidity and mortality rates of 2.9% and 0%, respectively [8]. Our program does not offer adolescent bariatric surgery secondary to its unique challenges. Centers providing this must include the resources to provide specialty care in relation to adolescent psychology, family counseling, anesthesiology, and appropriate equipment.

Body Mass Index, Gender, and Preoperative Weight Loss

The size of a patient and the distribution of adipose tissue can greatly influence the difficulty of performing bariatric surgery. Surgical field exposure in patients with android adiposity can be significantly limited by hepatomegaly and increased visceral fat [9, 10]. This limitation can translate into increased postoperative complications with data from the USA indicating an increased risk of 2% for every increase in BMI point and data from Germany demonstrating a 1.16-fold increase for every five BMI points [5, 6]. Additionally, elevated waist-to-hip ratio is associated with increased surgical difficulty in bariatric surgery and, in colorectal surgery, is a better predictor of morbidity and mortality than is BMI [11, 12]. Although male gender has not consistently been recognized as a risk factor for postoperative complications, men tend to have higher body mass indices and more central obesity compared to female patients, so it is not surprising that male gender may carry a higher risk for postoperative complications, including mortality [6, 13].

Fortunately, preoperative weight loss has been demonstrated to reduce both liver volume and intra-abdominal adipose tissue with a resultant decrease in perioperative blood loss, operative time, length of stay, and overall complication rates [14–19]. During a 4-week low-calorie diet in morbidly obese women, the intrahepatic fat content can decrease by 50%, with the majority of volume change occurring in the first 2 weeks [20]. However, patients with very large livers can obtain an additional 20% decrease after the initial 2 weeks, and therefore longer preoperative diets may be beneficial in this subgroup [15].

Within our group, we begin educating patients regarding the benefits of preoperative weight loss at our presurgical seminar, and we have found some patients will begin losing weight from that time forward. All patients receive education from our on-site dietitians regarding food choices and associated nutrients, understanding nutrition labels, and vitamin supplementation. We will individualize the length of our preoperative very low-calorie diet (VLCD, 800 calories/day) based on BMI, central adiposity, and amount of weight loss from the patient's historical high. All patients placed on the VLCD are monitored for renal function with blood urea nitrogen and creatinine (BUN/Cr) checked after the first 5–7 days of therapy, and patients who are on a diuretic will have their dose cut in half at the start of the diet. Patients with renal insufficiency are monitored much more closely with the potential of decreasing the amount of protein consumed during the diet, further reduction in diuretics, and increased fluid intake.

Health and Functional Status and the Edmonton Obesity Staging System

The patient's overall well-being is a predictor of outcomes following bariatric surgery with multiple risk factors being associated with increased morbidity and mortality including a history of deep venous thrombosis/pulmonary embolism, bleeding disorders, obstructive sleep apnea, hypertension, dyspnea, chronic obstructive pulmonary disease, impaired functional status, chronic renal insufficiency requiring dialysis, low preoperative serum albumin, congestive heart failure, and increased American Society of Anesthesiologists (ASA) classification [5, 21–27]. Indeed, preoperative functional status is the strongest predictor of postsurgical inpatient morbidity and mortality [2]. The Edmonton obesity staging system (EOSS) incorporates many of these risk factors, divides patients into five stages (0–4), and has been shown to be more accurate in predicting all-cause mortality in overweight and obese patients compared to standard anthropometric-based classification schemes (Figs. 34.1 and 34.2) [28]. Although hyperglycemia has not been demonstrated as a separate risk factor for increased morbidity and mortality following bariatric surgery specifically, it has been identified in postsurgical patients to cause increased cardiovascular,

Criteria for assigning Edmonton Obesity Staging System score [17]

EOSS	0	1	2		
Definition	No apparent risk factors, physical symptoms, psychopathology, functional limitations, and/or mpairment of well-being related to obesity.	Presence of obesity-related subclinical risk factors, mild physical symptoms, mild functional limitations, and/or mild impairment of well-being.	Presence of established obesity-related chronic disease, moderate limitations in activities of daily living and/or well-being.	Established end-organ damage, significant psychopathology, significant functional limitation, and/or impairment of well-being	Severe (potentially end-stage) disabilities from obesity-related chronic diseases, severe disabling psychopathology, severe functional limitations, and/or severe impairment of well-being
		E.g., borderline hypertension, impaired fasting glucose levels, elevated levels of liver enzymes, intermittent gastroesophageal reflux disease, dyspnea on moderate exertion, occasional aches and pains, fatigue.	*E.g. hypertension, type 2 diabetes, sleep apnea. osteoarthritis, gastroesophageal reflux disease, polycystic ovary syndrome.*	*E.g., history of angina, coronary heart disease, congesitve heart failure, cerebrovascular disease, renal failure*	*E.g., tracheostomy in hypoventilation, wheelchair after amputation.*
Fasting glucose (mmol/L)	<5.6	5.6–6.9	≥7.0 or self report of diabetes, or treatment with insulin or antidiabetic agents		
Blood pressure (mm Hg)	< 130/80	SBP 130–139.9 DBP 85–89.9	≥BP 140/90		
LDL (mmol/L)	< 3.4	3.4–4.0	≥4.1		
Total cholesterol (mmol/L)	< 5.2	5.2–6.1	≥6.2		
HDL cholesterol (mmol/L)	> 1.6	1.0–1.6	<1.0		
Triglycerides (mmol/L)	< 1.7	1.7–2.3	>2.3		
Liver disease	No self-report of any liver condition, normal liver enzymes	Elevated liver enzymes but no self-report of liver disease	Elevated liver enzymes and self-report of liver disease		
Kidney disease: GFR (mL/min/m²)	GFR ≥90	GFR 60–89.9	GFR 30–59.9	GFR <30	
Osteoarthritis	No history of joint or back pain	Occasional joint or back pain	Self-report of osteoarthritis		
Physical health	No functional or ADL limitation	Functional impairment but no ADL limitations	ADL limitations		

ADL = activity of daily living; BP = blood pressure; DBP = diastolic blood pressure; EOSS = Edmonton Obesity Staging System; GFR = glomerular filtration rate; HDL = high-density lipoprotein; LDL = low-density lipoprotein; SBP = systolic blood pressure

EOSS for Postoperative Outcome and 30-Day Mortality / Surgery for Obesity and Related Diseases 12 (2016) 1847-1855

Fig. 34.1 Criteria for assigning Edmonton obesity staging system score. (From Chiappetta et al. [31])

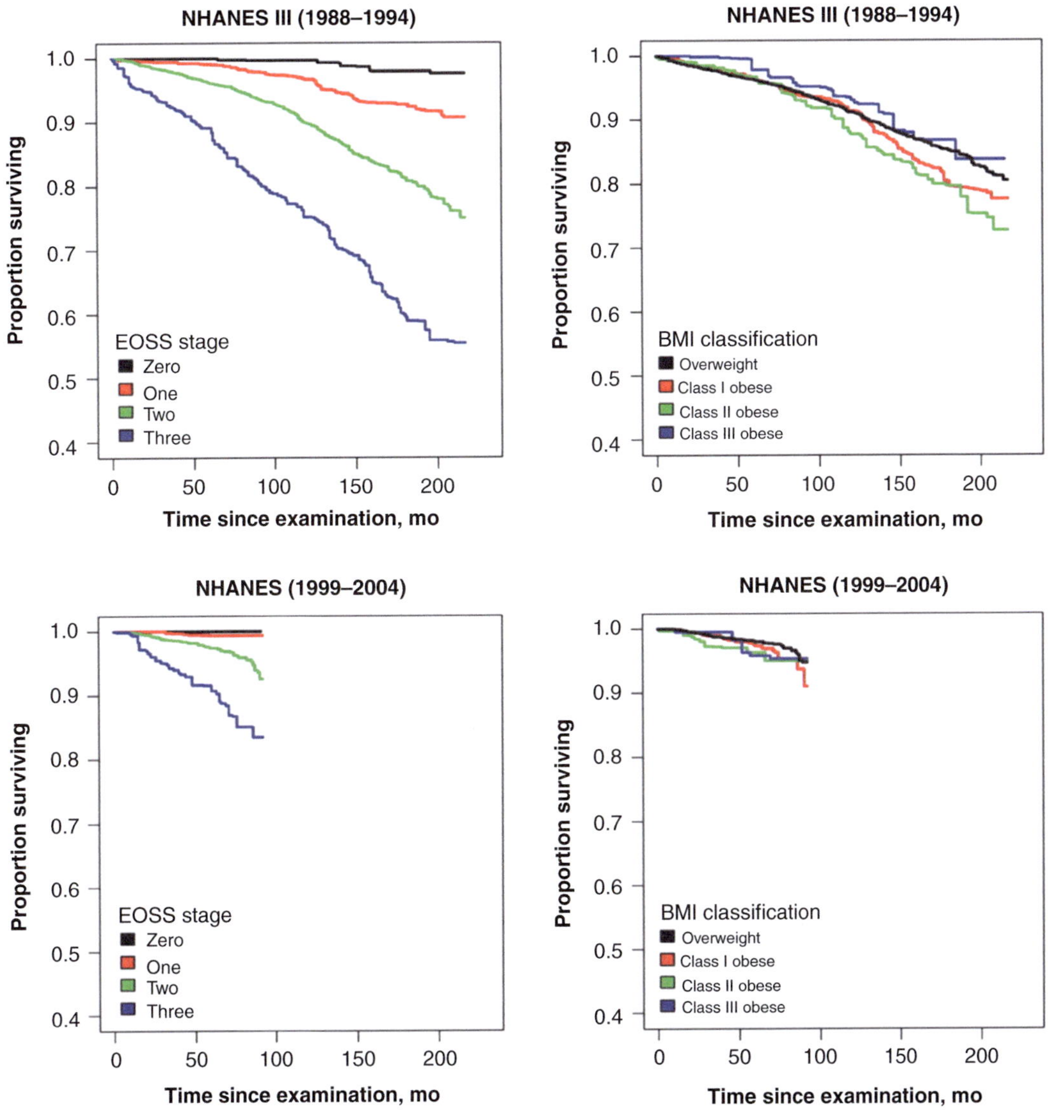

Fig. 34.2 Comparison of staging system and anthropometric classification scheme for predicting all-cause mortality among people with overweight and obesity. *BMI* body mass index, *EOSS* Edmonton obesity staging system, *NHANES* National Health and Human Nutrition Examination Surveys. (From Padwal et al. [28])

respiratory, neurologic, and infectious morbidity as well as mortality and is incorporated into the EOSS [29, 30]. By obtaining data regarding the patient's overall health and functional status, the EOSS has also been shown to predict patients at increased risk for 30-day postoperative morbidity and mortality [31].

Secondary to the complexity of assessing the degree of physiologic derangements in the bariatric surgery patient, our multidisciplinary team includes bariatricians who determine the need for additional testing above and beyond the typical history, physical, and laboratory evaluation. Additionally, they attempt to improve the patient's baseline well-being prior to surgery by utilizing recommendations from the American Society of Metabolic and Bariatric Surgery (ASMBS) clinical practice guidelines, such as improving preoperative glycemic control. Our center also has on-site exercise physiologists who provide education and training to patients with impaired physical functioning in an attempt to improve this preoperatively. For patients with more severe limitations, we may also refer for preoperative rehabilitation and conditioning [32].

Obstructive Sleep Apnea, Atelectasis, and Preoperative Pulmonary Training

Morbidly obese patients are at increased risk for a variety of postoperative pulmonary complications including atelectasis, pneumonia, laryngospasm, respiratory distress, impaired gas exchange, and the need for re-intubation, which may result in prolonged length of hospitalization and increased morbidity and mortality [33–35]. Multiple mechanisms involved in the physiologic changes associated with reduced pulmonary function in the morbidly obese are related to reduction in lung volumes, impaired ventilation/perfusion ratios, increased work of breathing, and hypoxemia [36, 37].

Additionally, increasing BMI is associated with increased prevalence of obstructive sleep apnea (OSA), with an overall prevalence rate in bariatric surgery patients ranging from 70% to 94% and severe OSA ranging from 20% to 50% of those patients [38–46]. Given the high frequency of OSA in the obese population, all patients being evaluated for bariatric surgery should be screened for this comorbidity. A cross-sectional comparison of four OSA screening questionnaires (Berlin, Epworth Sleepiness Scale, STOP, and STOP-Bang) verified against polysomnography demonstrated various sensitivities and specificities [47]. Within our practice, any patient with observed apnea, loud snoring, daytime sleepiness, frequent nighttime urination, or morning headaches receives testing with polysomnography and is treated accordingly.

Although morbidly obese patients are at increased risk for postoperative pulmonary complications, there is currently no evidence to recommend preoperative pulmonary function tests in the asymptomatic patient [48–50]. However, postoperative atelectasis develops in up to 90% of patients with normal lungs following intubation, can exceed 20% of lung volume in obese patients, and can persist for several weeks [51, 52]. Obesity and its associated increased intraabdominal pressure and upper displacement of the diaphragm, along with decreased chest wall compliance from excess adiposity, results in a decrease in functional residual capacity [53, 54]. Reports documenting the benefits of postoperative deep breathing with associated 3–5 s breath hold demonstrated a lower incidence of atelectasis (27% vs. 42%), with a further 12% reduction in patients who received preoperative instruction in deep breathing exercises [55]. A recent cross-sectional study demonstrated that preoperative deep breathing exercises and incentive spirometry increased thoracoabdominal mobility [56]. Furthermore, a meta-analysis demonstrated that incentive spirometry, intermittent positive pressure breathing, and deep breathing exercises appeared to be more effective than no physical therapy for preventing postoperative pulmonary complications following upper abdominal surgery [57]. We have incorporated preoperative incentive spirometer training in our program because it is low-cost and minimally labor intensive and mandates patient involvement. This training in conjunction with improved preoperative exercise tolerance and early postoperative ambulation has been beneficial in limiting our postoperative pulmonary complications.

Cardiovascular Evaluation

Obesity is an independent risk factor for hypertension, coronary artery disease (CAD), myocardial infarction, congestive heart disease, and atrial fibrillation [58, 59]. Secondary to these, coronary artery disease remains one of the most common etiologies of postoperative morbidity and mortality for the bariatric surgery patient [60]. Currently, there are no published guidelines for the preoperative cardiac evaluation prior to bariatric surgery, but given the prevalence of CAD in obese patients, the workup should be the same as for any high-risk surgical patient.

A detailed history and physical with assessment of functional status, exercise tolerance, and history of chest pain must be completed. All patients with any signs of cardiac disease should undergo an electrocardiogram (ECG) [61, 62]. Referral for a stress test (either dobutamine or exercise) is individualized based on symptoms and findings on the ECG, and any patient with an abnormal stress test is referred to a cardiologist. The routine use of echocardiography in the bariatric patient does not alter perioperative management and should be confined to patients with known heart disease [63].

Renal Disease

Obesity is associated with hypertension, hyperglycemia, dyslipidemia, inflammation, and atherosclerosis, which can each independently contribute to renal dysfunction. In addition, the increased prevalence of chronic kidney disease (CKD) has paralleled the increase in obesity rates [64, 65]. Patients with android obesity are at a higher risk for renal insufficiency independent of BMI, dyslipidemia, hypertension, and hyperglycemia [66]. Fortunately, bariatric surgery-induced weight loss has demonstrated improvement in renal function, although malabsorption and hyperoxaluria associated with malabsorptive procedures (roux-en-Y gastric bypass, and biliopancreatic diversion ± duodenal switch) can lead to further renal dysfunction [67, 68].

The evaluation for renal disease includes a detailed history and lab work consisting of BUN/Cr levels. Patients with documented CKD typically will already have a relationship with a nephrologist, which can be valuable in the preoperative preparation of the bariatric surgery patient. With appropriate preoperative optimization of renal function and education regarding the risk of renal failure following surgery, renal insufficiency of any degree is not an absolute contraindication for bariatric surgery. We have successfully performed surgery on patients with end-stage CKD requiring dialysis and those with renal transplants. As mentioned previously, alteration in preoperative VLCD is required for patients with CKD, including adjustment of diuretics, lower protein goals, and additional monitoring.

GERD, *H. pylori*, and Preoperative EGD

There is considerable debate regarding the need for preoperative evaluation of the upper gastrointestinal tract. A significant portion of bariatric patients have gastroesophageal reflux disease (GERD), which has been demonstrated as a risk factor for pathologic findings on esophagogastroduodenoscopy (EGD). Additionally, both GERD and obesity are known risk factors for esophageal cancer [69, 70]. Moreover, although there is debate regarding the impact of *H. pylori* infection on postoperative outcomes, *H. pylori* occurs in 9–61% of bariatric patients with regional variation [71, 72]. The American Society for Gastrointestinal Endoscopy (ASGE), the Society of Gastrointestinal and Endoscopic Surgeons (SAGES), and the ASMBS jointly developed a guideline for the use of upper endoscopy in bariatric patients, recommending evaluation on all symptomatic patients and indicating a possible role in asymptomatic patients [73]. Indeed, up to 65% of asymptomatic patients will have findings on EGD, including a 0.5–1% incidence of carcinoma in bariatric patients [74, 75]. Even in patients who are symptomatic, there may be no correlation between symptoms and pathologic results [74]. Although barium swallow can evaluate for hiatal hernias and gross lesions, it is limited in its ability to identify mucosal abnormalities, while studies investigating EGD demonstrate abnormal findings in 5–90% of patients [76–78]. Additionally, some authors advocate biopsy of macroscopically normal appearing mucosa since microscopic findings can be present (including the presence of *H. pylori*) [79]. The preoperative identification of a hiatal hernia allows for appropriate education, operative consent, and scheduling, but does not reduce the operative time compared to intraoperative identification alone [76]. Although there are economic costs and risks associated with performing an EGD, the overall complication rate is low at 0.22% [80]. Given the high prevalence of pathologic findings (even in normal appearing mucosa), some of which can alter surgical decision-making, and the low risk of complications, we recommend the routine use of preoperative screening EGD with biopsies of any suspicious areas and the antrum to evaluate for *H. pylori* or other microscopic conditions. Any condition diagnosed on preoperative EGD is treated or evaluated further prior to proceeding with surgery. Within our group, we have unfortunately had patients develop esophageal carcinoma after a vertical sleeve gastrectomy, a roux-en-Y gastric bypass, and a biliopancreatic diversion with duodenal switch, and therefore, a preoperative EGD can also serve as a baseline evaluation.

Nonalcoholic Fatty Liver Disease

Obesity and metabolic syndrome are risk factors for nonalcoholic fatty liver disease (NAFLD), which encompasses a spectrum of severity from simple steatosis to cirrhosis. Up to 90% of bariatric surgery patients have some form of NAFLD, with a prevalence of nonalcoholic steatohepatitis (NASH) in up to 35% of these patients [81–83]. Unfortunately, 32–53% of patients with NASH will develop progressive liver fibrosis [84, 85]. Fortunately, bariatric surgery has demonstrated improvement in liver function, resolution of NASH in up to 82% of patients, as well as possibly clearing sinusoidal fibrosis [86–88]. Despite these studies, both a Cochrane review and a meta-analysis indicate that the evidence is too limited to make recommendations that bariatric surgery is an effective treatment for NASH [81, 89]. Although NASH has not been associated with increased perioperative morbidity or mortality, hepatic dysfunction has been, and therefore these patients must be considered at a higher risk [90]. The data regarding compensated cirrhosis (i.e., cirrhosis without hepatic dysfunction) are not completely clear but seem to indicate that bariatric surgery can be performed relatively safely [91]. However, the mortality rate in patients with decompensated cirrhosis carries an odds ratio of 21.2 higher than non-cirrhotic patients and should be considered an absolute contraindication for bariatric surgery.

Since physical examination findings of a cirrhotic or enlarged liver are difficult to determine in the obese population, NAFLD is typically determined by a detailed history of fatty liver, NASH, cirrhosis, hepatitis, jaundice, and alcohol dependence as well as laboratory evaluation of albumin, alanine aminotransferase, aspartate aminotransferase, and bilirubin. Patients with evidence of hepatic dysfunction should also have a prothrombin time/international normalized ratio (PT/INR) evaluated, as well as a hepatic ultrasound with probable biopsy, and be counseled to avoid potentially hepatotoxic substances such as alcohol and acetaminophen. Referral to a gastroenterologist for further evaluation and management is also warranted. If patients with hepatic dysfunction are deemed to be appropriate candidates for bariatric surgery, malabsorptive procedures should be avoided secondary to the risk of protein malabsorption and worsening of hepatic function, which can result in complete hepatic failure [92].

Mental Health Disorders and Socioeconomic Deprivation

There is an increased prevalence of mood disorders, depression, and binge eating disorder among bariatric patients (23%, 19%, and 17%, respectively) compared to estimates of the US population (10%, 8%, and 1–5%, respectively) [93, 94]. The true incidence within bariatric surgery practices may actually be higher since patients with uncontrolled disorders, such as current substance dependence, severe depression, psychosis, suicidal ideation, and untreated eating disorders, typically do not proceed to surgery. Secondary to this, the ASMBS recommends routine preoperative review of patients' mental health conditions, with most authors recommending a more comprehensive mental health examination, including clinical interviews conducted by mental health professionals with bariatric experience and the use of formal psychological testing if desired [95–97]. Patients with psychological issues require a more time and resource-intensive preoperative evaluation resulting in a longer preoperative duration to surgery [98]. With appropriate identification and treatment of mental health disorders, it appears that these do not interfere with postoperative weight loss as demonstrated in a meta-analysis and a systematic review of the literature [93, 99]. Additionally, severely obese patients with depression appear to gain psychological benefits from bariatric surgery including a reduction in the prevalence, frequency, and severity of depressive symptoms postoperatively [93, 100–103]. However, the bariatric team must also educate and monitor patients for postoperative mental health problems, such as addiction transference and resultant alcoholism or loss of control eating in patients with a history of binge eating disorder.

Although socioeconomic deprivation should not be a final determinant in eligibility for bariatric surgery, evidence suggests that outcomes after bariatric surgery are influenced by self-esteem, cognitive function, support networks, and socioeconomic stability [99, 104]. Bariatric centers must be aware of the unique challenges that need to be addressed for these patients, such as poor social networks and support, financial limitations, and knowledge deficits. Each of these factors can decrease access to care, but with appropriate support, postsurgical weight loss outcomes can be equivalent to non-deprived groups [105]. It is imperative that the entire multidisciplinary team is involved in the evaluation process since poor patient selection and education can result in increased workload postoperatively [106].

For all patients, we encourage involvement of family and friends in the process, but for those with poor social networks and support, we help the patient establish and strengthen these areas. Financial limitations can be addressed with local support (donations from individuals, institutions, or charities) and regional and national programs. Knowledge deficits are addressed based on the areas of weakness and can involve additional visits with any member of our team and must be corrected prior to proceeding with surgery. Our in-office behaviorists and psychologists not only perform the preoperative behavioral evaluation and postoperative education, but they also serve as resources for patients who require additional mental health support both pre- and postoperatively. We also recommend both preoperative and lifelong postoperative attendance at our behavioral education groups and surgical support groups where a multitude of topics are addressed, including cognitive behavioral therapy skills, body image, shame reduction, coping with obesity stigma, etc. Additionally, we will pair past patients with new patients to develop a mentor-mentee relationship, which we have found to be very beneficial. Although most of these efforts are carried out face to face in our office, we have been introducing social media in our ongoing education and support groups, which the patients report is very convenient and useful.

Substance Abuse

Substance abuse may be present in up to 25% of patients seeking bariatric surgery with high-risk psychiatric profiles including 14% with tobacco dependency, 16% with alcohol abuse, and 2% with illicit drug use [96, 97]. Substance abuse among bariatric surgery candidates results in program congestion secondary to patients having a decreased likelihood of making it to surgery [106].

Tobacco abuse has been associated with an increase in postsurgical complications including myocardial infarction, delayed wound healing, pneumonia, and mortality [107, 108]. The pathophysiologic effects of tobacco use include an increase in heart rate, blood pressure, and oxygen demand secondary to decreased blood flow from vasoconstriction, narrowing of small airways, reduction in immune responses, and increased risk of thrombosis [109–112]. In bariatric surgery specifically, smoking is associated with a twofold increase in mortality and a 1.5 times higher 30-day complication rate including venous thromboembolism, which remains elevated for at least 6 months postoperatively [113–115]. Secondary to these issues, the evidence-based bariatric surgery guidelines recommend tobacco cessation at least 6 weeks preoperatively and provide support for long-term abstinence [116]. It is our practice to require all patients to stop the use of tobacco and nicotine, as demonstrated by a negative nicotine urinalysis prior to proceeding with bariatric surgery. Additionally, we educate patients on the negative effects of secondhand smoke and encourage patients to distance themselves from this exposure.

Worldwide, cannabis is the most widely used illicit drug, and unfortunately it carries risk factors both similar to and unique from tobacco use [117]. Inhaled marijuana smoke is associated with inflammation and atypia of airway epithelium accompanied by symptoms of chronic bronchitis, including a sore throat and cough [118, 119]. Patients with pre-existing cardiac disease have an increased risk of myocardial infarction in the hour following cannabis smoking, and even brief exposure to secondhand smoke results in impaired vascular endothelial function [120, 121]. Cannabis also has additive effects with anti-cholinergics and central nervous system depressants, resulting in increased sedation, dizziness or lightheadedness, muscle weakness, dry mouth, and confusion [122, 123]. Although infrequent, tachycardia and postural hypotension can occur in patients with cardiovascular disease [122]. Secondary to the potential complications and side effects associated with cannabis use, we require all recreational users to have three negative random urine screens over a 6-month time frame. For patients who have a clear medical need for cannabis, we discuss the risk and benefits of continuing versus discontinuing this therapy and strongly encourage cessation.

The exact prevalence of alcohol use disorders (AUD, previously alcohol dependence and alcohol abuse) in patients seeking bariatric surgery is unknown but ranges from that of the general population to as high as 16% in high-risk psychiatric patients [96, 124]. Although a current diagnosis of AUD is considered a contraindication to bariatric surgery, the history of this diagnosis is not. However, patients with a history of AUD may be at increased risk for relapsing to alcohol use following roux-en-Y gastric bypass procedures, which typically presents greater than 2 years postoperatively [124, 125]. This association has not been seen in patients undergoing adjustable gastric banding or vertical sleeve gastrectomy. Within our practice, any patient with an active diagnosis of AUD is put on hold, provided resources to stop drinking, and is required to be alcohol-free for 6 months prior to surgery.

Interestingly, patients with a history of preoperative treatment for substance abuse lost more weight 2 years postoperatively following a roux-en-Y gastric bypass compared to those who had not required treatment (79% versus 67%) [126]. Therefore, a history of substance abuse should not be a contraindication to bariatric surgery, but rather may actually be a prognosticator of improved outcomes secondary to previous success with long-term behavioral changes.

Preoperative Laboratory Evaluation

Successful management of the bariatric patient's postoperative nutrition begins with a strong preoperative educational program, thorough assessment of nutritional status, and follow-up to reinforce important principals associated with long-term weight loss maintenance. While it is important to evaluate a patient's readiness for change, realistic goal setting, and general nutritional knowledge, standard laboratory assessment is critical. It is our practice to require all bariatric surgery candidates be screened with a comprehensive panel of laboratory studies to assess their baseline health and nutritional status. Routine labs consist of fasting blood glucose, lipid panel, kidney function, liver profile, thyroid-stimulating hormone (TSH), parathyroid hormone (PTH), complete blood count (CBC), urinalysis, and select vitamin levels (see below). This information may then be used to optimize their preoperative health by modifying medications or starting new medications to treat comorbid conditions or restore vitamin deficiencies.

Diabetes: Glycemic Control

Preoperative glycemic control should be optimized with the help of a diabetes comprehensive care plan as described by the American Association of Clinical Endocrinologists (AACE) in 2011 [127]. Measures include healthy dietary patterns, medical nutrition therapy, physical activity, and, as needed, pharmacotherapy. In the end, a shorter duration and better preoperative glycemic control is associated with a higher rate of T2D remission after bariatric surgery [128]. Reasonable treatment targets include a hemoglobin A1c value of 6.5–7.0% or less, a fasting blood glucose level of ≤110 mg/dL, and a 2-h postprandial blood glucose concentration of ≤140 mg/dL. However, clinical judgment should be considered in patients with microvascular or macrovascular complications, extensive comorbidities, or long-standing, treatment-resistant diabetes. A more liberal preoperative hemoglobin A1c target of 7–8% may be appropriate in this population, and, on a rare occasion, patients with extremely treatment-resistant T2D may only be able to obtain a level less than 10%. Nevertheless, an elevated preoperative A1c in patients undergoing RYGB is associated with elevated postoperative hyperglycemia, which, in turn, is independently associated with higher rates of wound infections, acute renal failure, and reduced T2D remission rates [129]. Baseline C-peptide levels are a surrogate for beta islet pancreatic cell mass and are commonly elevated in T2D, and remission rates after RYGB were positively correlated with preoperative C-peptide levels. Although we do not routinely check this biomarker, it may be used to assist in the selection and counseling of patients with obesity-related T2D that are most likely to benefit from bariatric surgery [130].

Thyroid Disease

Subclinical hypothyroidism and increased TSH levels are associated with severe obesity. It is also widely known that TSH levels decrease after bariatric surgery and significant weight loss [131–135]. Although routine screening for primary hypothyroidism in obese patients is not recommended per the American Thyroid Association, appropriate testing should proceed with at-risk patients based on clinical presentation, family history of thyroid disease, or the presence of other autoimmune disorders such as rheumatoid arthritis and type 1 diabetes [136]. Nevertheless, many insurance companies in the USA require TSH testing before proceeding with bariatric surgery, which is our standard practice.

Lipids

A fasting lipid panel should be obtained for all obese patients considering bariatric surgery. Currently within the USA, most insurance require a 6–12-month presurgical medical weight loss program, and therefore, treatment should be initiated for the management of dyslipidemia and prevention of atherosclerosis. Improvement in serum lipid levels after bariatric surgery has been well documented, but results are often variable and incomplete and are not simply due to weight loss. Changes in gastrointestinal absorption and altered dietary patterns contribute to lowering low-density lipoprotein and total cholesterol while raising high-density lipoprotein levels. Therefore, the need for lipid-lowering medications, such as statins, should be periodically evaluated and not be stopped unless clearly indicated [137].

Pregnancy

All premenopausal women considering bariatric surgery should be screened for pregnancy with a urine human chorionic gonadotropin on the day of surgery. Current pregnancy is an absolute contraindication for bariatric surgery and should be avoided for 12–18 months postoperatively. This has been supported by numerous reviews and position statements related to the harmful effects of various deficiencies on the developing fetus, including iron, calcium, vitamin B12, folic acid, and vitamin D, as well as teratogens such as vitamin A [138–140]. Therefore, all women of reproductive age should be counseled on both barrier and pharmacologic contraceptive choices prior to surgery. Many bariatric surgery practices routinely advise patients to stop taking combined hormonal oral contraceptives for a period of time before surgery until at least 30 days postoperatively due to the relative increased risk of venous thromboembolism (VTE). During that time frame, we recommend the use of barrier contraceptives due to the inconsistency of pharmacokinetics in obese women, especially after malabsorptive procedures (RYGB, BPD-DS). Our group has recently recommended the ongoing use of both oral hormonal and barrier contraceptives during the perioperative period due to the risk of VTE in morbidly obese women who experience unintended pregnancy compared to nonpregnant women taking oral contraceptives. For the women who become pregnant after bariatric surgery, they should be monitored for appropriate weight gain, nutritional supplementation, and fetal health. Nutritional surveillance should include screening for deficiencies in iron, folate, vitamin B_{12}, calcium, and fat-soluble vitamins every trimester.

Biochemical Monitoring for Nutrition Status

Establishing baseline laboratory values for all potential bariatric surgery candidates is critical, especially in patients who proceed with a malabsorptive operation (Fig. 34.3a, b). This information becomes important when trying to distinguish between pre-existing deficiencies, postoperative complications, and noncompliance with recommended nutrient supplementation. Numerous biologic processes are dependent upon vitamins and minerals as essential factors and cofactors in the regulation of body size. They help in the modulation of appetite, hunger, nutrient absorption, metabolic rate, fat and sugar metabolism, thyroid and adrenal function, glucose homeostasis, and neural activities. A growing body of literature has documented several micronutrient deficiencies that may actually be more prevalent in overweight and obese adults and children. This may seem paradoxical in light of the typical excess caloric intake associated with obesity. Poor dietary selection and habits coupled with reduced vitamin and mineral contents of processed foods can lead to micronutrient deficiencies among the general population. Increased adiposity itself may also contribute to altered fat-soluble vitamin metabolism, such as vitamin D. Therefore, adequate preoperative micronutrient repletion is not only important for good health but for weight loss success and longevity. The following sections discuss potential signs, symptoms, and treatment or supplementation of micronutrient deficiencies as they relate to bariatric surgery.

Vitamin B_{12} and Folate

Both vitamin B_{12} (cobalamin) and folate (folic acid) are involved in the maturation of red blood cells, and chronic deficiency can lead to macrocytic anemia. Among the most commonly performed bariatric operations, RYGB patients are at most risk. They experience a significant decrease in hydrochloric acid production, resulting in a decreased conversion of pepsinogen to pepsin, which is necessary for the release of vitamin B_{12} from protein [141]. The reduced availability of intrinsic factor (IF) only compounds the problem as it is a glycoprotein produced by parietal cells that is required for absorptions of cobalamin in the terminal ileum. A reduction in hydrochloric acid and subsequently vitamin B_{12} is not as prevalent in patients who undergo adjustable gastric banding (AGB), vertical sleeve gastrectomy (VSG), and biliopancreatic diversion with duodenal switch (BPD-DS). This is because AGB patients retain full use of the exocrine and endocrine properties of the gastric mucosa while VSG and BPD-DS patients retain the use of a larger gastric volume, better tolerance of animal proteins, and greater pepsin and gastric acid production, which allows increased availability and interaction of IF with pouch contents.

Several medications commonly taken by bariatric patients may elevate their preoperative risk of deficiency by altering vitamin B_{12} absorption and liver stores. Of patients taking metformin for impaired glucose tolerance or T2D, 10–30% present with reduced vitamin B_{12} absorption [142]. The high incidence of GERD in obese patients translates to prevalent use of proton pump inhibitors (PPIs), which may increase the potential risk of developing vitamin B_{12} deficiency.

a

Suggested Biochemical Monitoring Tools for Nutrition Status

Vitamin/mineral	Screening	Normal range	Additional laboratory indexes	Critical range	Preoperative deficiency	Postoperative deficiency	Comments
B_1 (thiamin)	Serum thiamin	10–64 ng/mL	↓ RBC transketolase ↑ Pyruvate	Transketolase activity >20% Pyruvate >1 mg/dL	15-29%; more common in African Americans and Hispanics; often associated with poor hydration	Rare, but occurs with RYGB, AGB, and BPD/DS	Serum thiamin responds to dietary supplementation but is poor indicator of total body stores
B_6 (pyridoxine)	PLP	5–24 ng/mL	RBC glutamic pyruvate Oxaloacetic transaminase	PLP <3 ng/ML	Unknown	Rare	Consider with unresolved anemia; diabetes could influence values
B_{12} (cobalamin)	Serum B_{12}	200–1000 pg/mL	↑ Serum and urinary MMA ↑ Serum tHcy	Serum B_{12} <200 pg/ML deficiency <400 pg/ML suboptimal sMMA >0.376 μmol/ μMMA >3.6 μmol/ mmol CRT tHcy > 13.2 μmol/L	10–13%; may occur with older patients and those taking H_2 blockers and PPIs	Common with RYGB in absence of supplementation, 12–33%	When symptoms are present and B_{12} 200–250 pg/mL, MMA and tHcy are useful; serum B_{12} may miss 25–30% of deficiency cases
Folate	RBC folate	280–791 ng/mL	Urinary FIGLU Normal serum and urinary MMA ↑ Serum tHcy	RBC folate <305 nmol/L deficiency, <227 nmol/L anemia	Uncommon	Uncommon	Serum folate reflects recent dietary intake rather than folate status; RBC folate is a more sensitive marker Excessive supplementation can mask B_{12} deficiency in CBC; neurologic symptoms will persist
Iron	Ferritin	Males: 15–200 ng/mL Females: 12–15p ng/mL	↓ Serum iron ↑ TIBC	Ferritin <20 ng/mL Serum iron <50 μg/dL TIBC >450 μg/dL	9–16% of adult women in general population are deficient	20–49% of patients; common with RYGB for menstruating women (51%), and patients with super obesity (49–52%)	Low Hgb and Hct are consistent with iron deficiency anemia in stage 3 or stage 4 anemia; ferritin is an acute phase reactant and will be elevated with illness and/or inflammation; oral contraceptives reduce blood loss for menstruating females
Vitamin A	Plasma retinol	20–80 μg/dL	RBP	Plasma retinol <10 μg/dL	Uncommon; up to 7% in some studies	Common (50%) with BPD/DS after 1 yr up to 70% at 4 yr; may occur with RYGB/AGB	Ocular finding may suggest diagnosis

L Aills et al/ Surgery for Obesity and Related Diseases 4 (2008) S73-S108

Fig. 34.3 (**a**, **b**) Suggested biochemical monitoring for nutrition status. (© Jeanne Blankenship, MS RD. Used with permission)

L Arills et al/ Surgery for Obesity and Related Diseases 4 (2008) S73-S108

b

Continued

Vitamin/mineral	Screening	Normal range	Additional laboratory indexes	Critical range	Preoperative deficiency	Postoperative deficiency	Comments
Vitamin D	25(OH)D	25–40 ng/mL	↓ Serum phosphors ↑ Alkaline phosphors ↑ Serum PTH ↓ Urinary clacium	Serum 25(OH)D <20 ng/mL suggests deficiency 20–30 mL suggests insufficiency	Common; 60–70%	Common with BOD/DS after 1 yr; may occure with RYGB; prevalence unknown	With deficiency, serum calcium may be low or normal; serum phosphorus may decrease, serum alkaline phosphatase increases; PTH elevated
Vitamin E	Plasma alpha tocopherol	5–20 μg/mL	Plasma lipids	<5 μg/mL	Uncommon	Uncommon	Low plasma alpha tocopherol to plasma lipids (0.8 mg/g total lipid) should be used with hyperlipidemia
Vitamin K	PT	10–13 seconds	↑ DCP ↓ Plasma phylloquinone	Variable	Uncommon	Common with BPD/DS after 1 yr	PT is not a sensitive meaure of vitamin K status
Zinc	Plasma zinc	60–130 μg/dL	↓ RBC zinc	Plasma zinc <70 μg/dL	Uncommon, but increased risk of low levels associated with obesity	Common with BPD/DS after 1 yr; may occur with RYGB	Monitor albumin levels and interpret zinc accordingly, albumin is primary binding protein for zinc; no reliable method of determining zinc status is available; plasma zinc is method generally used; studies cited in this repot did not adequately describe methods of zinc analysis
Protein	Serum albumin Serum total protein	4–6 g/dL 6–8 g/dL	↓ Serum prealbumin (transthyretin)	Albumin <3.0 g/dL Prealbumin <20 mg/dL	Uncommon	Rare, but can occur with RYGB, AGB, and BPD/DS if protein intake is low in total intake or indispensable amino acids	Half-life for prealbumin is 2–4 d and reflects changes in nutritional status sooner than albumin, a nonspecific protein carrier with a half-life of 22 d

RYGB = Roux-en-Y gastric bypass; AGB = adjustable gastric banding; BPD/DS = biliopancreatic diversion/ducdenal switch; PLP = pyridoxal-5′ - phosphate; RBC = red blood cell; MMA = methylmalonic acid; tHcy = total homocysteine; CRT = creatinine; PPIs = protein pump inhibitors; FIGLU = formiminoglutamic acid; CBC = complete blood count; TIBC = total iron binding capacity; Hgb = hemoglobin; Hct = hematocrit; RPB = retinol binding protein; PTH = parathyroid hormone; 25(OH)D = 25.hydroxyvitamin D; PT = prothrombin time; DCP = des-gamma-carboxypromthrombin.

In general, laboratory values should be reviewed annually or as indicated by clinical presentation. Laboratory normal values vary among laboratory setting and are method dependent. This chart provdes a brief summary of monitoring tools. See the Appendix for additional detail and diagnostic tools.

Fig. 34.3 (continued)

Some vitamin B_{12}-deficient patients may develop significant symptoms such as polyneuropathy, paresthesia, and permanent neural impairment including delusions, hallucination, and overt psychosis [143]. Catastrophic consequences of undetected chronic deficiency are too great to forego supplementation. Therefore, we recommend both preoperative and annual postoperative screening among all bariatric patients but especially those undergoing RYGB. Both patient compliance and practitioner preference can be taken into consideration when choosing the doses of daily, weekly, or monthly supplementation. It can be given parenterally, via nasal sprays, sublingual preparations, and intramuscular injections. Oral supplementation with 350–500 μg/d may prevent most postoperative vitamin B_{12} deficiency in RYGB patients [144, 145].

It is common knowledge that folic acid deficiency or failing to consume the recommended dietary intake of 400 μg/d among pregnant women is associated with a greater risk of fetal neural tube defects. Despite the pervasiveness of folate-fortified grain products, the increasing popularity of high-protein/low-carbohydrate diets may exacerbate this risk. Boylan et al. found that 56% of preoperative RYGB patients were deficient in folic acid [146]. Since the majority of patients remains asymptomatic or has subclinical symptoms, the consequences of failing to identify folate deficiency are potentially much greater for women than men. Folate absorption occurs preferentially in the proximal small bowel, but it can occur along the entire length of the small bowel with postoperative brush border adaptation. Folate deficiency is preventable with supplementation that provides 200% of the recommended daily value (800 μg/d) or corrected with 1000 μg/d [147].

Iron

Iron deficiency has been reported in nearly 50% of morbidly obese preoperative candidates [148]. Symptoms of fatigue and a diminished capacity to exercise are often experienced when total body iron stores are depleted and erythropoiesis is impaired. Women of child-bearing age comprise the majority of bariatric surgeries performed each year in the USA. Iron deficiency as a result of menstrual losses should be considered and addressed given that oral contraceptives alone can decrease blood loss by as much as 60% [149]. Screening for iron status should begin with measuring serum iron and total iron-binding capacity. Serum ferritin is an acute phase reactant and should not be used to diagnose deficiency since it can fluctuate with age, inflammation, and infection. Hemoglobin and hematocrit should be obtained as part of a complete blood count; however, they reflect the later stages of iron deficiency anemia. Pre-existing iron deficiency anemia should be factored into the surgeon's discussion with the patient regarding the selection of an appropriate bariatric surgery. For instance, the reports of iron deficiency after RYGB range from 20% to 49%, since the duodenum and proximal jejunum where iron is most efficiently absorbed are bypassed [150]. The problem of decreased absorption is often magnified by reduced intake of iron-rich foods such as red meats, enriched grains, and vegetables, due to poor tolerance by RYGB patients postoperatively.

Calcium and Vitamin D

Similar to iron, calcium is absorbed preferentially in the duodenum and proximal jejunum; however, its absorption is facilitated by vitamin D in an acidic environment. Vitamin D is absorbed more distally in the jejunum and ileum. While it is important to consider the elevated risk of deficiency in patients undergoing malabsorptive operations, attention must be focused on early identification and treatment in the preoperative setting. For instance, vitamin D deficiency has been found in 60–80% of morbidly obese preoperative candidates [148, 151–153]. This results in a cascade of reduced dietary calcium absorption and increased calcitriol which causes metabolic changes that may also favor fat accumulation [154–156]. Even though low vitamin D levels are associated with decreased dietary calcium absorption, it does not always equate to a reduction in serum calcium.

Calcium homeostasis is maintained by an upregulation of PTH with downstream effects on the kidney, liver, and the skeletal system in the form of bone resorption. Measurable calcium deficiency is often not expected until osteoporosis has severely depleted the skeleton of calcium stores.

Observational studies and clinical trials alike show that calcium malnutrition and hypovitaminosis D can predispose patients to a variety of common chronic diseases, such as skeletal disorders, malignancies (colon, breast, and prostate), chronic inflammation and autoimmune diseases (e.g., type 1 diabetes mellitus, inflammatory bowel disease, multiple sclerosis, rheumatoid arthritis), metabolic disorders (metabolic syndrome and hypertension), and peripheral vascular disease [157, 158]. Treatment for vitamin D deficiency can consist of 50,000 IU of ergocalciferol taken orally, once weekly, for 8 weeks [148]. Standard multivitamins containing 1200 mg of daily calcium and 400–800 IU of vitamin D may not provide adequate protection in the postoperative setting against increasing PTH and bone resorption [159, 160]. Supratherapeutic dosing of calcium citrate and vitamin D is often required because deficits in vitamin D, calcium, and potentially secondary hyperparathyroidism will result in osteopenia, osteoporosis, and ultimately osteomalacia [161]. It is our practice to correct hypovitaminosis D preoperatively with 2000–10,000 IU of ergocalciferol daily and adjust the dose postoperatively as needed based on regular assessment of laboratory values. In addition to medical therapy, patient should be encouraged to participate in weight-bearing physical exercise; increase the dietary intake of calcium and vitamin D-rich foods, moderate sun exposure, and smoking cessation; and reduce intake of alcohol, caffeine, and phosphoric acid to promote strong and healthy bones.

Vitamins A, E, and K and Zinc

The risk of fat-soluble vitamin deficiencies among preoperative bariatric surgery patients remains relatively low. Few studies have investigated preoperative fat-soluble vitamin deficiencies, but Madan et al. investigated vitamin and trace minerals before and after RYGB and found vitamin A was deficient in only 7% of patients prior to surgery [162]. Boylan et al. found 23% of RYGB patients had low vitamin E levels prior to surgery [146]. Routine screening for zinc deficiency should be reserved for the postoperative setting as well, unless there are signs of hair loss, pica, altered sense of taste (dysgeusia), or in male patients with hypogonadism or erectile dysfunction. To summarize, more effort should be put into appropriate screening for the signs and symptoms of vitamin A, E, K, and zinc deficiencies in the postoperative care of patients undergoing malabsorptive procedures, particularly the BPD-DS. Even though the RYGB, VSG, and AGB may have variable effects on the digestion, absorption, and transport of fat-soluble vitamins, they do not result in a 72% decrease in fat absorption as seen with the BPD-DS [163].

Protein

Few studies have investigated the rate of preoperative protein deficiency in bariatric surgery patients. Overall, it is very unlikely, but it would be unwise to assume that it does not exist altogether among morbidly obese patients, given the popularity of food faddism and the often disordered eating pattern observed in the morbidly obese. With a half-life of 3 weeks, preoperative albumin levels (normal range 3.5–5.0 g/dL) should suffice as an indicator of long-term protein status. If needed, diagnosis of protein malnutrition (PM) can be supported with additional laboratory testing of serum transferrin (half-life 8–10 days), retinol-binding protein (half-life 12 h), or prealbumin (half-life 2 days). The concomitant anemia often seen in the setting of PM or protein-energy malnutrition can be due to iron, vitamin B_{12}, folate, and/or copper deficiency [150].

Venous Thromboembolism Prophylaxis

Deep vein thrombosis (DVT) occurs in 0.3–2.2% of post-bariatric surgery patients with an approximate 1% incidence of pulmonary embolism (PE) [25, 164–168]. Unfortunately, despite attempts at reducing these complications, PE remains one of the leading causes of 30-day postoperative mortality representing 17–20.7% of post-bariatric surgery mortalities [60, 169]. Patient-related risk factors for VTE include increasing age, male sex, increasing BMI (37% increased risk with each ten point increase in BMI), history of VTE, and smoking [60, 114, 115, 168, 170]. Additionally, procedure-related risk factors include open procedure, operative time >3 h, postoperative RYGB leak, and procedure type including revision surgery [114, 167, 171]. Analysis of data from a state-wide registry including 27,000 patients stratified patients into low- (<1%), medium- (1–4%), and high-risk (>4%) categories and identified that 97% of patients fell in the low-risk category [168].

Strategies to reduce VTE rates include lower extremity compression devices (LECD), early postsurgical ambulation, and chemoprophylaxis. In a Cochrane review and meta-analysis, the use of LECD reduced the risk of DVT by >60% compared to no prophylaxis [172–174]. The data regarding the direct impact of early ambulation on VTE reduction are limited since this strategy has not been studied in isolation. The use of chemoprophylaxis with either unfractionated heparin (UFH) or low-molecular-weight heparin (LMWH) has demonstrated risk reductions in VTE rates of 47% and 71%, respectively but also demonstrated an increased risk of bleeding complications in 57% with UFH and relative risk of hemorrhage of 2.03 with LMWH [174, 175]. Unfortunately, data are limited to suggest the superiority of UFH compared to LMWH, and the appropriate VTE prophylaxis dosing continues to be debated. Although most studies focus on LMWH and have evaluated standard- versus adjusted-dose regimens, there is significant heterogeneity in the study groups, and the relatively small size of the cohorts limits their power [176–180].

Based on recommendations from the Michigan Bariatric Surgery Collaborative (MBSC), our current practice for low-risk patients is to give enoxaparin 40 mg subcutaneously 2 h preoperatively and then 30 mg twice a day while hospitalized. For moderate- and high-risk patients, we discharge on 40 mg subcutaneously once or twice daily, respectively, for 30 days. Patients on lifelong anticoagulation for a history of DVT/PE are typically transitioned off their oral medication and onto enoxaparin preoperatively, and then the process is reversed postoperatively. We have intermittently utilized postoperative oral factor Xa inhibitors with success, but there are limited data related to their use. The use of inferior vena cava (IVC) filters as PE prophylaxis has fallen out of favor, and the combined VTE prophylaxis guidelines of the AACE, the Obesity Society, and the ASMBS indicate that its risks may outweigh its benefits [61]. Our group abandoned the use of IVC filters in 2010 after data from the MBSC suggested increased complications, including mortality, associated with their use [181].

Antibiotic Prophylaxis

Following the introduction of laparoscopic bariatric surgery with the resultant smaller incisions, shorter hospital length of stay, and minimal blood loss, the incidence of surgical site infections (SSI) has decreased to approximately 4% [182–184]. The organisms causing SSI following bariatric surgery are most commonly Gram-positive (*staphylococci* and *streptococci*), but can be Gram-negative or anaerobic [185, 186]. Per the Antimicrobial Prophylaxis in Surgery guidelines jointly developed by the American Society of Health-System Pharmacists (ASHP), the Infectious Diseases Society of America (IDSA), the Surgical Infection Society (SIS), and the Society for Healthcare Epidemiology of America (SHEA), cefazolin 2 g intravenously (3 g if weight >120 kg) within 60 min of incision is adequate for low-risk patients undergoing gastrointestinal surgery [187]. However, cephamycins have improved anaerobic coverage, with cefoxitin having the greatest activity against *B. fragilis*, and therefore have also become a common prophylactic agent in bariatric surgery [188]. For those patients with an allergy to cephalosporins or severe allergy to penicillin (e.g., IgE mediated), clindamycin or vancomycin with an aminoglycoside or aztreonam or fluoroquinolone should be utilized [187]. Given variations in regional pathogens and antimicrobial resistance, choice of antibiotic prophylaxis should be driven by local population susceptibility profiles.

It is our protocol to utilize cefoxitin 2 g IV 30–60 min prior to incision with intraoperative repeat dosing every 2 h for extended procedures. For patients with allergies to cephalosporins or anaphylactic reactions to penicillin, we use clindamycin 900 mg and gentamicin with adjusted dose to BMI and renal function, intravenously. We previously continued patients on antibiotics for the first 24 h postoperatively but found an increased rate of oral candidiasis and, after switching to only preoperative and intraoperative dosing, found no change in our SSI infection rates but a decrease in the incidence of oral candidiasis.

Consents

The informed consent is more than a document the patient signs but rather is a dynamic process that represents the education a patient receives regarding the options for treatment and the risks and benefits of each of these options [189]. When done appropriately, the informed consent can have positive effects on physician-patient relationships and communication with more realistic expectations, increased patient sense of empowerment and satisfaction, and potentially decrease medical errors and malpractice claims [190–194]. Our process of informed consent begins with an initial educational seminar (available both online and in-person) and ongoing education from all segments of our multidisciplinary team including handouts and a presurgical informed consent seminar and is completed in the preoperative holding area. The typical patient within our program will receive this information at least three separate times throughout the process, with some patients requiring even more attention. We have found that the additional effort invested in the preoperative education pays dividends in increased patient satisfaction and reduced malpractice claims.

Reoperative Surgery

With the significant number of bariatric surgeries performed worldwide and their associated complications including failed weight loss, reoperative surgery is becoming much more common. Additionally, patients with a history of an antireflux procedure who meet criteria for a bariatric operation represent a significant surgical challenge. In addition to all the risk factors discussed above, these patients have the added challenge of altered surgical anatomy and scarring and may also have protein-calorie and micronutrient deficiencies. The evaluation of the reoperative surgery patient typically requires a detailed history and physical with specific attention to signs and symptoms of complications from their previous procedure(s), review of previous operative notes, extended laboratory testing to assess nutrient levels, additional imaging modalities for appropriate identification of the altered anatomy, and appropriate nutrient supplementation to address deficiencies. In-depth education is required to guide the patient toward appropriate expectations with the procedure. The complexities of these reoperations are associated with higher postoperative complication rates. Reoperative procedures should only be performed by experienced bariatric surgeons [195].

Within our group, we have four experienced bariatric surgeons who perform our complex reoperative procedures and will assist each other for extremely complex operations. With each new surgeon we add to our group, we provide a mentorship throughout their first year of practice and will assist them as they develop the skills required for reoperative procedures, including a backup surgeon who is on-call to assist with complex emergent surgeries. It has been our experience that patients will seek treatment for a specific complication (i.e., chronic marginal ulcer) with the unspoken desire for additional weight loss. Patients who present for additional bariatric surgery after a "failed" VSG, RYGB, or BPD±DS undergo an extensive evaluation as discussed above and, if an anatomic abnormality is not detected, are enrolled into our 6-month revision surgery protocol. This protocol involves monthly educational visits with recommendations from a bariatrician with the possible addition of weight loss medication, dietitian for review of their daily food diary, behaviorist for ongoing counseling, and exercise physiologist for review of their daily exercise diary. It has been our experience that this protocol is effective in determining which patients have a behavioral component to their weight regain and prevents the vast majority from undergoing a high-risk, low-benefit reoperative procedure. Although our desire is to help all patients with morbid obesity, our experience has demonstrated that some patients have "metastatic" or "terminal" obesity and, similar to stage IV cancer, cannot be treated successfully with surgery.

Hospital Standards for Optimal Care of the Metabolic and Bariatric Surgery Patient

The ACS and the ASMBS have jointly published the latest standards manual for the Metabolic and Bariatric Surgery Accreditation and Quality Improvement Program (MBSAQIP) for 2016. This collaborative effort outlines the necessary resources for the optimal care of the metabolic and bariatric surgery patient in the USA. This comprehensive focus on patient safety has been supported in the literature with a large-scale study (n = 277,760) demonstrating in-hospital mortality rates at non-accredited centers to be more than three times higher than accredited centers (0.22% vs. 0.06%) [196]. The following discussion summarizes the basic requirements of a hospital-based bariatric surgery program ranging from staffing personnel to hospital facilities and equipment [197].

Staffing and Services

A bariatric center must have procedures in place that employ an integrated health approach to the metabolic and bariatric surgery patient. The team is typically led by an actively practicing surgeon as the metabolic and bariatric surgery (MBS) director. Administrative assistance is provided by a designated MBS coordinator. The MBS coordinator manages the accreditation process and compliance with MBSAQIP requirements through maintenance of policies, patient education, outcomes data collection, quality improvement process, and education of relevant staff in the various aspects of bariatric patient care with a focus on patient safety. The team should include registered nurses, advanced practice nurses or other physician extenders, registered dietitians, psychologists, psychiatrists, social workers, and physical or exercise therapists. Specialized designation may also be pursued, such as Certified Bariatric Nurses (CBN) certification. Recovery room staff should be experienced in difficult ventilator support. Nurses working on the floor or unit should be experienced in respiratory care, management of nasogastric tubes, intraabdominal drains, ambulation of the morbidly obese patient, knowledge of common perioperative complications, and early recognition of intravascular volume depletion, cardiac, diabetic, and vascular problems. Comprehensive bariatric centers must also be able to provide anesthesia services, critical or intensive care unit (CCU/ICU) services, comprehensive endoscopy services, and on-site diagnostic and interventional radiology services. Specialists in cardiology, pulmonology, rehabilitation, and psychiatry should be readily available as well.

Operating Room and Hospital Facilities

The MBSAQIP requires facilities to have a full line of equipment and instruments for the care of patients who undergo metabolic and bariatric surgery. Furniture and equipment must be able to accommodate patients within the weight limits established by the center (e.g., 750 lbs). Staff must be trained to use appropriate patient movement and transfer systems without injury to the patient or themselves. The following list includes but is not limited to equipment and instruments needed in the care of bariatric patients:

- Examination tables
- Operating room tables
- Radiological tables and facilities
- Fluoroscopic technologies
- Medical imaging equipment for diagnostic purposes
- Surgical instruments (specifically designed stapling instruments, retractors, and appropriately long instruments)
- Intensive care unit (ICU) equipment
- Crash carts
- Blood pressure cuffs
- Sequential compression device sleeves

Additional facility requirements must also be considered and should be constructed to accommodate morbidly obese patients.

- Doorways
- Chairs
- Beds
- Scales
- Gowns
- Floor-mounted or floor-supported toilets
- Shower rooms
- Wheelchairs
- Walkers

Conclusion

Bariatric surgery is the most successful treatment of obesity and its comorbidities with complication rates that have decreased significantly over the past decade and a half. The development of bariatric multidisciplinary teams, dedicated centers, proper equipment, and thorough training of laparoscopic bariatric surgeons in the appropriate patient selection, workup, and preoperative preparation has led to these improvements. Novice bariatric surgeons would be wise to select patients with low-risk profiles to gain the necessary experience prior to performing surgery on higher-risk patients. Reoperative surgery with its significantly higher risks should only be performed by seasoned surgeons at facilities with the necessary resources to deal with complex complications.

References

1. Karra E, Chandarana K, Batterham RL. The role of peptide YY in appetite regulation and obesity. J Physiol. 2009;587(pt 1):19–25.
2. Khan MA, Grinberg R, Johnson S, et al. Perioperative risk factors for 30-day mortality after bariatric surgery: is functional status important. Surg Endosc. 2013;27(5):1772–7.
3. Gastrointestinal surgery for severe obesity: National Institutes of Health consensus development conference statement. Am J Clin Nutr 1992;55(2 Suppl):615S–619S.
4. Gupta PK, Franck C, Miller WJ, et al. Development and validation of a bariatric surgery morbidity risk calculator using the prospective, multicenter NSQIP dataset. JACS. 2011;212(3):301–9.
5. Sanni A, Perez S, Medbery R, et al. Postoperative complications in bariatric surgery using age and BMI stratification: a study using ACS-NSQIP data. Surg Endosc. 2014;28:3302–9.
6. Stroh C, Weiner R, Wolff S, et al. Influences of gender on complication rate and outcome after roux-en-y gastric bypass: data analysis of more than 10,000 operations from the German Bariatric surgery Registry. Obes Surg. 2014;24:1625–33.
7. O'Keefe KL, Kemmeter PR, Kemmeter KD. Bariatric surgery outcomes in patients aged 65 years and older at an American Society for Metabolic and Bariatric Surgery Center of Excellence. Obes Surg. 2010;20(9):1199–205.
8. Nguyen NT, Karipineni F, Masoomi H. Increasing utilization of laparoscopic gastric banding in the adolescent: data from academic medical centers, 2002–2009. Am Surg. 2011;11:1510–4.
9. Fris RJ. Preoperative low energy diet diminishes liver size. Obes Surg. 2004;4(9):1165–70.
10. Owers CE, Abbas Y, Ackroyd R, et al. Perioperative optimization of patients undergoing bariatric surgery. J Obes. 2012;2012:781546.
11. Lee WJ, Wang W, Chen TC, et al. Clinical significance of central obesity in laparoscopic bariatric surgery. Obes Surg. 2003;13(6):921–5.
12. Kartheuser AH, Leonard DF, Penninckx F, et al. Waist circumference and waist/hip ratio are better predictive risk factors for mortality and morbidity after colorectal surgery than body mass index and body surface area. Ann Surg. 2013;258(5): 722–30.
13. Tymitz K, Kerlakian G, Engel A, et al. Gender differences in early outcomes following hand-assisted laparoscopic Roux-en-Y gastric bypass surgery:

gender differences in bariatric surgery. Obes Surg. 2007;17:1588–91.
14. Edholm D, Kullberg J, Haenni A, et al. Preoperative 4-week low-calorie diet reduces liver volume and intrahepatic fat, and facilitates laparoscopic gastric bypass in morbidly obese. Obes Surg. 2011;21:345–50.
15. Coles SL, Dixon JB, Marks P, et al. Preoperative weight loss with a very-low-energy diet: quantitation of changes in liver and abdominal fat by serial imaging. Am J Clin Nutr. 2006;84:304–11.
16. Liu RC, Sabnis AA, Forsyth C, et al. The effects of acute preoperative weight loss on laparoscopic Roux-en-Y gastric bypass. Obes Surg. 2005;15:1396–402.
17. Huerta S, Dredar S, Hayden E, et al. Preoperative weight loss decreases the operative time of gastric bypass at a Veterans Administration Hospital. Obes Surg. 2008;18:508–12.
18. Alami RS, Morton JM, Schuster R, et al. Is there a benefit to preoperative weight loss in gastric bypass patients? A prospective randomized trial. Surg Obes Relat Dis. 2007;3:141–6.
19. Benotti PN, Still CD, Wood GC, et al. Preoperative weight loss before bariatric surgery. Arch Surg. 2009;144:1150–5.
20. Edholm D, Kullberg J, Karlsson FA, et al. Changes in liver volume and body composition during 4 weeks of low calorie diet before laparoscopic gastric bypass. Surg Obes Relat Dis. 2015;11:602–6.
21. Sjöström L, Narbro K, Sjöström CD, et al. Effects of bariatric surgery on mortality in Swedish obese subjects. N Engl J Med. 2007;357(8):741–52.
22. Nandipati K, Lin E, Husain F, et al. Factors predicting the increased risk for return to the operating room in bariatric patients: a NSQIP database study. Surg Endosc. 2013;27(4):1172–7.
23. Turgeon NA, Perez S, Mondestin M, et al. The impact of renal function on outcomes of bariatric surgery. J Am Soc Nephrol. 2012;23(5):885–94.
24. Lancaster RT, Hutter MM. Bands and bypasses: 30-day morbidity and mortality of bariatric surgical procedures as assessed by prospective, multicenter, risk-adjusted ACS-NSQIP data. Surg Endosc. 2008;22(12):2554–63.
25. Adams TD, Gress RE, Smith SC, et al. Long-term mortality after gastric bypass surgery. N Engl J Med. 2007;357(8):753–61.
26. Davis MM, Slish K, Chao C, Cabana MD. National trends in bariatric surgery 1996–2002. Arch Surg. 2006;141(1):71–4. disc 75
27. Hutter MM, Randall S, Khuri SF, et al. Laparoscopic versus open gastric bypass for morbid obesity; a multicenter, prospective, risk-adjusted analysis from the National Surgical quality Improvement Program. Ann Surg. 2006;243(5):657–62. disc 662-6
28. Padwal RS, Pajewski NM, Allison DB, Sharma AM. Using the Edmonton obesity staging system to predict mortality in a population-representative cohort of people with overweight and obesity. CMAJ. 2011;183(14):E1059–66.
29. Duncan AE, Abd-Elsayed A, Maheshwari A, et al. Role of intraoperative and postoperative blood glucose concentrations in predicting outcomes after cardiac surgery. Anesthesiology. 2010;112(4):860–71.
30. Doenst T, Wijeysundera D, Karkouti K, et al. Hyperglycemia during cardiopulmonary bypass is an independent risk factor for mortality in patients undergoing cardiac surgery. J Thorac Cardiovasc Surg. 2005;130(4):1144–50.
31. Chiappetta S, Stier C, Squillante S, et al. The importance of the Edmonton Obesity Staging System in predicting postoperative outcome and 30-day mortality after metabolic surgery. Surg Obes Relat Dis. 2016;12:1847–55.
32. Clinical Practice Guidelines for the Perioperative Nutritional, Metabolic, and Nonsurgical Support of the Bariatric Surgery Patient. Published. 2013. Last accessed 4/30/17. https://asmbs.org/resources/clinical-practice-guidelines-for-the-perioperative-nutritional-metabolic-and-nonsurgical-support-of-the-bariatric-surgery-patient.
33. Rothen HU, Sporre B, Engberg G, et al. Airway closure, atelectasis and gas exchange during general anaesthesia. Br J Anaesth. 1998;81:681–6.
34. Wightman JA. A prospective survey of the incidence of postoperative pulmonary complications. Br J Surg. 1968;55:85–91.
35. Lawrence VA, Dhanda R, Helsenbeck SG, et al. Risk of pulmonary complications after elective abdominal surgery. Chest. 1996;110:744–50.
36. Pasulka PS, Bistrian BR, Benotti PN, et al. The risks of surgery in obese patients. Ann Intern Med. 1986;104:540–6.
37. Wei YF, Wu HD. Candidates for bariatric surgery; morbidly obese patients with pulmonary dysfunction. J Obes. 2012;1:1–6.
38. O'Keeffe T, Patterson EJ. Evidence supporting routine polysomnography before bariatric surgery. Obes Surg. 2004;14(1):23–6.
39. Lopez PP, Stefan B, Schulman CI, Byers PM. Prevalence of sleep apnea in morbidly obese patients who presented for weight loss surgery evaluation: more evidence for routine screening for obstructive sleep apnea before weight loss surgery. Am Surg. 2008;74(9):834–8.
40. Aguiar IC, Freita WR Jr, Santos IR, et al. Obstructive sleep apnea and pulmonary function in patients with severe obesity before and after bariatric surgery: a randomized clinical trial. Multidiscip Respir Med. 2014;9:43–51.
41. De Menezes Duarte RL, Magalhaes-da-Silveira FJ. Factors predictive of obstructive sleep apnea in patients undergoing pre-operative evaluation for bariatric surgery and referred to a sleep laboratory for polysomnography. J Bras Pneumol. 2015;41(5):440–8.

42. Farinholt GN, Carr AD, Chang EJ, Ali MR. A call to arms: obese men with more severe comorbid disease and underutilization of bariatric operations. Surg Endosc. 2013;27(12):4556–63.
43. Ravesloot MJ, Van Maanen JP, Hilgevoord AA, et al. Obstructive sleep apnea is underrecognized and underdiagnosed in patients undergoing bariatric surgery. Eur Arch Otorhinolaryngol. 2012;269(7):1865–71.
44. Daltro C, Gregorio PB, Alves E, et al. Prevalence and severity of sleep apnea in a group of morbidly obese patients. Obes Surg. 2007;17(6):809–14.
45. Sareli AE, Cantor CR, Williams NN, et al. Obstructive sleep apnea in patients undergoing bariatric surgery- a tertiary center experience. Obes Surg. 2011;23(3):316–27.
46. Lee YH, Johan A, Wong KK, et al. Prevalence and risk factors for obstructive sleep apnea in a multiethnic population of patients presenting for bariatric surgery in Singapore. Sleep Med. 2009;10(2):226–32.
47. El-Sayed IH. Comparison of four sleep questionnaires for screening obstructive sleep apnea. Egypt J Chest Dis Tuberc. 2012;61(4):433–41.
48. MeChanick JI, Youdim A, Jones DB, et al. Bariatric surgery clinical practice guidelines. Endocr Pract. 2013;19:337–72.
49. Qaseem A. Risk assessment for and strategies to reduce perioperative pulmonary complications for patients undergoing non-cardiothoracic surgery: a guideline from the American College of Physicians. Ann Inter Med. 2006;144:575–80.
50. Clavellina-Gaytan D, Velazquez-Fernandez D, Del-Villar E, et al. Evaluation of spirometric testing as a routine preoperative assessment in patients undergoing bariatric surgery. Obes Surg. 2015;25:530–6.
51. Poelaert J, Szegedi L, Blot S, et al. Prevention of postoperative pulmonary problems starts intraoperatively. In: Annual updates in intensive care and emergency medicine. 2013. p. 539–52.
52. Kelkar KV. Post-operative pulmonary complications after non-cardiothoracic surgery. Indian J Anaesth. 2015;59(9):599–605.
53. Fonseca-Junior SJ, Sá CGADB, Rodrigues PAF, et al. Physical exercise and morbid obesity: a systematic review. Arq Bras Cir Dig. 2013;26:67–73.
54. Wrzesinski A, Correia JM, Fernandes TMB, et al. Complications requiring hospital management after bariatric surgery. Arq Bras Cir Dig. 2015;28:3–6.
55. Bartlett RH, Brennan ML, Gazzaniga AB, Hanson EL. Studies on the pathogenesis and prevention of postoperative pulmonary complications. Surg Gynecol Obstet. 1973;137(6):925–33.
56. Veloso APLR, Cusmanich KG. Evaluation of the thoracoabdominal mobility of obese subjects in prebariatric surgery. Arq Bras Cir Dig. 2016;29(Sup. 1):39–42.
57. Thomas JA, McIntosh JM. Are incentive spirometry, intermittent positive pressure breathing, and deep breathing exercises effective in the prevention of postoperative pulmonary complications after upper abdominal surgery? A systematic overview and meta-analysis. Phys Ther. 1994;74(1):3.
58. Must A, Spadano J, Coakley EH, et al. The disease burden associated with overweight and obesity. JAMA. 1999;282(16):1523–9.
59. Klein S, Burke LE, Bray GA, et al. American Heart Association Council on Nutrition, Physical Activity, and Metabolism. Clinical implications of obesity with specific focus on cardiovascular disease: a statement for professionals from the American Heart Association Council on Nutrition, Physical Activity, and Metabolism: endorsed by the American College of Cardiology Foundation. Circulation. 2004;110(18):2952–67.
60. Omalu BI, Ives DG, Buhari AM, et al. Death rates and causes of death after bariatric surgery for Pennsylvania residents, 1995 to 2004. Arch Surg. 2007;142(10):923–8. disc 929
61. Mechanick JI, Youdim A, Jones DB, et al. American Association of Clinical Endocrinologists; Obesity Society; American Society for Metabolic & Bariatric Surgery (2013) Clinical practice guidelines for the perioperative nutritional, metabolic, and nonsurgical support of the bariatric surgery patient – 2013 update: cosponsored by American Association of Clinical Endocrinologists, The Obesity Society, and American Society for Metabolic & Bariatric Surgery. Obesity. 2013;21:S1–27.
62. Feely MA, Collins CS, Daniels PR, et al. Preoperative testing before noncardiac surgery: guidelines and recommendations. Am Fam Physician. 2013;87(6):414–8.
63. Michalopoulou T, Aponte EM, Ruiz-Majoral A, et al. Role of echocardiography in bariatric surgery: preoperative assessment of non-cardiopathic morbidly obese patients. J Anaesth Clin Res. 2015; 6:493.
64. Hall ME, do Carmo JM, da Silva AA, et al. Obesity, hypertension, and chronic kidney diseas. Int J Nephrol Renov Dis. 2014;7:75–88.
65. Hall JE, Henegar JR, Dwyer TM, et al. Is obesity a major cause of chronic renal disease? Adv Ren Replace Ther. 2004;11(1):41–54.
66. Gomez P, Ruilope LM, Barrios V, et al. FATH Study Group Prevalence of renal insufficiency in individuals with hypertension and obesity/overweight: the FATH study. J Am Soc Nephrol. 2006;17(12 Suppl 3):S194–200.
67. Fenske WK, Dubb S, Bueter M, et al. Effect of bariatric surgery-induced weight loss on renal and systemic inflammation and blood pressure: a 12-month prospective study. Surg Obes Relat Dis. 2013;9(4):559–68.
68. Matlaga BR, Shore AD, Magnuson T, et al. Effect of gastric bypass surgery on kidney stone disease. J Urol. 2009;181(6):2573–7.
69. Sutherland V, Kuwada T, Gersin K, et al. Impact of bariatric surgery on hiatal hernia repair outcomes. Am Surg. 2016;82(8):743–7.

70. Che F, Nguyen B, Cohen A, Nguyen NT. Prevalence of hiatal hernia in the morbidly obese. Surg Obes Relat Dis. 2013;9(6):920–4.
71. Erim T, Cruz-Correa MR, Szomstein S, et al. Prevalence of Helicobacter pylori seropositivity among patients undergoing bariatric surgery: a preliminary study. World J Surg. 2008;32: 2021–5.
72. Kuper MA, Kratt T, Kramer KM, et al. Effort, safety, and finding of routine preoperative endoscopic evaluation of morbidly obese patients undergoing bariatric surgery. Surg Endosc. 2010;28(8):1996–2001.
73. ASGE, SAGES, ASMBS Guideline. The role of endoscopy in the bariatric patient. GI Endo. 2015;81(5):1063–72.
74. Ng JY, Cheng AKS, Kim G, et al. Is elective gastroscopy prior to bariatric surgery in an Asian cohort worthwhile? Obes Surg. 2016;26(9):2156–60.
75. Wolter S, Duprée A, Miro J, et al. Upper gastrointestinal endoscopy prior to bariatric surgery-mandatory or expendable? An analysis of 801 cases. Obes Surg. 27:1938–43. Published online: 27 Feb 2017
76. Goitein D, Sakran N, Rayman S, et al. Barium swallow for hiatal hernia detection is unnecessary prior to primary sleeve gastrectomy. Surg Obes Relat Dis. 2017;13:138–43.
77. Schirmer B, Erenoglu C, Miller A. Flexible endoscopy in the management of patients undergoing Roux-en-Y gastric bypass. Obes Surg. 2002;12:634–8.
78. Madan AK, Speck KE, Hiler ML. Routine preoperative upper endoscopy for laparoscopic gastric bypass: is it necessary? Am Surg. 2004;70:684–6.
79. Muñoz R, Ibáñez L, Salinas J, et al. Importance of routine preoperative upper GI endoscopy: why all patients should be evaluated? Obes Surg. 2009;19:427–31.
80. Goudra B, Nuzat A, Singh PM, et al. Association between type of sedation and the adverse events associated with gastrointestinal endoscopy: an analysis of 5 years' data from a tertiary center in the USA. Clin Endosc. 2017;50(2):161–9.
81. Chalasani N, Younossi Z, Lavine JE, et al. The diagnosis and management of non-alcoholic fatty liver disease: practice guideline by the American Association for the Study of Liver Diseases, American College of Gastroenterology, and the American Gastroenterological Association. Hepatology. 2012;55(6):2005–23.
82. Bellentani S, Scaglioni F, Marino M, Bedogni G. Epidemiology of non-alcoholic fatty liver disease. Dig Dis. 2010;28(1):155–61.
83. Reha JL, Lee S, Hofmann LJ. Prevalence and predictors of nonalcoholic steatohepatitis in obese patients undergoing bariatric surgery: a Department of Defense experience. Am Surg. 2014;80(6):595–9.
84. Fassio E, Alvarez E, Domı'nguez N, Landeira G, Longo C. Natural history of nonalcoholic steatohepatitis: a longitudinal study of repeat liver biopsies. Hepatology. 2004;40:820–6.
85. Sorrentino P, Tarantino G, Conca P, et al. Silent non-alcoholic fatty liver disease-a clinical-histological study. J Hepatol. 2004;41:751–7.
86. Dixon JB, Bhathal PS, Hughes NR, O'Brien PE. Nonalcoholic fatty liver disease: improvement in liver histological analysis with weight loss. Hepatology. 2004;39(6):1647–54.
87. Alizai PH, Wendl J, Roeth AA, et al. Functional liver recovery after bariatric surgery – a prospective cohort study with the LiMAx test. Obes Surg. 2015;25(11):2047–53.
88. Silverman EM, Sapala JA, Appelman HD. Regression of hepatic steatosis in morbidly obese persons after gastric bypass. Am J Clin Pathol. 1995;104:23–31.
89. Chavez-Tapia NC, Tellez-Avila FI, Barrientos-Gutierrez T, et al. Bariatric surgery for non-alcoholic steatohepatitis in obese patients. Cochrane Database Syst Rev. 2010;1:CD007340.
90. Brolin RE, Bradley LJ, Taliwal RV. Unsuspected cirrhosis discovered during elective obesity operations. Arch Surg. 1998;113:84–8.
91. Jan A, Narwaria M, Mahawar K. A systematic review of bariatric surgery in patients with liver cirrhosis. Obes Surg. 2015;25(8):1518–26.
92. D'Albuquerque LAC, Gonzalez AD, Wahle RC, et al. Liver transplantation for subacute hepatocellular failure due to massive steatohepatitis after bariatric surgery. Liver Transpl. 2008;14:881–5.
93. Dawes AJ, Maggard-Gibbons M, Maher AR, et al. Mental health conditions among patients seeking and undergoing bariatric surgery: a meta-analysis. JAMA. 2016;315(2):150–63.
94. Kessler RC, Chiu WT, Demler O, et al. Prevalence, severity, and comorbidity of 12-month DSM-IV disorders in the National Comorbidity Survey Replication. Arch Gen Psychiatry. 2005;62(6):617–27.
95. Lemont D, Moorehead MK, Parish MS, et al. Suggestions for the pre-surgical psychological assessment of bariatric surgery candidates: American Society for Bariatric Surgery. 2004. https://asmbs.org/wp/uploads/2014/05/psychpresurgicalassessment.pdf.
96. Beauchowitz A, Gonder-Frederick LA, Olbrisch ME, et al. Psychosocial evaluation of bariatric surgery candidates; a survey of present practices. Psychosom Med. 2005;65(5):825–32.
97. Santry HP, Chin MH, Cagney KA, et al. The use of multidisciplinary teams to evaluate bariatric surgery patients: results from a national survey in the U.S.A. Obes Surg. 2006;16(1):59–66.
98. Batayyah E, Sharma G, Aminian A, et al. The role of the multidisciplinary conference in the evaluation of bariatric surgery candidates with a high-risk psychiatric profile. Bariatric Surg Pract Patient Care. 2015;10(4):156–9.
99. Livhits M, Mercado C, Yermilov I, et al. Preoperative predictors of weight loss following bariatric surgery: systematic review. Obes Surg. 2012;22(1):70–89.
100. Buchwald H, Estok R, Fahrbach K, et al. Weight and type 2 diabetes after bariatric surgery:

systematic review and meta-analysis. Am J Med. 2009;122(3):248–56.
101. Christou NV, Lieverman M, Sampalis F, Sampalis JS. Bariatric surgery reduces cancer risk in morbidly obese patients. Surg Obes Relat Dis. 2008;4(6):691–5.
102. Kokkinos A, Alexiadou K, Liasko C, et al. Improvement in cardiovascular indices after Roux-en-Y gastric bypass or sleeve gastrectomy for morbid obesity. Obes Surg. 2013;23(1):31–8.
103. Maggard-Gibbons M, Maglione M, Livhits M, et al. Bariatric surgery for weight loss and glycemic control in nonmorbidly obese adults with diabetes: a systematic review. JAMA. 2013;309(21):2250–61.
104. Wali A, Ashrafian H, Schofield KL, et al. Is social deprivation associated with weight loss outcomes following bariatric surgery? A 10-year single institutional experience. Obes Surg. 2014;24(12):2126–32.
105. Fysekidis M, Catheline JM, Kouacou N, et al. Socioeconomic deprivation remains a significant barrier in the choice of bariatric surgery even when full medical expense coverage is present. Surg Obes Relat Dis. 2016;12:1403–9.
106. Diamant A, Cleghorn MC, Milner J, et al. Patient operational factors affecting wait times in a bariatric surgery program in Toronto: a retrospective cohort study. CMAJ Open. 2015;3(3):E331–7.
107. Furlong C. Smoking cessation and its effects on outcomes of surgical interventions. London Health Observatory and Barnet PCT. 2005. www.LHO.org.uk.
108. Krueger JK, Rohrich RJ. Clearing the smoke: the scientific rationale for tobacco abstention with plastic surgery. Plast Reconstr Surg. 2001;108(4):1063–73.
109. Rejali M, Rejali AR, Zhang L, et al. Effects of nicotine on the cardiovascular system. Vasc Dis Prev. 2005;2:135–44.
110. Ngaage DL, Martins E, Orkell E, et al. The impact of the duration of mechanical ventilation on the respiratory outcome in smokers undergoing cardiac surgery. Cardiovasc Surg. 2002;10(4):345–50.
111. Warner DO. Preoperative smoking cessation: the role of the primary care provider. Mayo Clin Proc. 2005;80:252–8.
112. Cole CW, Hill GB, Farzad E, et al. Cigarette smoking and peripheral arterial occlusive disease. Surgery. 1993;114(4):753–7.
113. Zhang W, Mason EE, Renquist KE, et al. Factors influencing survival following surgical treatment of obesity. Obes Surg. 2005;15(1):43–50.
114. Gonzalez R, Haines K, Nelson L, et al. Predictive factors of thromboembolic events in patients undergoing Roux-en-Y gastric bypass. Surg Obes Relat Dis. 2006;2(1):30–5. disc 35–6
115. Steele K, Schweitzer M, Prokopowicz G, et al. The long-term risk of venous thromboembolism following bariatric surgery. Obes Surg. 2011;21(9):1371–6.
116. Blackburn GL, Hutter MM, Harvey AM, et al. Expert panel on weight loss surgery: executive report update. Obesity. 2009;17(5):842–62.
117. Leggett T. United Nations Office on Drugs and Crime A review of the world cannabis situation. Bull Narc. 2006;58(1–2):1–155.
118. Sarafian TA, Habib N, Oldham M, et al. Inhaled marijuana smoke disrupts mitochondrial energetics in pulmonary epithelial cells in vivo. Am J Physiol Lung Cell Mol Physiol. 2006;290(6):L1202–9.
119. Ware MA, Wang T, Shapiro S, et al. Smoked cannabis for chronic neuropathic pain: a randomized controlled trial. CMAJ. 2010;182(14):E694–701.
120. Mittleman MA, Lewis RA, Maclure M, et al. Triggering myocardial infarction by marijuana. Circulation. 2001;103(23):2805–9.
121. Wang X, Derakhshandeh R, Liu J, et al. One minute of marijuana secondhand smoke exposure substantially impairs vascular endothelial function. JAHA. 2016;5:1–10.
122. Grant I, Atkinson JH, Gouaux B, Wilsey B. Medical marijuana: clearing away the smoke. Neurol J. 2012;6:18–25.
123. Pertwee RG. Cannabinoids and multiple sclerosis. Mol Neurobiol. 2007;36(1):45–59.
124. Suzuki J, Haimovici F, Chang G. Alcohol use disorders after bariatric surgery. Obes Surg. 2012;22(2):201–7.
125. Spadola CE, Wagner EF, Dillon FR, et al. Alcohol and drug use among postoperative bariatric patients: a systematic review of the emerging research and its implications. Alcohol Clin Exp Res. 2015;39(9):1582–601.
126. Clark MM, Balsiger BM, Sletten CD, et al. Psychosocial factors and 2-year outcome following bariatric surgery for weight loss. Obes Surg. 2003;13(5):739–45.
127. Handelsman Y, Mechanick JI, Blonde L, et al. American Association of Clinical Endocrinologists Medical Guidelines for Clinical Practice for developing a diabetes mellitus comprehensive care plan. Endocr Pract. 2011;17(Suppl 2):1–52.
128. Hall TC, Pellen MGC, Sedman PC, et al. Preoperative factors predicting remission of type 2 diabetes mellitus after Roux-en-Y gastric bypass surgery for obesity. Obes Surg. 2010;20:1245–50.
129. Perna M, Romagnuolo J, Morgan K, et al. Preoperative hemoglobin A1c and postoperative glucose control in outcomes after gastric bypass for obesity. Surg Obes Relat Dis. 2012;6: 686–90.
130. Lee W-J, Chong K, Ser K-H, et al. C-peptide predicts the remission of type 2 diabetes after bariatric surgery. Obes Surg. 2012;2:293–8.
131. Moulin de Moraes CM, Mancini MC, Edna de Melo M, et al. Prevalence of subclinical hypothyroidism in a morbidly obese population and improvement after weight loss induced by Roux- en-Y gastric bypass. Obes Surg. 2005;15:1287–91.
132. Raftopoulos Y, Gagne DJ, Papasavas P, et al. Improvement of hypothyroidism after laparoscopic Roux-en-Y gastric bypass for morbid obesity. Obes Surg. 2004;14:509–13.

133. Chikunguwo S, Brethauer S, Nirujogi V, et al. Influence of obesity and surgical weight loss on thyroid hormone levels. Surg Obes Relat Dis. 2007;3:631–6.
134. Fierabracci P, Pinchera A, Marinelli S, et al. Prevalence of endocrine diseases in morbidly obese patients scheduled for bariatric surgery: beyond diabetes. Obes Surg. 2011;21:54–60.
135. Jankovic D, Wolf P, Anderwald C-H, et al. Prevalence of endocrine disorders in morbidly obese patients and the effects of bariatric surgery on endocrine and metabolic parameters. Obes Surg. 2012;22: 62–9.
136. Garber J, Cobin RH, Gharib H, et al. Clinical practice guidelines for hypothyroidism in adults: cosponsored by American Association of Clinical Endocrinologists and the American Thyroid Association. Endocr Pract. 2012;11:1–207.
137. Perna M, Baker M, Byrne TK, et al. Statins and the bariatric patient: characterization and perioperative effects of statin therapy in the gastric bypass patient. Am Surg. 2011;77:44–7.
138. American College of Obstetricians and Gynecologists. ACOG practice bulletin no.105: bariatric surgery and pregnancy. Obstet Gynecol. 2009;113:1405–13.
139. Kominiarek MA. Pregnancy after bariatric surgery. Obstet Gynecol Clin N Am. 2010;37:305–20.
140. Magdaleno R, Pereira BG, Chaim EA, et al. Pregnancy after bariatric surgery: a current view of maternal, obstetrical and perinatal challenges. Arch Gynecol Obstet. 2012;285:559–66.
141. Ponsky TA, Brody F, Pucci E. Alterations in gastrointestinal physiology after Roux-en-Y gastric bypass. J Am Coll Surg. 2005;201:125–31.
142. Bauman WA, Shaw S, Jayatilleke K, et al. Increased intake of calcium reverses: the B-12 malabsorption induced by metformin. Diabetes Care. 2000;23:1227–31.
143. Smith CD, Herkes SB, Behrns KE, et al. Gastric acid secretion and vitamin B-12 absorption after vertical Roux-en-Y gastric bypass for morbid obesity. Ann Surg. 1993;218:91–6.
144. Brolin RE, Gorman JH, Gorman RC, et al. Are vitamin B-12 and folate deficiency clinically important after Roux-en-Y gastric bypass? J Gastrointest Surg. 1998;2:436–42.
145. Rhode BM, Tamim H, Gilfix MB. Treatment of vitamin B-12 deficiency after gastric bypass surgery for severe obesity. Obes Surg. 1995;5:154–8.
146. Boylan LM, Sugerman HJ, Driskell JA. Vitamin E, vitamin B-6, vitamin B-12, and folate status of gastric bypass surgery patients. J Am Diet Assoc. 1988;88:579–85.
147. Brolin RE, Gorman RC, Milgrim LM, Kenler HA. Multivitamin prophylaxis in prevention of post-gastric bypass vitamin and mineral deficiencies. Int J Obes. 1991;15:661–7.
148. Flancbaum L, Belsley S, Drake V, et al. Preoperative nutritional status of patients undergoing Roux-en-Y gastric bypass for morbid obesity. J Gastrointest Surg. 2006;10:1033–7.
149. Wood RJ, Ronnenberg AG. Iron. In: Shils ME, Shike M, Ross AC, Caballero B, Cousins RJ, editors. Modern nutrition in health and disease. 10th ed. Philadelphia: Lippincott Williams & Wilkins; 2006.
150. Aills L, Blankenship J, Buffington C, et al. ASMBS allied health nutritional guidelines for the surgical weight loss patient. Surg Obes Relat Dis. 2008;4:S73–S108.
151. Buffington CK, Walker B, Cowan GS, et al. Vitamin D deficiency in the morbidly obese. Obes Surg. 1993;3:421–4.
152. Ybarra J, Sanchez-Hernandez J, Vich I, et al. Unchanged hypovitaminosis D and secondary hyperparathyroidism in morbid obesity alter bariatric surgery. Obes Surg. 2005;15:330–5.
153. Carlin AM, Rao DS, Meslemani AM, et al. Prevalence of vitaminosis D depletion among morbidly obese patients seeking bypass surgery. Surg Obes Relat Dis. 2006;2:98–103.
154. El-Kadre LJ, Roca PR, de Almeida Tinoco AC, et al. Calcium metabolism in pre and postmenopausal morbidly obese women at baseline and after laparoscopic Roux-en-Y gastric bypass. Obes Surg. 2004;14:1062–6.
155. Schrager S. Dietary calcium intake and obesity. J Am Board Fam Pract. 2005;18:205–10.
156. Zemel MB, Richards J, Mathis S, et al. Dairy augmentation of total and central fat loss in obese subjects. Int J Obes. 2005;29:391–7.
157. Peterlik M, Cross HS. Vitamin D and calcium deficits predispose for multiple chronic diseases. Eur J Clin Investig. 2005;35:290–304.
158. Holik MF. The vitamin D epidemic and its health consequences. J Nutr. 2005;135:2739S–48S.
159. Goode LR, Brolin RE, Chowdry HA, Shapes SA. Bone and gastric bypass surgery: effects of dietary calcium and vitamin D. Obes Res. 2004;12:40–7.
160. Coates PS, Fernstrom JD, Fernstrom MH, Schauer PR, Greenspan SL. Gastric bypass surgery for morbid obesity leads to an increase in bone turnover and a decrease in bone mass. J Clin Endocrinol Metab. 2004;89:1061–5.
161. Golder WS, O'Dorsio TM, Dillon JS, Mason EE. Severe metabolic bone disease as a long-term complication of obesity surgery. Obes Surg. 2002;12:685–92.
162. Madan AK, Orth WS, Tichansky DS, Ternovits CA. Vitamin and trace mineral levels after laparoscopic gastric bypass. Obes Surg. 2006;16:603–6.
163. Scopinaro N, Adami GF, Marinari GM, et al. Biliopancreatic diversion. World J Surg. 1998;22:936–46.
164. Stein PD, Matta F. Pulmonary embolism and deep venous thrombosis following bariatric surgery. Obes Surg. 2013;23(5):663–8.
165. Froehling DA, Daniels PR, Mauck KF, et al. Incidence of venous thromboembolism after

bariatric surgery: a population-based cohort study. Obes Surg. 2013;23(11):1874–9.
166. Winegar DA, Sherif B, Pate V, Demaria EJ. Venous thromboembolism after bariatric surgery performed by Bariatric Surgery Center of Excellence Participants: analysis of the Bariatric Outcomes Longitudinal Database. Surg Obes Relat Dis. 2011;7(2):181–8.
167. Jamal MH, Corcelles R, Shimizu H, et al. Thromboembolic events in bariatric surgery: a large multi-institutional referral center experience. Surg Endosc. 2015;29(2):376–80.
168. Finks JF, English WJ, Carlin AM, et al. Predicting risk for venous thromboembolism with bariatric surgery: results from the Michigan bariatric surgery collaborative. Ann Surg. 2012;255(6):1100–4.
169. Smith MD, Patterson E, Wahed AS, et al. 30-day mortality after bariatric surgery: independently adjudicated causes of death in the Longitudinal Assessment of Bariatric Surgery. Obes Surg. 2011;21(11):1687–92.
170. Masoomi H, Buchberg B, Reavis KM, et al. Factors predictive of venous thromboembolism in bariatric surgery. Am Surg. 2011;77(10):1403–6.
171. Chan MM, Hamza N, Ammori BJ. Duration of surgery independently influences risk of venous thromboembolism after laparoscopic bariatric surgery. Surg Obes Relat Dis. 2013;9(1):88–93.
172. Sachdeva A, Dalton M, Amaragiri SV, Lees T. Elastic compression stockings for prevention of deep vein thrombosis. Cochrane Database Syst Rev. 2010;7:CD001484.
173. Urbankova J, Quiroz R, Kucher N, Goldhaber SZ. Intermittent pneumatic compression and deep vein thrombosis prevention. A meta-analysis in postoperative patients. Thromb Haemost. 2005;94(6):1181–5.
174. Gould MK, Garcia DA, Wren SM, et al. Prevention of VTE in non-orthopedic surgical patients. Antithrombotic therapy and prevention of thrombosis, 9th ed: American College of chest physicians evidence-based clinical practice guidelines. Chest. 2012;141(2 Suppl):e227S–77S.
175. Mismetti P, Laporte S, Darmon JY, et al. Meta-analysis of low molecular weight heparin in the prevention of venous thromboembolism in general surgery. Br J Surg. 2001;88(7):913–30.
176. Imberti D, Baldini E, Pierfranceschi MG, et al. Prophylaxis of venous thromboembolism with low molecular weight heparin in bariatric surgery: a prospective, randomised pilot study evaluating two doses of parnaparin (BAFLUX study). Obes Surg. 2014;24(2):284–91.
177. Chlysta WJ, Iffland PH, Haller NA. Review of BMI-based pharmacologic protocols for the prevention of venous thromboembolism in bariatric surgery patients. Bariatric Surg Pract Patient Care. 2014;9(3):91–6.
178. Borkgren-Okonek MJ, Hart RW, Pantano JE, et al. Enoxaparin thromboprophylaxis in gastric bypass patients: extended duration, dose stratification, and antifactor Xa activity. Surg Obes Relat Dis. 2008;4(5):625–31.
179. Singh K, Podolsky ER, Um S, et al. Evaluating the safety and efficacy of BMI-based preoperative administration of low-molecular-weight heparin in morbidly obese patients undergoing Roux-en-Y gastric bypass surgery. Obes Surg. 2012;22(1):47–51.
180. Ojo P, Asiyanbola B, Valin E, Reinhold R. Post discharge prophylactic anticoagulation in gastric bypass patient – how safe? Obes Surg. 2008;18(7):791–6.
181. Birkmeyer NJ, Share D, Baser O, et al. Preoperative placement of inferior vena cava filters and outcomes after gastric bypass surgery. Ann Surg. 2010;252(2):313–8.
182. Nguyen NT, Goldman C, Rosenquist CJ, et al. Laparoscopic versus open gastric bypass: a randomized study of outcomes, quality of life, and costs. Ann Surg. 2001;234(3):279–89.
183. Schauer PR, Ikramuddin S, Gourash W, et al. Outcomes after laparoscopic Roux-en-Y gastric bypass for morbid obesity. Ann Surg. 2000;232(4):515–29.
184. Higa KD, Boone KB, Ho T. Complications of the laparoscopic Roux-en-Y gastric bypass: 1,040 patients – what have we learned? Obes Surg. 2000;10(6):509–13.
185. Christou NV, Jarand J, Sylvestre JL, McLean AP. Analysis of the incidence and risk factors for wound infections in open bariatric surgery. Obes Surg. 2004;14(1):16–22.
186. Chopra TCK, Dhar S, Deborah T, et al. Epidemiology and outcomes associated with surgical site infection (SSI) following bariatric surgery. Expert Rev Pharmacoecon Outcomes Res. 2010;10(3):317–28.
187. Bratzler DW, Dellinger EP, Olsen KM, et al. Clinical practice guidelines for antimicrobial prophylaxis in surgery. Am J Health-Syst Pharm. 2013;70(3):195–283.
188. Wexler HM. Bacteroides: the good, the bad, and the nitty-gritty. Clin Microbiol Rev. 2007;20(4):593–621.
189. Jones JW, McCullough LB, Richman BW. Informed consent: it's not just signing a form. Thorac Surg Clin. 2005;15(4):451–60.
190. Greenfield S, Kaplan S, Ware JE Jr. Expanding patient involvement in care. Effects on patient outcomes. Ann Intern Med. 1985;102(4):520–8.
191. Stewart MA. Effective physician-patient communication and health outcomes: a review. CMAJ. 1995;152(9):1423–33.
192. Chen JY, Tao ML, Tisnado D, et al. Impact of physician-patient discussions on patient satisfaction. Med Care. 2008;46(11):1157–62.
193. Iversen MD, Daltroy LH, Fossel AH, et al. The prognostic importance of patient pre-operative

expectations of surgery for lumbar spinal stenosis. Patient Educ Couns. 1998;34(2):169–78.

194. Levinson W, Roter DL, Mullooly JP, et al. Physician-patient communication. The relationship with malpractice claims among primary care physicians and surgeons. JAMA. 1997;277(7): 553–9.
195. Brethauer SA, Kothari S, Sudan R, et al. Review article systematic review on reoperative bariatric surgery American Society for Metabolic and Bariatric Surgery Revision Task Force. Surg Obes Relat Dis. 2014;10:952–72.
196. Jafari MD, Jafari F, Young MT, et al. Surg Endosc. 2013 Dec;27(12):4539–46.
197. Standards Manual. Resources for optimal care of the metabolic and bariatric surgery patient. 2016. https://www.facs.org/quality-programs/mbsaqip/standards. Accessed: 5/5/17.

Medical Management of Obesity

35

Marianela Aguirre Ackermann

Introduction

The genetic-environment combination is central to the genesis of obesity. Obesity emerged as one of the major health problems during the last century, from the enormous environmental changes that the world experienced. The environmental factors favoring a positive energy balance and weight gain include, on the one hand, increased availability of food, particularly high-calorie foods and increased portion sizes [1]. On the other hand, decreased movement, with less time of physical activity at work and the replacement of physical activity in leisure time with sedentary activities such as watching TV and the use of electronic devices [2]. Other factors considered to contribute to the obesity epidemic are use of drugs that have weight gain as a side effect, reduction in variability of ambient temperatures, sleep debt, increasing maternal age, greater fecundity among people with higher adiposity, assortative mating, endocrine disruptors, microorganisms, epigenetics and intrauterine and intergenerational effects [3]. These and many other factors, combined with medical innovations that have reduced mortality and prolonged life, laid the foundation for the obesity epidemic.

Weight loss produces multiple benefits, including improved risk factors, disease prevention, functional improvement and self-esteem. Increased weight loss produces greater benefits, but even the loss of only 5–10% of weight has been shown to produce significant improvements in many conditions [4].

The central strategies for any weight loss effort are lifestyle change, eating plan and increased physical activity. In those patients with difficulties in weight loss, the use of approved weight management drugs coupled with lifestyle changes is appropriate. Surgical management can produce remarkable health improvement and reduce mortality for patients with severe obesity.

However, surgery is not a procedure to be used in all patients but only in selected patients. On the other hand, patients before and after surgery should perform treatment for obesity and achieve lifestyle changes. In this chapter we will review the current nonsurgical approach to obesity.

Components of Running a Successful Medical Weight Management Practice

A structured lifestyle intervention program designed for weight loss (lifestyle therapy) consisting of a healthy meal plan, physical activity, and behavioral interventions should be available to patients who are being treated for overweight or obesity [5].

M. A. Ackermann
Obesity and Diabetes Department, Centro CIEN - Endocrinology, Obesity and Nutrition Center, Corrientes, Buenos Aires, Misiones, Formosa, Argentina

R. Lutfi et al. (eds.), *Global Bariatric Surgery*, https://doi.org/10.1007/978-3-319-93545-4_35

Table 35.1 Elements for comprehensive lifestyle intervention

Element	Recommendation
Reduced calorie diet	Effective methods to reduce calories:
	Set a caloric goal (1200–1500 kcal/day for women, 1500–1800 kcal/day for men, adjusted for body weight)
	Specify a caloric deficit (500–750 kcal/day)
	Restrict/reduce intake of certain food types to create energy deficit
	Consider patient preferences and health status when identifying a diet. A variety of approaches can produce weight loss
Increased physical activity	Aerobic activity >150 min/week for weight loss
	Resistance training to preserve lean mass 200–300 min/week aerobic activity to maintain weight loss
Behavioral intervention	Ideal:
	Face-to-face sessions (>14 with a trained interventionist over the first 6 months)
	Maintain efforts over 1 year
	Incorporate strategies such as goal setting and self-monitoring
	Alternatives:
	Telephone or electronic counseling with a trained interventionist
	Commercial weight loss programs
	Tend to produce less weight loss tan face-to-face counseling
	Maintenance: Continued contact (once monthly) with a trained interventionist

From: Jensen et al. [9]

Primary care professionals often provide general recommendations for weight loss, but they are usually not trained to offer intensive treatments for obesity because they receive minimal training in obesity, nutrition, and exercise [6, 7]. One of the most important barriers is the well-documented negative attitude of physicians toward obese patients, and low levels of emotional rapport in primary care visits with overweight and obese patients may weaken the patient-physician relationship, diminish patients' adherence to recommendations, and decrease the effectiveness of behavior change counseling [8].

Also, the approaches in which it is performed only recommendations result in very limited weight loss, which may frustrate both patients and their physicians. Therefore, it is essential to have more training in primary care physicians so that they can adequately refer obese patients to teams that have the tools to perform safe treatments with scientific approval of overweight and obesity.

The cornerstone for the treatment of an obese patient is an intervention with interdisciplinary strategies that involve multiple components, to achieve a better integral lifestyle. The term interdisciplinary refers to the simultaneous implementation of three strategies: *behavioral training, changes in dietary plan to reduce energy intake, and an increase in physical movement* (Table 35.1).

Multicomponent interventions are the treatment of choice [10]:

(a) When instituting a treatment in an overweight-obese person, it is important to verify that health professionals working in weight management interventions have relevant competencies and have had training in the management of these patients.
(b) Take into account the following considerations:
   - Individual preferences and sociocultural circumstances
   - The experiences and results of previous treatments
   - The level of risk of the person, based on BMI, waist circumference, and comorbidities
(c) Document the agreed goals and actions and the results.
(d) Provide support according to the needs of the individual and be attentive to changes over time.
(e) Provide information using standard language. Take into account the person:

- Age, stage of life, ethnicity, and gender
- Cultural needs and social and economic circumstances

(f) Praise progress in behaviors—even small ones—at every opportunity, to encourage the person through the difficult process of changing established behaviors.

(g) Give patients relevant information on obesity in general, related health risks, realistic targets for weight loss, the distinction between losing weight and maintaining weight loss, and the importance of developing skills for both; advise them that the change from losing weight to maintenance typically happens after 6–9 months of treatment. It is also important to focus on behavioral goals (increased physical activity and healthier eating) rather than a particular body weight.

(h) It is important to explain treatment options and—if the patient has indication—surgical treatments.

(i) If a person does not feel this is the right time for them to take action, the treating professional should explain that advice and support will be available in the future whenever they need it. Also, provide contact details so that the person can get in touch when they are ready.

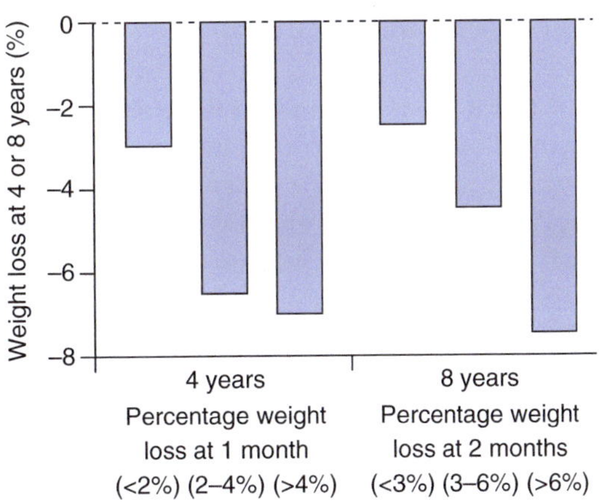

Fig. 35.1 Factors that predict weight loss in the LOOK AHEAD study [11]. (From Bray et al. [12])

One of the largest and longest randomized evaluations supporting the efficacy of implementation of lifestyle intervention in obesity treatment is the LOOK AHEAD. Overweight/obese individuals assigned at intensive lifestyle intervention (ILI) lost 4.7% of initial body weight at year 8, compared with 2.1% for participants assigned to usual care (DSE). At year 8, 50% of ILI and 37% of DSE participants achieved a mean loss ≥5% of initial weight. Nearly 40% of ILI participants who lost ≥10% of initial weight at year 1 maintained this loss at 8 years, and 50% of participants who lost ≥5% maintained this loss at 8 years, revealing that long-term weight control is possible with continued practice of skills taught in intensive lifestyle interventions [11]. An interesting aspect of this study is that the initial rate of weight loss in the first and second months of ILI was positively associated with weight loss at 4 and 8 years (Fig. 35.1). This suggests that early weight loss may be a useful indicator of long-term success. Achievement of >2% weight loss at month 1 or >6% weight loss at month 2 increased the likelihood of achieving a clinically significant weight loss at year 8, compared to those losing <2% at month 1 and <3% at month 2, respectively [13].

Taking into account that the success of obesity treatment programs is the long-term maintenance of lost weight, these findings demonstrate the importance of participants having a good start in a lifestyle intervention.

The problem of long-term interdisciplinary intensive approaches such as LOOK AHEAD is its high cost. That is why other alternatives are evaluated either as support for treatment or for long-term maintenance. Web-based programs are a potential medium for supporting weight loss because of their accessibility and wide reach. A Randomized Control Trial (RCT) evaluated the effects of a web-based component of a weight loss service in an overweight/obese population at risk of cardiovascular disease (CVD) using a control group [14]. More intervention group participants lost ≥5% of their baseline body weight at 3 months (34% vs 3%, $P < 0.001$) and 6 months (41% vs 18% $P = 0.047$), but not at 12 months (22% vs 21%, $P = 0.95$) versus control group. Although the intervention group had high attrition levels, this study provides evidence that a web-based program can be used at least to initiate treatment for weight loss and lower CVD risk up to 3–6 months.

Behavioral Modification

The oldest report of the use of BT in the management of obesity came out around 1967 [15]. Comprehensive lifestyle interventions usually provide a structured behavior change program that includes regular self-monitoring of food intake, physical activity, and weight. These same behaviors are recommended to maintain lost weight, with the addition of frequent (i.e., weekly or more often) monitoring of body weight [9].

Behavioral therapy is a central aspect of lifestyle change intervention, as it provides patients with techniques to implement dietary recommendations and physical activity and to incorporate them as their own habits [16].

Among these recommendations is the recording of food intake (through writing or photos), physical activity performed, and weight. Self-monitoring provides personal accountability and allows for greater awareness of how behaviors are impacting weight [17].

Self-weighing is a simple way to perform self-monitoring, which has been shown to be useful for self-monitoring and self-regulation of body weight. Self-weighing provides information by acting as a suggestive indicator of how changes in eating and exercise behavior are influencing weight. It acts as a tool so that the patient can consider making small adjustments in his behavior according to the evolution of the weight that he registers himself. This allows for better self-regulation as small changes in body weight can be identified and resolved, likely leading to greater self-efficacy and empowerment over one's ability to regulate their body weight.

The National Weight Control Registry (NWCR) is a study that included individuals who have maintained a required minimum weight loss of 13.6 kg for 5 years. The authors identified a large sample of individuals who were highly successful at maintaining weight loss; within the behaviors that had the successful ones, 75% of the NWCR subjects weigh themselves at least once a week [18]. In another study, weight loss maintainers reported that they currently perform more weight-controlling behaviors than those who had regained weight or controls: 55% of maintainers weigh themselves at least once a week, compared with 35.7% of regainers [19].

On-site (face-to-face, group or individual), comprehensive, high-intensity lifestyle interventions (14 or more contacts in first 6 months) represent the standard for behavioral weight [9]. However, registration can be facilitated by smartphone applications, counters, web-based weight loss graph, weekly emails with tailored feedback, and cell-connected scales. Patients can review their progress two to four times a month, with an interview with a trained professional who evaluates progress and provides motivational, objective, and problem-solving training [20].

The Diabetes Prevention Program (DPP) is an excellent example of a comprehensive behavioral intervention [21]. More than 3200 overweight or obese subjects with impaired glucose tolerance were randomly assigned to placebo, metformin, or an intensive lifestyle intervention (ILI) designed to induce and maintain a 7 kg reduction in initial weight, and the primary outcome was the reduction in the incidence of type 2 diabetes (DM2).

Participants in the lifestyle change group attended 16 individual counseling sessions (with a nutritionist) for the first 24 weeks and then had contact at least every 2 months for the remainder of the 4-year study. Subjects were given a hypocaloric and low-fat eating plan and 150 min/week of physical activity (mainly fast walking). The study was stopped after an average of 2.8 years; up to that point, participants in lifestyle changes had achieved an average loss of 5.6 kg, compared to significantly lower losses of 2.1 kg for metformin and 0.1 kg for placebo.

The lifestyle intervention, compared to the placebo and metformin groups, reduced the risk of developing DM2 by 58% and 31%, respectively, which led to the early termination of the study to provide the modification of the style of life to the other two groups.

At 10-year follow-up, it was found that, in comparison with placebo, lifestyle intervention maintained a 34% reduction in the risk of developing DM2, although the latter had regained most of the weight lost [22].

Components of Behavioral Interventions

- *Diet*: Behavioral weight control typically prescribes a calorie target to induce a loss of about 1% of the weight per week. As we will see in this chapter, a variety of different interventions can be incorporated in behavioral treatment considering that all diets will produce weight loss, regardless of their macronutrient composition, if a consistent caloric deficit is achieved.
- *Include the following strategies in behavioral interventions*:
  - *Self-monitoring of behavior and progress*: The record of the type and amount of foods and beverages consumed is a central component of behavioral treatment. The goal is to increase awareness of behaviors needing change, not trying to catch a patient in an inconsistency. Self-monitoring helps patients identify patterns in their eating, select targets for reducing intake, and track progress in meeting goals. More frequent self-monitoring is associated with greater weight loss [23, 24].
  - *Stimulus control*: The food "enters" through the senses. Stimulus control teaches patients to manage external cues from food, which are perceived through sight or smell. Also, to manage the times, places, and events associated with feeding [25].
  - *Goal setting*: Behavioral treatment helps patients make concrete, objective, and tangible changes in diet, in movement, and in managing everyday situations. Goal setting clearly identifies the behavior to be changed and stipulates when, where, and how it will be carried out. However, change is a process. Patients periodically review the progress made in meeting the objectives with the support of their food and activity records [26].
  - *Slowing rate of eating*: Slow eating may be associated with reduced energy intake; the evidence shows that eating at a physiologically moderate pace leads to a more pronounced anorexigenic gut peptide response than eating fast [27]. Techniques include concentrating on tastes, pausing in between meals, and drinking water in between meals.
  - *Social support*: Provides patients motivation for lifestyle change, role models, enhancement of self-acceptance, and confidence feelings. Enhancing social support by including spouses and family members is one of the best ways to accomplish this. A meta-analysis has concluded that including family members led to an additional 3 kg weight loss compared to programs that did not include family members [28].
  - *Problem-solving*: Problem-solving skills help patients analyze the challenges they face in adhering to their eating plan and activity requirements.
  - *Assertiveness*: Assertiveness training includes learning to say "no."
  - *Behavioral contracting*: Patients agree with the therapist one or more healthy behaviors they commit to perform for the next session and then translate it in writing. Healthy behaviors chosen should be short term, realistic, simple, somewhat challenging, but possible. For example, increase the days a week by walking, add a vegetable dish to lunch or dinner, or start having breakfast [29].
  - *Reinforcement of changes*: Rather than reinforcing successful outcomes, it is important to reward good behaviors.
  - *Cognitive restructuring (modifying thoughts)*: Assists patients in identifying and changing unhealthy beliefs about themselves.
  - *Stress management*: Teaches patients to use cognitive behavioral strategies to lessen and relieve negative affective states.
  - *Relapse prevention*: Teaches patients that lapses are normal, expected, and manageable by developing behavior strategies to cope with and prevent them. Relapse prevention involves helping patients understand that to err is human. Interventionists can help patients anticipate the situations when lapses may occur; the goal is not specifically to prevent all lapses, but to prevent them from becoming relapses [29].

The "Clinical Practice Guidelines" [5] for patients with obesity from AACE/ACE (American Association of Clinical Endocrinologists and American College of Endocrinology) give these guidelines on behavioral therapy:

- Lifestyle-enhancing treatment should include behavioral interventions that increase adherence to a reduced-calorie meal schedule and increased movement.
- Behavioral intervention should be performed by a multidisciplinary team that includes physicians, dietitians, health educators, fitness trainers, and psychologists.
- Psychologists and psychiatrists should participate in treatment when, in addition, overweight patients suffer from eating disorders, depression, anxiety, psychosis, and other psychological problems that may affect the effectiveness of lifestyle intervention programs.
- Behavioral lifestyle intervention and support should be intensified if patients do not achieve a 2.5% weight loss in the 1st month of treatment. As mentioned earlier, initial weight reduction is a key factor for long-term treatment success.
- The behavioral approach should teach the management of the different possible situations for each person, as well as problem-solving skills, and should evaluate the results during the change process.
- Behavioral lifestyle intervention must be adapted to the characteristics of each person: ethnic, cultural, socioeconomic, etc.

Weight regain is frequent after a patient completes a lifestyle intervention program. The continued long-term support (weekly, monthly, in person, or by telephone) is the most effective behavioral method for preventing weight regain, but it is infrequent, because of several causes. One of them is that is not widely available. Another, the dropout in the treatment of obesity is high. In the event of failure to obtain weight loss, or not continuing to lose weight, patients generally do not sustain treatment [16, 30].

It is important to note that the maintenance phase is an active phase of the treatment. The weight is not maintained only with what has already been learned. The most commonly used behavioral resources for the maintenance of lost weight are occasional or frequent monitoring of food intake and physical activity, as needed; weekly monitoring of weight; and curriculum of behavioral change including problem-solving, cognitive restructuring, relapse prevention, and regular feedback from a trained interventionist [31]. Therefore, it is important to include within the behavioral treatment strategies for dealing with weight regain. And during the process of change in the treatment of obesity, transmit to the patient that the important thing is consistency, not perfection.

Dietary Strategies for Weight Loss

Which Dietary Strategies Are Effective for Weight Loss?

One diet is "THE diet"? When we are selecting a diet for weight loss, we need to take several considerations. One of the most important aspects in the selection of the diet is that it achieves the patient's adherence.

Basically there are two strategies used in the development of the diet plan for weight loss:

- Based on the energy value (calories)
- Based on macronutrients (proteins, carbohydrates, fats)

The diet must have less calories than is required daily to generate a negative calorie balance. Any of the following methods can be used to reduce calorie intake [32]:

- Reduction of 500/750 kcal below daily requirements.
- Prescribe 1200–1500 kcal/day for women and 1500–1800 kcal/day for men. The selection should be adjusted for personal body weight.
- Prescribe a calorie-restricted diet, based on each patient's individuality, health status, and personal preferences.
- While restricting a particular group of foods (e.g., high-carbohydrate foods or high-fat

foods) could be considered a method to restrict calories, there is no evidence that avoiding a food group is more beneficial in the long term, than include it in the correct portions. Finally, it is the caloric deficit that provides the weight loss.

Randomized controlled trials often involve hundreds or thousands of subjects prescribed to follow different diet regimens, with investigators providing instructions and support to participants on how to eat the prescribed diets. However, there is little evidence that people actually adhere to the diet prescriptions. The weight decrease curve in the studies is not linear. After a few weeks, it does not reflect the targeted energy deficit resulting in pounds lost. This is the effect of metabolic adaptation and mainly suboptimal dietary adherence [33].

Such studies actually test the effects of different *diet prescriptions* rather than the effects of different diets. As an alternative, controlled feeding studies can provide more useful physiological information, but *diet adherence* is often poor in outpatient studies even when participants are provided with all of their food [34]. That is why food studies are required to properly control physiological diets and measure effects, but these studies are very expensive and labor intensive, making them typically small in size.

We will analyze the available evidence of different dietary approaches in the management of obesity.

There is no doubt that in the short term, diets with fewer calories and diets with higher protein content are the ones that achieve greater weight loss. However, long-term differences are minimal or nonexistent.

A meta-analysis of 48 RCTs (N = 7286 individuals) shows that all types of diets are the same. In the analysis adjusted for diet class, all treatments were superior to no diet at 6-month follow-up. At 12-month follow-up, the estimated average weight losses of all diet classes compared with no diet were 1–2 kg less than after 6-month follow-up. The results show that both the low-carbohydrate and low-fat diets were associated with average weight losses of approximately 8 kg at 6 months and 6–7 kg at 12 months compared with no diet. Although statistical differences existed among several of the diets, the differences were small [35].

These findings support the recommendations for weight loss in that most calorie-reducing diets result in clinically important weight loss—as long as the diet is maintained [16].

Several organizations have published guideline recommendations for weight management in patients who are overweight or obese [9, 36, 37]. In general, guidelines recommend lifestyle and behavioral modifications as the foundation of weight loss (Table 35.2). In some they specifically recommend a caloric gap, for example, Scottish Guidelines recommend that dietary interventions for weight loss should be calculated to produce a 600 kcal/day energy deficit, and programs should be tailored to the dietary preferences of the individual patient [38]. Although this can produce meaningful weight loss, long-term and sustainable weight loss is difficult to achieve for most patients, and alternative options such as medications should be considered.

Table 35.2 Lifestyle interventions, physical activity, and dietary approaches (NICE 2014)

Multicomponent interventions are the treatment of choice
Weight management strategies should include behavior change strategies to increase people's physical activity levels or decrease inactivity and improve eating behaviors
People should have relevant information on realistic targets for weight loss (5–10% of original weight)
To prevent obesity, most people may need to do 45–60 min of moderate intensity activity a day, particularly if they do not reduce their energy intake. Advise people who have been obese and have lost weight that they may need to do 60–90 min of activity a day to avoid regaining weight
The main requirement of a dietary approach is that total energy intake should be less than energy expenditure
Diets with 600 kcal/day deficit (600 kcal fewer than is needed to stay the same weight) or that reduce energy intake by reducing fat content in combination with expert support and intensive follow-up are recommended for sustainable weight loss

From: Stegenga et al. [37]

Table 35.3 Association of macronutrient composition on health and weight loss efficacy [5, 39–42]

Macronutrient change	Effect
Low carbohydrate	Benefits
	Improved glycemic status and HDL cholesterol
	Improved TGL
	Improved satiety
	Disadvantages
	Increased LDL cholesterol
	Ketosis
	Excess of protein intake: risk in kidney disease, liver disease, diabetes, gout
	Low in fiber
	Low in vitamins and minerals (C, D, A, B1, B5, B6, folic acid, Ca, Mg, K, Zn, Cu)
	No incremental effect on weight loss (some studies show more short-term weight loss)
Moderate carbohydrate-moderate protein	Improved body composition, lipid, post-prandial insulin response
	No incremental effect on weight loss
Low fat	Beneficial effects on lipids
	Benefits on lipids replacing with unsaturated fat
	Improved renal function
	No incremental effect on weight loss
Mediterranean diet	Reduces cardiometabolic risk factors
	Reduces metabolic syndrome
	Reduces markers of inflammation
	Decreased risk certain cancers
	Improves hepatic steatosis and insulin sensitivity
	Improves renal function
	Reduces mortality
	No incremental effect on weight loss

Very Low Calorie Diets: Which Is Their Place?

Treatment with a very-low-calorie diet (VLCD; ≤800 kcal/day) is associated with substantial initial weight loss but also greater weight regain compared with weight loss achieved through a more moderate restriction in energy intake [39].

Several organizations have expressed in guidelines regarding VLCD. NICE recommended do not routinely use VLCD to manage obesity. Do not use excessively restrictive and nutritionally unbalanced diets, because they are ineffective in the long term and can be harmful [37].

Only consider VLCD as part of a multicomponent weight management strategy for people who are obese and who have a clinically assessed need to lose weight rapidly (e.g., those who need joint replacement surgery or who are seeking fertility services). The maximum time that should be followed is 12 weeks (continuously or intermittently), and people following the diet are given ongoing clinical support.

Before starting people on a VLCD as part of a multicomponent weight management strategy, it is important to consider counseling and assess for eating disorders or other psychopathology, explain the risks and benefits, and tell patient that this is not a long-term weight management strategy. And it is important to provide a long-term multicomponent strategy to help people maintain their weight after the use of a very-low-calorie diet (see Table 35.3).

Macronutrients: What About Proteins?

The macronutrient composition of meals has less impact on weight loss than adherence rates in most patients. Although, in certain patient populations, modifying macronutrient composition may be considered to optimize adherence, eating patterns, weight loss, metabolic profiles, risk factor reduction, and/or clinical outcomes [5].

While low-fat diets were popular in the latter part of the twentieth century, carbohydrate restriction has regained popularity in recent years. Dietary carbohydrate restriction has been sustained to cause endocrine adaptations that promote body fat loss more than dietary fat restriction, with proponents claiming that the resulting decreased insulin secretion causes elevated release of free fatty acids from adipose tissue, increased fat oxidation and energy expenditure, and greater body fat loss than restriction of dietary fat [40, 43].

Hall et al. investigated adults with obesity that selectively restricted dietary carbohydrate versus fat. Cutting carbohydrates increased net fat oxidation, while equal calorie fat restriction had no effect. However, cutting fat resulted in more body fat loss than cutting carbohydrates as measured by metabolic balance. Mathematical model simulations predicted small long-term differences in body fat [44].

In overweight people, low-carbohydrate diets can produce more rapid and greater short-term (less than 6 months) weight reductions than other dietary prescriptions [45]. However, longer-term studies (more than 12 months) show only a small difference (typically around 1 kg) between “high”- and “low”-carbohydrate weight-reducing diets and suggest that compliance with dietary advice rather than macronutrient composition is the main determinant of weight loss [41].

Why was long-term weight loss so poor, regardless of the type of diet prescribed? This question has been hotly debated for decades. One key reason is that adherence to the diets decreases with the course of treatment time. Weight loss studies achieve a maximum weight loss after about 6–8 months, followed by weight regain [46].

Energy balance calculations suggest that at the point of maximum weight loss, diet adherence has already been substantially reduced [47, 48].

RCT comparing different types of diets shows huge differences, but very little evidence has been published about the effects of the prescribed diets over the long term. A major problem is that accurate assessment of diet adherence in outpatient studies is very limited, although new methods are being developed [48].

What is surprising is that in the long run, the same pattern of weight loss is repeated, regardless of the diet used [46]. Much more research is needed to determine factors that affect diet adherence and thereby help maintain weight loss over the long term [49]. What seems to be clear is that long-term diet adherence is extremely bad, irrespective of what type of diet is prescribed [42].

And, as weight loss occurs, energy requirements decrease out of proportion to the reduction accounted for in lowered weight. Consequently, targeted energy intake needs to be decreased if continued weight loss is to be achieved, as well as for the maintenance of lost weight.

The appeal of abundant highly palatable food that influences eating patterns can make caloric restriction an unachievable goal for many individuals and does not seem to be a problem of “lack of will.” Powerful biological forces propel the body to regain lost weight. In obese patients who have achieved weight loss, clinical data suggest the presence of compensatory mechanisms that may lead to weight regain. One study reported that obese patients who underwent a 10-week weight loss program had significantly lower levels of the saciogenic peptides leptin, PYY, CCK, insulin, and amylin and significant increases in the orexigenic peptide ghrelin levels from baseline. These differences persisted at 1 year and were accompanied by significant increases in appetite and preoccupation with food [50].

Physical Activity

Increased physical activity is one of the essential components of the comprehensive approach to life changes in the management of obesity.

Recommendations typically prescribe a gradual and progressive increase in physical activity (e.g., rapid walking) to reach a minimum goal of at least 150 min/week (30 min or more/day, at least 5 days per week) [10, 32]. Beyond weight loss, achieving this goal brings additional benefits to health. However, some guidelines [38] recommend prescribe in overweight and obese individuals a higher volume of physical activity, equal to approximately 1800–2500 kcal/week (225–300 min/week of moderate intensity physical activity).

For maintenance of lost weight, more exercise is needed, at least 60–90 min a day [32, 37, 51].

The type of physical activity (e.g., aerobic vs resistance or high intensity vs low intensity) does not seem to affect overall weight loss, but as more intensive activity produces similar weight loss with a reduced time commitment, this might be preferable to some; it would therefore seem appropriate to recommend programs that are acceptable to patients [52].

In a meta-analysis of three small RCTs, weight loss at 12 months was significantly greater with physical activity than control. Physical activity (minimum of 45 min, three times per week) combined with diet results in significantly greater weight loss at 12 months than diet alone. Median weight change across three studies was a loss of 5.60 kg for physical activity and diet and a loss of 4.10 kg for diet alone [53].

The recommendations from NICE for physical activity for adults include encourage patients to increase their level of physical activity even if they do not lose weight as a result, because of the other health benefits it can bring (e.g., reduced risk of type 2 diabetes and cardiovascular disease) [37]. Also, encourage adults to build up to the recommended activity levels for weight maintenance, using a managed approach with agreed goals. Recommend types of physical activity, including activities that can be incorporated into everyday life, such as brisk walking, gardening, or cycling, supervised exercise programs, and other activities, such as swimming, aiming to walk a certain number of steps each day, or stair climbing.

The recommendations from AACE 2016 are [5]:

- Voluntary aerobic physical activity progressing to >150 min/week performed on 3 to 5 separate days per week.
- Resistance exercise: single-set repetitions involving major muscle groups, two to three times per week.
- Reduce sedentary behavior.
- Individualize program based on preferences and take into account physical limitations.

Physical activity alone, however, contributes minimally to weight loss in the short term. Individuals who engage in high levels of physical activity in the absence of dietary restriction lose small amounts of weight. In a RCT with 120 sedentary overweight adults, the objective was determine the effects of the amount of exercise on body weight, in 8 months of treatment [54]. Patients were divided into three groups with different amounts and intensity of exercise, and subjects were counseled not to change their diet. It was found a dose-response relationship between the amount of weekly exercise and the amount of weight change. However, weight loss with physical exercise without dietary support was minimal. The patients with high amount/vigorous intensity lost 3.5 kg, patients with low amount/moderate intensity lost 1.3 kg, and patients with low amount/vigorous intensity lost 1.1 kg. Control group gained 1.1 kg in 8 months. So, in the short term, physical activity alone contributes minimally to weight loss. In the absence of caloric reduction, people lose little weight despite adhering to high levels of physical activity.

Nevertheless, although physical activity is effective in the short term in controlled settings, the activities and their benefits are not readily sustained, as was found comparing the 1- and 4-year results in the LOOK AHEAD study [11].

Pharmacotherapy

Weight loss is difficult for most patients, and the patient's desire to restrict food and energy intake is counteracted by adaptive biological responses to weight loss [55, 56]. Pharmacotherapy for overweight and obesity is an interesting strategy but should be used as an adjunct to lifestyle therapy and not alone.

A systematic review and clinical guidance of the Endocrine Society promotes the concept that, for patients with obesity, *medicating for chronic diseases should be with a weight centric focus* [31]. Both, the AHA/ACC/TOS Guidelines and the Endocrine Society Guidelines recommend that medications be considered as an adjunct to lifestyle or behavioral interventions in patients with a BMI ≥30 kg/m^2 or patients with a BMI ≥27 kg/m^2 plus one or more associated comorbid medical conditions (e.g., hypertension, dyslipidemia, diabetes) [9, 36].

FDA approval of weight loss medications requires demonstration of at least a 5% mean weight loss after 1 year of treatment and at least 35% of patients treated achieving a 5% weight loss [57].

Although there have been limited medications available in the past, there are currently six medication options available—namely, phentermine, orlistat, lorcaserin, phentermine/topiramate ER, naltrexone/bupropion, and liraglutide—the latter four of which have been approved by the Food and Drug Administration (FDA) within the past 4 years for chronic weight management.

Significant differences exist between the medications in regard to efficacy, safety, adverse effects, precautions, dosing, and costs.

Guideline recommendations provide minimal guidance on patient-specific decision-making for drug selection [58]. Nevertheless, several guiding principles should be followed when prescribing drugs for weight loss [36].

First, effective lifestyle support for weight loss should be provided during their use. These medications work to reinforce the patient's attempts to change eating behaviors and produce an energy deficit.

Second, the prescriber and patient should be familiar with the drug and its potential side effects.

Third, unless clinically meaningful weight loss occurs after 3–4 months (generally defined as loss of more than 4–5% of total body weight in patients without diabetes; in patients with obesity and diabetes, loss of more than 3% of total body weight can be considered satisfactory), a new treatment plan should be implemented.

No one medication is effective in every patient just as not every patient is appropriate for every medication.

These are the recommendations of the AACE 2016 [5] about the pharmacotherapy of obesity:

- The addition of pharmacotherapy produces greater weight loss and weight loss maintenance compared with lifestyle therapy alone.
- The concurrent initiation of lifestyle therapy and pharmacotherapy should be considered in patients with weight-related complications that can be ameliorated by weight loss.

Mechanisms of Action of Pharmacological Agents

With the exception of orlistat, medications indicated for obesity target appetite mechanisms. The medications available for obesity treatment work primarily in the arcuate nucleus to stimulate the POMC neurons, which promote satiety [36].

Five medications have been approved in the USA for chronic weight management, and three of these have also been approved in the European Union. Phentermine is available only in the USA (for short-term use). For chronic use, orlistat, naltrexone SR/bupropion SR, and liraglutide are available both in the USA and European Union. And lorcaserin and phentermine/topiramate ER are available only in the USA (Table 35.4) [12].

Every patient is appropriate for every medication.

Phentermine is a sympathomimetic drug with cardiostimulatory properties. Approved in 1960s for short-term use (3 months), it has only been studied in short-term trials and is a controlled substance in the USA. It has misuse potential (albeit small) and small risk of primary pulmonary hypertension, thus making its use for managing a chronic disease less than ideal.

Mechanism of Action Inhibits Na-dependent NE transporter. Reduces NE uptake. Inhibits serotonin and dopamine reuptake

Table 35.4 Medications for weight management: mechanism of action, dosing, and results [12]

Drug	Mechanism of action	Mean % weight loss placebo	drug
Phentermine 15–30 mg orally	Sympathomimetic	Not stated in label	Not stated in label
Orlistat 120 mg orally three times a day before meals	Pancreatic lipase inhibitor	−2.6%[a]	−6.1%[a]
Lorcaserin 10 mg orally twice a day	5-HT_xserotonin agonist with little affinity for other serotoninergic receptors	−2.5%	−5.8%
Phentermine/topiramate ER 7.5 mg/46 mg or 15 mg/92 mg orally indicated as rescue (requires titration)	Sympathomimetic anticonvulsant (GABA receptor modulation, carbonic anhydrase inhibition, glutamate antagonism)	−1.2%	−7.8% (mid-dose) −9.8% (full dose)
Naltrexone SR/bupropion SR 32 mg/360 mg orally (Requires titration)	Opioid receptor antagonist; dopamine and noradrenaline reuptake inhibitor	−1.3%	−5.4%
Liraglutide 3.0 mg injection (Requires titration)	GLP-1 receptor agonist	−3%	−7.4% (full dose)

From Bray et al. [12]
Information is from US product labels, except where noted. The data supporting these tables are derived from prescribing information labeling approved by the US Food and Drug Administration
ER extended release, *SR* sustained release
[a]Assuming the average patient in the orlistat and placebo groups weighed 100 kg at baseline

Dosing 15–30 mg/day

Contraindications Anxiety disorders (agitated states), history of heart disease, uncontrolled HTA, seizure, MAO (monoamine oxidase) inhibitors, pregnancy and breastfeeding, hyperthyroidism, glaucoma, history of drug abuse, sympathomimetic amines

Adverse Effects Dry mouth, headache, insomnia, constipation, anxiety. Cardiovascular: palpitation, tachycardia, elevated BP, ischemic events. Central nervous system: overstimulation, restlessness, dizziness, insomnia, euphoria, dysphoria, tremor, headache, psychosis. Gastrointestinal: dryness of the mouth, unpleasant taste, diarrhea, constipation, other gastrointestinal disturbances. Allergic: urticaria. Endocrine: impotence, changes in libido

Although phentermine is FDA approved for weight loss, it is not approved for long-term use.

The problem is that once the drug is stopped, the risk of weight regain is high. One approach that has been tried to avoid this situation is intermittent therapy [59]. Although this approach appears to work, it is not a logical way to prescribe given what is understood about the effects of weight loss medications on weight regulation. The question then is whether or not it is reasonable to prescribe phentermine off-label long term. Phentermine is currently the most widely prescribed weight loss medication, and it is likely that much of this prescribing is off-label [36].

Orlistat is a pancreatic lipase inhibitor that blocks absorption of 30% of ingested fat when eating a 30% fat diet [60].

Dosing Starts 120 mg daily and ranges 120 mg/day 120 mg TID

Contraindications Orlistat is one of the safest drugs in this category and is approved for use in adolescents [61]. Also, the study XENDOS of 4 years of duration supports its long-term safety and efficacy and shows that orlistat reduces the development of diabetes mellitus in people with prediabetes [62]. However the drug's gastrointestinal side effects (flatulence, diarrhea, bloating, cramping, abdominal pain) limit its popularity with patients. Other contraindications are chronic malabsorption syndrome, pregnancy and breastfeeding, and cholestasis.

Table 35.5 Cardiovascular outcomes with anti-obesity drugs [70–72]

Drug	LDL	HDL	TGL	SBP	A1C
Phen/Top CR	↓	↑	↓	↓	↓
Lorcaserin	↓	–	↓	↓/–	↓
Nal/Bupr SR	–	↑	↓	↑	↓
Liraglutide	↓	↑	↓	↓	↓

Advice/Precautions Advise daily multivitamin, monitor fat-soluble vitamins, and decrease levels of cyclosporin if co-administered.

In recent years, four medications have reached the market in the USA:

- Lorcaserin (*Belviq*) [63, 64]
- A combination of phentermine/topiramate extended release (ER) (*Qsymia*) [65, 66]
- A combination of naltrexone sustained release (SR)/bupropion SR (*Contrave*) [67, 68]
- Liraglutide 3 mg (*Saxenda*) [69]

These drugs are required by regulatory agencies in the USA and European Union to present data to approximate or exceed 5% greater weight loss than placebo and to show positive effects on various risk factors and disease markers. Also, the studies must have included more than 2500 patients, and all of these drugs must show evidence of no increase in cardiovascular risk (Table 35.5), and they were studied with a suicidality rating scale [73].

Lorcaserin is a specific 5-HT 2c serotonin receptor agonist, with little affinity for other serotoninergic receptors.

Mechanism of Action It increases satiety via alpha-MSH and POMC neuron activation.

Dosing 10 mg BID

Contraindications Congestive heart failure, depression. Pregnancy and breastfeeding. Use with caution: SSRI, SNRI/MAO inhibitors, St John's wort, triptans, bupropion, dextromethorphan

The drug should not be used with monoamine oxidase inhibitors because of the risk of serotonin syndrome. It has not been studied with serotonin reuptake inhibitors, serotonin-norepinephrine reuptake inhibitors, or other serotonergic drugs, and extreme caution should be used in combining it with those drugs.

Adverse Effects Nasopharyngitis, headache, nausea, dizziness, fatigue, priapism

The combination of phentermine and topiramate as an ER formulation uses lower doses of both drugs (7·5 mg of phentermine and 46 mg of topiramate at the recommended dose) than are usually prescribed when either drug is used as alone.

Mechanism of Action It combines GABA receptor modulation (topiramate) plus norepinephrine-releasing agent (phentermine). This medication is associated with greater mean weight loss than other available medications.

Dosing 3.75/23–15/92 mg/day

Contraindications Pregnancy and breastfeeding. Cardiovascular disease (MI, atrial fibrillation, arrhythmia, uncontrolled HTA). Hyperthyroidism, seizures, anxiety, panic attacks. Nephrolithiasis, Glaucoma. The combination is also contraindicated with MAO inhibitors and with sympathomimetic amines.

Topiramate is associated with fetal toxic effects (oral clefts). A pregnancy test before initiation of therapy, and monthly thereafter, is recommended.

Adverse Effects Dry mouth, restlessness, insomnia, palpitations, constipation. Paresthesias, dysgeusia, somnolence, cognitive impairment. A rare side effect of topiramate is acute myopia with glaucoma, and that is the reason of the contraindication in glaucoma.

The combination of naltrexone SR/bupropion SR was approved in the USA in 2014 and in the European Union in 2015.

Mechanism of Action Bupropion is a mild reuptake inhibitor of dopamine and noradrenaline. Naltrexone, an opioid receptor antagonist, has minimum effect on weight loss on its own.

Naltrexone is thought to block the inhibitory effects of opioid receptors activated by the β-endorphin released in the hypothalamus that stimulates feeding, thus allowing the inhibitory effects of α-melanocyte stimulating hormone to reduce food intake.

Dosing 8/90–32/360 mg/day

Contraindications Seizure disorders. Uncontrolled HTA, anorexia nervosa or bulimia, drug or alcohol withdrawal, MAO inhibitors.

Adverse Effects Naltrexone SR/bupropion SR can increase blood pressure, and therefore the combination should only be prescribed to patients with controlled hypertension, and the patient's blood pressure should be monitored in the early weeks of therapy. Nausea, constipation, headache, vomiting, dizziness. Tolerability issues, chiefly nausea on initiating the drug, mandate a dose escalation over 4 weeks.

Liraglutide is a GLP-1 agonist with a 97% homology to GLP-1 which extends its circulating half-life. It has been used for management of diabetes at doses of up to 1.8 mg, given by injection. It is now approved in the USA and European Union for chronic weight management.

Mechanism of Action Acylated human GLP-1 receptor agonist

Dosing 0.6–3 mg/day. Injectable. The dose can be increased by 0.6 mg per week up to a maximum of 3.0 mg. If side effects such as nausea develop during dose escalation, the dose should not be increased further until tolerated.

Contraindications Pancreatitis. Medullary thyroid cancer. MEN type II. Gastroparesis. GLP-1 agonists are associated with thyroid C cell tumors in animals, but this has not been shown with certainty in humans. Liraglutide should not be prescribed in patients with family or personal history of medullary thyroid cancer or multiple endocrine neoplasia.

Adverse Effects Nausea has been one of the principal complaints in patients injecting this drug, and a slow dose escalation over 5 weeks is prescribed. Nausea may improve with time. There is also a small but significant increase in heart rate, but blood pressure tends to fall. Acute pancreatitis, gall bladder disease, and hypoglycemia in diabetics are safety issues that require managing if they occur [69].

How to Choose a Medication: Adverse Effects Versus Efficacy

Khera R et al. published recently a systematic review and meta-analysis to compare weight loss and adverse events among drug treatments for obesity [74]. For this meta-analysis, researchers identified 28 randomized trials that involved 29,018 patients (median age, 46; median baseline body mass index, 36.1 kg/m^2); in all trials, one or more of the five approved medications were compared with placebo. Excess weight loss over placebo at 1 year was 8.8 kg for phentermine-topiramate, 5.3 kg for liraglutide, 5.0 kg for naltrexone-bupropion, 3.2 kg for lorcaserin, and 2.6 kg for orlistat. The likelihood of participants discontinuing because of adverse events was highest with liraglutide (odds ratio, 2.95) and lowest with lorcaserin (OR, 1.34) compared with placebo. In conclusion the results of this review show that phentermine-topiramate might be the best choice to optimize weight loss success with a low adverse-event rate.

The best balance of weight loss success and lack of adverse events seems to reside with phentermine-topiramate [74].

When to Refer Patients to Bariatric Surgery?

Bariatric surgery is the most effective treatment for severe obesity. It achieves substantial and sustained weight loss, comorbidity resolution, and improvements in quality of life and is associated with extended life span [75–77]. Also, it's a cost-effective treatment [78].

A lot of professional societies that represent physicians who manage severely obese patients—the American College of Cardiology/American Heart Association [16], the American Association of Clinical Endocrinologists [5], the Obesity Society [79], the American Society for Metabolic and Bariatric Surgery [79], and the American Academy of Family Physicians (AAFP) [80]—recommend bariatric surgery referral and evaluation for morbidly obese patients considered appropriate surgical candidates. Despite these data, 1% of severely obese US adults undergo bariatric surgery annually [81].

In a qualitative study, primary care physicians (PCPs) were asked to discuss prioritization of treatment for a severely obese patient with multiple comorbidities and considerations regarding bariatric surgery referral [82]. Five factors made PCPs hesitate to refer patients for bariatric surgery: (1) wanting to "do no harm," (2) questioning the long-term effectiveness of bariatric surgery, (3) limited knowledge about bariatric surgery, (4) not wanting to recommend bariatric surgery too early, and (5) not knowing if insurance would cover bariatric surgery.

So, decision-making by PCPs for severely obese patients seems to underprioritize obesity treatment and overestimate bariatric surgery risks. Many of the concerns expressed by PCPs about bariatric surgery can be addressed through education and improved communication with bariatric surgery teams and patients.

Furthermore, discussions about medical and surgical weight management options should be provided early in the course of the patient's disease. Such discussions not only inform patients about the health risks of ongoing obesity but also provide knowledge about risks, benefits, and outcomes of treatments. Support that facilitate shared decision-making could help providers optimize care for individuals with severe obesity.

Finally, the current practice environment makes it difficult and frustrating for health team to medically manage severe obesity successfully. Although PCPs believe that bariatric surgery is effective, they have concerns about its long-term benefits. Severe obesity care can be substantially improved with improvements in communication, PCP and patient education, establishment of standardized metrics, and additional research. These are potentially high-impact areas from a public health perspective and should be prioritized.

Treatment Algorithm

Currently, a BMI-centric approach represents the most commonly employed algorithm for care (Table 35.6).

The advancements in therapy and understanding of the relationship between BMI and obesity-related complications call for a reexamination of this approach. This approach emphasizes the identification and staging of complications, and treatment paradigm directed at patients who would derive the most benefit from weight loss.

Therefore, the first step is to *evaluate the patient for the presence and severity of obesity complications* in order to develop an appropriate therapeutic strategy. In patients with cardiometabolic disease or risk factors, the objective of weight loss therapy is to reduce risk of future T2DM and CVD and to treat patients with overt

Table 35.6 National Heart, Lung, and Blood Institute guide to selecting treatment for overweight and obesity [83]

	BMI category				
Treatment	25–26.9	27–29.9	30–34.9	35–39.9	≥40
Lifestyle (diet, physical activity, behavior)	Yes	Yes	Yes	Yes	Yes
Pharmacotherapy	No	Only with comorbidities	Yes	Yes	Yes
Surgery[a]	No	No	No. only LAGB approved with ≥1 comorbidity[a]	Only with comorbidities	Yes

Adapted from Ref. [83]

[a]US Food and Drug Administration (FDA)-approved Lap Band surgery for patients with BMI of at least 30 and one weight-related medical condition (February 2011)

Table 35.7 Edmonton obesity staging system [85]

Stage	Cardiometabolic and mechanical disease complications	Functional impact
0	No risk factors	No functional impairments or impairments in well-being
1	"Subclinical risk factors": prediabetes, metabolic syndrome, NAFLD, borderline hypertension, dyspnea, or moderate exertion	Mild functional limitations and impairment of well-being, mild psychopathology, occasional aches and pains
2	Established chronic disease: T2DM, hypertension, sleep apnea, PCOS, osteoarthritis, GERD	Moderate limitations in activities of daily living, moderate impairment of well-being, and/or moderate psychopathology (e.g., anxiety disorder)
3	Established end organ damage: myocardial infarction, heart failure, strokes, diabetes vascular complications, incapacitating osteoarthritis	Significant functional limitations and/or impairment of well-being
4	Severe end-stage disabilities	Severe limitations and impairment of well-being, severe disabling psychopathology

Adapted from Sharma and Kushner [85]
GERD gastroesophageal reflux disease, *NAFLD* nonalcoholic fatty liver disease, *PCOS* polycystic ovary syndrome, *T2DM* type 2 diabetes mellitus

diabetes, hypertension, and dyslipidemia. The clinician should evaluate patients for the metabolic syndrome and prediabetes, as this effectively identifies individuals at high risk for future diabetes and CVD. The initial evaluation should also screen for other disease entities that will benefit from weight loss, including nonalcoholic fatty liver disease (NAFLD) and sleep apnea. Finally, obese patients should be evaluated for mechanical complications such as problematic degenerative joint disease, GERD, stress incontinence, and immobility/disability [84].

Current Obesity Staging Systems

There are two paradigms that have been developed for comprehensive clinical staging of obesity according to the severity of comorbidities that can be used to guide the modality and intensity of therapy.

Edmonton Obesity Staging System

In 2009 Sharma and Kushner from the University of Alberta proposed complementing the existing system using a simple staging framework that provides an indication of obesity-related disease extent and severity [85]. The proposed EOSS (Edmonton obesity staging system) establishes five stages (0 through 4) that integrate the severity of obesity-related complications together with an assessment of the adverse functional impact imposed by complications on the well-being and functional status of the patient. EOSS was the first cogent complications-centric strategy that went beyond BMI level and emphasized obesity-related complications as a basis for the intensity of weight loss therapy (Table 35.7).

Cardiometabolic Disease Staging System

Garvey and coworkers [86] have proposed CMDS as a guide for treatment of obesity.

CMDS is a single staging system that provides a strong predictor of diabetes, CVD mortality, and all-cause mortality independent of BMI. CMDS assigns patients to one of five risk categories using quantitative parameters available to the clinician, including waist circumference, SBP and DBP, fasting blood levels of glucose, triglycerides, and HDL-C, as well as the 2-h oral glucose tolerance test (OGTT) value. With advancement of CMDS from stages 0 to 4, there is a progression of risk for both diabetes and all-cause and CVD mortality (Table 35.8).

Individuals in stage 0 have no risk factors (i.e., metabolically healthy obese) and exhibit minimal rates of incident diabetes and all-cause and CVD

Table 35.8 Cardiometabolic disease staging

Stage	Descriptor	Criteria
0	Metabolically healthy	No risk factors
1	One or two risk factors	Have one or two of the following risk factors:
		(a) High waist circumference (≥88 cm in women; ≥ 102 cm in men; and ≥80 cm in Southeast Asian women and ≥90 in Southeast Asian men)
		(b) Elevated blood pressure (systolic ≥130 mmHg and/or diastolic ≥85 mmHg) or on antihypertensive medication
		(c) Reduced serum HDL cholesterol (<1.0 mmol/l or 40 mg/dl in men; <1.3 mmol/l or 50 mg/dl in women)
		(d) Elevated fasting serum triglycerides (>1.7 mmol/l or 150 mg/dl)
2	Metabolic syndrome or prediabetes	Have only one of the following three conditions in isolation:
		(a) Metabolic syndrome based on three or more of four risk factors: high waist circumference, elevated blood pressure, reduced HDLC, and elevated triglycerides
		(b) Impaired fasting glucose (fasting glucose ≥5.6 mmol/l or 100 mg/dll)
		(c) Impaired glucose tolerance (2-h glucose ≥7.8 mmol/l or 140 mg/dll)
3	Metabolic syndrome and prediabetes	Have any two of the following three conditions:
		(a) Metabolic syndrome
		(b) IFG
		(c) IGT
4	T2DM and/or CVD	Have T2DM and/or CVD:
		(a) T2DM (fasting glucose ≥126 mg/dll or 2-h glucose ≥200 mg/dll or an antidiabetic therapy)
		(b) Active CVD (angina pectoris or status after a CVD event such as acute coronary artery syndrome, stent placement, coronary artery bypass, thrombotic stroke, non-traumatic amputation due to peripheral vascular disease)

Adapted from Guo et al. [92]

mortality. Patients with one or two risk factors (waist, blood pressure, HDL, or triglycerides) comprise stage 1; these patients do not meet criteria for either metabolic syndrome or prediabetes, but exhibit increased risk of future diabetes. In stage 2, patients meet criteria for only one of the following: metabolic syndrome (three or four of the following risk factors: waist circumference, blood pressure, HDL, triglycerides), or impaired fasting glucose (IFG), or impaired glucose tolerance (IGT). Stage 3 describes patients who meet criteria for any two out of three: metabolic syndrome, IFG, and IGT. Stage 4 represents the highest severity stage of CMDS and includes patients with overt T2DM and/or CVD and considers T2DM as CVD equivalent due to the high risk of future CVD events conferred by T2DM even in the absence of known CVD.

The table shows the basic elements of a complications-centric approach to obesity treatment. The presence and severity of complications that can be ameliorated by weight loss are the critical determinants for the selection of treatment modality and intensity. The BMI cutoff of 27 kg/m^2 reflects the US Food and Drug Administration indication threshold for medications at which point expanded treatment options are available to the clinician.

Several Guides of Scientific Societies Have Proposed Algorithms of Treatment

This is the algorithm proposed by the AHA/ACC/TOS Obesity Guideline 2013 (Fig. 35.2) [9]:

- They recommend treatment if BMI >30 or BMI 25–30 with additional risk factors (e.g., diabetes, prediabetes, hypertension, dyslipidemia, elevated waist circumference) or other obesity-related comorbidities.
- All patients for whom weight loss is recommended should be referred for *comprehensive lifestyle intervention*. By expert opinion, if the weight and lifestyle history indicates that the

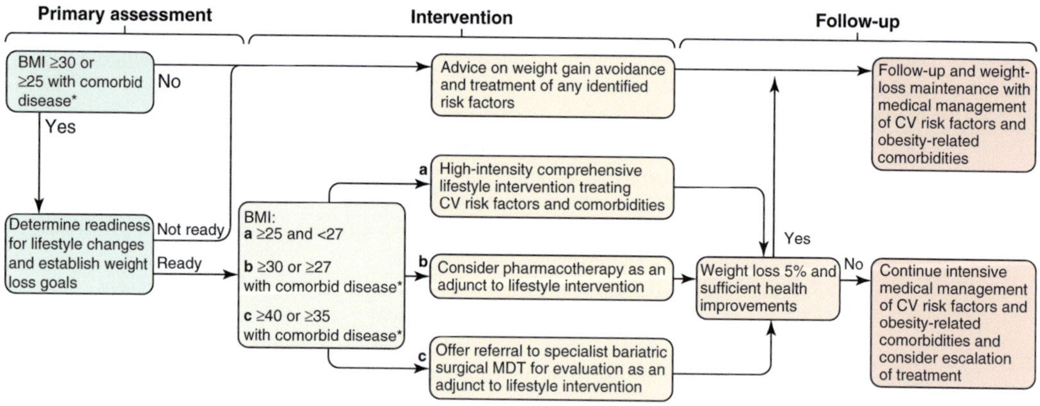

Fig. 35.2 Obesity management flow. Summarized from AHA/ACC/TOS 2013 [87]. (From Beamish et al. [87])

patient has NEVER participated in a comprehensive lifestyle intervention program, it is recommended that he or she be encouraged to undertake such a program prior to adding adjunctive therapies. This recommendation may be modified by the availability of comprehensive lifestyle intervention or by patient factors, such as medical conditions that warrant earlier initiation of *more intensive treatment.*

- If the patient has been unable to lose weight or sustain weight loss with comprehensive lifestyle intervention and they have a BMI ≥30 or ≥27 with comorbidity, *adjunctive therapies may be considered.*
- Patients who are candidates for *obesity drug treatment or bariatric surgery*, whose weight and lifestyle history indicates a history of being unable to lose weight or sustain weight loss, may be offered the option to add pharmacotherapy at the time of initiation of a lifestyle intervention program (BMI ≥30 or ≥27 with comorbidity) or to be referred for evaluation for bariatric surgery (BMI ≥40 or BMI ≥35 with comorbidity) (expert opinion).

Similarly, The AACE/ACE Guidelines for Medical Care of Patients with Obesity [5] recommend algorithm according to BMI and stages of disease. Stages are determined using criteria specific to each obesity-related complication: stage 0 = no complication, stage 1 = mild to moderate, and stage 2 = severe.

- All patients with BMI ≥25 have either overweight or obesity stage 0 or higher, depending on the initial clinical evaluation for presence and severity of complications. The diagnoses of overweight/obesity stage 0, obesity stage 1, and obesity stage 2 are not static, and disease progression may warrant more aggressive weight loss therapy in the future.
- BMI 25–29,9 kg/m^2 Overweight stage 0 (no complications): lifestyle therapy.
- BMI ≥27 is consistent with the recommendations established by the US Food and Drug Administration for weight loss medications.
- BMI >30 kg/m^2 Obesity stage 0 (no complications): lifestyle therapy. Consider weight loss medications if lifestyle therapy fails to prevent progressive weight gain (BMI >27).
- BMI >25 kg/m^2 Obesity stage 1 (one or more mild to moderate complications): Consider weight loss medications if lifestyle therapy fails to achieve therapeutic target or initiate concurrently with lifestyle therapy (BMI >27).
- BMI >25 kg/m^2 Obesity stage 2 (at least one severe complication): Add weight loss medication concurrently with lifestyle therapy (BMI >27). Consider bariatric surgery (BMI >35).

Based on the algorithm of AACE/ACE Guidelines, Sunil Daniel et al. proposed COTA [84] (comprehensive complications-centric obesity treatment algorithm), a complications-based clinical staging of obesity to guide treatment modality and intensity. In this way, they had incorporated the comprehensive approach pioneered by the EOSS, and they added cardiometabolic disease staging (CMDS) as a quantitative approach to assessing severity of cardiometabolic disease and the attendant risk of T2DM and CVD, together with the broad-based evaluation of all other key complications that can be treated with weight loss.

Figure 35.3 illustrates the three steps of a complications-centric model for the management of obesity. In step 1, a comprehensive approach to the identification and staging of obesity-related complications is depicted using quantitative measures wherever possible. Step 2 indicates that weight loss therapy can be intensified, whether involving lifestyle therapy or medications or bariatric surgery options. Step 3 reflects the observation that there is a dose-response relationship between the amount of weight loss and the degree of improvement for multiple complications (GERD, gastroesophageal reflux disease; OSA, obstructive sleep apnea).

Finally, and using EOSS, the Italian Society for Obesity (SIO) [88] proposed recently a simpler and interesting algorithm (Fig. 35.4). At each intersection a color code identifies the proposed preferred treatment option. Obviously, treatment options are not mutually exclusive but have to be understood as additive.

And what is the role of bariatric surgery in the main guidelines of patient management?

Role of bariatric surgery within medical guidelines:

- International Diabetes Federation (2011) [89]

This position statement recommended that bariatric surgery is an appropriate treatment for people with type 2 diabetes (T2DM) and obesity (BMI ≥35 kg/m^2) not achieving recommended targets with medical therapies, especially where other obesity-related comorbidities exist.

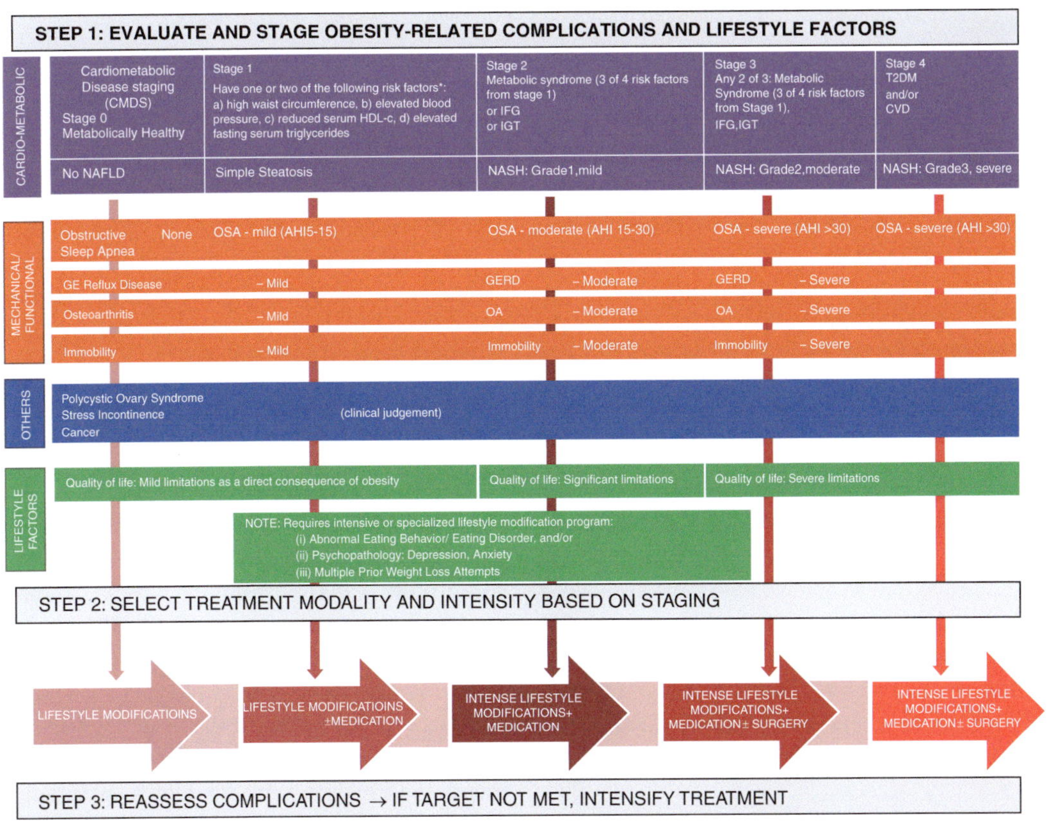

Fig. 35.3 Comprehensive obesity treatment algorithm (COTA). (From Daniel et al. [84])

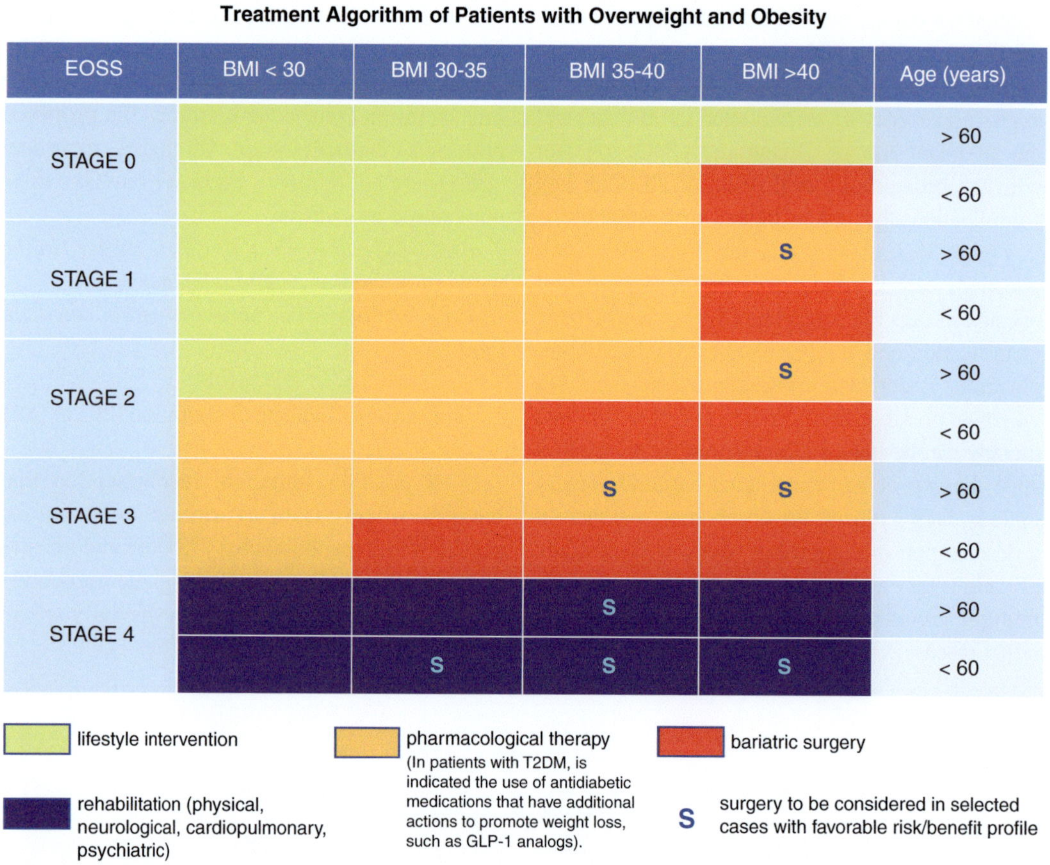

Fig. 35.4 SIO management algorithm for patients with overweight or obesity. (From Santini et al. [88])

- AHA–ACC–TOS (American Heart Association, American College of Cardiology, The Obesity Society) Guideline for the Management of Overweight and Obesity in Adults (2013) [9]

This guideline advises that bariatric surgery could be an appropriate option to improve health in adults with a BMI >40 kg/m^2 (or BMI ≥35 kg/m^2 with obesity-related comorbid conditions), who are motivated to lose weight but have not responded to behavioral treatment (with or without pharmacotherapy) with sufficient weight loss to achieve targeted health outcome goals. Referral of these patients to an experienced bariatric surgeon for consultation and evaluation is recommended.

- American Association of Clinical Endocrinologists and American College of Endocrinology [90]

This statement advised that bariatric surgery should be considered in patients with severe obesity and obesity-related complications including T2DM if the BMI is ≥35 kg/m^2.

- American Diabetes Association [91]

They use the term "metabolic surgery." Three recommendations were made regarding metabolic surgery for individuals with obesity and T2DM. Firstly, metabolic surgery should be recommended to treat type 2 diabetes in appropriate surgical candidates with BMI ≥40 kg/m^2 (BMI ≥37.5 kg/m^2 in Asian Americans), regardless of the level of glycemic control or complexity of glucose-lowering regimens, and in adults with BMI 35.0–39.9 kg/m^2 (32.5–37.4 kg/m^2 in Asian Americans) when hyperglycemia is inadequately controlled despite lifestyle and optimal medical therapy.

Secondly, metabolic surgery should be considered for adults with type 2 diabetes and BMI 30.0–34.9 kg/m^2 (27.5–32.4 kg/m^2 in Asian Americans) if hyperglycemia is inadequately controlled despite optimal medical control by either oral or injectable medications (including insulin). Thirdly, patients with T2DM who have undergone bariatric surgery need lifelong lifestyle support and medical monitoring.

Conclusions

Obesity is a chronic medical condition that requires a comprehensive approach for successful management. According to principles of chronic disease management, healthcare professionals should work collaboratively with patients to determine appropriate therapeutic strategies that address obesity, specifically considering a patient's disease status in addition to their individual needs, preferences, and attitudes regarding treatment. A central role and responsibility of healthcare professionals in this process is to inform and educate patients about their treatment options. To manage obesity as a chronic disease, clinicians should be prepared to employ an array of interventions to help patients face the physiological and behavioral challenges of weight loss and to provide ongoing and adaptable treatment to support the successful achievement of long-term weight and health goals.

Once it has been determined that treatment for obesity is indicated and that a person is ready to initiate therapy, the provider should work with that individual to develop an appropriate, patient-centered treatment plan. For each patient, the potential benefit of reducing obesity-associated risk should be evaluated against the risk associated with the intervention.

The principal goals of obesity management—improvement in body weight and composition, health, and quality of life—are achieved through interventions that help patients lose and maintain weight. Sustained weight loss of 5–10% yields significant health benefits and is recommended as an initial goal.

Behavioral change is central and all affected patients should receive counseling on nutrition and physical activity. Comprehensive lifestyle management is the base of obesity treatment, whereas pharmacotherapy and bariatric surgery are adjunct therapies that are indicated for use in combination with lifestyle management. Available agents are able to help patients achieve, on average, 5–15% weight loss, which usually leads to significant improvements in many obesity-associated comorbid conditions, including diabetes, hyperlipidemia, hypertension, and others. In patients with indication, it is important to consider bariatric surgery: it should not be the last resort.

Although current recommendations for the management of adult obesity provide general guidance regarding safe and proper implementation of lifestyle, pharmacological, and surgical interventions, healthcare professionals need awareness of specific evidence-based information that supports individualized clinical application of these therapies. More specifically, healthcare professionals should be up-to-date on approaches that promote successful lifestyle management and be knowledgeable about newer weight loss pharmacotherapies and bariatric surgery, so they can offer patients with obesity a wide range of options to personalize their treatment.

References

1. Popkin BM, Hawkes C. Sweetening of the global diet, particularly beverages: patterns, trends, and policy responses. Lancet Diabetes Endocrinol. 2016;4:174–86.
2. Church TS, Thomas DM, Tudor-Locke CT. Trends over 5 decades in U.S. occupation-related physical activity and their associations with obesity. PLoS One. 2011;6(5):e19657.
3. Mc Allister EJ, Dhurandhar N, Keith S. Ten putative contributors to the obesity epidemic. Crit Rev Food Sci Nutr. 2009;49:868–913.
4. Allison DB, Downey M, Atkinson RL. Obesity as a disease: a white paper on evidence and arguments commissioned by the Council of the Obesity Society. Obesity (Silver Spring). 2008;16:1161–77.
5. Garvey T, Mechanick JI, Brett EM. American Association of Clinical Endocrinologists and American College of Endocrinology Comprehensive Clinical Practice Guidelines for medical care of patients with obesity. Endocr Pract. 2016;22(Suppl 3):1–203.

6. Wadden TA, Butryn ML, Hong PS, Wadden TA. Behavioral treatment of obesity in patients encountered in primary care settings: a systematic review. JAMA. 2014;312:1779–91.
7. Antognoli EL, Seeholzer EL, Gullett H. Primary care resident training for obesity, nutrition, and physical activity counseling. Health Promot Pract. 2017;18(5):672–80.
8. Gudzune KA, Beach MC, Roter DL. Physicians build less rapport with obese patients. Obesity (Silver Spring). 2013;21(10):2146–52.
9. Jensen MD, Ryan DH, Donato KA, Apovian CM, Ard JD, Comuzzie AG, Hu FB, Hubbard VS, Jakicic JM, Kushner RF, Loria CM, Millen BE, Nonas CA, Pi-Sunyer FX, Stevens J, Stevens VJ, Wadden TA, Wolfe BM, Yanovski SZ. Guidelines (2013) for managing overweight and obesity in adults. Obesity. 2014;22(S2):S1–S410.
10. National Institute for Health and Care Excellence (UK). National Institute for Health and Clinical Excellence: guidance. Obesity: identification, assessment and management of overweight and obesity in children, young people and adults: partial update of CG43. National Clinical Guideline Centre (UK). 2014.
11. Look AHEAD Research Group. Eight-year weight losses with an intensive lifestyle intervention: the look AHEAD study. Obesity (Silver Spring). 2014;22(1):5–13.
12. Bray GA, Frühbeck G, Ryan DH. Management of obesity. Lancet. 387(10031):1947–56.
13. Unick JL, Neiberg RH, Hogan PE. Weight change in the fi rst 2 months of a lifestyle intervention predicts weight changes 8 years later. Obesity (Silver Spring). 2015;23:1353–6.
14. Watson S, Woodside JV, Ware LJ. Effect of a web-based behavior change program on weight loss and cardiovascular risk factors in overweight and obese adults at high risk of developing cardiovascular disease: randomized controlled trial. J Med Internet Res. 2015;17(7):e177.
15. Stuart R. Behavioral control of overeating. Behav Ther. 1967;5:357–65.
16. Association ACoCH. Task force on Practice Guidelines, Obesity Expert Panel, 2013. Expert panel report: guidelines (2013) for the management of overweight and obesity in adults. Obesity (Silver Spring). 2014;22(Suppl 2):S41–410.
17. Baker RC, Kirschenbaum D. Self-monitoring may be necessary for successful weight control. Behav Ther. 1993;24(3):377–94.
18. Klem ML, Wing RR, MT MG. A descriptive study of individuals successful at long-term maintenance of substantial weight loss. Am J Clin Nutr. 1977;66(2):239–46.
19. Mc Guire M, Wing RR, Klem ML. Behavioral strategies of individuals who have maintained long-term weight losses. Obes Res. 1999;7(4):334–41.
20. Steinberg D, Tate D, Bennett G. The efficacy of a daily self-weogjomg weight loss intervention using smart scales and e-mail. Obesity (Silver Spring). 2013;21(9):1789–97.
21. Knowler WC, Barrett-Connor E, Fowler SE. Diabetes Prevention Program Research Group Reduction in the incidence of type 2 diabetes with lifestyle intervention or metformin. N Engl J Med. 2002;346(6):393–403.
22. Knowler WC, Fowler SE, Hamman RF. Diabetes Prevention Program Research Group. 10-year follow-up of diabetes incidence and weight loss in the Diabetes Prevention Program Outcomes Study. Lancet. 2009;374(9702):1677–86.
23. Wadden TA, Berkowitz RI, Womble LG. Randomized trial of lifestyle modification and pharmacotherapy for obesity. N Engl J Med. 2005;353(20):2111–21120.
24. Wing RR, Tate D, Gorin A. A self-regulation program for maintenance of weight loss. N Engl J Med. 2006;355(15):1563–71.
25. Brownell KD. The LEARN program for weight management. Dallas: American Health Publishing Company; 2004. ISBN-10: 1878513419; ISBN-13: 978-1878513410
26. Alamuddin N, Wadden TA. Behavioral treatment of the patient with obesity. Endocrinol Metab Clin N Am. 2016;45(3):565–80.
27. Kokkinos A, le Roux CW, Alexiadou K. Eating slowly increases the postprandial response of the anorexigenic gut hormones, peptide YY and glucagon-like peptide-1. J Clin Endocrinol Metab. 2010;95(1):333–7.
28. Avenell A Broom J, Brown TJ. Systematic review of the long-term effects and economic consequences of treatments for obesity and implications for health improvement. Health Technol Assess. 2004;8(21):III–V.
29. Foreyt JP, Johnston C. Behavior modification and cognitive therapy. In: Mechanick J, editor. Lifestyle medicine a manual for clinical practice. Cham: Springer International Publishing; 2016. Chapter 14, p. 129–34.
30. Perri MG, Limacher MC, Durning PE. Extended-care programs for weight management in rural communities: the treatment of obesity in undeserved rural settings (TOURS) randomized trial. Arch Intern Med. 2008;168(21):2347–54.
31. Heymsfield SB, Wadden T. Mechanisms, pathophysiology, and management of obesity. N Engl J Med. 2017;376(3):254–66.
32. Ryan D, Heaner M. Guidelines (2013) for managing overweight and obesity in adults. Obesity. 2014;22(suppl 2):S1–3.
33. Leibel RL, Rosenbaum M, Hirsch J. Changes in energy expenditure resulting from altered body weight. N Engl J Med. 1995;332(10):621–8.
34. Das SK, Gilhooly CH, Golden JK. Long-term effects of 2 energy-restricted diets differing in glycemic load on dietary adherence, body composition, and metabolism in CALERIE: a 1-y randomized controlled trial. Am J Clin Nutr. 2007;85(4):1023–30.
35. Johnston BC, Kanters S, Bandayrel K. Comparison of weight loss among named diet programs in overweight and obese adults: a meta-analysis. JAMA. 2014;312(9):923–33.
36. Apovian CM, Aronne LJ, Bessesen DH. Pharmacological management of obesity: an

Endocrine Society clinical practice guideline. J Clin Endocrinol Metab. 2015;100(2):342–62.
37. Stegenga H, Haines A, Jones K, Wilding J. Identification, assessment, and management of overweight and obesity: summary of updated NICE guidance. BMJ. 2014;349:g6608. https://doi.org/10.1136/bmj.g6608.
38. Logue J, Thompson L, Romanes F. Scottish Intercollegiate Guidelines Network. Guidelines: management of obesity: summary of SIGN guideline. BMJ. 2010;340.; 7744(27):474–7.
39. Tsai AG, Wadden TA. The evolution of very-low-calorie diets: an update and meta-analysis. Obesity (Silver Spring). 2006;14(8):1283–93.
40. Westman EC, Feinman RD, Mavropoulos JC. Low-carbohydrate nutrition and metabolism. Am J Clin Nutr. 2007;86:276–84.
41. Tobias DK, Chen M, Manson JE, Ludwig DS, Willett W, Hu FB. Effect of low-fat diet in-terventions versus other diet interventions on long-term weight change in adults: a systematic review and meta-analysis. Lancet Diabetes Endocrinol. 2015;3(12):968–79.
42. Hall K. Prescribing low-fat diets: useless for long-term weight loss? Lancet Diabetes Endocrinol 2015; Published Online S2213-8587 (15) 00413-1.
43. Ludwig DS, Friedman MI. Increasing adiposity: consequence or cause of overeating? JAMA. 2014;311(21):2167–8.
44. Hall K, Bemis T, Brychta R. Calorie for calorie, dietary fat restriction results in more body fat loss than carbohydrate restriction in people with obesity. Cell Metab. 2015;22(3):427–36.
45. Hession M, Rolland C, Kulkarni U. Systematic review of randomized controlled trials of low-carbohydrate vs. low-fat/low-calorie diets in the management of obesity and its comorbidities. Obes Rev. 2009;10(1):36–50.
46. Franz MJ, VanWormer JJ, Crain AL. Weight-loss outcomes: a systematic review and meta-analysis of weight-loss clinical trials with a minimum 1-year follow-up. J Am Diet Assoc. 2007;107(10):1755–67.
47. Hall KD, Sacks G, Chandramohan D. Quantification of the effect of energy imbalance on bodyweight. Lancet. 2011;378(9793):826–37.
48. Sanghvi A, Redman LM, Martin CK. Validation of an inexpensive and accurate mathematical method to measure long-term changes in free-living energy intake. Am J Clin Nutr. 2015;102(2):353–8.
49. MacLean PS, Wing RR, Davidson T. NIH working group report: innovative research to improve maintenance of weight loss. Obesity (Silver Spring). 2015;23(1):7–15.
50. Sumithran P, Prendergast LA, Delbridge E. Long-term persistence of hormonal adaptations to weight loss. N Engl J Med. 2011;365(17):1597–604.
51. National Institute for Health and Clinical Excellence: Guidance. Obesity: identification, assessment and management of overweight and obesity in children, young people and adults. London: National Clinical Guideline Centre (UK). National Institute for Health and Care Excellence (UK); 2014. nice.org.uk/guidance/cg189.
52. Ross R, Hudson R, Stotz PJ. Effects of exercise amount and intensity on abdominal obesity and glucose tolerance in obese adults: a randomized trial. Ann Intern Med. 2015;162(5):325–34.
53. National Institute for Health and Clinical Excellence (NICE). Obesity: the prevention, identification, assessment and management of overweight and obesity in adults and children. London: NICE; 2006. Available from url: http://guidance.nice.org.uk/CG43.
54. Slentz CA, Duscha BD, Johnson JL. Effects of the amount of exercise on body weight, body composition, and measures of central obesity: STRRIDE–a randomized controlled study. Arch Intern Med. 2004;164(1):31–9.
55. Hinkle W, Cordell M, Leibel R. Effects of reduced weight maintenance and leptin repletion on functional connectivity of the hypothalamus in obese humans. PLoS One. 2013;8:e5914.
56. Rosembaum M, Hirsch J, Gallagher DA. Long-term persistence of adaptive thermogenesis in subjects who have maintained a reduced body weight. Am J Clin Nutr. 2008;88(4):906–12.
57. Pucci A, Finer N. New medications for treatment of obesity: metabolic and cardiovascular effects. Can J Cardiol. 2015;31(2):142–52.
58. Nuffer W, Trujillo JM, Megyeri JA. Comparison of new pharmacological agents for the treatment of obesity. Ann Pharmacother. 2016;50(5):376–88.
59. Weintraub M, Sundaresan PR, Madan M. Long-term weight control study. II (weeks 34 to 104). An open-label study of continuous fenfluramine plus phentermine versus targeted intermittent medication as adjuncts to behavior modification, caloric restriction, and exercise. Clin Pharmacol Ther. 1992;51(5):595–601.
60. Sjöström L, Rissanen A, Andersen T. Randomised placebo-controlled trial of orlistat for weight loss and prevention of weight regain in obese patients. Lancet. 1998;352(9123):167–72.
61. Chanoine JP, Hampl S, Jensen C. Effect of orlistat on weight and body composition in obese adolescents: a randomized controlled trial. JAMA. 2005;293(23):2873–83.
62. Torgerson JS, Hauptman J, Boldrin MN. XENical in the prevention of diabetes in obese subjects (XENDOS) study: a randomized study of orlistat as an adjunct to lifestyle changes for the prevention of type 2 diabetes in obese patients. Diabetes Care. 2004;27(1):155–61.
63. Smith SR, Weissman NJ, Anderson CM. Behavioral Modification and Lorcaserin for Overweight and Obesity Management (BLOOM) Study Group. Multicenter, placebo-controlled trial of lorcaserin for weight management. N Engl J Med. 2010;363(3):245–56.
64. Fidler MC, Sanchez M, Raether B, for the BLOSSOM Clinical Trial Group. A one-year randomized trial of lorcaserin for weight loss in obese and overweight adults: the BLOSSOM trial. J Clin Endocrinol Metab. 2011;96(10):3067–77.

65. Aronne LJ, Wadden TA, Peterson C. Evaluation of phentermine and topiramate versus phentermine/topiramate extended-release in obese adults. Obesity (Silver Spring). 2013;21(11):2163–71.
66. Allison DB, Gadde KM, Garvey WT. Controlled-release phentermine/topiramate in severely obese adults: a randomized controlled trial (EQUIP). Obesity (Silver Spring). 2010;20(2):330–42.
67. Apovian CM, Aronne L, Rubino D, COR-II Study Group. A randomized, phase 3 trial of naltrexone SR/bupropion SR on weight and obesity-related risk factors (COR-II). Obesity (Silver Spring). 2013;21(5):935–43.
68. Wadden TA, Foreyt JP, Foster GD. Weight loss with naltrexone SR/bupropion SR combination therapy as an adjunct to behavior modification: the COR-BMOD trial. Obesity (Silver Spring). 2011;19(1):110–20.
69. Astrup A, Carraro R, Finer N. Safety, tolerability and sustained weight loss over 2 years with the once-daily human GLP-1 analog, liraglutide. Int J Obes (Lond). 2012;36(6):843–54.
70. Gadde KM, Allison DB, Ryan DH. Effects of low-dose, controlled-release, phentermine plus topiramate combination on weight and associated comorbidities in overweight and obese adults (CONQUER): a randomised, placebo-controlled, phase 3 trial. Lancet. 2011;377(9774):1341–52.
71. Crane J, McGowan B. The GLP-1 agonist, liraglutide, as a pharmacotherapy for obesity. Ther Adv Chronic Dis. 2016;7(2):92–107.
72. Rueda-Clausen CF, Padwal RS, Sharma AM. New pharmacological approaches for obesity management. Nat Rev Endocrinol. 2013;9:467–78.
73. Giddens JM, Sheehan KH, Sheehan DV. The Columbia suicidality severity rating scale (C-SSRS): has the gold standard become a liability? Innov Clin Neurosci. 2014;11(9–10):66–80.
74. Khera R, Murad MH, Chandar AK. Association of pharmacological treatments for obesity with weight loss and adverse events: a systematic review and meta-analysis. JAMA. 2016;315(22):2424.
75. Chang SH, Stoll CR, Song J. The effectiveness and risks of bariatric surgery: an updated systematic review and meta-analysis 2003–2012. JAMA Surg. 2014;149(3):275–87.
76. Schauer PR, Bhatt DL, Kirwan JP for the STAMPEDE Investigators. Bariatric surgery versus intensive medical therapy for diabetes – 5-year outcomes. N Engl J Med. 2017;376(7):641–51.
77. Arterburn DE, Weidenbacher H, Maciejewski ML. Association between bariatric surgery and long-term survival. JAMA. 2015;313(1):62–70.
78. Wang BC, Furnback W. Modelling the long-term outcomes of bariatric surgery: a review of cost-effectiveness studies. Best Pract Res Clin Gastroenterol. 2013;27(6):987–95.
79. Mechanick J, Youdim A, Jones DB. AACE/TOS/ASMBS guidelines clinical practice guidelines for the perioperative nutritional, metabolic, and nonsurgical support of the bariatric surgery patient—2013 update: cosponsored by American Association of Clinical Endocrinologists, The Obesity Society and American Society for Metabolic & Bariatric Surgery. Obesity (Silver Spring). 2013;21(0 1):S1–27.
80. Mc Kinney L, Skolnik N, Chrusch A. Diagnosis and management of obesity. American Academy of Family Physicians. 2013. http://www.aafp.org/dam/AAFP/documents/patient_care/fitness/obesity-diagnosis-management.pdf.
81. Nguyen NT, Masoomi H, Magno CP. Trends in use of bariatric surgery 2003–2008. J Am Coll Surg. 2011;213(2):261–6.
82. Funk LM, Jolles SA, Greenberg CC. Primary care physician decision making regarding severe obesity and bariatric surgery: a qualitative study. Surg Obes Relat Dis. 2016;12(4):893–901.
83. Pi-Sunyer FX, Aronne LJ, et al. The practical guide: identification, evaluation, and treatment of overweight and obesity in adults. Bethesda: National Heart, Lung, and Blood Institute; 2000.
84. Daniel S, Soleymani T, Garvey WT. A complications-based clinical staging of obesity to guide treatment modality and intensity. Curr Opin Endocrinol Diabetes Obes. 2013;20(5):377–88.
85. Sharma AM, Kushner RF. A proposed clinical staging system for obesity. Int J Obes (Lond). 2009;33(3):289–95.
86. Garvey WT. New tools for weight-loss therapy enable a more robust medical model for obesity treatment: rationale for a complications-centric approach. Endocr Pract. 2013;19(5):864–74.
87. Beamish AJ, Olbers T, Kelly AS, Inge TI. Cardiovascular effects of bariatric surgery. Nat Rev Cardiol. 2016;13:730–43. https://doi.org/10.1038/nrcardio.2016.162.
88. Santini F, Busetto L, Cresci B, Sbraccia P. SIO management algorithm for patients with overweight or obesity: consensus statement of the Italian Society for Obesity (SIO). Eat Weight Disord. 2016;21:305–7. https://doi.org/10.1007/s40519-016-0279-3.
89. Dixon JB, Zimmet P, Alberti KG. International Diabetes Federation Taskforce on Epidemiology and Prevention. Bariatric surgery: an IDF statement for obese type 2 diabetes. Diabet Med. 2011;28(6):628–42.
90. Handelsman Y, Bloomgarden ZT, Grunberger G. American Association of Clinical Endocrinologists and American College of Endocrinology – clinical practice guidelines for developing a diabetes mellitus comprehensive care plan. Endocr Pract. 2015;21(Suppl 1):1–87.
91. American Diabetes Association. Standards of medical care in diabetes 2017. Diabetes Care. 2017;40(Supp 1):S11.
92. Guo F, Moellering DR, Garvey WT. The progression of cardiometabolic disease: validation of a new cardiometabolic disease staging system applicable to obesity. Obesity. 2014;22(1):110–8.

Metabolic Surgery, Reality or Myth: Scientific Side of Obesity Pathophysiology and Management

36

Emma Rose McGlone and Ahmed R. Ahmed

Introduction

Etymologically, the term 'bariatric surgery' means surgery to reduce weight, deriving from the Greek 'baros' (heavy). It is clear however that most bariatric operations have dramatic effects on type 2 diabetes mellitus and other metabolic conditions, many of which occur independently of weight loss. Weight loss may be regarded as just one of several clinical outcomes that result from the systemic changes in nutrient metabolism conferred by operations such as Roux-en-Y gastric bypass (RYGB): hence these operations can be considered examples of 'metabolic surgery'.

This chapter will outline the existing evidence that bariatric procedures have clinical outcomes independent of weight loss and may therefore be termed 'metabolic'. It will then outline current understanding of the main mechanisms by which weight loss-independent changes in metabolism are conferred: caloric restriction, gut hormones, bile acids and the gut microbiome (summarised in Fig. 36.1). Finally, it will consider potential limits to the notion that bariatric surgery is purely metabolic.

E. R. McGlone
Department of Endocrinology and Investigative Medicine, Imperial College London, London, UK
e-mail: e.mcglone@imperial.ac.uk

A. R. Ahmed (✉)
Department of Bariatric Surgery, St Mary's Hospital, Imperial College London, London, UK
e-mail: ahmed.ahmed@imperial.nhs.uk

'Bariatric' or 'Metabolic': Mere Semantics?

The concept of metabolic surgery is not new. In 1978 William Buchwald and Richard Varco published the book *Metabolic Surgery*, a practice they defined as 'the operative manipulation of a normal organ system to achieve a biological result for a potential health gain' [1]. From this broad perspective, bariatric surgery is one part of metabolic surgery, a much larger field that also includes operations as diverse as partial ileal bypass for primary hypercholesterolaemia [2], oophorectomy for hormone-sensitive breast cancers [3] and deep brain stimulation for refractory depression [4].

More recently, Professor Rubino proposed that 'gastrointestinal metabolic surgery' should be characterised by its 'intent to treat diabetes and obesity from the perspective of a metabolic illness as opposed to traditional bariatric surgery intended as mere weight-reduction' [5]. This change in emphasis from weight-reduction to treatment of metabolic disease has profound ramifications for the goals and expectations of patients and care providers regarding this branch of surgery. A striking example of this was shown in an elegant study of two otherwise identical surgical programs run from the same medical centre in the USA, one entitled 'bariatric surgery' and the other 'metabolic surgery', which attracted patients with significantly different demographics [6]. The former attracted patients with a higher BMI, whereas

R. Lutfi et al. (eds.), *Global Bariatric Surgery*, https://doi.org/10.1007/978-3-319-93545-4_36

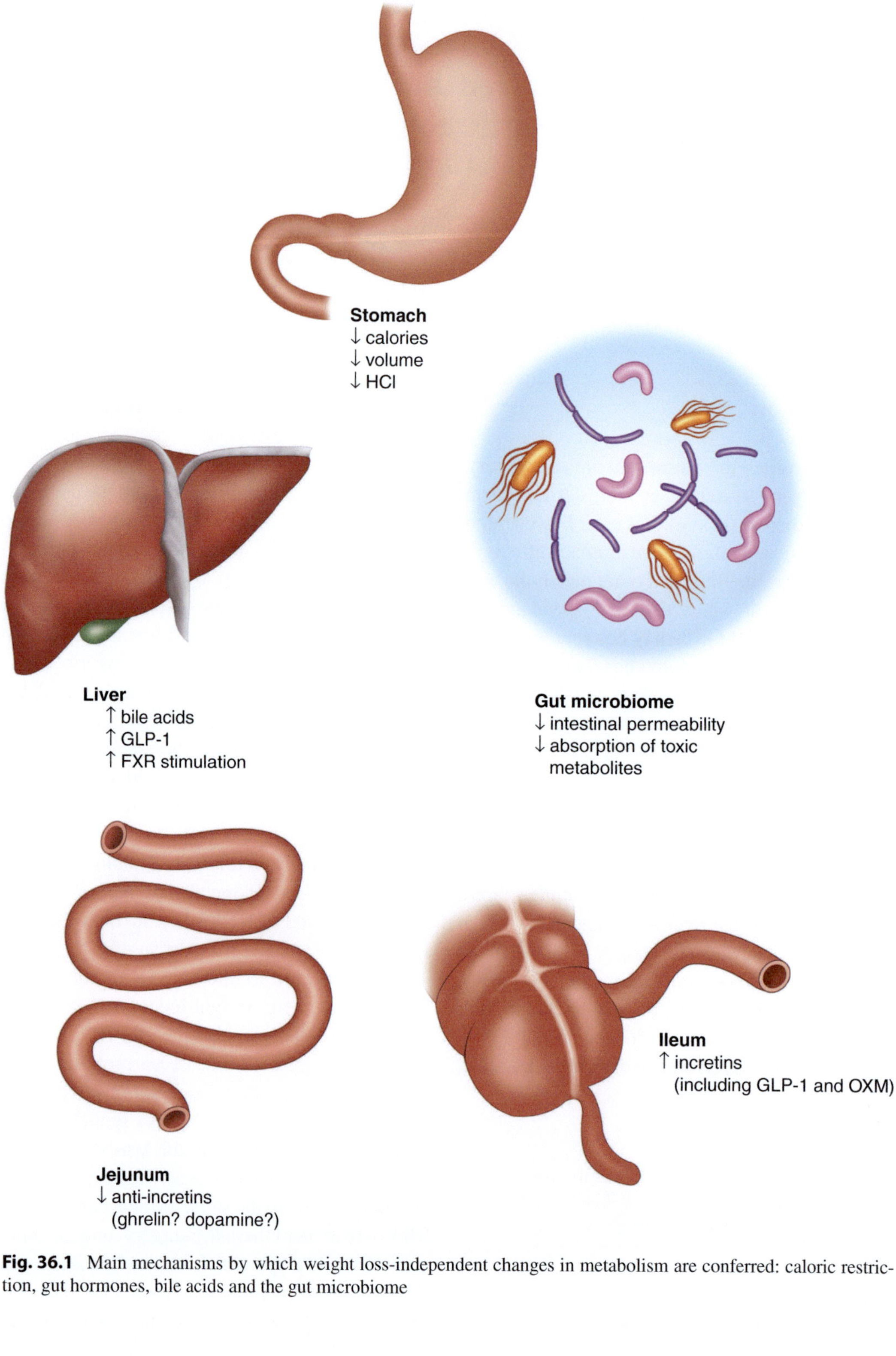

Fig. 36.1 Main mechanisms by which weight loss-independent changes in metabolism are conferred: caloric restriction, gut hormones, bile acids and the gut microbiome

the latter attracted patients with higher rates of diabetes and cardiovascular disease. A focus on metabolic health as the primary outcome of surgical intervention informs changes in eligibility criteria to reflect the value of surgery in diabetes [7] and opens the door to the potential use of surgical procedures to treat diabetes and related conditions in the nonobese [8].

Metabolic Surgery: For Better and for Worse

In the early development of bariatric surgery, the metabolic consequences of intestinal manipulation to achieve weight loss were dramatic, mostly problematic, and a significant drive for evolution of the specialism. For example, the jejunoileal bypass was developed as an alternative to the ileal bypass with jejunocolic anastomosis, due to the severe electrolyte imbalance and diarrhoea experienced with the latter procedure [9, 10]. Resulting morbidity was often so severe as to require reversal of these early bariatric procedures.

Positive metabolic sequelae of bariatric surgery were also quickly apparent, however. Buchwald and Varco's jejunoileal bypass was found not only to induce significant weight loss, but also to significantly improve hyperlipidaemia [11]. These effects on hyperlipidaemia are not explained by weight loss alone, as a less extensive ileal bypass [2] has been shown to improve long-term lipid profile without significant change in weight.

The most dramatic effect of bariatric surgery on metabolic disease, its ability to restore normal glycaemic control in type 2 diabetes, has been known for over 30 years [12]. The speed of normalisation of blood sugars – far before any significant weight loss – was noted in early reports, and at that time early diabetes resolution was proposed to occur due to reduction of caloric intake [13]. The superiority of bariatric surgery over conservative measures in improving diabetes was reported in the mid-1990s [14] and has subsequently been confirmed in several large randomised controlled trials and meta-analyses [15–18].

As well as improvement in diabetes and hyperlipidaemia, bariatric surgery is associated with long-term reduction in overall mortality, due to decreased myocardial infarction, stroke and cancer death [19]. Reduction in cardiovascular events following bariatric surgery (stroke and myocardial infarction) is not associated with degree of weight loss, implying that again this benefit occurs through other mechanisms [20]. Bariatric surgery is associated with reduced overall cancer incidence in obese women; again, this effect is not correlated with weight loss [21]. The effect of bariatric surgery on cancer mortality varies according to cancer type. Colorectal cancer is the only known malignancy where the risk of being diagnosed with the disease seems to increase after obesity surgery. In fact, mortality from rectal cancer increases threefold in patients that have had bariatric surgery [22]. Again, this would suggest that effects of bariatric surgery on cancer risk are not solely due to weight loss.

The strong association between Billroth II gastrojejunostomy and late metabolic complications including bone disease and anaemia was recognised from the mid-twentieth century [23]. Although the mechanisms behind these complications were difficult to elucidate, comparison with similar procedures led researchers to deduce that certain severe nutritional deficiencies were due to duodenal bypass, for example, although Billroth I (direct anastomosis of proximal stomach to pylorus) was noted to cause milk intolerance and osteopenia, it did not cause vitamin D deficiency and osteomalacia [24]. Fracture risk increases after bariatric surgery, associated with accelerated bone turnover, a phenomenon which appears to be in part but not entirely weight loss dependent [25, 26].

The relationship of liver disease with obesity and its response to surgery is complex. Nonalcoholic fatty liver disease is extremely common in obesity and responds well to weight loss including that induced by RYGB [27, 28]. Interestingly after bariatric surgery, there is initially a transient increase in liver fat, probably due to increased circulating free fatty acids released from adipose tissue lipolysis as insulin sensitivity improves

[29]. Improvement in liver enzymes correlates reasonably well with extent of weight loss [30], although findings of the recent LEAN trial of liraglutide suggest that some of the beneficial effects of GLP-1 agonism on steatosis are weight loss independent [31]. Other conditions improved by bariatric surgery potentially through mechanisms distinct from weight loss include male and female fertility [32, 33]and obstructive sleep apnoea [34].

Caloric Restriction as a Mediator of Metabolic Surgery

The beneficial effects of bariatric surgery on glucose homeostasis in the immediate post-operative period are in part due to the customary severe caloric restriction. Patients with diabetes administered a very low calorie diet (VLCD) as inpatients experienced similar improvements in hepatic insulin secretion in response to intravenous glucose administration to those undergoing RYGB over a 3-week period [35]. In this study, although all patients lost weight, the improvement in glucose metabolism was not correlated with weight loss. Changes conferred by acute caloric restriction are largely due to decrease in liver fat, which occurs very rapidly and improves insulin sensitivity, followed by decrease in pancreatic fat, which occurs over a few weeks and improves B cell function [36, 37].

Gut Hormones as Mediators of Metabolic Surgery

Although caloric restriction improves insulin secretion and sensitivity to an intravenous glucose stimulus, augmentation of incretin gut hormones post-bariatric surgery plays an important role in attenuation of post-prandial blood sugar peaks. The incretin effect refers to the additional insulin secretion conferred by oral glucose in excess of that stimulated by an equivalent intravenous glucose load; the incretin effect accounts for around 50% of post-prandial insulin secretion [38, 39].

The best studied and most therapeutically tractable incretin hormone is glucagon-like peptide 1 (GLP-1), so-called because it derives from the same precursor as glucagon 'proglucagon' and is structurally related [40]. GLP-1 is secreted from the enteroendocrine L cells of the terminal ileum in response to the presence of luminal nutrients. The most important metabolic effect of GLP-1 is to stimulate pancreatic insulin secretion; additionally it slows gastric emptying, elicits satiety, reduces food intake and reduces weight [41]. It also inhibits glucagon release, contributing to improved glucose tolerance [42].

Post-prandial GLP-1 is augmented after bariatric operations that accelerate delivery of nutrients to the small bowel (e.g. RYGB), but not after gastric banding or caloric restriction [43, 44]. This elevation in post-prandial GLP-1, which occurs within days of surgery and lasts for at least 10 years [45, 46], is associated with an increase in the incretin effect in patients post-RYGB [47]. Administration of the specific GLP-1 receptor antagonist exendin (9–39) in patients post-RYGB diminishes the augmentation of insulin secretion post-prandially by 43% [39]. This evidence would strongly suggest that enhanced GLP-1 secretion is responsible for at least part of the improvement in diabetes seen after bariatric surgery.

Another gut hormone which is augmented post-prandially after bariatric surgery is oxyntomodulin (OXM), a dual glucagon and GLP-1 receptor agonist, also released from L cells in response to nutrients. OXM reduces food intake and gastric emptying in humans. As a weak agonist of the GLP-1 receptor, OXM generates a small incretin effect, [44, 48] although it is likely to be much less important than GLP-1 for weight loss-independent diabetes improvements in humans [49].

Although subcutaneously injected GLP-1 agonists are licensed for use in diabetes, their effects on glucose control are modest at approximately 1% reduction in HbA1C over 26 weeks [50]. Maximal dose is limited by side-effects of nausea and vomiting. The far more dramatic effects induced by endogenously secreted GLP-1 are likely due to the fact that GLP-1 is extensively degraded by dipeptidyl peptidase 4 (DPP4) and therefore levels in the portal circulation are much higher than peripheral levels in the post-prandial post-RYGB patient [36].

'Foregut' and 'Hindgut' Hypotheses

RYGB and BPD are complex procedures, resulting in several anatomical and functional changes: these include reduction in stomach volume; exclusion of the 'foregut', duodenum and part of the small bowel; and accelerated delivery of poorly digested nutrients to the 'hindgut' – distal ileum. Correspondingly, an improvement in glucose control post-surgery could theoretically derive from one of three changes: firstly, a reduced caloric intake due to a smaller stomach (or exclusion of hormonal or other signalling factors usually secreted by the excluded stomach in response to nutrient stimuli); secondly, exclusion of factors usually produced by the foregut in response to nutrient stimuli (the 'foregut hypothesis'); or thirdly, augmentation of factors produced by the hindgut in response to accelerated delivery of nutrient stimuli (the 'hindgut hypothesis'). Of these latter 'hindgut hypothesis' mediators, GLP-1 and the other incretins are examples. Theoretical mediators of the 'foregut hypothesis' would worsen glucose tolerance and so they are named 'anti-incretins'.

To investigate the importance of the different components of these complex procedures, Professor Rubino performed a series of experiments on a rat model of nonobese type 2 diabetes [51, 52]. Duodenojejunal bypass (DJB), in which there is no reduction in stomach volume but bypass of the duodenum and proximal jejunum, led to significant improvements in glucose profile compared to sham operated rats [52]. Interestingly, the two groups of rats ate the same quantity and gained weight at the same rate. This experiment provides good evidence that glucose tolerance is improved post-RYGB due to mechanisms beyond reduction of stomach volume, reduced caloric consumption and weight loss. Indeed in the same experiment, a control group of rats treated with caloric restriction experienced less improvement in glucose homeostasis despite losing more weight than the DJB-treated rats.

In order to investigate whether the mechanism responsible for improved glucose tolerance post-surgery is exclusion of the duodenum and proximal jejunum (the 'foregut hypothesis') or rapid delivery of nutrients to the terminal ileum (the 'hindgut hypothesis'), Rubino next compared DJB with gastrojejunal anastomosis (GJ) [51]. The latter procedure simply consists of anastomosis between the stomach and proximal jejunum, with the result that just as in DJB nutrients are delivered rapidly to the terminal ileum (preserving any potential increase in incretin release due to enhanced nutrient delivery to the terminal ileum, as proposed by the hindgut hypothesis), but a small amount will pass through the duodenum allowing stimulation of any potential anti-incretins (preventing any effects attributable to the foregut hypothesis). Rats undergoing DJB and GJ had similar post-operative food intake post-operatively and lost comparable amounts of weight. DJB-treated rats, however, had markedly improved glucose tolerance in comparison to both controls and GJ-treated diabetic animals. This finding would support the foregut hypothesis, as exclusion of the foregut in this experiment is necessary to improve diabetes in diabetic rats.

Further experiments in rats using anatomical variants to unpick relative contributions of the foregut and hindgut to glucose metabolism revealed that resection or bypass of jejunum, but not ileum, improves insulin sensitivity in nonobese diabetic rats, again supporting the hypothesis that anti-incretins are secreted from the foregut [53]. In this experiment, DJB and ileectomy were surprisingly not associated with increased post-prandial GLP-1, leaving the authors to conclude that the effects on glucose homeostasis must be due to putative anti-incretin factors. In contrast, GLP-1 is known to rise dramatically post-prandially after RYGB. It has therefore been proposed that manipulation of stomach anatomy is in some way important for incretin response, rather than that it occurs simply due to an increased delivery of nutrients to the distal small bowel [54]. This would help to explain why sleeve gastrectomy (where there is no small bowel bypass) and RYGB produce similar early improvements in glucose tolerance and increased secretion of post-prandial GLP-1 [55].

Additional evidence that incretins are not the whole story derives from experiments in genetically modified mice that lack the GLP-1 receptor. These mice nonetheless experience improvements in glucose homeostasis and reduced body weight following RYGB [56], which would imply that GLP-1 is dispensable for improved diabetes post-RYGB. Furthermore, in nondiabetic patients after RYGB, blockade of the GLP-1 receptor with exendin 9–39 does alter glucose and insulin profile after a standardised meal, but appears not to alter overall disposition index (composite of insulin secretion and insulin sensitivity) [39, 57], again suggesting that effective glucose control post-bypass does not solely rely on GLP-1 action.

On the other hand, GLP-1 is implicated in the pathogenesis of post-prandial hyperinsulinaemic hypoglycaemia (PHH), a condition that affects a small proportion of patients post-RYGB. These patients experience hypoglycaemia due to dramatically elevated insulin post-prandially compared to asymptomatic post-RYGB controls, which is associated with higher post-prandial GLP-1 peak and can be blocked with exendin 9–39 [58]. This would suggest that PPH is dependent on GLP-1. Proponents of the foregut hypothesis claim that PHH is in fact relatively uncommon, which suggests that there are control mechanisms in place to prevent excessive stimulation of B cells and insulin secretion in response to GLP-1 [59]. Although severe PPH requiring hospitalisation is rare, however, the incidence of mild symptomatic PPH may affect as many as one-third of patients post-RYGB or sleeve gastrectomy [60]. It appears to be less common following sleeve gastrectomy than RYGB [60], so given that the foregut is not bypassed in the former condition, this might support a role of anti-incretins in preventing the complication.

What Are 'Anti-incretins'?

In spite of the persuasive evidence that the foregut may produce substances that are 'diabetogenic', acting to suppress insulin and increase glucagon and generally counteracting the effects of the incretins, the nature of these substances has not been identified [59]. In order to positively confirm their existence, Salinari et al. examined jejunal extracts from insulin-resistant humans and diabetic mice and demonstrated that they secrete proteins which impair insulin signalling in skeletal muscle cells in vitro [61].

One contender for an anti-incretin is ghrelin, an orexigenic hormone secreted from the stomach and proximal small bowel, which has an inhibitory effect on glucose-stimulated insulin release in humans [62] and from pancreatic B cells in vitro [63]. There is evidence from some studies that ghrelin is suppressed post-RYGB for up to 2 years [64], although other researchers have detected no change [65]. Mathematical modelling indicates that ghrelin changes are unlikely to be solely responsible for the remission of diabetes post-bariatric surgery [66], although ghrelin could perhaps be one of several anti-incretins.

Recently gastrointestinal dopamine has been proposed to be a chief anti-incretin, on the basis that it is secreted by the foregut and can prevent the effect of incretins on beta cell insulin secretion in vitro [67]. This is an exciting area that merits further investigation. Positively identifying physiological anti-incretins would potentially enable their inhibition to medically treat diabetes and/or their stimulation to treat PPH.

Sleeve Gastrectomy

Sleeve gastrectomy is highly effective for weight loss and resolution of metabolic comorbidities [68]. Specific mechanisms that have been proposed for the efficacy of sleeve include the 'gastric hypothesis', which relates a reduction in gastric hydrochloric acid release to decrease in secretion of gastric releasing peptide and increased GLP-1 release [69]. Another possible mechanism is due to faster delivery of nutrients to distal small gut, leading to increased GLP-1 and PYY secretion [70].

Bile Acids as Mediators of Metabolic Surgery

Bariatric procedures disrupt physiological enterohepatic circulation of bile acids, resulting in changes in overall levels and nature of circulating bile acids [71]. In particular, RYGB increases fasting and post-prandial circulating levels of bile acids and alters relative proportions of different types of bile acid in circulation and luminally [71, 72].

Bile acids stimulate GLP-1 secretion from L cells in the distal gut via their action on TGR5 receptors [73]. Infused into the jejunum with a glucose load, the potent TGR5 agonist taurocholic acid increases circulating GLP-1 and improves glucose tolerance in healthy volunteers [74]. In nondiabetics and fasting obese diabetics, rectal taurocholate is associated with increases in GLP-1 and insulin secretion and decreases in plasma glucose [75, 76].

Surgical experiments involving bile diversion support the notion that bile acids are important stimuli of improved glucose tolerance following metabolic surgery, albeit an effect largely mediated through gut hormones. In obese rats, a catheter inserted from the common bile duct to the mid-distal jejunum results in weight loss, improved glucose tolerance, higher post-prandial GLP-1 levels and less hepatic steatosis [77]. In a mouse model of obesity, comparison of bile acid diversion from the gallbladder to the duodenum (i.e. sham), jejunum or ileum reveals that only the latter procedure results in sustained weight loss and sustained improvements in glucose homeostasis [78]. In this study the observed weight loss was slightly greater than that observed in control mice treated with RYGB, which would imply that bile acid diversion is a very important contributor to the effects of RYGB. It was also higher than that observed in mice pair-fed to the ileum bile acid diversion group, confirming that bile acid diversion has metabolic effects independent of caloric restriction.

Changes in bile acids may also improve glucose metabolism independently of gut hormones. One proposed mechanism is due to their ability to act as Farnesoid X receptor (FXR) agonists. Hepatic FXR stimulation inhibits hepatic gluconeogenesis; adipose stimulation of FXR leads to improvements in insulin sensitivity; and intestinal FXR stimulation leads to release of FGF19 (FGF 15 in mice), which also inhibits hepatic gluconeogenesis [72]. Evidence that bile acid stimulation of FXR is important for effects of bariatric surgery comes from FXR knockout mice, which do not experience the sustained weight loss after sleeve gastrectomy observed in wild type controls [79]. Additionally, although FXR knock out mice have lower fasting blood glucose compared to wildtype, after SG their fasting glucose increases rather than decreases as in wildtype, and there is no improvement in their overall glucose homeostasis [79].

Bile acid circulation is a crucial component of overall lipid metabolism [80]. Bile acids excreted in faeces are replaced by synthesis from cholesterol in the liver, which can be a significant source of cholesterol elimination. Total circulating cholesterol improves after bariatric surgery; however, this does not appear to be associated with an increase in faecal bile acids [81, 82]. It may therefore be a result of weight loss or caloric restriction rather than bile acid diversion. Similarly, bile acids regulate hepatic fatty acid and triglyceride synthesis, but at present there is limited evidence that the beneficial effects of metabolic surgery on hepatic steatosis are directly related to changes in bile acid circulation [71].

Gut Microbiome as a Mediator of Metabolic Surgery

After RYGB, the gut microbiome changes towards higher levels of proteobacteria and lower levels of firmicutes [82, 83]. Microbiome changes are associated with changes in bile acid circulation bidirectionally, as bile acids are transformed by intestinal bacteria, and changes in bile acid composition will alter conditions affecting relative species of bacterial growth [84]. It is likely that changes in the gut microbiome in obesity and following bariatric surgery are secondary to changes in dietary intake, bile acid circulation and/or gut hormone milieu rather than direct consequences of surgery. Nonetheless, faecal transplant experiments demonstrate that transfer of gut microbiota from humans or mice that have undergone RYGB to unoperated mice reduces recipients' fat mass [83, 85]. This is associated with a lower respiratory quotient, indicating more energy production from fat rather than carbohydrate [83].

Other mechanisms via which a change in gut microbiome might improve metabolic health include a decrease in absorption of toxic metabolites such as choline and ethanol metabolites [86]. These are not only produced in greater quantities by dysregulated gut microbiota, but an unhealthy gut microbiome is also associated with increased intestinal permeability, which facilitates their absorption [87]. These factors contribute to the development of obesity-associated steatohepatitis [88]. Further research is required to determine whether changes in the gut microbiome following bariatric surgery independently account for substantial metabolic effects.

Is There a Limit to 'Metabolic' Surgery?

In this chapter we have outlined evidence that bariatric procedures such as gastric bypass work through mechanisms independent to weight loss, to cause resolution of diabetes and other metabolic disorders. For these operations to be considered 'truly' metabolic, rather than bariatric, it has been argued that they should cause resolution of metabolic disorder even in nonobese patients [89]. Although evidence from nonobese cohorts is to date very limited, the metabolic effects of bariatric surgery in the nonobese appear to be modest [90], with some indication that they are inferior to results seen in the morbidly obese [91]. A recent meta-analysis of bariatric procedures in 290 patients with a BMI of under 30 (mean 26 kg/m^2), all of which were either bypass-type operations or SG, demonstrated an overall HbA1C reduction of 1.88% with a major complication rate of 6.2% [8]. Although further research is required to confirm the value of bariatric surgery as a treatment for metabolic disorder in the nonobese, it is highly likely that maximal effect of such operations is achieved through a combination of weight loss-dependent and weight loss-independent means. Perhaps, then, these procedures are best termed 'bariatric/metabolic' surgery.

Conclusion

The ability of bariatric surgery to alter metabolism via mechanisms independent of weight loss is certainly a reality and has been demonstrated for many obesity-related conditions. The mechanisms by which bariatric surgery produces these effects include reduced caloric intake, alteration of gut hormones and other signalling molecules, bile acid circulation and the gut microbiome. These factors are interlinked and depend on operation type, which presents some challenges to achieving a complete understanding.

Better understanding of the metabolic effects of surgery and the mechanisms through which they occur will enable the development of new surgical strategies, and potentially the tailoring of surgical strategies to each individual's unique profile of metabolic disorder. Ways of predicting response to bariatric surgery are still very crude: better understanding of mechanism may well lead to more physiological and accurate methods [92]. Furthermore, understanding of the mechanisms by which metabolic effects occur will enable us to develop non-surgical alternatives, for example, gut hormone analogues [93], with consequent risk reduction for a relatively high-risk cohort of patients. It may also lead to the use of medications as targeted adjuncts for non-responders [94]. Metabolic surgery, medicine and science are closely intertwined in this fast-evolving and exciting field.

References

1. Buchwald H. Metabolic surgery: a brief history and perspective. Surg Obes Relat Dis Elsevier. 2010;6(2):221–2.
2. Buchwald H, Stoller DK, Campos CT, Matts JP, Varco RL. Partial ileal bypass for hypercholesterolemia. 20- to 26-year follow-up of the first 57 consecutive cases. Ann Surg. Lippincott, Williams, and Wilkins; 1990;212(3):318–29; discussion 329–31.
3. Love RR. Adjuvant surgical oophorectomy plus tamoxifen in premenopausal women with operable hormone receptor-positive breast cancer: a global treatment option. Clin Breast Cancer. 2016;16(4):233–7.
4. Buchwald H. The evolution of metabolic/bariatric surgery. Obes Surg. Springer US. 2014;24(8):1126–35.
5. Rubino F. From bariatric to metabolic surgery: definition of a new discipline and implications for clinical practice. Curr Atheroscler Rep. Springer US. 2013;15(12):369.
6. Rubino F, Shukla A, Pomp A, Moreira M, Ahn SM, Dakin G. Bariatric, metabolic, and diabetes surgery: what's in a name? Ann Surg. 2014;259(1):117–22.

7. Frühbeck G. Bariatric and metabolic surgery: a shift in eligibility and success criteria. Nat Rev Endocrinol. Nature Research. 2015;11(8):465–77.
8. Baskota A, Li S, Dhakal N, Liu G, Tian H. Bariatric surgery for type 2 diabetes mellitus in patients with BMI <30 kg/m^2: a systematic review and meta-analysis. Folli F, editor. PLoS One. Public Library of Science; 2015;10(7):e0132335.
9. Buchwald H, Buchwald JN. Evolution of operative procedures for the management of morbid obesity 1950–2000. Obes Surg. 2002;12(5):705–17.
10. Scott HW, Law DH, Sandstead HH, Lanier VC, Younger RK. Jejunoileal shunt in surgical treatment of morbid obesity. Ann Surg. Lippincott, Williams, and Wilkins. 1970;171(5):770–82.
11. Buchwald H, Varco RL. A bypass operation for obese hyperlipidemic patients. Surgery. 1971;70(1):62–70.
12. Ackerman NB. Observations on the improvements in carbohydrate metabolism in diabetic and other morbidly obese patients after jejunoileal bypass. Surg Gynecol Obstet. 1981;152(5):581–6.
13. Pories WJ, Swanson MS, MacDonald KG, Long SB, Morris PG, Brown BM, et al. Who would have thought it? An operation proves to be the most effective therapy for adult-onset diabetes mellitus. Ann Surg. Lippincott, Williams, and Wilkins. 1995;222(3):339–50; discussion 350–2.
14. MacDonald KG, Long SD, Swanson MS, Brown BM, Morris P, Dohm GL, et al. The gastric bypass operation reduces the progression and mortality of non-insulin-dependent diabetes mellitus. J Gastrointest Surg. 1997;1(3):213–20; discussion 220.
15. Courcoulas AP, Belle SH, Neiberg RH, Pierson SK, Eagleton JK, Kalarchian MA, et al. Three-year outcomes of bariatric surgery vs lifestyle intervention for type 2 diabetes mellitus treatment: a randomized clinical trial. JAMA Surg Am Med Assoc. 2015;150(10):931–40.
16. Mingrone G, Panunzi S, De Gaetano A, Guidone C, Iaconelli A, Nanni G, et al. Bariatric-metabolic surgery versus conventional medical treatment in obese patients with type 2 diabetes: 5 year follow-up of an open-label, single-centre, randomised controlled trial. Lancet Elsevier. 2015;386(9997):964–73.
17. Ribaric G, Buchwald JN, McGlennon TW. Diabetes and weight in comparative studies of bariatric surgery vs conventional medical therapy: a systematic review and meta-analysis. Obes Surg Springer US. 2014;24(3):437–55.
18. Colquitt JL, Pickett K, Loveman E, Frampton GK. Surgery for weight loss in adults. Colquitt JL, editor. Cochrane Database Syst Rev. Chichester, UK: John Wiley & Sons, Ltd. 2014 8;(8):CD003641.
19. Sjöström L. Review of the key results from the Swedish Obese Subjects (SOS) trial – a prospective controlled intervention study of bariatric surgery. J Intern Med. 2013;273(3):219–34.
20. Sjöström L, Peltonen M, Jacobson P, Sjöström CD, Karason K, Wedel H, et al. Bariatric surgery and long-term cardiovascular events. JAMA Am Med Assoc. 2012;307(1):56–65.
21. Sjöström L, Gummesson A, Sjöström CD, Narbro K, Peltonen M, Wedel H, et al. Effects of bariatric surgery on cancer incidence in obese patients in Sweden (Swedish Obese Subjects Study): a prospective, controlled intervention trial. Lancet Oncol Elsevier. 2009;10(7):653–62.
22. Tao W, Konings P, Hull MA, Adami H-O, Mattsson F, Lagergren J. Colorectal cancer prognosis following obesity surgery in a population-based cohort study. Obes Surg Springer US. 2016;7:1–7.
23. Mitchell AB, Glass D, and Gill AM. Bone disease after gastrectomy. Br Med J. BMJ Group; 1972;1(5798):461.
24. Fukuda M, Shibata H, Hatakeyama K, Yamagishi Y, Soga J, Koyama S, et al. Difference in calcium metabolism following Billroth-I and Billroth-II procedures for gastric and duodenal ulcers. Jpn J Surg. 1979;9(4):295–303.
25. Yu EW. Bone metabolism after bariatric surgery. J Bone Miner Res. 2014;29(7):1507–18.
26. Ivaska KK, Huovinen V, Soinio M, Hannukainen JC, Saunavaara V, Salminen P, et al. Changes in bone metabolism after bariatric surgery by gastric bypass or sleeve gastrectomy. Bone. 2016;95:47.
27. Clark JM, Alkhuraishi ARA, Solga SF, Alli P, Diehl AM, Magnuson TH. Roux-en-Y gastric bypass improves liver histology in patients with non-alcoholic fatty liver disease. Obes Res Blackwell Publishing Ltd. 2005;13(7):1180–6.
28. Hassanian M, Al-Mulhim A, Al-Sabhan A, Al-Amro S, Bamehriz F, Abdo A, et al. The effect of bariatric surgeries on nonalcoholic fatty liver disease. Saudi J Gastroenterol. Medknow Publications. 2014;20(5):270–8.
29. Papadia F, Marinari GM, Camerini G, Adami GF, Murelli F, Carlini F, et al. Short-term liver function after biliopancreatic diversion. Obes Surg Springer. 2003;13(5):752–5.
30. Burza MA, Romeo S, Kotronen A, Svensson P-A, Sjöholm K, Torgerson JS, et al. Long-term effect of bariatric surgery on liver enzymes in the Swedish Obese Subjects (SOS) study. Targher G, editor. PLoS One. Public Library of Science. 2013;8(3):e60495.
31. Armstrong MJ, Gaunt P, Aithal GP, Barton D, Hull D, Parker R, et al. Liraglutide safety and efficacy in patients with non-alcoholic steatohepatitis (LEAN): a multicentre, double-blind, randomised, placebo-controlled phase 2 study. Lancet. Elsevier. 2016;387(10019):679–90.
32. Rosenblatt A, Faintuch J, Cecconello I. Abnormalities of reproductive function in male obesity before and after bariatric surgery-a comprehensive review. Obes Surg Springer US. 2015;25(7):1281–92.
33. Eid GM, McCloskey C, Titchner R, Korytkowski M, Gross D, Grabowski C, et al. Changes in hormones and biomarkers in polycystic ovarian syndrome treated with gastric bypass. Surg Obes Relat Dis. 2014;10(5):787–91.
34. Ashrafian H, le Roux CW, Rowland SP, Ali M, Cummin AR, Darzi A, et al. Metabolic surgery and

obstructive sleep apnoea: the protective effects of bariatric procedures. Thorax. BMJ Publishing Group Ltd and British Thoracic Society. 2012;67(5):442–9.
35. Jackness C, Karmally W, Febres G, Conwell IM, Ahmed L, Bessler M, et al. Very low-calorie diet mimics the early beneficial effect of Roux-en-Y gastric bypass on insulin sensitivity and β-cell function in type 2 diabetic patients. Diabetes. American Diabetes Association. 2013;62(9):3027–32.
36. Knop FK, Taylor R. Mechanism of metabolic advantages after bariatric surgery: it's all gastrointestinal factors versus it's all food restriction. Diabetes Care. American Diabetes Association. 2013;36 Suppl 2(Supplement_2):S287–91.
37. Lim EL, Hollingsworth KG, Aribisala BS, Chen MJ, Mathers JC, Taylor R. Reversal of type 2 diabetes: normalisation of beta cell function in association with decreased pancreas and liver triacylglycerol. Diabetologia. Springer. 2011;54(10):2506–14.
38. Preitner F, Ibberson M, Franklin I, Binnert C, Pende M, Gjinovci A, et al. Gluco-incretins control insulin secretion at multiple levels as revealed in mice lacking GLP-1 and GIP receptors. J Clin Invest American Society for Clinical Investigation. 2004;113(4):635–45.
39. Salehi M, Prigeon RL, D'Alessio DA. Gastric bypass surgery enhances glucagon-like peptide 1-stimulated postprandial insulin secretion in humans. Diabetes. American Diabetes Association. 2011;60(9):2308–14.
40. Nadejda Bozadjieva JAW, Bernal-Mizrachi E. Glucagon. Pancreapedia: the exocrine pancreas knowledge base. Michigan Publishing, University of Michigan Library; 2014:1–12.
41. Scott RV, Tan TM, Bloom SR. Can Bayliss and Starling gut hormones cure a worldwide pandemic? J Physiol. 2014;592(23):5153–67.
42. Jørgensen NB, Dirksen C, Bojsen-Møller KN, Jacobsen SH, Worm D, Hansen DL, et al. Exaggerated glucagon-like peptide 1 response is important for improved β-cell function and glucose tolerance after Roux-en-Y gastric bypass in patients with type 2 diabetes. Diabetes. 2013;62(9):3044–52.
43. Usinger L, Hansen KB, Kristiansen VB, Larsen S, Holst JJ, Knop FK. Gastric emptying of orally administered glucose solutions and incretin hormone responses are unaffected by laparoscopic adjustable gastric banding. Obes Surg. Springer. 2011;21(5):625–32.
44. Laferrère B, Swerdlow N, Bawa B, Arias S, Bose M, Olivan B, et al. Rise of oxyntomodulin in response to oral glucose after gastric bypass surgery in patients with type 2 diabetes. J Clin Endocrinol Metab. 2010;95(8):4072–6.
45. Dar MS, Chapman WH, Pender JR, Drake AJ, O'Brien K, Tanenberg RJ, et al. GLP-1 response to a mixed meal: what happens 10 years after Roux-en-Y gastric bypass (RYGB)? Obes Surg Springer. 2012;22(7):1077–83.
46. le Roux CW, Welbourn R, Werling M, Osborne A, Kokkinos A, Laurenius A, et al. Gut hormones as mediators of appetite and weight loss after Roux-en-Y gastric bypass. Ann Surg. 2007;246(5):780–5.
47. Laferrère B, Heshka S, Wang K, Khan Y, McGinty J, Teixeira J, et al. Incretin levels and effect are markedly enhanced 1 month after Roux-en-Y gastric bypass surgery in obese patients with type 2 diabetes. Diabetes Care. American Diabetes Association. 2007;30(7):1709–16.
48. Day JW, Ottaway N, Patterson JT, Gelfanov V, Smiley D, Gidda J, et al. A new glucagon and GLP-1 co-agonist eliminates obesity in rodents. Nat Chem Biol Nature Publishing Group. 2009;5(10):749–57.
49. Cohen MA, Ellis SM, le Roux CW, Batterham RL, Park A, Patterson M, et al. Oxyntomodulin suppresses appetite and reduces food intake in humans. J Clin Endocrinol Metab Endocrine Society. 2003;88(10):4696–701.
50. Prasad-Reddy L, Isaacs D. A clinical review of GLP-1 receptor agonists: efficacy and safety in diabetes and beyond. Drugs Context. 2015;4:212283–19.
51. Rubino F, Forgione A, Cummings DE, Vix M, Gnuli D, Mingrone G, et al. The mechanism of diabetes control after gastrointestinal bypass surgery reveals a role of the proximal small intestine in the pathophysiology of type 2 diabetes. Ann Surg. 2006;244(5):741–9.
52. Rubino F, Marescaux J. Effect of duodenal-jejunal exclusion in a non-obese animal model of type 2 diabetes: a new perspective for an old disease. Ann Surg. 2004;239(1):1–11.
53. Salinari S, le Roux CW, Bertuzzi A, Rubino F, Mingrone G. Duodenal-jejunal bypass and jejunectomy improve insulin sensitivity in Goto-Kakizaki diabetic rats without changes in incretins or insulin secretion. Diabetes. American Diabetes Association. 2014;63(3):1069–78.
54. Patel RT, Shukla AP, Ahn SM, Moreira M, Rubino F. Surgical control of obesity and diabetes: the role of intestinal vs. gastric mechanisms in the regulation of body weight and glucose homeostasis. Obesity (Silver Spring). 2014;22(1):159–69.
55. Romero F, Nicolau J, Flores L, Casamitjana R, Ibarzabal A, Lacy A, et al. Comparable early changes in gastrointestinal hormones after sleeve gastrectomy and Roux-En-Y gastric bypass surgery for morbidly obese type 2 diabetic subjects. Surg Endosc. Springer. 2012;26(8):2231–9.
56. Mokadem M, Zechner JF, Margolskee RF, Drucker DJ, Aguirre V. Effects of Roux-en-Y gastric bypass on energy and glucose homeostasis are preserved in two mouse models of functional glucagon-like peptide-1 deficiency. Mol Metab. 2014;3(2):191–201.
57. Shah M, Law JH, Micheletto F, Sathananthan M, Dalla Man C, Cobelli C, et al. Contribution of endogenous glucagon-like peptide 1 to glucose metabolism after Roux-en-Y gastric bypass. Diabetes. American Diabetes Association. 2014;63(2):483–93.
58. Salehi M, Gastaldelli A, D'Alessio DA. Blockade of glucagon-like peptide 1 receptor corrects postprandial hypoglycemia after gastric bypass. Gastroenterology. Elsevier. 2014;146(3):669–680.e2.

59. Kamvissi V, Salerno A, Bornstein SR, Mingrone G, Rubino F. Incretins or anti-incretins? A new model for the "entero-pancreatic axis". Horm Metab Res. © Georg Thieme Verlag KG. 2015;47(1):84–7.
60. Lee CJ, Clark JM, Schweitzer M, Magnuson T, Steele K, Koerner O, et al. Prevalence of and risk factors for hypoglycemic symptoms after gastric bypass and sleeve gastrectomy. Obesity (Silver Spring). 2015;23(5):1079–84.
61. Salinari S, Debard C, Bertuzzi A, Durand C, Zimmet P, Vidal H, et al. Jejunal proteins secreted by db/db mice or insulin-resistant humans impair the insulin signaling and determine insulin resistance. Federici M, editor. PLoS One. Public Library of Science. 2013;8(2):e56258.
62. Tong J, Prigeon RL, Davis HW, Bidlingmaier M, Kahn SE, Cummings DE, et al. Ghrelin suppresses glucose-stimulated insulin secretion and deteriorates glucose tolerance in healthy humans. Diabetes. Am Diab Assoc. 2010;59(9):2145–51.
63. Damdindorj B, Dezaki K, Kurashina T, Sone H, Rita R, Kakei M, et al. Exogenous and endogenous ghrelin counteracts GLP-1 action to stimulate cAMP signaling and insulin secretion in islet β-cells. FEBS Lett. 2012;586(16):2555–62.
64. Malin SK, Samat A, Wolski K, Abood B, Pothier CE, Bhatt DL, et al. Improved acylated ghrelin suppression at 2 years in obese patients with type 2 diabetes: effects of bariatric surgery vs standard medical therapy. Int J Obes. Nature Publishing Group. 2014;38(3):364–70.
65. Cummings DE. Endocrine mechanisms mediating remission of diabetes after gastric bypass surgery. Int J Obes. Nature Publishing Group. 2009;33(Suppl 1):S33–40.
66. Toghaw P, Matone A, Lenbury Y, De Gaetano A. Bariatric surgery and T2DM improvement mechanisms: a mathematical model. Theor Biol Med Model. BioMed Central. 2012;9(1):16.
67. Chaudhry S, Bernardes M, Harris PE, Maffei A. Gastrointestinal dopamine as an anti-incretin and its possible role in bypass surgery as therapy for type 2 diabetes with associated obesity. Minerva Endocrinol. NIH Public Access. 2016;41(1):43–56.
68. Schauer PR, Bhatt DL, Kirwan JP, Wolski K, Aminian A, Brethauer SA, et al. Bariatric surgery versus intensive medical therapy for diabetes – 5-year outcomes. N Engl J Med. Massachusetts Medical Society. 2017;376(7):641–51.
69. First-phase insulin secretion, insulin sensitivity, ghrelin, GLP-1, and PYY changes 72 h after sleeve gastrectomy in obese diabetic patients: the gastric hypothesis. Springer; 2011;25(11):3540–50. Available from: http://link.springer.com/10.1007/s00464-011-1755-5.
70. Shabbir A, Dargan D. The success of sleeve gastrectomy in the management of metabolic syndrome and obesity. J Biomed Res. 2015;29(2):93–7.
71. Penney NC, Kinross J, Newton RC, Purkayastha S. The role of bile acids in reducing the metabolic complications of obesity after bariatric surgery: a systematic review. Int J Obes. Nature Publishing Group. 2015;39(11):1565–74.
72. Kaska L, Sledzinski T, Chomiczewska A, Dettlaff-Pokora A, Swierczynski J. Improved glucose metabolism following bariatric surgery is associated with increased circulating bile acid concentrations and remodeling of the gut microbiome. World J Gastroenterol. 2016;22(39):8698–719.
73. Thomas C, Gioiello A, Noriega L, Strehle A, Oury J, Rizzo G, et al. TGR5-mediated bile acid sensing controls glucose homeostasis. Cell Metab. 2009;10(3):167–77.
74. Wu T, Bound MJ, Standfield SD, Jones KL, Horowitz M, Rayner CK. Effects of taurocholic acid on glycemic, glucagon-like peptide-1, and insulin responses to small intestinal glucose infusion in healthy humans. J Clin Endocrinol Metab. Endocrine Society Chevy Chase, MD. 2013;98(4):E718–22.
75. Adrian TE, Gariballa S, Parekh KA, Thomas SA, Saadi H, Kaabi Al J, et al. Rectal taurocholate increases L cell and insulin secretion, and decreases blood glucose and food intake in obese type 2 diabetic volunteers. Diabetologia. Springer. 2012;55(9):2343–7.
76. Wu T, Bound MJ, Standfield SD, Gedulin B, Jones KL, Horowitz M, et al. Effects of rectal administration of taurocholic acid on glucagon-like peptide-1 and peptide YY secretion in healthy humans. Diabetes Obes Metab Blackwell Publishing Ltd. 2013;15(5):474–7.
77. Kohli R, Setchell KD, Kirby M, Myronovych A, Ryan KK, Ibrahim SH, et al. A surgical model in male obese rats uncovers protective effects of bile acids post-bariatric surgery. Endocrinology. Endocrine Society Chevy Chase, MD. 2013;154(7):2341–51.
78. Flynn CR, Albaugh VL, Cai S, Cheung-Flynn J, Williams PE, Brucker RM, et al. Bile diversion to the distal small intestine has comparable metabolic benefits to bariatric surgery. Nat Commun Nature Publishing Group. 2015;6:7715.
79. Ryan KK, Tremaroli V, Clemmensen C, Kovatcheva-Datchary P, Myronovych A, Karns R, et al. FXR is a molecular target for the effects of vertical sleeve gastrectomy. Nature. Nature Research. 2014;509(7499):183–8.
80. Martinez-Augustin O, Sanchez de Medina F. Intestinal bile acid physiology and pathophysiology. World J Gastroenterol. Baishideng Publishing Group Inc. 2008;14(37):5630–40.
81. Bhutta HY, Rajpal N, White W, Freudenberg JM, Liu Y, Way J, et al. Effect of Roux-en-Y gastric bypass surgery on bile acid metabolism in normal and obese diabetic rats. Covasa M, editor. PLoS One. Public Library of Science. 2015;10(3):e0122273.
82. Li JV, Ashrafian H, Bueter M, Kinross J, Sands C, le Roux CW, et al. Metabolic surgery profoundly influences gut microbial-host metabolic cross-talk. Gut BMJ Publishing Group Ltd and British Society of Gastroenterology. 2011;60(9):1214–23.
83. Tremaroli V, Karlsson F, Werling M, Ståhlman M, Kovatcheva-Datchary P, Olbers T, et al. Roux-en-Y

gastric bypass and vertical banded gastroplasty induce long-term changes on the human gut microbiome contributing to fat mass regulation. Cell Metab. 2015;22(2):228–38.

84. Ridlon JM, Kang DJ, Hylemon PB, Bajaj JS. Bile acids and the gut microbiome. Curr Opin Gastroenterol. 2014;30(3):332–8.
85. Liou AP, Paziuk M, Luevano J-M, Machineni S, Turnbaugh PJ, Kaplan LM. Conserved shifts in the gut microbiota due to gastric bypass reduce host weight and adiposity. Sci Transl Med. American Association for the Advancement of Science. 2013;5(178):178ra41.
86. Stojsavljević S, Gomerčić Palčić M, Virović Jukić L, Smirčić Duvnjak L, Duvnjak M. Adipokines and proinflammatory cytokines, the key mediators in the pathogenesis of nonalcoholic fatty liver disease. World J Gastroenterol. Baishideng Publishing Group Inc. 2014;20(48):18070–91.
87. Kelly JR, Kennedy PJ, Cryan JF, Dinan TG, Clarke G, Hyland NP. Breaking down the barriers: the gut microbiome, intestinal permeability and stress-related psychiatric disorders. Front Cell Neurosci Frontiers. 2015;9(2):392.
88. Luther J, Garber JJ, Khalili H, Dave M, Bale SS, Jindal R, et al. Hepatic injury in nonalcoholic steatohepatitis contributes to altered intestinal permeability. Cell Mol Gastroenterol Hepatol. 2015;1(2):222–32.
89. Cordera R, Adami GF. From bariatric to metabolic surgery: looking for a "disease modifier" surgery for type 2 diabetes. World J Diabetes. 2016;7(2):27–33.
90. Astiarraga B, Gastaldelli A, Muscelli E, Baldi S, Camastra S, Mari A, et al. Biliopancreatic diversion in nonobese patients with type 2 diabetes: impact and mechanisms. J Clin Endocrinol Metab. Endocrine Society Chevy Chase, MD. 2013;98(7):2765–73.
91. Scopinaro N, Camerini G, Papadia F, Andraghetti G, Cordera R, Adami GF. Long-term clinical and functional impact of biliopancreatic diversion on type 2 diabetes in morbidly and non-morbidly obese patients. Surg Obes Relat Dis. Elsevier. 2016;12(4):822–7.
92. Tharakan G, Scott R, Szepietowski O, Miras AD, Blakemore AI, Purkayastha S, et al. Limitations of the DiaRem score in predicting remission of diabetes following Roux-En-Y Gastric Bypass (RYGB) in an ethnically diverse population from a single institution in the UK. Obes Surg Springer US. 2016;10:1–5.
93. Troke RC, Tan TM, Bloom SR. The future role of gut hormones in the treatment of obesity. Ther Adv Chronic Dis SAGE Publications. 2014;5(1):4–14.
94. Miras A. The effects of liraglytide in controlling blood sugar and weight in poor-responders to bariatric surgery. Available at: https://doi.org/10.1186/ISRCTN13643081, accessed 3rd July 2018.

37 Is Type 2 Diabetes a Surgical Disease?

Kai Tai Derek Yeung and Ahmed R. Ahmed

Introduction

Type 2 diabetes mellitus (T2DM) affects and will continue to affect more and more people across the globe. It is a complex disease process leading to significant morbidity, mortality and burden on healthcare systems.

Traditionally treatment is achieved through lifestyle modifications and medication. There is an ever increasing range of medications being made available to help achieve glycaemic control and modification of risk factors. However, only 10% of patients ever achieve these goals [1]. Weight loss and T2DM remission or improvement achieved with low calorie diets and lifestyle modification are rarely still present after 1–5 years [2].

This led to a search for alternative therapies, and recently the GI tract has become a target of interest in the management of T2DM. Bariatric surgery began with the sole intent of weight loss. However, the observation of complete or partial remission of T2DM has led to a new discipline of "metabolic surgery" [3].

Bariatric/metabolic surgery is effective at improving outcomes in obese patients and in those with obesity-related diseases. In particular, with type 2 diabetes mellitus (T2DM), glycaemic control is achieved rapidly before weight loss and is sustained. Recently the emergence of level 1 evidence supporting the superiority of surgery over intense medical therapy for diabetes has changed and continues to change many minds that doubted the benefit of surgery in diabetic patients.

We are only beginning to understand the metabolic effects of surgery. Many still think this is due to dietary restriction and weight loss leading to improvement in diabetes; there is, however, much more to it than this. In this chapter we will examine what is known about surgery for T2DM.

When Did the Idea First Appear?

The first observation of T2DM improvement was seen in patients who underwent the Billroth II procedure for gastric cancer or gastric ulcers. Not only did the ulcer improve but in diabetic patients, even those who were nonobese showed improvement in their diabetic control [4].

In 1987, Pories and his team published an article in the Annals of Surgery titled "The control of diabetes mellitus (NIDDM) in the morbidly obese with the Greenville gastric bypass". They reported 86/88 patients with NIDDM became

K. T. D. Yeung
Department of Bariatric Surgery, St Mary's Hospital, London, UK
e-mail: k.yeung@nhs.net

A. R. Ahmed (✉)
Department of Bariatric Surgery, St Mary's Hospital, Imperial College London, London, UK
e-mail: ahmed.ahmed@imperial.nhs.uk

R. Lutfi et al. (eds.), *Global Bariatric Surgery*, https://doi.org/10.1007/978-3-319-93545-4_37

euglycaemic within 4 months post-operatively [5]. It was hypothesised then that normalisation of glucose metabolism may not just be related to weight loss and restriction.

Several years later in 1992, he and his team went on to publish a paper title "Is type II diabetes (NIDDM) a surgical disease?" This was a continuation of his earlier work. The paper reported a much larger cohort of 515 morbidly obese patients undergoing the Greenville gastric bypass. 88.7% of patients remained or became euglycaemic post-operatively. It was proposed that NIDDM could be controlled in the severely obese by gastric bypass. They took it a step further to suggest that patients with severe NIDDM who were not severely obese may perhaps be considered for gastric bypass. One significant flaw at that point was the surgical technique involved an unacceptably high rate of staple line failure [6].

In 1995, over 14 years, the cohort grew to 608 morbidly obese patients. Surgical technique had improved with mortality and morbidity rates reduced to 1.5% and 8.5%, respectively. More importantly, long-term data published showed 82.9% of patients with NIDDM and 98.7% of patients with glucose impairment returned to euglycaemic levels [7]. "No other therapy has produced such durable and complete control of diabetes mellitus" was the conclusion of the authors.

Weight Loss and Metabolic Effect

We now know that glycaemic control occurs well before significant weight loss is achieved in the post-operative period. This leads to the question of what are the weight-independent antidiabetic mechanisms and how might we use this furthermore to our advantage to achieve desirable results.

Also worth noting is in the long run, failure of weight loss also does not necessary mean failed metabolic effects. Aminian et al. have demonstrated a modest 5–10% weight loss is already associated with a significant improvement in reduction of blood pressure, circulating triglycerides and decreased diabetic medication requirement. In their cohort, patients achieved <25% excess weight loss, but 65% still showed remission or clinical improvement of their diabetes [8].

What is incredibly interesting is that certain studies show that patients with type 2 diabetes, when subjected to calorie restriction strictly to the extent of those who underwent gastric bypass, show the same effect on insulin sensitivity and blood glucose [9].

Can Diabetes Be Surgically Cured?

Can diabetes be surgically cured? A retrospective study of 217 T2DM patients who underwent bariatric surgery and had at least 5-year follow-up [10] showed surgery induced a significant, sustainable remission and improvement of T2DM. There was also an improvement in other metabolic risk factors such as long-term control of lipid status and hypertension. Furthermore, diabetic nephropathy was shown to either regress or stabilise. Interestingly, it has also been suggested that in patients without diabetes, having bariatric surgery reduced the risk to developing T2DM by 96% [11].

Surgical Versus Medical Therapy: What Does the Evidence Say?

For a while, we have known conventional medical treatment only partially achieves glycaemic control and modification of subsequent risk factors. This has been the case despite new classes of drugs appearing on the market. Patients who were obese pose a further challenge to manage. This led to a search for alternative therapies.

In 2009 Buchwald and colleagues published a systematic review and meta-analysis of 621 studies which included 135,246 patients with the aim of determining the impact of bariatric surgery on T2DM. It was found that 78.1% of patients had complete resolution and 86.6% of patients had improvement or resolution of disease. This was also found to be sustained 2 years post-operatively [12].

Following on, in 2012, Mingrone et al. published an original article in the *New England*

Journal of Medicine of a non-blinded, randomised control trial comparing bariatric surgery versus conventional medical therapy for type 2 diabetes. At that point in time, there was a lack of level 1 clinical evidence to support surgery as an alternative treatment for T2DM. Their study randomised 60 patients with BMI >35 to gastric bypass, biliopancreatic diversion or medical therapy and was followed up for 24 months. The study reported no remissions in the medical group but an astonishing 75% and 95% remission in the gastric bypass and biliopancreatic diversion groups. Weight loss and reduction in lipids was much more significant in the surgical group. No operative deaths were reported. Additionally, there was no correlation between weight loss and normalisation of fasting glucose. This is consistent with previous studies that the effects that lead to resolution of T2DM are independent of weight loss [13].

The Swedish Obese Subjects (SOS) was a prospective long-running controlled intervention study of bariatric surgery. The investigators compared 2010 obese patients who underwent bariatric surgery to 2037 matched obese patients who received conventional medical therapy. A 2-year diabetes remission was 72% and 21% for surgical and medical therapy, respectively. At 10 years remissions were shown to be 12% compared to 37% in the surgical group. In this particular study, bariatric surgery was also associated with long-term reductions in overall mortality, myocardial infarction, stroke and cancer. High BMI was not predictive of favourable treatment effects [11].

Subsequently several systematic reviews and meta-analyses have been published. Ribaric and colleagues reported in their analysis of 16 papers, a 63.5 vs 15.6% overall T2DM remission rate when comparing surgery and conventional therapy [14].

Another systematic review and meta-analysis [15] looked at surgical versus medical therapy in T2DM patients with BMI less than 35. Five RCTs and 6 OCSs with 706 patients were included in this, and surgery was associated with a higher T2DM remission rate, higher rate of glycaemic control and lower HbA1c levels compared to medical therapy.

A further meta-analysis of 11 published RCTs [16] also concluded similarly with level 1A evidence that surgery showed superiority in T2DM remission, glycaemic control and lower HbA1c levels. Furthermore, the author also concludes this to be true in patients with BMI lower than 35.

Surgery in the Nonobese Group

It is currently suggested that surgery may have a role in patients with BMI less than 35 [17]. It is also considered safe with reported rates of 80% of patients achieving adequate glycaemic control and a low rate (3.2%) of complications [18]. Taking it a step further, there is suggestion that there may also be benefit in those patients with BMI less than 30 with drug refractory disease [19]. In fact, both the National Institute for Health and Care Excellence (NICE) in the UK and the International Diabetes Federation have stipulated the use of metabolic surgery in some cases of BMI>28 for instance in those of Southeast Asian descent [20].

For the time being, the general consensus is that long-term evaluation is still required in the nonobese group of T2DM patients.

Who Will Benefit? Predictive Factors of Remission

There is variability in the reported rate of T2DM remission at 1-year post-operatively (50–95%). A French retrospective analysis [21] found that a shorter duration of diabetes and good preoperative glycaemic control increased the rate of T2DM remission in that duration. The Swedish Obese Subjects study also confirmed short diabetes duration was associated with high remission and low relapse rates at both 2 and 10 years post-operatively [22]. Another long-term 5-year cohort study from Taiwan also reported a higher rate of T2DM remission in patient with early onset T2DM [23].

Others have demonstrated that young age, shorter diabetes duration, better glycaemic control and better B-cell function baseline BMI

<50, short duration of diabetes (<4 years), lower Hba1c, fasting glucose and the absence of insulin therapy are all factors that lead to more successful T2DM remission [21, 24].

A large-scale meta-analysis including 94 studies and 94,578 patients found bariatric surgery and T2DM remission rates were similar in patients with BMI >35 (72%) and <35 (71%). Effects of each procedure appeared independent of weight [25].

Interestingly, there appears to be an association between weight regain and recurrence of T2DM [26]. Metabolic failure rate was lower after RYGB compared to other procedures. Similarly, in the long history of T2DM, high preoperative HbA1c was found to be predictive of failure of improvement in the early post-operative course after bariatric surgery. Higher age and use of preoperative insulin or oral antidiabetic medication are also reported to be significant and independent predictors for less favourable metabolic outcome post-operatively [27].

In summary choosing the appropriate candidate is important: preoperative metabolic data can potentially help select those patients who are most likely to achieve remission.

Specific Procedures

Gastric Band

The first RCT looking at bariatric surgery vs best medical therapy was performed using the gastric band. In 2008, Dixon et al. reported a RCT comparing 60 patients who underwent adjustable gastric banding versus conventional therapy for T2DM. Seventy-three percent of patients in the surgical group achieved remission compared to only 13% in the conventional group [28].

Sleeve

Laparoscopic sleeve gastrectomy has become the most popular bariatric surgical procedure in the USA. In the fourth quarter of 2014, 60% of all bariatric procedures performed were sleeve gastrectomy [29]. This is echoed in institutions around the world. The most recent International Consensus Summit for sleeve gastrectomy reported a survey of 103 expert surgeons. Approximately 80% endorsed sleeve gastrectomy in patients with metabolic syndrome or BMI 30–35 with associated comorbidities [30]. Mihmanli and colleagues reported a cohort of 88 diabetic patients undergoing sleeve gastrectomy resulted in a 95% complete type 2 diabetes remission rate 1-year post-operatively. In the literature this rate stands at about 80% [31].

Mini-Gastric Bypass

Musella et al. reported outcomes of 974 patients from multiple centres in Italy who underwent mini-gastric bypass [32]. Eight hundred eighteen of these patients remained under follow-up, and at 60 months T2DM remission was achieved in 84% as was resolution of hypertension in 87%.

Another randomised trial comparing sleeve gastrectomy to mini-gastric bypass also concluded that although sleeve gastrectomy is effective at improving glycaemic control up to 5-year follow-up, mini-gastric bypass was more likely to achieve better glycaemic control [33].

A Chinese systematic review and meta-analysis reviewed 15 articles that compared mini-gastric bypass to RYGB, SG and LAGB. Weight loss was more significant with MGB and remission rates were shown to be higher or comparable to other procedures. However, the use of MGB as a metabolic procedure still needs to be further evaluated [34].

Which Is the Best Metabolic Procedure?

Table 37.1 summarises a variety of studies comparing various procedures along with intense medical therapy. What is clear is that surgical therapy along with medical therapy is far superior compared to intense medical therapy only. More and more long-term data is beginning to surface and the trends continue.

Table 37.1 A variety of studies comparing various procedures along with intense medical therapy

Author (et al.)	Year	Treatment groups	*N*	Time (months)	T2DM remission rates
Dixon [28]	2008	Med vs LAGB	30/30	24	13% med/73% LAGB
Mingrone [13]	2012	Med vs BPD vs RYGB	20/20/20	24	0% med/95%BPD/75% RYGB
Milone [48]	2013	LSG vs MGB	15/16	12	56% SG/68% MGB
Ikramuddin [49]	2013	IMT vs RYGB	60/60	12	19% IMT/44% RYGB
Courcoulas [50]	2015	ILM only vs (RYGB vs LAGB – combined with ILM)	61	36	0% ILM/40% RYGB/29% LAGB
Ikramuddin [51]	2016	IMT vs IMT&RYGB	60/60	36	0% IMT/19% IMT&RYBG
Purnell [52]	2016	RYBG vs LAGB	466/140	36	68% RYGB/30% LAGB
Schauer [41] (stampede)	2017	IMT vs RYGB vs LSG	50/50/50	60	5% IMT/29% RYGB/23% LSG

Med medical therapy, *LAGB* laparoscopic adjustable gastric band, *LSG* laparoscopic sleeve gastrectomy, *BPD* biliary pancreatic diversion, *IMT* intense medical therapy, *MGB* mini-gastric bypass

Gastric Bypass Versus Sleeve Gastrectomy?

There are several meta-analyses compared RYBG to SG. Yip et al. found that both RYBP and SG resulted in similar rates of early T2DM remission, 76 and 68% at 12 months and 81 and 80% at 36 months for RYGB and SG, respectively [35].

In their review of recent clinical trials up to 2014, Torgersen et al. reports both RYGB and sleeve gastrectomy to be well tolerated. No long-term conclusions were drawn. RYGB seemed to be more effective at resolution and remission to T2DM, even with high-risk patients. In terms of obesity-related comorbidities, both were similar in their rates of reduction except gastroesophageal reflux occurred more in sleeve gastrectomy patients. Mortality rates were similar [36].

A meta-analysis of 429 patients undergoing RYGB and 429 patients undergoing SG found similar efficacy of T2DM remission in non-randomised studies. In randomised control studies, however, SG has a lower effect compared to RYGB. Again it was reported that T2DM remission was not correlated with excess weight loss [37].

RYGB is suggested to achieve more durable glycaemic control compared to sleeve gastrectomy and medical therapy. Beta-cell function increases by 5.8-fold as well as other hormonal changes [38].

Mechanisms

The antidiabetic effect of metabolic surgery occurs before significant weight loss. We do not yet know the precise mechanism that lead to this effect, but it is thought to be multifactorial and will be discussed in a separate chapter.

Current and Recent Clinical Trials

There are currently many recently published randomised control trials. Many more are active and recruiting comparing metabolic surgery and medical therapy for type 2 diabetes.

CROSSROADS [39] looked at Roux-en-Y gastric bypass compared to intensive lifestyle and medical intervention for type 2 diabetics. Although small in scale 15 (RYGB) vs 17 (lifestyle and medical) patients, 1-year diabetes remission was 60% in the surgical group compared to 5.9% in the lifestyle and medical group. Weight loss and HbA1c reduction were also more successful in the surgical group.

STAMPEDE [40] is a randomised control trial comparing sleeve gastrectomy, Roux-en-Y gastric bypass and advanced medical therapy in 150 type 2 diabetics with BMI 27–42. The authors in their 1 year update that gastric bypass and sleeve gastrectomy were superior in achieving glycaemic control. The 3-year outcomes were published in the *New England Journal of Medicine*, at which point the surgical group still showed statistically significant and superior results. Thirty-eight percent (bypass), 24% (sleeve) and 5% (medical) of patients achieved an Hba1C of 6% or less. Weight reduction was again found to be superior in the surgical group as was quality of life.

The most recent 5-year outcomes from the STAMPEDE study were published in 2017 [41]. In the same cohort, 29% (bypass), 23% (sleeve) and 5% (medical) achieved an Hba1C of 6% or less. This study showed that the beneficial effects from surgery were durable and subsequently reduced the need for diabetics and cardiovascular medications. Furthermore, the authors also concluded that these effects were also evident in mildly obese patients (BMI 27–34).

The Rome trial [42] was a randomised control trial based in Italy published in the Lancet. The investigators compared 60 patients with a BMI over 35 and a minimum 5-year history of type 2 diabetes. The patients received either medical treatment, gastric bypass or biliopancreatic diversion. At 5 years, 50% of the surgical patients maintained diabetic remission compared to none of the medically treated patients. Interestingly, the authors also reported that within the surgical group, 53% of patients who has gastric bypass and 37% of patients who underwent biliopancreatic diversion had achieved diabetic remission at 2 years but had a degree of relapse by 5 years. Again, other associated factors such as plasma lipids and cardiovascular risk were significantly lower in the surgical groups.

The diabetes surgery study [43] published their 2-year outcomes of 5-year RCT. This study is looking at 120 patients assigned to either medical management or medical management along with gastric bypass. The primary outcome of this study was a trio of Hba1c <7%, LDL cholesterol <2.59 mmol/L and SBP <130 mmHg. At 24 months, the 43% of the surgical group achieved this compared to 14% in the medical group. In particular, glycaemic control was achieved in 75% vs 24% in the respective surgical and medical groups. Of note, the authors mention nutritional deficiencies occurred more commonly in the bypass group.

Another RCT from Pittsburgh [44] compared patients receiving 1 year of high-intensity weight loss intervention followed by low-level intervention for 2 years to surgical treatment (Roux-en-Y gastric bypass or laparoscopic adjustable gastric band) followed by 2 years of low-level weight loss intervention. Similarly, T2DM remission at 3 years was achieved in 40% of the RYGB group, 29% in LAGB and 0% in the non-surgical group.

These are only a few examples of trials looking at the surgical effect on type 2 diabetes. Many studies come to a similar conclusion that for now, surgical therapy seems superior in achieving glucose homeostasis when compared to medical and behavioural therapy.

Long-Lasting Effects

Following on from the SOS study described above, Sjostrom and colleagues went on to look at the long-term remission of type 2 diabetes with macrovascular (limbs, heart and brain) and microvascular complications (eyes, kidneys and peripheral nerves). They found that macrovascular complications were observed in 44.2/1000 person-years in the control group compared to 33.7/1000 person-years in the surgical group. Microvascular complications were found to be 41.8 and 20.6/1000 person-years in the respective control and surgical groups. At 15 years diabetes remission was at 6.5% and 30.4% for the control and surgical groups [45]. For now, this is the best long-term data published to date, and these findings require confirmation by randomised controlled trials.

There is no doubt more work needs to be put into establishing long-term effects of bariatric. In particular, long-term effects on micro- and macrovascular complications related to diabetes are clinically important. Most current published studies only follow up patients for 1–2 years or inconsistent long-term reporting of results. This statement was also reflected in a Cochrane review performed in 2014 [46].

Table 37.2 Although further studies are required to show long-term benefits, there is now enough evidence to support the inclusion of metabolic surgery amongst all interventions for the treatment of T2DM and obesity [47]

Metabolic surgery?	Glycaemic control	BMI (kg/m^2)
Recommended	Regardless of glycaemic control	≥40
Recommended	Inadequate glycaemic control despite lifestyle and medical therapy	35–39.9
Consider	Inadequate glycaemic control despite medical and injectable medications	30.0–34.9

2016 American Diabetes Association
Consider ancestry. For example, patients of Asian descent should have BMI threshold values reduced by 2.5 kg/m^2

So Where Are We Now?

The most recent consensus comes from the 3rd World Congress on Interventional therapies for Type 2 Diabetes and the 2nd Diabetes Surgery Summit (DSS-II). This international consensus conference included leading diabetes organisations and aimed at developing guidelines to the benefit and limitations for metabolic surgery for T2DM. Attendees included 48 international clinicians/scholars (25% surgeons).

A joint statement and algorithm conclude that although further studies are required to show long-term benefits, there is now enough evidence to support the inclusion of metabolic surgery amongst all interventions for the treatment of T2DM and obesity [47]. The algorithm in Table 37.2 was suggested.

Conclusion

We should be considering bariatric/metabolic surgery as one of the options along with lifestyle and medical therapy to treat patients with T2DM. More high-quality long-term follow-up data is also required, but for now all evidence points to surgical intervention being much more effective than any existing medical treatment in certain patient groups.

The gut must be seen a metabolic organ and has a big role to play in glucose haemostasis. There is no doubt that further understanding on the precise and important mechanisms are required. The next research objective is to identify these processes, by then not only will surgical techniques be refined to target these areas, but it will open doors to other therapeutic options.

References

1. De Block C, Van Gaal L. Bariatric surgery to treat type 2 diabetes. Curr Opin Endocrinol Diabetes Obes. 2012;19(5):352–8.
2. Scheen A, Van Gaal L. Weight management in type 2 diabetes: current and emerging approaches to treatment. Diabetes Care., [online]. 2015;38(6):1161–72.
3. Petry T, Caravatto P, Cohen R. Metabolic surgery for type 2 diabetes in patients with a BMI of <35 kg/m^2: a surgeon's perspective. Obes Surg. 2013;23(6):809–18.
4. Magovern G, Sancetta A, Friedman M. The amelioration of diabetes mellitus following subtotal gastrectomy. Surg Gynecol Obstet., [online]. 1955;100(2):201–4.
5. Swanson M, Meelheim H, Flickinger E, Card J, Pories W. The control of diabetes mellitus (NIDDM) in the morbidly obese with the greenville gastric bypass. Ann Surg. 1987;206(3):316–23.
6. Card J, O'Brien K, Brown B, Long S, Leggett-Frazier N, Morgan E, Swanson M, Khazanie P, May H, Barakat H, Sinha M, Dohm G, Flickinger E, Macdonald K, Pories W. Is type II diabetes mellitus (NIDDM) a surgical disease? Ann Surg. 1992;215(6):633–43.
7. Dohm L, Dolezal J, Israel G, deRamon R, Barakat H, Brown B, Morris P, Long S, MacDonald K, Swanson M, Pories W. Who would have thought it? An operation proves to be the most effective therapy for adult-onset diabetes mellitus. Ann Surg. 1995;222(3):339–52.
8. Brethauer S, Schauer P, Kirwan J, Corcelles R, Augustin T, Jamal M, Aminian A. Failed surgical weight loss does not necessarily mean failed metabolic effects. Diabetes Technol Ther. 2015;17(10):682–4.
9. Abbasi J. Unveiling the "magic" of diabetes remission after weight-loss surgery. JAMA. 2017;317(6):571–4.
10. Schauer P, Chand B, Kroh M, Rogula T, Kirwan J, Kashyap S, Kennedy L, Mackey J, Batayyah E, Romero-Talamás H, Aminian A, Brethauer S. Can diabetes be surgically cured? Long-term metabolic effects of bariatric surgery in obese patients with type 2 diabetes mellitus. Ann Surg. 2013;258:1.
11. Sjöström L. Review of the key results from the Swedish obese subjects (SOS) trial – a prospective controlled intervention study of bariatric surgery. J Intern Med. 2013;273(3):219–34.

12. Sledge I, Bantle J, Pories W, Jensen M, Banel D, Fahrbach K, Estok R, Buchwald H. Weight and type 2 diabetes after bariatric surgery: systematic review and meta-analysis. Am J Med. 2009;122(3):248–256.e5.
13. Rubino F, Ghirlanda G, Castagneto M, Pomp A, Nanni G, Leccesi L, Iaconelli A, Guidone C, De Gaetano A, Panunzi S, Mingrone G. Bariatric surgery versus conventional medical therapy for type 2 diabetes. N Engl J Med. 2012;366(17):1577–85.
14. McGlennon T, Buchwald J, Ribaric G. Diabetes and weight in comparative studies of bariatric surgery vs conventional medical therapy: a systematic review and meta-analysis. Obes Surg. 2013;24(3):437–55.
15. Nawroth P, Büchler M, Fischer L, Diener M, Helfert S, Vit G, Billeter A, Kenngott H, Warschkow R, Senft J, Müller-Stich B. Surgical versus medical treatment of type 2 diabetes mellitus in nonseverely obese patients. Ann Surg. 2015;261(3):421–9.
16. Cohen R, Cummings D. Bariatric/metabolic surgery to treat type 2 diabetes in patients with a BMI <35 kg/m^2. Diabetes Care. 2016;39(6):924–33.
17. Qiu M, Jiang D, Zhang W, Shan C, Rao W. A meta-analysis of short-term outcomes of patients with type 2 diabetes mellitus and BMI ≤35 kg/m^2 undergoing roux-en-Y gastric bypass. World J Surg. 2014;39(1):223–30.
18. Hu R, Qu S, Liu C, Zhao W, Zhang Z, Gong W, Feng X, Zhang S, He M, Huang Y, Ye Z, Yang Z, Chen L, Li Q. Metabolic effects of bariatric surgery in type 2 diabetic patients with body mass index < 35 kg/m^2. Diabetes Obes Metab. 2011;14(3):262–70.
19. Folli F, Tian H, Liu G, Dhakal N, Li S, Baskota A. Bariatric surgery for type 2 diabetes mellitus in patients with BMI <30 kg/m^2: a systematic review and meta-analysis. PLoS One. 2015;10(7):e0132335.
20. NICE. Obesity: Identification, assessment and management. 2014. [online] Available at: https://www.nice.org.uk/guidance/cg189. Accessed 15 Jan 2017.
21. Thivolet C, Gouillat C, Laville M, Simon C, Espalieu P, Disse E, Ferrand-Gaillard C, Robert M. Predictive factors of type 2 diabetes remission 1 year after bariatric surgery: impact of surgical techniques. Obes Surg. 2013;23(6):770–5.
22. Sjöström L, Peltonen M, Jacobson P. Association of bariatric surgery with long term remission of type 2 diabetes and with microvascular and macrovascular complications. JAMA. 2014;311(22):2297–304.
23. Chen J, Lee Y, Chong K, Wu C, Ser K, Chen S, Lee W, Aung L. Bariatric surgery for patients with early-onset vs late-onset type 2 diabetes. JAMA Surg. 2016;151:798–805.
24. Yang T, Xu J, Wu Y, Ma N, Han G, Zhang J, Hui Y, Yin D, Xu N, Yan Y, Wang G. Predictive factors of type 2 diabetes mellitus remission following bariatric surgery: a meta-analysis. Obes Surg. 2014;25(2):199–208.
25. Mingrone G, Carnicelli A, De Gaetano A, Panunzi S. Predictors of remission of diabetes mellitus in severely obese individuals undergoing bariatric surgery. Ann Surg. 2015;261(3):459–67.
26. Ferraz A, Zeve J, Araujo-Junior J, Silva L, Lins D, Campos J. Metabolic surgery, weight regain and diabetes re-emergence. Arq Bras Cir Dig. 2013;26:57–62.
27. Wichelmann C, Germer C, Seyfried F, Bender G, Hartmann D, Thalheimer A, Jurowich C. Improvement of type 2 diabetes mellitus (T2DM) after bariatric surgery—who fails in the early postoperative course? Obes Surg. 2012;22(10):1521–6.
28. Anderson M, Bailey M, Proietto J, Skinner S, Schachter L, Chapman L, Playfair J, O'Brien P, Dixon J. Adjustable gastric banding and conventional therapy for type 2 diabetes: a randomized controlled trial. JAMA. 2008;299(3):316–23.
29. Esteban Varela J, Nguyen N. Laparoscopic sleeve gastrectomy leads the U.S. utilization of bariatric surgery at academic medical centers. Surg Obes Relat Dis. 2015;11(5):987–90.
30. Gagner M, Hutchinson C, Rosenthal R. Fifth international consensus conference: current status of sleeve gastrectomy. Surg Obes Relat Dis. 2016;12(4):750–6.
31. Altuntas Y, Ozturk F, Oba S, Sayin P, Isil C, Bostanci O, Kaya C, Demir U, Bozkurt E, Isil R, Mihmanli M. Postoperative effects of laparoscopic sleeve gastrectomy in morbid obese patients with type 2 diabetes. Springerplus. 2016;5:497.
32. Musella M, Susa A, Greco F, De Luca M, Manno E, Di Stefano C, Milone M, Bonfanti R, Segato G, Antonino A, Piazza L. The laparoscopic mini-gastric bypass: the Italian experience: outcomes from 974 consecutive cases in a multicenter review. Surg Endosc. 2013a;28(1):156–63.
33. Lee W, Chong K, Lin Y, Wei J, Chen S. Laparoscopic sleeve gastrectomy versus single anastomosis (mini-) gastric bypass for the treatment of type 2 diabetes mellitus: 5-year results of a randomized trial and study of incretin effect. Obes Surg. 2014;24(9):1552–62.
34. Min Z, Yu B, Zhang P, Zhuang B, Xu M, Ye M, Huang A, Quan Y. Efficacy of laparoscopic mini gastric bypass for obesity and type 2 diabetes mellitus: a systematic review and meta-analysis. Gastroenterol Res Pract., [online]. 2015;2015:152852.
35. Murphy R, Plank L, Yip S. Gastric bypass and sleeve gastrectomy for type 2 diabetes: a systematic review and meta-analysis of outcomes. Obes Surg., [online]. 2013;23(12):1994–2003. Available at: https://www.ncbi.nlm.nih.gov/pubmed/23955521 [Accessed 26 Aug 2016].
36. Forse R, Osmolak A, Torgersen Z. Sleeve gastrectomy and roux en Y gastric bypass: current state of metabolic surgery. Curr Opin Endocrinol Diabetes Obes. 2014;21(5):352–7.
37. Rosenthal R, Szomstein S, Park S, Menzo L, Kim H, Cho J. Effect of sleeve gastrectomy on type 2 diabetes as an alternative treatment modality to roux-en-Y gastric bypass: systemic review and meta-analysis. Surg Obes Relat Dis : Off J Am Soc Bariatric Surg[online]. 2015;11(6):1273–80.
38. Kashyap S, Kirwan J, Schauer P, Brethauer S, Nissen S, Bhatt D, Pothier C, Abood B, Wolski K, Samat A, Malin S. Improved acylated ghrelin suppression at 2

years in obese patients with type 2 diabetes: effects of bariatric surgery vs standard medical therapy. Int J Obes. 2013;38(3):364–70.
39. Flum D, Foster-Schubert K, Kratz M, Landers J, Bock S, Chan C, Stewart S, Kuzma J, Westbrook E, Arterburn D, Cummings D. Gastric bypass surgery vs intensive lifestyle and medical intervention for type 2 diabetes: the CROSSROADS randomised controlled trial. Diabetologia. 2016;59(5):945–53.
40. Kashyap S, Nissen S, Kim E, Pothier C, Aminian A, Navaneethan S, Brethauer S, Wolski K, Kirwan J, Bhatt D, Schauer P. Bariatric surgery versus intensive medical therapy for diabetes – 3-year outcomes. N Engl J Med. 2014;370(21):2002–13.
41. Schauer P, Bhatt D, Kirwan J, Wolski K, Aminian A, Brethauer S, Navaneethan S, Singh R, Pothier C, Nissen S, Kashyap S. Bariatric surgery versus intensive medical therapy for diabetes – 5-year outcomes. N Engl J Med. 2017;376(7):641–51.
42. Rubino F, Bornstein S, Castagneto M, Nanni G, Iaconelli A, Guidone C, De Gaetano A, Panunzi S, Mingrone G. Bariatric–metabolic surgery versus conventional medical treatment in obese patients with type 2 diabetes: 5 year follow-up of an open-label, single-centre, randomised controlled trial. Lancet. 2015;386(9997):964–73.
43. Korner J, Wang Q, Laqua P, Bainbridge H, Olofson A, Schone J, Belani K, Ahmed L, Vella A, Jensen M, Sarr M, Chuang L, Chong K, Jeffery R, Inabnet W, Leslie D, Connett J, Thomas A, Bantle J, Lee W, Billington C, Ikramuddin S. Roux-en-Y gastric bypass for diabetes (the diabetes surgery study): 2-year outcomes of a 5-year, randomised, controlled trial. Lancet Diabetes Endocrinol. 2015;3(6):413–22.
44. Courcoulas A, Belle S, Neiberg R, Pierson S, Eagleton J, Kalarchian M, DeLany J, Lang W, Jakicic J. Three-year outcomes of bariatric surgery vs lifestyle intervention for type 2 diabetes mellitus treatment. JAMA Surg. 2015;150(10):931.
45. Carlsson L, Sjöholm K, Svensson P, Wedel H, Taube M, Sjöström E, Näslund I, Lönroth H, Karason K, Carlsson B, Bouchard C, Anveden Å, Andersson-Assarsson J, Ahlin S, Jacobson P, Peltonen M, Sjöström L. Association of Bariatric surgery with long-term remission of type 2 diabetes and with microvascular and macrovascular complications. JAMA. 2014;311(22):2297.
46. Frampton G, Loveman E, Pickett K, Colquitt J. Surgery for weight loss in adults. Cochrane Database Syst Rev. 2014. [online] Available at: http://www.ncbi.nlm.nih.gov/pubmed/25105982. Accessed 26 Aug 2016.
47. Cummings D, Taroncher-Oldenburg G, Kaplan L, Amiel S, Herman W, Sadikot S, Ji L, Del Prato S, Zimmet P, Alberti K, Schauer P, Eckel R, Nathan D, Rubino F. Metabolic surgery in the treatment algorithm for type 2 diabetes: a joint statement by international diabetes organizations. Diabetes Care. 2016;39(6):861–77.
48. Musella M, Savastano S, Lupoli R, Gaudioso D, Taffuri C, Bianco P, Maietta P, Leongito M, Minno D, Milone M. Bariatric surgery and diabetes remission: sleeve gastrectomy or mini-gastric bypass? World J Gastroenterol., [online]. 2013b;19(39):6590–7.
49. Ikramuddin S, Korner J, Lee W, Connett J, Inabnet W, Billington C, Thomas A, Leslie D, Chong K, Jeffery R, Ahmed L, Vella A, Chuang L, Bessler M, Sarr M, Swain J, Laqua P, Jensen M, Bantle J. Roux-en-Y gastric bypass vs intensive medical management for the control of type 2 diabetes, hypertension, and hyperlipidemia. JAMA. 2013;309(21):2240.
50. Jakicic J, Lang W, DeLany J, Kalarchian M, Eagleton J, Pierson S, Neiberg R, Belle S, Courcoulas A. Three-year outcomes of bariatric surgery vs lifestyle intervention for type 2 diabetes mellitus treatment. JAMA Surg. 2015;150(10):931.
51. Ikramuddin S, Korner J, Lee W, Bantle J, Thomas A, Connett J, Leslie D, Inabnet W, Wang Q, Jeffery R, Chong K, Chuang L, Jensen M, Vella A, Ahmed L, Belani K, Olofson A, Bainbridge H, Billington C. Durability of addition of roux-en-Y gastric bypass to lifestyle intervention and medical management in achieving primary treatment goals for uncontrolled type 2 diabetes in mild to moderate obesity: a randomized control trial. Diabetes Care. 2016;39(9):1510–8.
52. Wolfe B, Courcoulas A, Flum, Cummings D, McCloskey C, Staten M, Garcia L, Mitchell J, Dakin G, Pomp A, Pories W, Pender J, Wahed A, Selzer F, Purnell J. Type 2 diabetes remission rates after laparoscopic gastric bypass and gastric banding: results of the longitudinal assessment of Bariatric surgery study. Diabetes Care., [online]. 2016;39(7):1101–7.

38 Biliary Disease and Bariatric Surgery

Mariano Palermo, Pablo Acquafresca, Flávio Coelho Ferreira, Cinthia Barbosa de Andrade, and Josemberg Campos

Cholelithiasis

It is known that the rapid weight loss is a predisposing factor to develop biliary lithiasis. The physiopathology is related with a supersaturation of bile with cholesterol, bile stasis, and increase in mucin concentration in bile. Therefore after any bariatric procedure (but gastric bypass specially), where a rapid weight loss occur, this can become a threat. Furthermore the treatment can be challenger because of the anatomical changes due to the bariatric procedure [1].

Diverse kind of protocols exist: prophylactic surgery (simultaneous cholecystectomy and gastric bypass in every patients, whether they have or not cholelithiasis) [2, 3], elective (simultaneous cholecystectomy with conventional gastric bypass in the patients with asymptomatic cholelithiasis) [4, 5], and conventional (cholecystectomy only in the presence of cholelithiasis with symptoms) [6, 7].

The incidence of cholelithiasis post gastric bypass is estimated around 37%. Almost 50% developed disease in the first year of monitoring and 60% in the first 6 months. Meanwhile the patients undergoing sleeve gastrectomy have an incidence of cholelithiasis of 27%, being most of the cases developed in the first and a half year [8].

Compared with the general population, the obese have high levels of serum cholesterol, determining a higher incidence of lithiasis, which is further increased in the patient population undergoing a bariatric procedure. The latter is linked to several factors, among which stands out the large weight loss (especially in the first 6 months after surgery) which favors a significant mobilization of cholesterol from adipose tissue reservoir and reduced production of bile salts and phospholipids to the gallbladder.

Furthermore, after bariatric surgery, a decrease in the gallbladder motility due to nerve damage, a deficit in phospholipids and contraction-stimulating proteins, and an increase of mucin secretion toward the gallbladder occur, leading to an acceleration of the nucleation process. This predominance of cholesterol over the bile salt and phospholipids in bile promotes the formation of gallstones [9, 10].

Other factors that promote the formation of lithiasis post-surgery, such as decreased motility by altering vagal innervation derived from the surgical process, are present in some cases but are not constant. Instead, rapid weight loss (more

M. Palermo (✉)
Department of Bariatric Surgery, Centro Cien–Diagnomed, Buenos Aires, Argentina

Department of Surgery, DAICIM Foundation, Buenos Aires, Argentina

P. Acquafresca
Department of Surgery, DAICIM Foundation, Buenos Aires, Argentina

F. C. Ferreira · C. B. de Andrade · J. Campos
Department of Surgery, Federal University of Pernambuco (UFPE), Recife, PE, Brazil

R. Lutfi et al. (eds.), *Global Bariatric Surgery*, https://doi.org/10.1007/978-3-319-93545-4_38

than 50% of excess weight lost 3 months after laparoscopic RYGB) is the only predictor of gallbladder disease present in every study [11].

Regarding prophylactic surgery (cholecystectomy in patients without gallbladder stones), the majority of surgeons concur that a watchful waiting should be taken and only perform the bariatric procedure, because the number of patients that will develop symptomatic cholelithiasis is low (around 6–8% of them) and this leads to an elevated number of patients exposed to an unnecessary procedure with potential complications [4, 11]. Laparoscopic cholecystectomy in bariatric patients may be challenging due to suboptimal port placement and difficult body habitus. Furthermore, it is accompanied by potential risks such as lengthening of operative time, increased morbidity, and prolonged hospitalization. Serious complications have been reported as high as 2–3% of cases [12].

Some studies have shown that an elective approach (simultaneous cholecystectomy only in the patients with cholelithiasis) may be favored because of better short-term outcomes with significantly lower rates of mortality, morbidity, reinterventions, and shorter hospital when compared with patients that had concomitant cholecystectomy. However, the long-term biliary morbidity requiring subsequent cholecystectomy was not clear in this study [6].

But other papers have shown that the rate of subsequent cholecystectomy after RYGB is low (6.8%), being the main cause for the subsequent cholecystectomy of the uncomplicated biliary disease, while choledocholithiasis and biliary pancreatitis occurred very rarely. It's estimated that the rate of subsequent cholecystectomy due to biliary colic or gallbladder dyskinesia is 5.3%; cholecystitis, 1.0%; choledocholithiasis, 0.2%; and biliary pancreatitis, 0.2%.

Furthermore about 95% of the subsequent cholecystectomies are performed laparoscopically with a very low conversion rate, and the risk to suffer a complication from a subsequent cholecystectomy is extremely low (0.1%) for all patients without concomitant cholecystectomy during RYGB. Therefore, a routine concomitant cholecystectomy cannot be recommended when weighting the observed low long-term morbidity against the known potential detrimental effect on the short-term outcome [6, 7].

On the other hand, when talking about patients with asymptomatic gallbladder stone, currently there is no consensus in the treatment in patients undergoing weight loss surgery. Asymptomatic gallstones (silent gallstones) represent a dilemmatic approach. The natural history of asymptomatic gallstones suggests that many affected individuals will remain asymptomatic. Recent trend analysis in gastric bypass patients suggests that concomitant cholecystectomy should be considered only in symptomatic gallstones [7].

The use of ursodeoxycholic acid (UDCA) also has been proposed as a preventive measure for the gallstone formation. The UDCA is a bile acid that dissolves gallstones by decreasing biliary cholesterol secretion to lower bile cholesterol saturation and by decreasing biliary glycoprotein secretion to lower biliary nucleating factors. It was reported that the oral dose of 600 mg UDCA following gastric bypass for 6 months or even until gallstone formation was associated with decreased rate of gallstone formation [13, 14]. However, the cost-effectiveness of the treatment is a matter of debate because even though the use of UDCA lessened the costs of concurrent cholecystectomy and reduced the hospital stay along with logical cost raise in selective cholecystectomy, the prescription of UDCA tends to be unaffordable as an additional cost.

Due to the previously exposed, it is possible to conclude that cholecystectomy should be performed only in patients with cholelithiasis and symptoms. Regarding patients with silent cholelithiasis, the surgeon must evaluate every case in particular, but it's admissible to choose a conservative management, follow up the patient, and, in case of developing symptoms, perform the cholecystectomy.

Choledocholitiasis

The presence of gallstones in the common bile duct (CBD) although is a rare complication after RYGB (around 0.2% of the bariatric patients) [7]

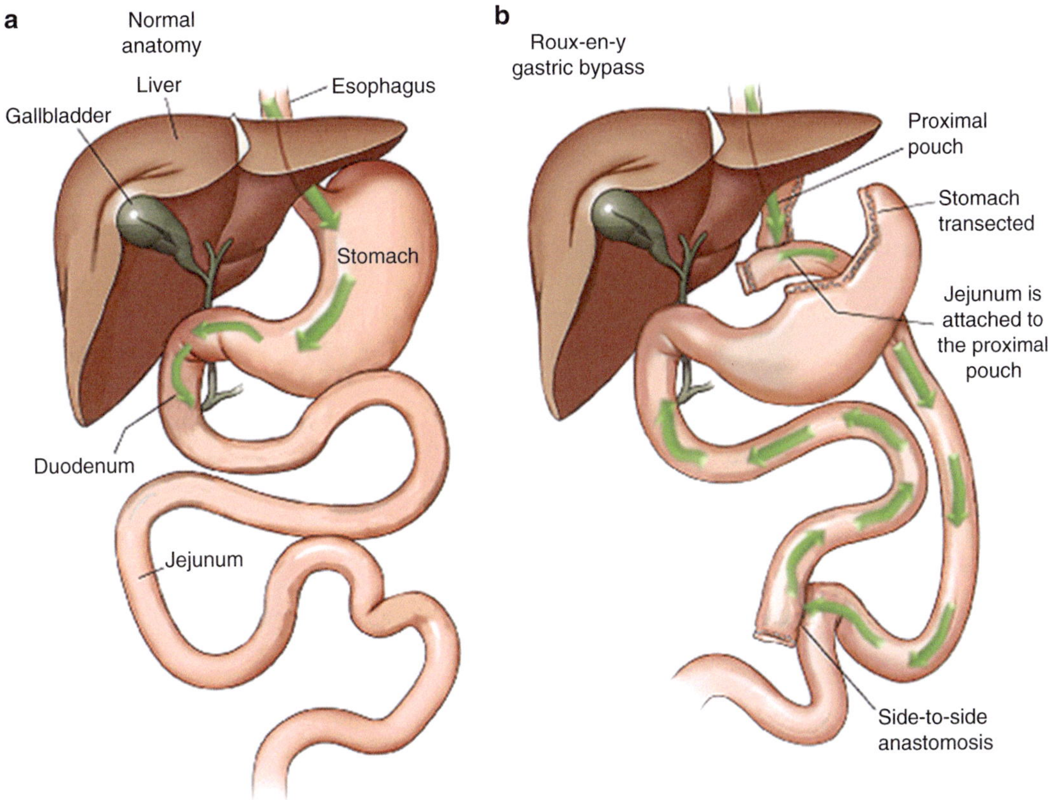

Fig. 38.1 (**a**) Green arrow showing the endoscopy path to the ampulla in normal anatomy. (**b**) Green arrow showing the endoscopy path to the ampulla in altered anatomy by gastric bypass

represents an important challenge due to the anatomical modifications of the gastrointestinal tract (Fig. 38.1).The duodenum remains adjacent to the surgically excluded stomach. Therefore, for the endoscopist, accessing the ampulla is technically very difficult. The endoscope must pass through the mouth, esophagus, gastric pouch, Roux limb, and then return retrograde through the afferent limb to reach the ampulla. This total length may easily exceed 300 cm, making almost impossible for traditional endoscopy access to the papilla to perform an endoscopic retrograde cholangiopancreatography (ERCP).

This leads to having to pursue other methods to reach the papillae for the resolution of choledocholitiasis. Which of these methods should we choose must be based on the surgeon experience, the equipment available, and the location of the stone. But whatever the method, a special training is needed on endoscopy, percutaneous surgery, and laparoscopy.

The methods that have been described can be listed as follows:

- Laparoscopy-assisted transgastric ERCP (LAT-ERCP)
- Balloon enteroscopy-assisted ERCP (BEA-ERCP)
- Percutaneous biliary drainage with subsequent trans-fistula treatment
- Laparoscopic exploration of common bile duct

Due to the long anatomical route required to reach the biliopancreatic limb in patients with RYGB, a solution that has been found is to access the excluded stomach through laparoscopy and insert the endoscope through a gastrotomy, thus allowing performance of an ERCP in a traditional way. The success rate of this procedure has been shown to be superior to BEA-ERCP. Biliary cannulation rates up to 100% have been described and are associated with a significantly shorter endoscopic procedure time, but not a shorter total procedure time (laparoscopy plus ERCP) [15–17].

In this procedure a standard laparoscopic access to the abdominal cavity is performed with insertion of four trocars, then the greater curve of the antrum is mobilized, and a gastrotomy and purse-string suture are fashioned on the anterior side of the greater curvature of the gastric remnant near the antrum (Fig. 38.2). An additional 15 mm or 18 mm trocar must be placed in the left upper quadrant and inserted into the gastrotomy in the center of the purse-string suture (Fig. 38.3). This purse string has to be tightly fixed around the trocar to prevent loss of insufflation pressure, and the gastrotomy should be made as lateral as possible along the greater curvature to permit smooth intubation of the pylorus. It's also recommended to occlude the biliopancreatic limb with an intestinal clamp to prevent over-insufflation of the small bowel that blocks the perioperative visualization.

Finally, a side-viewing endoscope is introduced through the 15 mm or 18 mm trocar secured into the gastrotomy, and ERCP can be performed under fluoroscopic guidance (Fig. 38.4). After the removal of the scope and the trocar, the purse string is tied and the gastrotomy incision sutured (Fig. 38.5). Described by Manoel Galvao-Neto from Brazil.

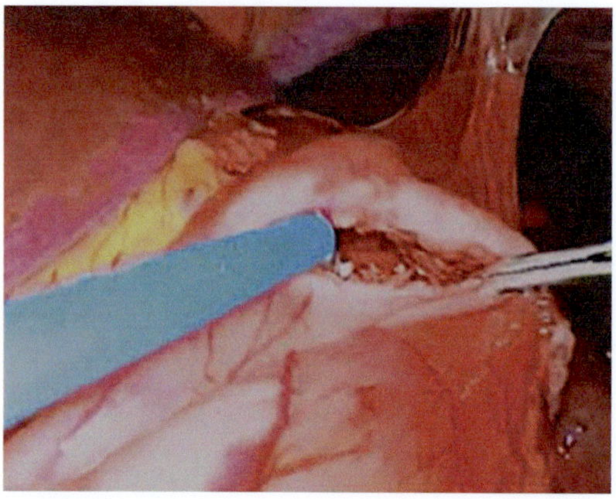

Fig. 38.2 Formation of a gastrotomy on the anterior wall of the greater curvature of the gastric remnant

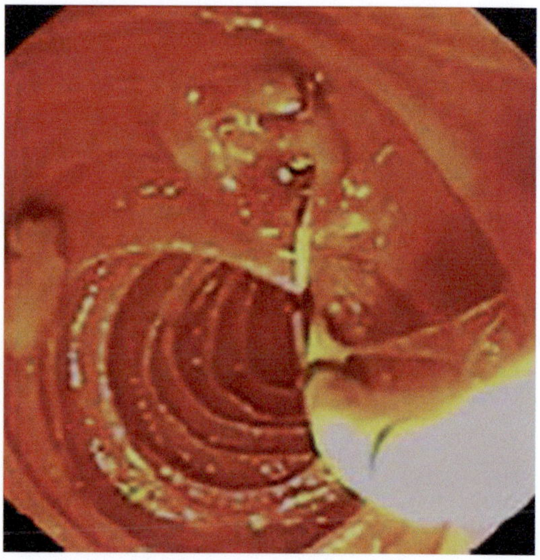

Fig. 38.4 ERCP with sphincterotomy and stone extraction

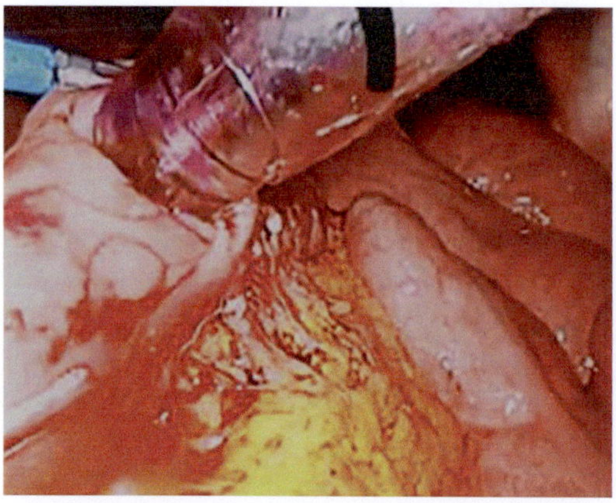

Fig. 38.3 Insertion of a 15 mm trocar into the gastric remnant through the gastrotomy

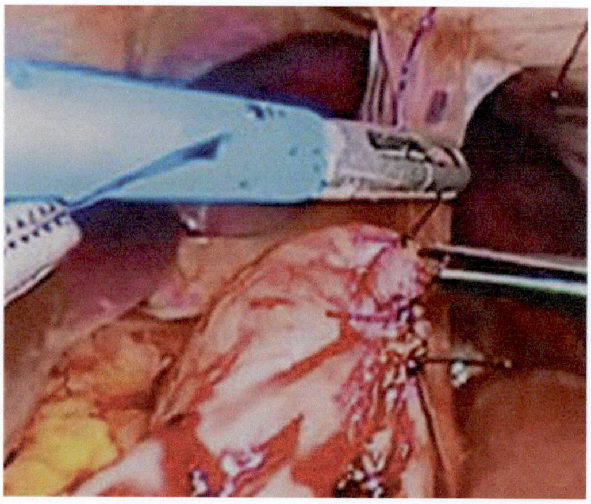

Fig. 38.5 Suture of the gastrotomy incision

In case of patients with gallbladder in situ, delaying the definitive cholecystectomy until ERCP is performed is considered to be the safest option because in case of a difficult cannulation of the papilla, a guidewire can be inserted into the cystic duct to perform a *rendezvous* technique in order to achieve the cannulation. In this technique the guidewire that was inserted through the cystic duct is then moved into the main biliary duct and passed through the papilla. Therefore, the flexible wire is taken by the endoscopist and used as a guide to enter the papilla.

Performance of the LAT-ERCP technique is influenced by the presence of postoperative adhesions which renders the transgastric access more difficult, sometimes being necessary to perform a minilaparotomy to achieve the transgastric access. This is expected in case of a history of open surgery, multiple laparoscopic interventions, and previous peritonitis or abscess formation.

When the need for repeat ERCP is anticipated during the first LAT-ERCP procedure, a gastrostomy tube can be inserted through the gastrotomy incision into the lumen of the stomach. Repeat ERCP can be performed percutaneously after the surgical gastrostomy tract has matured (Fig. 38.6) [18].

The LAT-ERCP, although it's a complex procedure, in experimented hands allows to successfully treating the choledocholitiasis with a biliary cannulation rates up to 100% and a low rate of complications like pancreatitis or post-sphincterotomy bleeding. In no case a leak of the gastrostomy suture was described (Fig. 38.7) [16–19].

The second option that we have to treat choledocholitiasis in patients with RYGB is the BEA-ERCP. The major advantage of balloon-assisted over conventional enteroscopy is the ability to reduce loops of small bowel which facilitates advancement of the endoscope in patients after Roux-en-Y reconstruction. In patients with Roux-en-Y anatomy, success rates varying from 60% to 90% for reaching the biliopancreatic limb and successful ERCP ranging from 46% to 80% have been reported [20–29], clearly inferior to the suc-

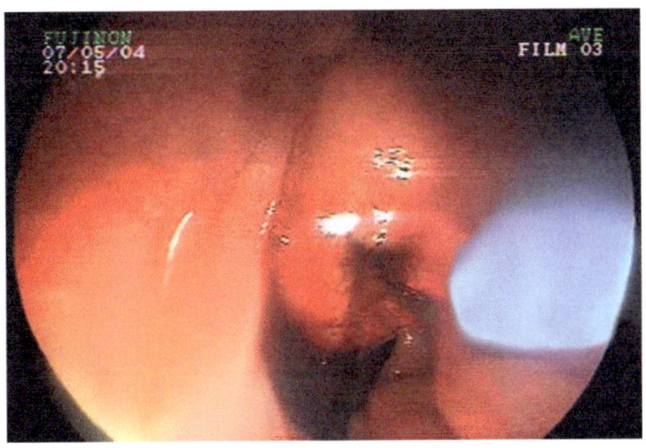

Fig. 38.7 Endoscopic view of papillotomy

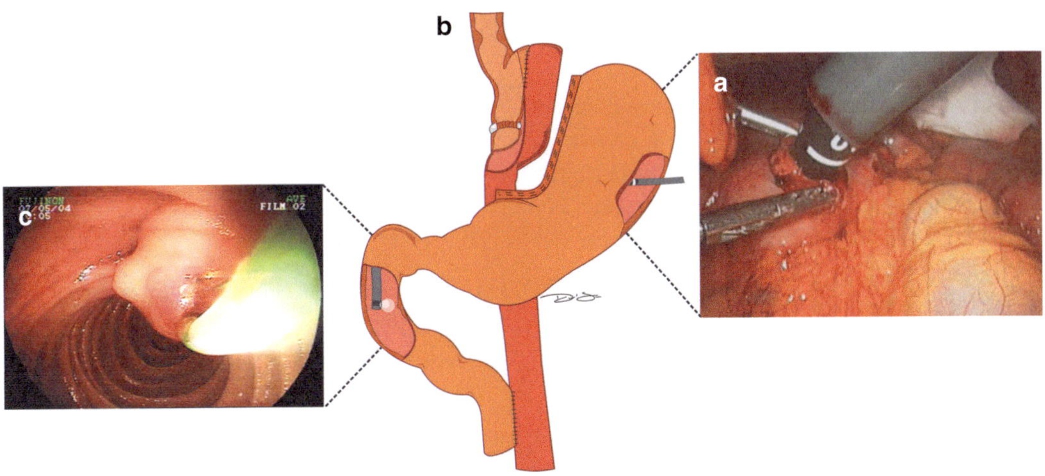

Fig. 38.6 (**a**) Introduction of the gastrotomy duodenoscope, (**b**) schematic drawing of access to the duodenum through the excluded stomach, (**c**) endoscopic view via cannulation of the papilla

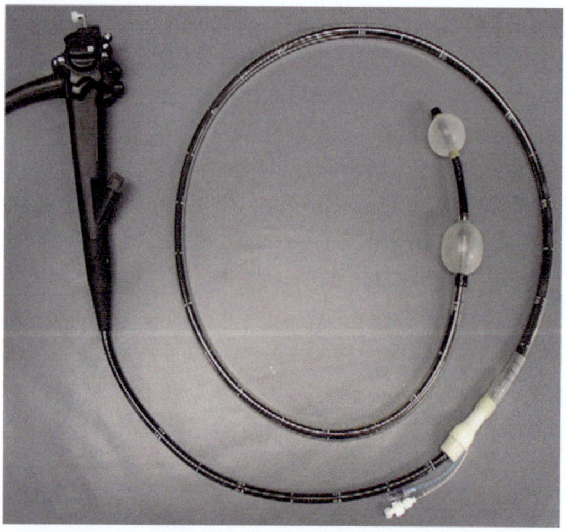

Fig. 38.8 Double-balloon endoscope

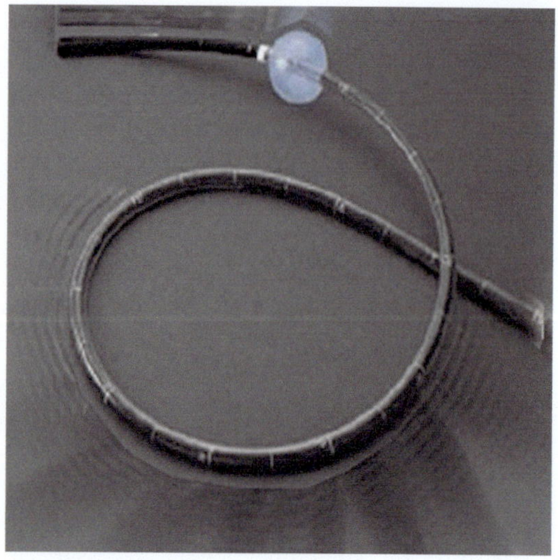

Fig. 38.9 Single-balloon endoscope

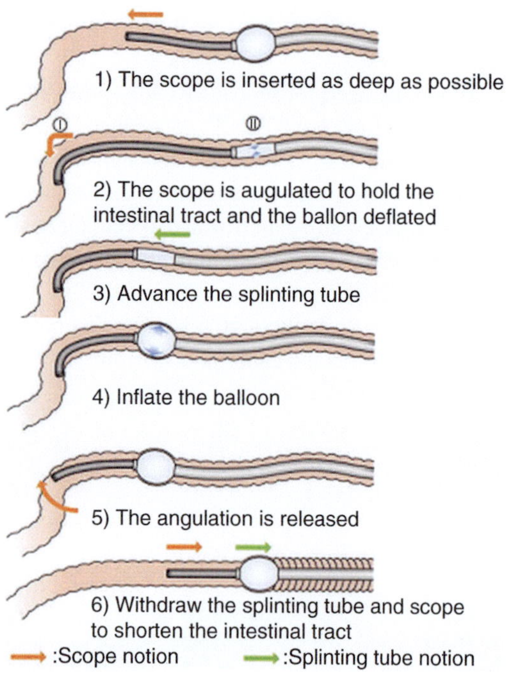

Fig. 38.10 Illustration of endoscopic technique with single balloon

cess rate of the LAT-ERCP. The devices that are used for the BEA-ERCP can consist in a single- or double-balloon system (Figs. 38.8 and 38.9).

The system is composed of a 200 cm, thin endoscope, with a 145 cm soft overtube. Latex balloons are attached to the end of the endoscope and to the end of the overtube. By using a series of inflations and deflations of the balloons, along with reductions, the endoscopist may advance the scope through the lumen in an “accordion-like” fashion and reach the distal small bowel [30] (Figs. 38.10 and 38.11).

The major problems that this technique must face are the long length of bowel that the scope must pass through and the acute angle of the afferent limb and Roux limb anastomosis which is also very difficult to navigate. Furthermore, attaching the balloon to the tip of the endoscope is often troublesome, and the balloon on the tip of the enteroscope can occasionally decrease the field of view if it becomes dislodged distally. It’s an invasive and time-consuming procedure, but on the other hand, the morbidity rate is low; especially for diagnostic procedures, the complication rate of diagnostic double-balloon endoscopies is 0.8% and of therapeutic procedures 4.3% [31].

Another important drawback of this technique is that the highest success rate is described in patients with hepaticojejunostomy, while the success rate in patients with native papilla tends to be lower due to the fact that the endoscope is forward viewing and the straight angle with which accessories can be advanced [21]. The cannulation rates of intact papilla using double-balloon enteroscope have ranged from 25% to 80% [20, 22, 23].

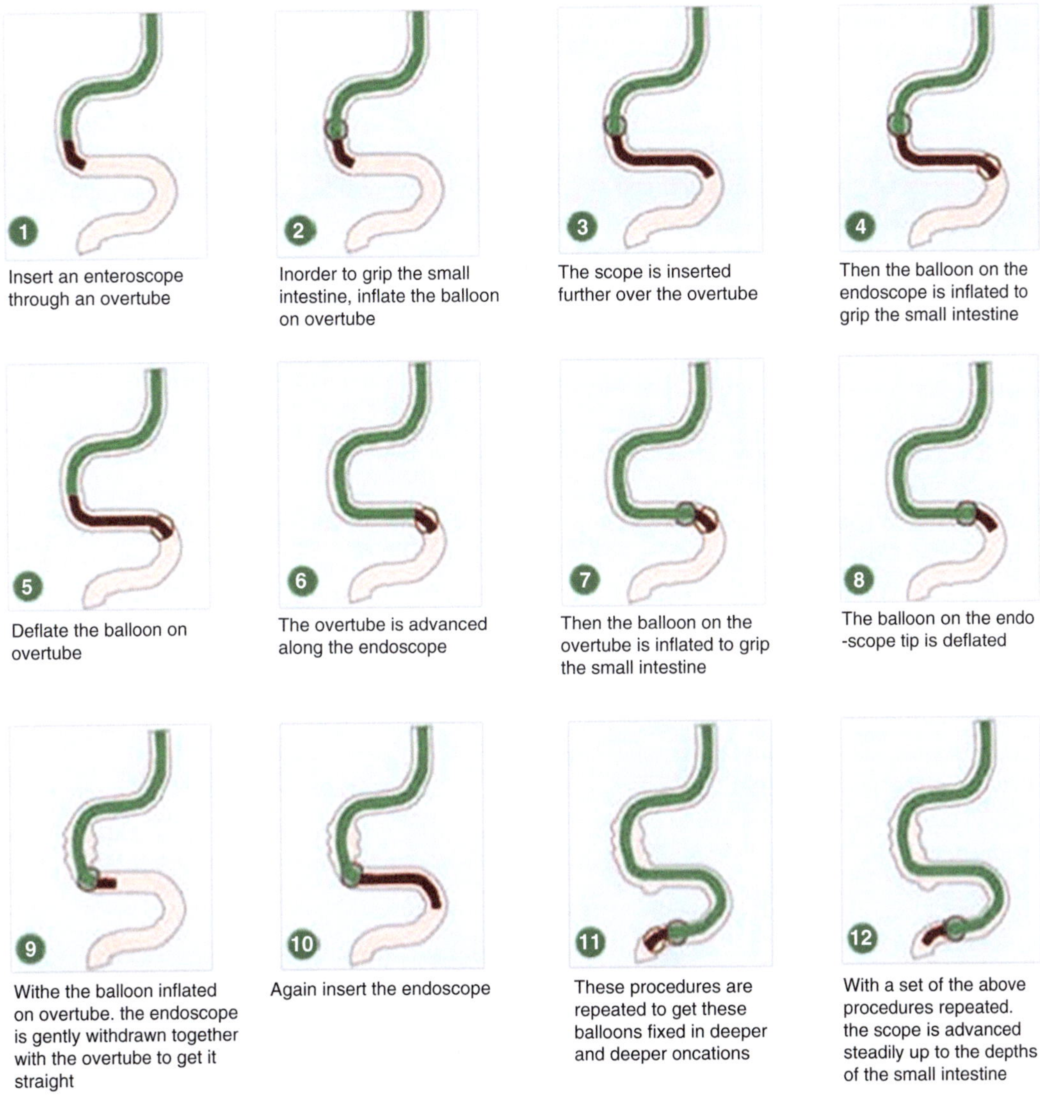

Fig. 38.11 Illustration of endoscopic technique with double balloon

There is also another problem; there is a limited availability of suitable equipment, as all accessories have to be of sufficient length. Unfortunately for double-balloon technique, there is a current trend in ERCP equipment to develop shorter rather than longer accessories. There is a lack of needle knifes, sphinctero-tomes, extraction balloons, lithotripsy devices, and retrieval baskets customized for the double-balloon system [32].

Due to the previously described, BEA-ERCP should not be considered as a first option when treating choledocholitiasis, especially if the physician is not an expert endoscopist. And if choledocholitiasis coexists with cholelithiasis, considering that the gallbladder will be removed, a laparoscopic approach (whether with a full laparoscopic resolution with CBD exploration or with a LAT-ERCP) is recommended.

The third option available to treat the lithiasis of the CBD is the percutaneous approach. With this technique, it is necessary first to perform a percutaneous biliary drainage, and later when the fistula between the biliary system and the skin is consolidated, a session to remove the stones can be performed.

The first step of the procedure consists in an ultrasound-guided puncture of the intrahepatic bile duct by using a 22G Chiba needle (Fig. 38.12), and then a percutaneous transhepatic cholangiogram should be performed to confirm the presence, location, number, and size of stones (Fig. 38.13). The choice whether to use a left-sided sub-xyphoid approach or a right-sided subcostal or intercostal approach must be based on individual and anatomic considerations, such as the position of the liver, bile duct anatomy (as seen on pre-procedural imaging), and number, position, and size of the bile duct stones.

The percutaneous transhepatic cholangiogram can be achieved in 98% of the patients with dilatation of the bile ducts and in 90% of those without dilatation [33].

Once we gain access to the biliary system with the Chiba needle, a guide wire must be introduced, and by using Seldinger technique, an 8 or 10Fr biliary drainage must be placed (Fig. 38.14).

After 7–10 days when the biliary system is decompressed, the symptoms of cholangitis (if were presents) are relieved, and the fistula starts to consolidate, it is possible to perform the treatment of the stones. By working through the biliary-cutaneous fistula, it is possible to push the stones into the duodenum or extracting them through the skin's hole. In order to achieve this, a standard percutaneous transluminal angioplasty balloon catheter is advanced beyond the stones and positioned across the papilla. Then

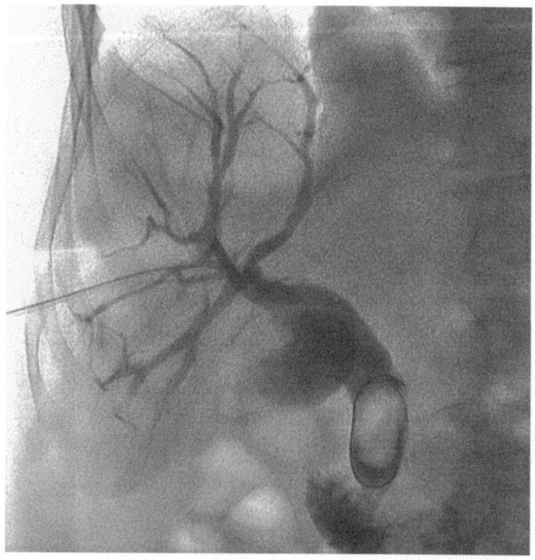

Fig. 38.13 Percutaneous transhepatic cholangiogram showing a big stone on distal common bile duct

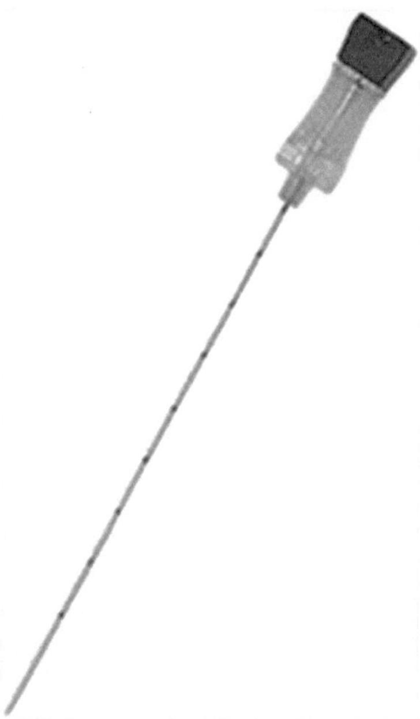

Fig. 38.12 22G Chiba needle

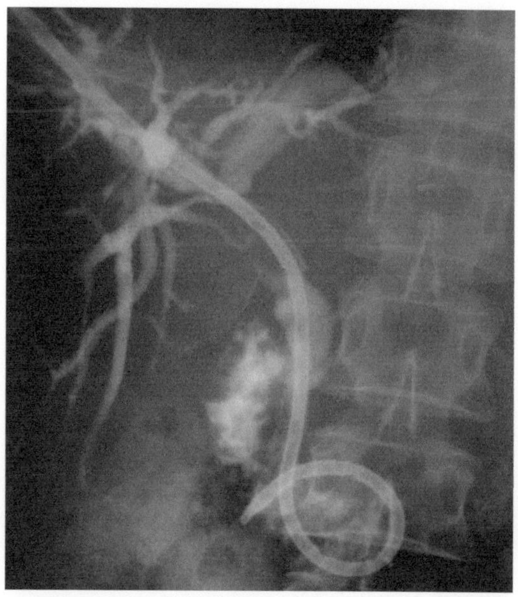

Fig. 38.14 Percutaneous biliary drainage with "pig-tail" in duodenum

the sphincter is dilated by an 8–12 mm balloon, depending of the size of the largest stone, until no waist could be seen in the balloon on fluoroscopy (Fig. 38.15). Once this is achieved, the balloon is deflated and the catheter withdrawn and positioned proximal to the stones. After reinflating the balloon, the stones are pushed forward through the dilated sphincter into the duodenum.

If the stone size exceeded 10 mm, mechanical lithotripsy with Dormia basket is recommended [34]. The stone fragments are then evacuated into the duodenum by using the balloon catheter or Dormia basket (Fig. 38.16).

If the stone's size is not too big, another option is to grab the stone with the Dormia basket and pull it out through the skin's hole. This maneuver could be dangerous if the stone is larger than the fistula diameter because the fistula could be damaged; thus, it is recommended to place a second (safety) wire through the papilla in order to preserve the biliary access.

When all the stones seem to have been extracted, cholangiography must be performed to confirm complete stone clearance. Then a biliary drainage is placed in the CBD.

After approximately 24 h later, a cholangiography must be performed to confirm CBD clearance, and if so, the external drain is removed. If residual stones are found, the procedure must be repeated until all stones are removed.

The success rate reported with this approach varies between 93% and 96%, and the complications vary between 4.7% and 6.7% [34–37]. The complications described include hemobilia, pancreatitis, cholangitis, pleural effusion due to a trans-pleural biliary drainage, and bile peritonitis due to fistula disruption.

The last option that is available to treat the choledocholitiasis is the laparoscopic approach with exploration of the CBD. In case we are treating a patient that has already been cholecistectomized, the laparoscopic approach should be considered as a second option, after the other minimal invasive approaches failed (endoscopic-percutaneous) as the patient's abdomen could be hostile due to adhesions which will make the CBD exploration difficult. But if the patient also has cholelithiasis and laparoscopic cholecystectomy must be performed, it is possible to do the treatment fully laparoscopic.

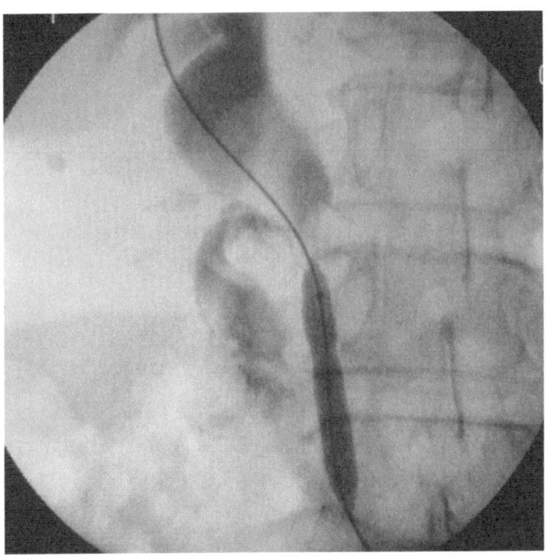

Fig. 38.15 Sphincter dilation with a 10 mm balloon. A waist can still be seen on the balloon

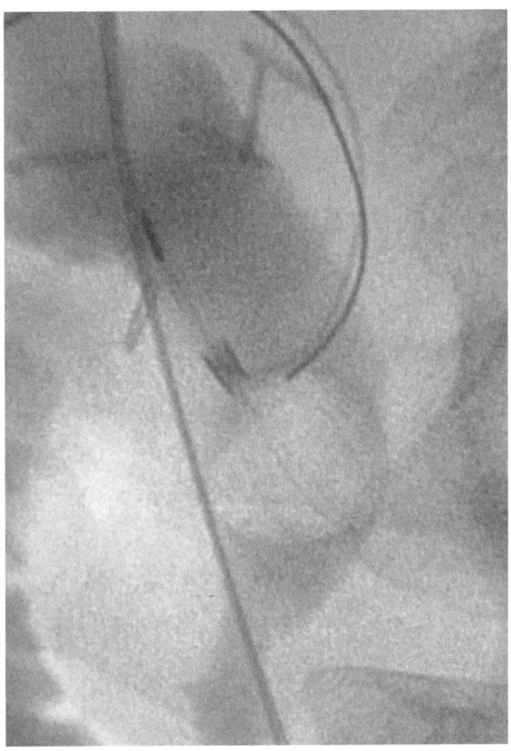

Fig. 38.16 A stone being grabbed with a Dormia basket

It is recommended to try first a transcystic approach to treat the stones. A technique similar to the percutaneous technique can be performed, and by introducing a percutaneous transluminal angioplasty balloon catheter through the cystic duct, the sphincter is dilated, and then, with the same balloon, the stone is pushed to the duodenum. It is also possible to do this maneuver with a Dormia basket through the cystic duct (Fig. 38.17). If this fails, one should consider opening the CBD and performing an exploration (Fig. 38.18).

If we decided to explore the CBD and after the stones' extraction we perform cholangiography and we are sure that there are no more stones and the bile duct is dilated, we can perform a primary closure of the CBD (Fig. 38.19). On the other hand, if the bile duct is thin, this measure is not so strongly recommended due to possible strictures at the suture site. In case we doubt the presence of more stones, we must place a T-tube in order to avoid a pressure increase inside the CBD and a bile leakage and, of course, to perform then a percutaneous approach through the T-tube to extract the remaining stones.

With the set of therapeutic tools mentioned previously, one should be able to face the prob-

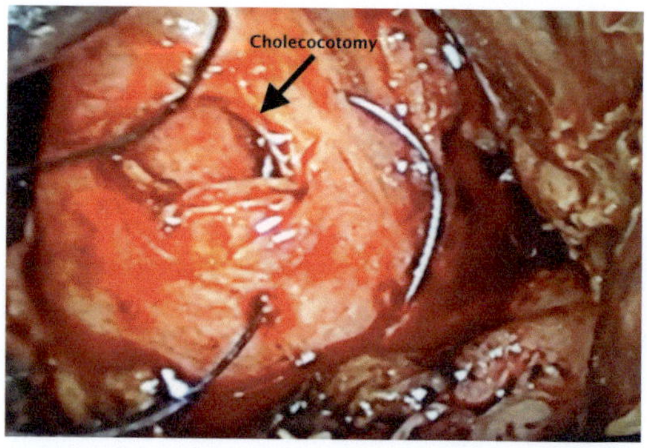

Fig. 38.19 Closure of the common bile duct after laparoscopic exploration

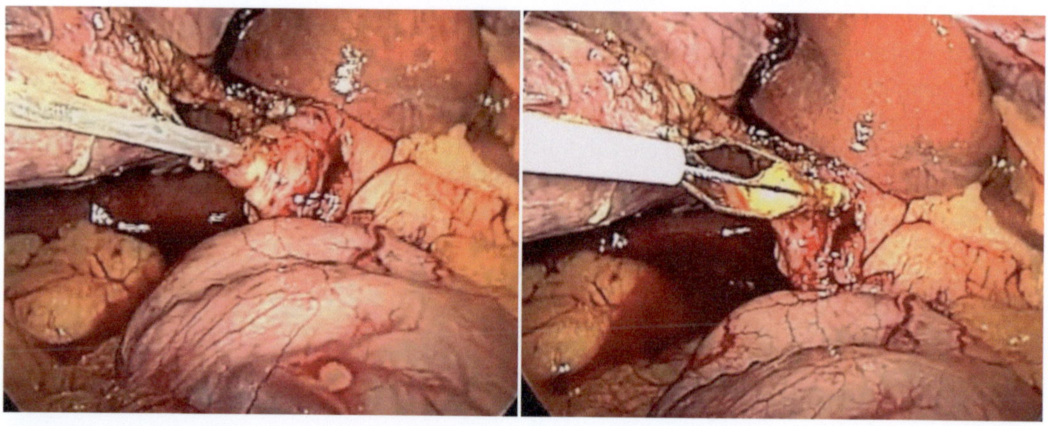

Fig. 38.17 A stone being pulled out with a Dormia basket through the cystic duct

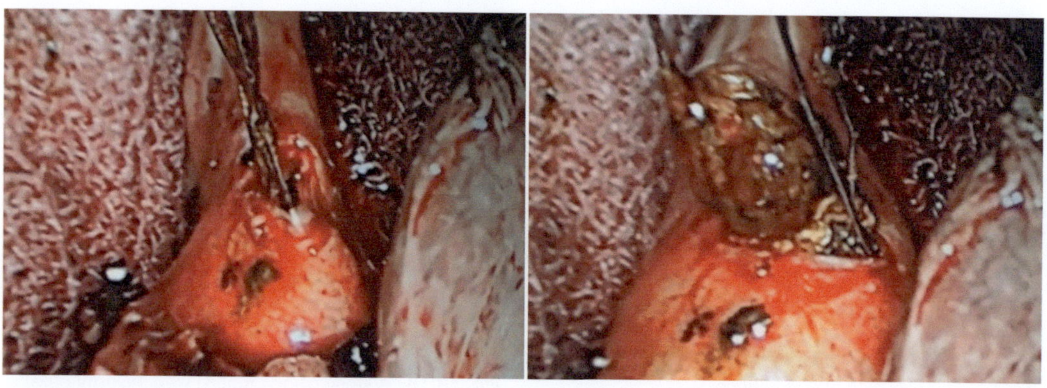

Fig. 38.18 A stone being removed with a Dormia basket through an incision on the CBD

lem of the choledocholitiasis. A proper training is needed in laparoscopic surgery, endoscopy, and percutaneous surgery due to the high technical difficulty of treating CBD stones in patients with Roux-en-Y anatomy. Which path to follow should be based on details of every case and personal experience with every mentioned technique; in the case of a lack of personal experience, it is strongly recommended to derivate these patients to a specialist.

References

1. Taha MIA, Malheiros CA, Freitas WR Jr, Puglia CR, Lacombe A. Fatores preditivos de colelitíase em obesos mórbidos após gastroplastia em Y de Roux. Rev Assoc Med Bras. 2006;52(6):430–4.
2. Nougou A, Suter M. Almost routine prophylactic cholecystectomy during laparoscopic gastric bypass is safe. Obes Surg United States. 2008;18(5):535–9.
3. Liem RK, Niloff PH. Prophylactic cholecystectomy with open gastric bypass operation. Obes Surg United States. 2004;14(6):763–5.
4. Tucker ON, Fajnwaks P, Szomstein S, Rosenthal RJ. Is concomitant cholecystectomy necessary in obese patients undergoing laparoscopic gastric bypass surgery? Surg Endosc Germany. 2008;22(11):2450–4.
5. Escalona A, Boza C, Munoz R, Perez G, Rayo S, Crovari F, et al. Routine preoperative ultrasonography and selective cholecystectomy in laparoscopic Roux-en-Y gastric bypass. Why not? Obes Surg United States. 2008;18(1):47–51.
6. Worni M, Guller U, Shah A, Gandhi M, Shah J, Rajgor D, et al. Cholecystectomy concomitant with laparoscopic gastric bypass: a trend analysis of the nationwide inpatient sample from 2001 to 2008. Obes Surg United States. 2012;22(2):220–9.
7. Warschkow R, Tarantino I, Ukegjini K, Beutner U, Guller U, Schmied BM, et al. Concomitant cholecystectomy during laparoscopic Roux-en-Y gastric bypass in obese patients is not justified: a meta-analysis. Obes Surg United States. 2013;23(3):397–407.
8. Ibarra E, Pascowsk M, Souza JM, Vega E, Duza GPM. Litiasis vesicular en pacientes sometidos a cirugía bariátrica: incidencia posquirúrgica según técnica. Pren Méd Argent. 2015;101(9):471–6.
9. Gustafsson U, Benthin L, Granstrom L, Groen AK, Sahlin S, Einarsson C. Changes in gallbladder bile composition and crystal detection time in morbidly obese subjects after bariatric surgery. Hepatology United States. 2005;41(6):1322–8.
10. Everhart JE. Contributions of obesity and weight loss to gallstone disease. Ann Intern Med United States. 1993;119(10):1029–35.
11. D'Hondt M, Sergeant G, Deylgat B, Devriendt D, Van Rooy F, Vansteenkiste F. Prophylactic cholecystectomy, a mandatory step in morbidly obese patients undergoing laparoscopic Roux-en-Y gastric bypass? J Gastrointest Surg United States. 2011;15(9):1532–6.
12. Strasberg SM, Hertl M, Soper NJ. An analysis of the problem of biliary injury during laparoscopic cholecystectomy. J Am Coll Surg United States. 1995;180(1):101–25.
13. Miller K, Hell E, Lang B, Lengauer E. Gallstone formation prophylaxis after gastric restrictive procedures for weight loss: a randomized double-blind placebo-controlled trial. Ann Surg United States. 2003;238(5):697–702.
14. Uy MC, Talingdan-Te MC, Espinosa WZ, Daez MLO, Ong JP. Ursodeoxycholic acid in the prevention of gallstone formation after bariatric surgery: a meta-analysis. Obes Surg United States. 2008;18(12):1532–8.
15. Schreiner MA, Chang L, Gluck M, Irani S, Gan SI, Brandabur JJ, et al. Laparoscopy-assisted versus balloon enteroscopy-assisted ERCP in bariatric post-Roux-en-Y gastric bypass patients. Gastrointest Endosc United States. 2012;75(4):748–56.
16. Lopes TL, Clements RH, Wilcox CM. Laparoscopy-assisted ERCP: experience of a high-volume bariatric surgery center (with video). Gastrointest Endosc United States. 2009;70(6):1254–9.
17. Bertin PM, Singh K, Arregui ME. Laparoscopic transgastric endoscopic retrograde cholangiopancreatography (ERCP) after gastric bypass: case series and a description of technique. Surg Endosc Germany. 2011;25(8):2592–6.
18. Tekola B, Wang AY, Ramanath M, Burnette B, Ellen K, Schirmer BD, et al. Percutaneous gastrostomy tube placement to perform transgastrostomy endoscopic retrograde cholangiopancreaticography in patients with Roux-en-Y anatomy. Dig Dis Sci United States. 2011;56(11):3364–9.
19. Snauwaert C, Laukens P, Dillemans B, Himpens J, De Looze D, Deprez PH, et al. Laparoscopy-assisted transgastric endoscopic retrograde cholangiopancreatography in bariatric Roux-en-Y gastric bypass patients. Endosc Int Open Germany. 2015;3(5):E458–63.
20. Chu Y-C, Yang C-C, Yeh Y-H, Chen C-H, Yueh S-K. Double-balloon enteroscopy application in biliary tract disease-its therapeutic and diagnostic functions. Gastrointest Endosc United States. 2008;68(3):585–91.
21. Koornstra JJ. Double balloon enteroscopy for endoscopic retrograde cholangiopancreaticography after Roux-en-Y reconstruction: case series and review of the literature. Neth J Med Netherlands. 2008;66(7):275–9.
22. Aabakken L, Bretthauer M, Line PD. Double-balloon enteroscopy for endoscopic retrograde cholangiography in patients with a Roux-en-Y anastomosis. EndoscopyGermany. 2007;39(12):1068–71.
23. Emmett DS, Mallat DB. Double-balloon ERCP in patients who have undergone Roux-en-Y surgery: a case series. Gastrointest Endosc United States. 2007;66(5):1038–41.
24. Moreels TG, Roth B, Vandervliet EJ, Parizel PM, Dutre J, Pelckmans PA. The use of the double-balloon

enteroscope for endoscopic retrograde cholangiopancreatography and biliary stent placement after Roux-en-Y hepaticojejunostomy. Endoscopy Germany. 2007;39(Suppl 1):E196–7.

25. Spahn TW, Grosse-Thie W, Spies P, Mueller MK. Treatment of choledocholithiasis following Roux-en-Y hepaticojejunostomy using double-balloon endoscopy. Digestion Switzerland. 2007;75:20–1.
26. Parlak E, Cicek B, Disibeyaz S, Cengiz C, Yurdakul M, Akdogan M, et al. Endoscopic retrograde cholangiography by double balloon enteroscopy in patients with Roux-en-Y hepaticojejunostomy. Surg Endosc Germany. 2010;24(2):466–70.
27. Moreels TG, Hubens GJ, Ysebaert DK, Op de Beeck B, Pelckmans PA. Diagnostic and therapeutic double-balloon enteroscopy after small bowel Roux-en-Y reconstructive surgery. Digestion Switzerland. 2009;80(3):141–7.
28. Kuga R, Furuya CKJ, Hondo FY, Ide E, Ishioka S, Sakai P. ERCP using double-balloon enteroscopy in patients with Roux-en-Y anatomy. Dig Dis Switzerland. 2008;26(4):330–5.
29. Wang AY, Sauer BG, Behm BW, Ramanath M, Cox DG, Ellen KL, et al. Single-balloon enteroscopy effectively enables diagnostic and therapeutic retrograde cholangiography in patients with surgically altered anatomy. Gastrointest Endosc United States. 2010;71(3):641–9.
30. Yamamoto H, Sekine Y, Sato Y, Higashizawa T, Miyata T, Iino S, et al. Total enteroscopy with a nonsurgical steerable double-balloon method. Gastrointest Endosc United States. 2001;53(2):216–20.
31. Mensink PBF, Haringsma J, Kucharzik T, Cellier C, Perez-Cuadrado E, Monkemuller K, et al. Complications of double balloon enteroscopy: a multicenter survey. Endoscopy Germany. 2007;39(7):613–5.
32. Joyce AM, Ahmad NA, Beilstein MC, Kochman ML, Long WB, Baron T, et al. Multicenter comparative trial of the V-scope system for therapeutic ERCP. Endoscopy Germany. 2006;38(7):713–6.
33. Gimenez ME, Berkowski DCP. Obstrucción biliar benigna. In: Gimenez M, Guimaraes M, Oleaga JSS, editors. Manual de técnicas intervencionistas guiadas por imágenes. Buenos Aires: Ediciones Journal; 2011. p. 119–38.
34. Kint JF, van den Bergh JE, van Gelder RE, Rauws EA, Gouma DJ, van Delden OM, et al. Percutaneous treatment of common bile duct stones: results and complications in 110 consecutive patients. Dig Surg Switzerland. 2015;32(1):9–15.
35. García-García L, Lanciego C. Percutaneous treatment of biliary stones: sphincteroplasty and occlusion balloon for the clearance of bile duct calculi. AJR Am J Roentgenol [Internet]. 2004;182(3):663–70. Available from: http://www.ncbi.nlm.nih.gov/pubmed/14975967
36. Szulman C, Gimenez M, Sierre S. Antegrade papillary balloon dilation for extrahepatic bile duct stone clearance: lessons learned from treating 300 patients. J Vasc Interv Radiol United States. 2011;22(3):346–53.
37. Gil S, de la Iglesia P, Verdu JF, de Espana F, Arenas J, Irurzun J. Effectiveness and safety of balloon dilation of the papilla and the use of an occlusion balloon for clearance of bile duct calculi. AJR Am J Roentgenol United States. 2000;174(5):1455–60.

39 Gastroesophageal Reflux Disease

Isaac C. Payne, Andrew C. Berry, and William O. Richards

Introduction

The prevalence of GERD is estimated to be between 10% and 20% in the Western world, with a higher predilection in developed countries [1]. Obesity itself has been shown to be an independent risk factor for GERD, with an observed dose-response relationship between frequency of heartburn or regurgitation and higher BMI [2]. A report of the US National Health and Education Survey (NHANES) found that approximately 66% of the US adult population is either overweight or obese, with this number on the rise annually [3]. Roughly 5% of the total global health-care cost is allocated toward treating obese patients, as there is clearly a rising economic burden associated with obesity. The direct health-care costs associated with GERD in all patient populations are estimated to be around \$9–\$10 billion annually. Indirect costs such as decrease in work productivity, disability, and absent workdays should also be considered [4–6]. Given the limited effectiveness of lifestyle modifications and medications, bariatric surgery has been shown to be the only modality with long-term sustained weight loss, reduction in morbidity, and improvement in all-cause mortality [7–9].

The evidence-based diagnostic and management algorithms for obese patients with GERD will be discussed in this chapter. Both the pathophysiology linking obesity and GERD and the diagnostic algorithm for GERD will be discussed. As many surgical and gastrointestinal societies are shifting toward episode payment models [10], there remains much debate about the role of preoperative hiatal hernia screening and preoperative endoscopy for bariatric surgery candidates. Discussion of the operation of choice for patients with GERD symptoms and management of hiatal hernias found incidentally during bariatric operations will be outlined below. We aim to provide a current, evidence-based analysis for obese patients and GERD, in regard to bariatric surgery options including an analysis of gastric bypass and sleeve gastrectomy.

I. C. Payne · W. O. Richards (✉)
Department of Surgery, University of South Alabama Medical Center, Mobile, AL, USA
e-mail: brichards@health.southalabama.edu

A. C. Berry
Department of Medicine, University of South Alabama Medical Center, Mobile, AL, USA

Relationship Between Obesity and Reflux (Pathophysiology Behind Increasing the Risk of GERD in This Population)

The natural anti-reflux anatomical mechanism is complex, consisting of the lower esophageal sphincter (LES), esophageal hiatus of the diaphragm, phrenoesophageal ligaments, and angle

R. Lutfi et al. (eds.), *Global Bariatric Surgery*, https://doi.org/10.1007/978-3-319-93545-4_39

of His. Associated complications of GERD include erosive esophagitis, stricture, Barrett's esophagus, and esophageal adenocarcinoma [11, 12]. Obesity is an independent risk factor for GERD, by as much as 50%, after adjusting for various co-founding variables [2]. A dose-response relationship between frequency of heartburn or regurgitation and higher BMI has been observed [2]. The pathophysiology behind obesity and its link to GERD is multifactorial including high intra-abdominal pressure, increased rate of hiatal hernia, more frequent transient LES relaxations (TLESR), slower esophageal acid clearance, and possible changes at the molecular level regarding adipokines and hormones [13, 14].

Following a linear trend, the higher the body mass index (BMI) and waist circumference, the greater the intragastric pressure and gastroesophageal pressure gradient (GEPG) [15]. The high-pressure gradient between the stomach and the esophagus likely contributes to a higher proportion of TLESRs with acid reflux due to an enlarged cross-sectional area at the gastroesophageal junction [16]. In the setting of obesity, manometry studies suggest that the pressure morphology within and across the esophagogastric junction is altered, as the intragastric pressure and the GEPG during the inspiratory respiratory phase increases. Obese patients also have shorter LES length. The higher postprandial intragastric pressure leads to more intense stimulation on both stretch and tension mechanoreceptors in the proximal stomach, which provokes more postprandial TLESRs in the setting of abdominal obesity [16–18]. Thus, LES dysfunction and TLERs may be one of the most important factors in functional integrity of the anti-reflux barrier in obesity.

Obese patients are over three times as likely to have hiatal hernias compared to nonobese individuals [19]. Some studies have identified the most important factor between GERD and increasing BMI was the presence of a hiatal hernia, further reinforcing hiatal hernia's link between obesity and GERD [20]. Along with increased intragastric pressure and gastroesophageal pressure gradients during inspiration, hiatal hernias increase the degree of reflux during TLESRs in the obese patient population. They also contribute to axial separation between the LES and the extrinsic crural diaphragm, thus decreasing the effectiveness of the mechanical anti-reflux barrier [21, 22].

Several investigators have raised the possibility that changes in the autonomic nervous system in obese patients increases GERD. Obese individuals have decreased parasympathetic activity while patients with pathologic esophageal acid exposure also have reduced parasympathetic activity. The vagus nerve contributes to the pathogenesis of GERD from its influences on esophageal peristalsis, LES function, and gastric motility [23]. Studies to date suggest that the autonomic abnormalities in these aforementioned patients are not generalized but are limited specifically to vagal dysfunction [23]. There has been much debate whether inflammation leads to parasympathetic dysfunction in the pathogenesis of GERD or vice versa. To date, impaired parasympathetic activity seems to be the primary factor in the pathophysiology of reflux, as the degree of esophageal inflammatory damage is unrelated to disturbances in parasympathetic function [24]. Most importantly, weight reduction, irrespective of route of loss, leads to an increase parasympathetic activity, further supporting the autonomic nervous system's role linking obesity to GERD [23].

Visceral abdominal fat in centrally obese individuals may cause dilation of intercellular spaces in the esophageal squamous epithelium and has been shown to be an early pathologic event in development of esophagitis [25]. Dilation of these spaces allows diffusion of HCl into the esophageal epithelium, facilitating injury, cytokine release, and destruction of normal epithelial integrity by tight junctions [26, 27]. Increased susceptibility of the esophageal epithelium to reflux-mediated injury and inflammation potentiates the development of esophageal metaplasia and neoplasia [26]. Central obesity is also associated with an impaired esophageal epithelial barrier, even in the absence of pathologic acid exposure levels [27].

Cell signaling proteins secreted by adipose tissue, adipokines, have been a hotly studied topic on GERD and obesity [28, 29]. Adipokines such as ghrelin, leptin, and adiponectin play a role in the body's sensing hunger and food intake. Though many of these studies still only involve animal models, levels of certain levels of adipokines have been implicated in GERD in the obese patient population. Rat models have shown increased secretion of peripheral ghrelin, secreted when the stomach is empty to stimulate appetite, and decreased ghrelin responsiveness. Meanwhile, in humans, ghrelin has been reported to be positively associated with Barrett's esophagus but inversely associated with GERD symptoms [30, 31]. Levels of leptin, the hormone that helps regulate energy balance by inhibiting hunger, have been found to be positively correlated with symptom score severity, weight, BMI, waist circumference, and total abdominal fat [32]. Adiponectin, released by adipose tissue and found to suppress inflammation, has been negatively correlated inversely correlated to BMI, and serum adiponectin levels were found to be lower in patients with erosive esophageal disease [33]. Further studies are necessary to decipher the clinical implications of the adipokines and their signaling pathways.

Diagnosing GERD (24pH, Manometry, Impedance, Endoscopy)

Society-based initiatives, such as the American Gastrological Association's (AGA) Roadmap to the Future of GI, provide physicians with means to deliver high-value care and to demonstrate quality [10]. Part of this roadmap includes episodic payment models, in which reimbursement payments to health-care providers are based on predetermined expected costs of a bundle or grouping of health-care services. Thus, the workup of GERD must be algorithmic and appropriate to the patient's presenting symptoms and risk factors. The consensus diagnostic algorithm for the diagnosis of GERD is outlined by the AGA and 2013 guidelines. The ASGE also provides a 2015 update on the specific role of endoscopy in GERD [1, 34, 35].

Current diagnostic tests for GERD include esophageal pH monitoring, impedance-pH monitoring (catheter-based or wireless) , manometry, or endoscopy. Many of these methods have their own respective pitfalls, such as patient discomfort, time of exam, deviation of daily lifestyle, lack of sensitivity, or cost of the procedure. The diagnosis of GERD is made using some combination of symptom presentation, ambulatory esophageal pH monitoring, endoscopy, and response to anti-secretory therapy. The sensitivity of heartburn and regurgitation for the presence of erosive esophagitis was found to be 30–76% and the specificity from 62% to 96% [36]. Thus, symptoms alone cannot diagnose GERD. If a likely GERD patient based on clinical symptoms does not present with alarm symptoms or at high risk for BE, an 8-week PPI trial is adequate to help establish the diagnosis. In the presence of typical GERD symptoms and the absence of alarm symptoms, empiric PPI therapy, and not initial EGD, remains the mainstay of therapy as the severity of GERD symptoms does not correlate with the degree of underlying esophageal damage [1, 37, 38]. PPI non-responders should undergo EGD as well as esophageal pH monitoring if EGD reveals no abnormalities. Patients with extra esophageal symptoms should undergo pH monitoring sooner in the diagnostic algorithm [1].

Ambulatory esophageal pH measures esophageal acid exposure over the course of a day and is the gold standard for diagnosis of GERD. However, it does not measure reflux of nonacid-gastric contents, particularly important when the patient is on PPI medications. Telemetry capsule pH monitoring has the advantages that the monitoring period is extended to 48 h and increased patient satisfaction from the lack of irritating nasal catheter. Catheter based and capsule pH monitoring does show good sensitivity (77–100%) and specificity (85–100%) in patients with erosive esophagitis; however, in those with endoscopy-negative reflux symptoms and when a diagnostic test is in need, the sensitivity is lower (<71%) [28]. Patients that proceed to endoscopy may or may not have mucosal damage, as about 50–60% of patients with abnormal reflux confirmed by pH monitoring do not have any evidence of mucosal damage [39, 40]. In addition, studies have shown that distal esophagus erythema predicts reflux disease in only 53% of patients [41]. In fact, endoscopic evidence of grade I and grade II esophagitis is quite nonspecific diagnostically because it has been seen in 25% of pH-negative patients [42].

However, in patients with suspected GERD who subsequently have persistent symptoms despite medical optimization of PPI therapy, some experts recommend intraluminal impedance-pH monitoring on PPI treatment to help decipher the symptom etiology and to assess the effect of PPIs [43]. Advantages of this methodology include the ability to differentiate refluxed acid from swallowed acidic beverages and correlate symptoms to measurement of acid and non-acid refluxate. However, utilization of this tool inevitably still requires physician oversight for interpretation, unlike the highly automated computer analysis generated for 24-h pH studies, and limitations in measurement of reflux event duration [43]. The difficulty in interpretation of esophageal impedance studies has greatly limited the adoption of the test in clinical practice, and it is our practice to study patients with 24-h esophageal pH off PPI therapy to diagnose GERD.

Esophageal manometry is of limited value in the primary diagnosis of GERD, as a motility abnormality or decreased LES pressure is far from adequate to establish a definitive diagnosis of GERD [1]. Manometry is used to aid in placement of transnasal pH-impedance probes. High-resolution manometry has been a novel advancement but cannot diagnose GERD on its own and mainly helps rule out other esophageal motility disorders in patients being evaluated for anti-reflux surgery [1].

What is the future in GERD diagnosis? Endoscopic-guided mucosal impedance may be an option.

This entails a single-channel impedance catheter, consisting of two 360°-circumferential sensing rings 3 mm in length spaced 2 mm apart mounted on a 2-mm-diameter catheter, passed through a standard upper endoscope. Endoscopic-guided mucosal impedance directly touches the lining of the esophagus at various locations to decipher changes in the epithelium due to reflux of acid and non-acid contents and, most importantly, can delineate GERD from non-GERD etiologies of symptoms without the need for prolonged and cumbersome ambulatory monitoring methods [44]. Studies so far have found that it only adds roughly 2 min to the endoscopy time [45]. Most importantly, mucosal impedance showed good predictive value that reliably distinguishes between GERD, non-GERD, and eosinophilic esophagitis (EoE) based on esophageal patterns of mucosal impedance [46]. Compared with wireless pH monitoring, mucosal impedance has demonstrated superior specificity and positive predictive value for predicting the presence of erosive esophagitis (95% and 96%, respectively, versus 64% and 40%, respectively) [46]. Another potential benefit may pertain to patients with refractory GERD symptoms, to determine if there is continued reflux or if symptoms are due to non-GERD conditions. Mucosal impedance can also inform clinicians whether PPI therapy is effective. Endoscopic-guided mucosal impedance has the potential to replace current pH and impedance-pH testing, but there remains a paucity of surgical outcome studies in patients who, based on mucosal impedance epithelium alteration changes, undergo surgery for GERD. Currently it is not widespread in public practice and very few institutions are teaching current GI following this technique [44]. However, endoscopic-guided mucosal impedance has the potential to quickly shift the paradigm for diagnosis of GERD.

All of the aforementioned diagnostic tests help objectively select which patients are best suited for anti-reflux surgery. According to the Society of American Gastrointestinal and Endoscopic Surgeons (SAGES), surgical procedures for GERD are highly effective in 85–93% of cases [47]. According to SAGES, surgical intervention may be appropriate in patients who have failed medical management, decide for surgery despite successful medical management, have complications of GERD such as Barrett's esophagus and/or peptic stricture, have medical complications attributable to a large hiatal hernia, or have "atypical" symptoms such as asthma, hoarseness, cough, chest pain, dental erosions or aspiration, and reflux documented on 24-h pH monitoring [47]. Many patients who fail anti-reflux medical therapy still opt for anti-reflux surgery, although long-term results may remain suboptimal [48]. As uncontrolled GERD can lead to BE and adenocarcinoma, appropriate selection for anti-reflux operations needs to be individualized for each operative candidate. Appropriate preoperative workup includes definitive diagnosis of GERD using esophageal pH or pathologic confirmation of esophagitis. Additional workup includes esophageal manometry and barium radiographs to exclude esophageal motility disorders such as achalasia or esophagogastric junction outflow obstruction (EGJOO) that can be confused with PPI unresponsive GERD and to determine the appropriate anti-reflux procedure to perform [10].

Screening for Hiatal Hernia and Preoperative Workup in Asymptomatic Patients for Bariatric Surgery

The American Society for Metabolic and Bariatric Surgery (ASMBS) published a position statement in 2011 on preoperative weight loss insurance-mandated requirements [49]. Since then, however, many providers have challenged the ongoing practice of insurance-mandated preoperative weight loss prior to surgical intervention. A 2016 ASMBS updated position statement calls into question this prior guideline and lack of evidence, causing even unnecessary delay of lifesaving treatment and leading to the progression of life-threatening comorbid conditions [50]. The most current ASMBS position states that patients seeking surgical treatment for clinically severe obesity should be evaluated by the provider based on comorbidities, initial BMI, and what constitutes failed weight loss efforts—not by insurance mandates [50]. As many societies are shifting toward episode payment models [10], what constitutes necessary preoperative workup in both the asymptomatic and symptomatic bariatric patient remains a highly debated topic of discussion globally.

In bariatric patients presenting with respective symptoms, be it GERD symptoms or other gastrointestinal or non-gastrointestinal symptoms, proper symptom-specific society and algorithm-based workup should ensue. Though the patient is obese and a potential bariatric candidate, the baseline symptom-specific workup should remain. The real dilemma presents in asymptomatic bariatric candidates. What, if any, preoperative workup should ensue, and how will the findings (or lack thereof) impact the bariatric course?

Current European Association for Endoscopic Surgery guidelines state that EGD, or upper GI series, is advisable for all bariatric procedures and strongly recommended for gastric bypass patients RYGB [51]. Meanwhile, the ASGE has recommended that EGD be performed in all symptomatic patients undergoing bariatric surgery and considered in all candidates [52]. In the American Society for Metabolic and Bariatric Surgery (ASMBS) guidelines, a GI evaluation (*H. pylori* screening in high-prevalence areas, gallbladder evaluation, and upper endoscopy) is part of the preoperative workup for bariatric surgery [52].

The rationale to consider upper GI endoscopy as part of the bariatric surgery preoperative workup seems plausible, as it can detect mucosal abnormalities, ulcerations, hiatal hernias, malignancies, and other anatomic abnormalities that will change the operative plan. However, additional preoperative workup adds additional cost and the question of what to do with any additional findings, let alone, additional procedure, and sedation risk. The current published guidelines suggest preoperative EGD in all symptomatic patients, but many studies have reported a lack of correlation of clinical symptoms with endoscopic findings [53–57], further questioning the clinical implications of further workup on symptoms alone. Studies have found that in all patients presenting for bariatric surgery (symptomatic or asymptomatic), between 60% and 80%, had clinically important lesions that affected surgical approach or necessitated medical treatment and thus surgical delay [54, 55]. Specifically, in the asymptomatic pre-bariatric population, roughly

20% of patients were found to have pathological or abnormal findings [55]. Asymptomatic patients undergoing RYGBP were found to have pathologic findings in 46% of cases, but <5% had clinical implications [56].

Clearly there is discordance in the literature about the recommendations regarding screening, stemming from study type, design, and patient population [57]. In one large survey sent to the British Obesity and Metabolic Surgery Society members in 49 large UK bariatric units (each with >5000 caseload/year) reported that 90% (44 of 49 units) included preoperative EGD routinely (15 units) or selectively (29 units) [58]. Only 10% (5 units) deemed preoperative EGD unnecessary in this patient population. Between 54% and 61% believed preoperative EGD to be necessary in patients with either family history GI cancer, pernicious anemia, or GERD symptoms. The results of the preoperative EGD resulted in 51% of the patients having a change in the operative plan, due to peptic ulcer (46%), hiatal hernia (43%), Barrett's esophagus (32%), or gastrointestinal stromal tumors (25%) [58]. A large recent meta-analysis analyzed the clinical significance of preoperative EGD in bariatric candidates. The number of patients undergoing a change in medical management and surgical management was 27.5% and 7.8%, respectively [59].

Though the preoperative EGD evaluation in asymptomatic patients remains a part of society-based guidelines, the notion of yet another procedure and the risks carried with it must be discussed. Patients presenting for bariatric surgery are complicated patients and have a higher probability of procedural-related and anesthesia adverse events secondary to cardiopulmonary comorbidities [53]. Due to the heavy demand caring for these patients, roughly 36% of centers utilizing preoperative endoscopy required an increase in hospital resources, beyond the actual cost of the additional procedure itself [58]. Though the studies have their own limitations, the data suggests 20–46% of asymptomatic preoperative bariatric candidates have endoscopic pathology [55, 56]. Thus, the absence of upper GI symptoms cannot adequately indicate absence of GI lesions and pathology. Though the society guidelines remain vague, roughly 90% of large bariatric centers utilize preoperative EGD in bariatric candidates, either routinely or selectively [58].

The decision on type of bariatric surgery is affected by preoperative comorbidities, such as GERD. Roux-en-Y gastric bypass is the preferred operation in morbidly obese patients with gastroesophageal reflux disease since laparoscopic sleeve gastrectomy can exacerbate postoperative reflux symptoms or cause de novo symptoms and may warrant revision surgery [60, 61]. However, laparoscopic sleeve gastrectomy (LSG) is favored by patients and by many surgeons due to its simplicity of operative technique, satisfactory weight loss outcomes, and resolution of obesity-related comorbidities [62–64]. Debate exists whether preoperative clinical assessment is sufficient to stratify bariatric candidates for one operation or another or what (if any) preoperative endoscopic or procedural assessment is warranted. For example, patients undergoing RYGB will undoubtedly have an inaccessible remnant stomach post procedure; thus, do these patients warrant special preoperative endoscopic consideration? Many feel that it does, as a concern with respect to screening premalignant and malignant disease persists. However, the incidence of malignancy at time of endoscopy, even in patients reporting dyspepsia (but without alarm symptoms), remains extremely low at 0.2% [65]. Thus preoperative screening EGD cannot be recommended based upon the extremely low incidence of malignancy.

Many bariatric centers have employed routes to offer preoperative EGD to all patients considering LSG. If patients had pre-existing GERD symptoms or evidence of hiatal hernia or reflux esophagitis on EGD, they were advised against LSG. As GERD symptoms alone can be very nonspecific, these patients were only denied LSG conjunction if endoscopic evidence of hiatal hernia or mucosal break were present. Madhok et al. hypothesized that those requiring pre-bariatric EGD would be better selected for LSG and less likely to have post-LSG reflux [66]. Their change in practice reduced the incidence in revision surgery for GERD symptoms from 8.5% to

1.8%. Regardless, in addition to the unaccounted patients with GERD responding to postoperative PPI, a small proportion still developed de novo GERD after LSG requiring revision surgery [66].

A few surgeons have proposed preoperative bariatric workup to include EGD and manometry. Moon and colleagues evaluated the preoperative LES pressures in all patients undergoing LSG and found that although most LSG patients with a competent LES pressure and preoperative GERD symptoms had their symptoms improved or resolved, 50% of patients with a low LES pressure developed GERD symptoms postoperatively after successful anatomic repair [66]. While interesting, the use of manometry cannot be recommended until others confirm the utility and cost-effectiveness [67].

Increased BMI is a strong independent predictor of hiatal hernia, which is an independent predictor of GERD [2]. In patients with moderate or large hiatal hernias, concomitant repair is performed at the time of the bariatric procedure to minimize post-procedural risk of GERD symptoms [68–70]. The necessity of preoperative EGD for hiatal hernia screening remains controversial. EGD is advantageous in estimating the size of a hiatal hernia compared to intraoperative methods. However, upper GI contrast studies more accurately and more cost-effectively detect the presence of hiatal hernias in the obese patient population [68]. The role of GI contrast studies in preoperative bariatric evaluation is not currently society-supported.

As episode payment models are the wave of the future [10], it remains imperative to include important preoperative endoscopy into each bundled pathologic workup and procedure set. Health-care providers not performing a thorough preoperative workup may be more prone to operating room anatomical surprises and subsequent procedural adjustments and outcomes. Just as importantly, episode payment models may limit reimbursement of these intraoperative modifications, such as repair of hiatal hernias if not identified on preoperative workup.

In summary, the literature supports preoperative EGD in patients with GERD or other foregut symptoms to identify esophagitis, presence, and size of hiatal hernias and exclude Barrett's esophagus. The bariatric surgeon can expect to modify their operative procedure, choose another procedure such as LRYGB over LSG in the case of erosive esophagitis, and plan an operative repair of the hiatal hernia especially when performing LSG. It is more difficult to make the case for EGD screening in the asymptomatic patients undergoing LSG because of the paucity of findings that would alter management of the patient. Even the patients undergoing LRYGB in which the argument is that the bypassed stomach will not be available for endoscopic evaluation, the argument for preoperative EGD is hard to justify because so few of these patients have findings that change operative approach, and the risks and cost of the procedure outweigh the potential benefits and changes to operative management. In our practice preoperative EGD is done only in symptomatic patients or in patients who have history of gastroesophageal surgery or family medical history of esophageal or gastric malignancy.

Surgical Considerations in Patients with GERD and Barrett's Esophagus

Patients suffering from concomitant morbid obesity and signs and symptoms consistent with gastroesophageal reflux disease (GERD) present a difficult surgical conundrum. More importantly, recent literature debates the surgical management in patients that are found to have concomitant hiatal hernia (HH) during preoperative workup or discovered incidentally during a weight loss procedure. This section will focus on surgical management options with these patient scenarios as well surgical approaches for obese patients with diagnosed Barrett's esophagus.

Surgical Considerations GERD in the Obese Population

There is considerable debate on the surgical management of morbidly obese patients that suffer from GERD with attendant HH. The surgical management of the obese population has been discussed, yet tailoring the operation to comorbidities, specifically GERD is paramount. Roux-en-Y gastric bypass (RYGBP) is recognized as the treatment of choice for obese patients with a history of GERD who desire a weight loss procedure [10, 68, 71, 72]. However, considering that laparoscopic sleeve gastrectomy (LSG) is the most performed bariatric procedure in many countries [73], there is conflicting literature on the role of LSG in patients with GERD with or without attendant HH.

Santonicola et al. discussed the effect of LSG with or without hiatal hernia on GERD [74]. In their study, all patients underwent a standardized questionnaire for GERD, a double-contrast barium swallow and upper gastrointestinal endoscopy prior to operation and 6 months postoperatively. Patients diagnosed preoperatively or intraoperatively with hiatal hernia underwent LSG + hiatal hernia repair (HHR). Those patients without HH underwent LSG. Reconstruction of the crus was always closed posteriorly with interrupted non-absorbable suture. In the group of patients that underwent LSG + HHR, 43% of the patients had persistence of GERD symptoms postoperatively, and 22.9% of the patients developed "de novo" GERD symptoms when there were no GERD symptoms preoperatively. In the LSG group who had no hiatal hernia, there was a statistically significant decrease in the prevalence of heartburn and regurgitation frequency-intensity scores postoperatively; however, 17% of the patients developed "de novo" GERD symptoms. The study concluded that LSG has a beneficial effect on relieving GERD symptoms, yet concomitant repair of HH when present did not produce improvement in GERD symptoms. Explanations for the development of "de novo" GERD or the exacerbation of GERD after LSG is multifactorial but not proven. Many authors have suggested the weakening of sling fibers during fundus mobilization and disrupting the angle of His may permit postoperative reflux symptoms [75]. In a large single institution study, Lyon et al. evaluated postoperative reflux symptoms after laparoscopic sleeve gastrectomy with liberal repair of diaphragmatic hiatal defects [76]. A cohort of 262 patients was prospectively studied, with preoperative evaluation for reflux included PPI use, GERD score, heartburn frequency, and severity. Ninety-two out of 262 patients did not have any hernia defect or weakness. The authors adopted a liberal approach to hiatal hernia repair. Anterior repair of the hiatus was performed in the setting of hiatal weakness defined as visible or instrument palpable anterior aperture between crura and stomach. Results of the cohort showed that patients undergoing hiatal intervention experienced a significant reduction in reflux frequency scores ($p = 0.30$) and clinical outcome scores. Conversely, the group that had no intervention had a non-significant increase in postoperative reflux frequency and PPI use. Interestingly, however, on long-term follow-up, there was a trend toward reflux symptoms returning. The authors recommend that crural defects should be repaired and that GERD need not be a contraindication to LSG.

Often consensus of expert opinion is helpful to determine the most reasonable way to treat patients. The 2012 International Sleeve Gastrectomy Expert Panel Consensus Statement recommends aggressive identification of hiatal hernia intraoperatively (83% agreement) and, if found, subsequent repair (82% agreement) [70]. At the current time, the evidence based upon the large series and the expert consensus panel overwhelming recommendation indicates that hiatal hernias should be diagnosed and repaired intraoperatively when they are found during the performance of LSG. The evidence and the experts conclude that repair of hiatal hernias diagnosed pre- or intraoperatively will reduce the propensity for severe GERD after LSG.

In contrast, laparoscopic Roux-en-Y gastric bypass has long been regarded as the treatment of choice for obese patients with reflux symptoms that desire a weight loss procedure. A large multicenter European study showed that in patients with GERD undergoing LRYGBP that 62% of the patients endorsed complete resolution of symptoms compared to 84% of patients with persistent GERD after LSG [60].

Despite conflicting reports on patient outcomes, a significant portion of bariatric surgeons will proceed with RYGBP in patients who suffer from GERD. However, these surgeons recognize the limitations of RYGBP in some patient populations, most notably inflammatory bowel disease and technical difficulty with abdominal adhesive disease. It seems reasonable for these surgeons to understand that overwhelming evidence supports the safety of LSG in couplet with HHR. A systemic review of literature by Mahawar et al. identified over 130 articles focused on LSG and GERD [77]. Of those, 20 described HHR with LSG. Results of the review demonstrated the safety of LSG in couplet with HHR and recommend the simultaneous procedure as an acceptable management strategy. In support of simultaneous LSG and HHR, the International Sleeve Gastrectomy Expert Panel Consensus statement recommended aggressive identification and repair hiatal hernia defects [70].

Technical aspects of the procedure are straightforward. After identifying a crural defect, surgeons will approach reconstruction of the hiatal defect first. Key points in the procedure include reduction of the hernia sac and stomach, circumferential dissection of the phrenoesophageal membranes, identification of both the left and right crus, and crural reconstruction. Although there are descriptions of anterior crural repair, posterior reconstruction with non-absorbable suture is regarded as standard practice [76, 78]. Posterior repair recreates the normal anatomic gastroesophageal angle and anti-reflux mechanism [77]. Using biologic mesh for reinforcement of the hiatal repair is acceptable when circumstances arise.

Treatment of Paraesophageal Hernia During Bariatric Procedures

When large paraesophageal hernias are encountered in the operating room, evidence supports the repair of hernia defects during weight loss surgery. Chaudhry et al. reported their results after simultaneous laparoscopic RYGBP with paraesophageal hernia repair (PEH) [79]. Fourteen patients underwent simultaneous laparoscopic RYGBP and PEH with a follow-up of 3 years. Results showed a significant improvement in reflux symptoms scores and quality of life measures. Importantly, the surgeons did not summon imaging studies to assess hernia recurrence as the patients were asymptomatic for PEH at follow-up. Mesh reinforcement was not utilized in this approach and hence not advocated. When crural tissues are tenuous, biologic mesh is recommended. Pham et al. reported his results of simultaneous laparoscopic paraesophageal hernia and sleeve gastrectomy in the morbidly obese [80]. Out of 23 patients that underwent combined LSG and PEH, 17 underwent posterior mesh reinforcement. After only a short-term follow-up of 6 months, data supported combined LSG and PEH with mesh reinforcement when indicated. Because preoperative EGD is often difficult to diagnose PEH, surgeons should anticipate intraoperative abnormalities including findings of PEH. The authors argue surgeons should possess the skillset for laparoscopic PEH in anticipation of these findings [80].

Future Surgical Options for Reflux Disease in Obese Population (the LINX Procedure)

Despite the reported efficacy of RYGBP or simultaneous LSG with HHR for obese patients with symptoms of GERD, new onset "de novo GERD" develops in up to 20% of patients [81]. Though PPIs have been effective treatments for this population, we must consider the scenario for patient's refractory to PPIs [82]. Operative conversion to RYGBP is an acceptable option for most patients who have severe medically refractory GERD after undergoing LSG. Performing fundoplication of the pouch with the retained stomach is not an alternative for most patients who previously underwent LSG or RYGBP.

The LINX [R] system for lower esophageal augmentation is a new innovative technique that has shown success in treating patients with GERD [83]. In this procedure the surgeon dissects the distal esophagus and implants the small ring of magnetic beads around the lower esophagus between the esophagus and posterior vagus nerve in order to augment the lower esophageal sphincter pressure and mechanically augment the anti-reflux barrier of the LES. The major advantage of the LINX R procedure in patients with GERD post-RYGB or post-LSG is that procedure can be performed in the absence of the fundus of the stomach by placing the magnetic beads around the lower esophageal sphincter, while in most patients after LRYGB or LSG, the absence of the gastric fundus limits the surgeon from performing a fundoplication [84]. Because of the advantages of the LINX R system, surgeons have applied this technique to patient's refractory to PPIs after LSG and RYGBP. One such study evaluated patients with refractory GERD following LSG and results showed that patients had significant improvement in their postoperative GERD score. The authors concluded that the LINX R magnetic sphincter device is a safe and effective option for patients with refractory GERD after LSG [85]. Likewise, application of the LINX R system for patients with GERD after RYGBP has been described as well. Hawasli et al. described a patient who experienced refractory GERD after RYGBP [86]. The patient underwent placement of a LINX R magnetic sphincter augmentation device. Postoperatively the patients reflux symptoms resolved and PPI use was discontinued. Quality of life scores improved after 6 weeks. Likewise, another case report described the successful application of magnetic sphincter augmentation for patients with recalcitrant GERD after LRYGBP**.** Largacha recommended the LINX R device as a safe alternative for this patient population [87]. The preliminary results of LINX R application to patient's refractory to PPIs after LSG or RYGBP appear to be an attractive safe alternative treatment.

Bariatric Surgery in Morbidly Obese Patients with Barrett's Esophagus

Barrett's esophagus in the morbidly obese population represents an interesting topic. Considering the overwhelming evidence in the association between GERD and morbid obesity, there is convincing literature for this population that supports a high rate of progression of reflux disease into development of Barrett's esophagus. Early reports highlighted that among obese patients with GERD, 18% display short-segment Barrett's esophagus, and 9% display long-segment Barrett's esophagus (LSBE) on endoscopic examination [88]. Follow-up studies confirmed that morbidly obese patients are three times more likely to develop Barrett's compared to normal weight individuals, and the odds of development of adenocarcinoma are 16.2 times higher than normal weight individuals [89–92].

Bariatric surgery has been proposed as a treatment for both the Barrett's and for the obesity and several institutions report regression of Barrett's esophagus after RYGBP. Early reports by Csendes showed that in patients with Barrett's esophagus and obesity, four (57%) patients with short-segment Barrett's esophagus (SSBE) and one (20%) of the patients with LSBE showed regression from intestinal metaplasia to cardiac mucosa [93, 94]. A review article on morbidly patients with BE conducted by Csendes and Braghetto in 2016 recommended that LRYGBP is the best surgical option for this patient population. Consensus among gastroenterologists and surgeons has been reached, recommending RYGB for morbidly obese individuals with severe GERD rather than anti-reflux procedures such as Nissen fundoplication [10].

The majority of bariatric surgeons (94.5%) consider BE to be a major contraindication for LSG [95]. They fear the development of "de novo" GERD or persistent GERD after LSG with risk of progression to adenocarcinoma. Gagner contends the development of de novo GERD in patients undergoing LSG is perhaps overstated [28]. Recent evidence estimates "de novo" GERD after LSG to be low, at 5% [96]. Gagner argues the hysteria of GERD and progression to adenocarcinoma after sleeve gastrectomy needs to be tempered as the benefits of LSG outweigh the potential risks [95]. However, the literature strongly supports LRYGBP as the first-line treatment for obese patients with Barrett's esophagus because of the ability to reduce both acid and non-acid refluxate and ameliorate symptoms and preserve the gastric remnant with an intact gastroepiploic vascular supply if the need for a gastric conduit after esophagectomy became necessary. On the other hand LSG is known to reduce LES pressure, increase reflux, and remove the stomach and gastroepiploic vascular arcade that would be used in reconstruction for esophagectomy. Therefore the literature does not support the performance of LSG in patients with Barrett's esophagus unless there is a comprehensive workup and informed decision is made by the patients of the potential risks of GERD exacerbation and progression of Barrett's. Future studies are necessary to define the role of LSG in the setting of obese patients with BE.

Conclusion

GERD is very common in the morbidly obese population and is an important consideration during the preoperative workup, operative planning, and intraoperative management. Preoperative endoscopy is indicated in the symptomatic patient with severe GERD, and the EGD will indicate changes needed in the operative plan. The consensus best operation for patients with severe GERD or Barrett's esophagus is the RYGB. Patients with less severe GERD who are undergoing LSG should have a concomitant hiatal hernia repair to reduce postoperative exacerbation of their GERD. For patients with medically refractory GERD post-LSG or post-RYGB, the placement of the LINX R magnetic beads around the lower esophagus appears to be safe and effective treatment and should be considered.

References

1. Katz PO, Gerson LB, Vela MF. Guidelines for the diagnosis and management of gastroesophageal reflux disease. Am J Gastroenterol. 2013;108:308–28.
2. El-Serag HB, Graham DY, Satia JA, Rabeneck L. Obesity is an independent risk factor for GERD symptoms and erosive esophagitis. Am J Gastroenterol. 2005;100(6):1243–50.
3. Ogden CL, Carroll MD, Curtin LR, McDowell MA, Tabak CJ, Flegal KM. Prevalence of overweight and obesity in the United States, 1999–2004. JAMA. 2006;295:1549–55.
4. Obesity: preventing and managing the global epidemic. Report of a WHO consultation. World Health Organ Tech Rep Ser. 2000;894:i–xii, 1–253.
5. Sandler RS, Everhart JE, Donowitz M, Adama E, Cronin K, Goodman C, et al. The burden of selected digestive diseases in the United States. Gastroenterology. 2002;122(5):1500–11.
6. Shaheen NJ, Hansen RA, Morgan DR, Gangarosa LM, Ringel Y, Thiny MT, et al. The burden of gastrointestinal and liver diseases, 2006. Am J Gastroenterol. 2006;101(9):2128–38.
7. Swedish Obese Subjects Study Scientific Group, Sjöström L, Lindroos AK, Peltonen M, Torgerson J, Bouchard C, Varlsson B, et al. Lifestyle, diabetes, and cardiovascular risk factors 10 years after bariatric surgery. N Engl J Med. 2004;351(26):2683–93.
8. Buchwald H, Avidor Y, Braunwald E, Jensen MD, Pories W, Fahrbach K, et al. Bariatric surgery: a systematic review and meta-analysis. JAMA. 2004;292(14):1724–37.
9. Puzziferri N, Roshek TB III, Mayo HG, Gallagher R, Belle SH, Livingston EH. Long-term follow-up after bariatric surgery: a systematic review. JAMA. 2014;312(9):934–42.
10. Vaezi MF, Brill JV, Mills MR, Bernstein BB, Ness RM, Richards WO, et al. An episode payment framework for gastroesophageal reflux disease. Gastroenterology. 2016;150(4):1019–25.
11. Poelmans J, Tack J. Extraoesophageal manifestations of gastro-oesophageal reflux. Gut. 2005;54(10):1492–9.
12. Trus TL, Hunter JG. Minimally invasive surgery of the esophagus and stomach. Am J Surg. 1997;173(3):242–55.
13. Hampel H, Abraham NS, El-Serag HB. Meta-analysis: obesity and the risk for gastroesophageal reflux disease and its complications. Ann Intern Med. 2005;143(3):199–211.
14. Wilson LJ, Ma W, Hirschowitz BI. Association of obesity with hiatal hernia and esophagitis. Am J Gastroenterol. 1999;94(10):2840–4.
15. Jung HS, Choi MG, Baeg MK, Lim CH, Kim JS, Cho YK, et al. Obesity is associated with increasing esophageal acid exposure in korean patients withgastroesophageal reflux disease symptoms. J Neurogastroenterol Motil. 2013;19(3):338–43.
16. Fass R. The pathophysiological mechanism of GERD in the obese patient. Dig Dis Sci. 2008;53:2300–6.
17. Fornari F, Madalosso CA, Farré R, Gurski RR, Thiesen V, Callegari-Jacques SM. The role of gastro-oesophageal pressure gradient and sliding hiatal hernia on pathological gastro-oesophageal reflux in severely obese patients. Eur J Gastroenterol Hepatol. 2010;22:404–11.
18. De Vries DR, Van Herwaarden MA, Smout AJ, Samsom M. Gastroesophageal pressure gradients in gastroesophageal reflux disease: relations with hiatal hernia, body mass index, and esophageal acid exposure. Am J Gastroenterol. 2008;103:1349–54.
19. Pandolfino JE, El-Serag HB, Zhang Q, Shah N, Ghosh SK, Kahrilas PJ. Obesity: a challenge to esophagogastric junction integrity. Gastroenterology. 2006;130:639–49.

20. Roman S, Pandolfino JE. Environmental – lifestyle related factors. Best Pract Res Clin Gastroenterol. 2010;24:847–59.
21. Tosato F, Marano S, Mattachione S, Luongo B, Paltrinieri G, Mingarelli V, et al. Surgical treatment of gastroesophageal reflux disease. In: Advances in endoscopic surgery: InTech; 2011;1:259–90.
22. Pandolfino JE, Shi G, Trueworthy B, Kahrilas PJ. Esophagogastric junction opening during relaxation distinguishes nonhernia reflux patients, hernia patients, and normal subjects. Gastroenterology. 2003;125:1018–24.
23. Devendran N, Chauhan N, Armstrong D, Upton AR, Kamath MV. GERD and obesity: is the autonomic nervous system the missing link? Crit Rev Biomed Eng. 2014;42(1):17–24. Review.
24. Dobrek L, Nowakowski M, Sygula A, Lipczynski A, Barylak H, Herman RM, et al. 24-hour heart rate variability in patients with gastroesophageal reflux disease. Folia Med Cracov. 2005;46(1–2):53–64.
25. Blevins CH, Shama AN, Johnson ML, Geno D, Gupta M, Bharucha AE, et al. Influence of reflux and central obesity on intercellular space diameter of esophageal squamous epithelium. United European Gastroenterol J. 2016;4(2):177–83.
26. He F, Peng J, Deng XL, et al. Mechanisms of tumor necrosis factor-alpha-induced leaks in intestine epithelial barrier. Cytokine. 2012;59:264–72.
27. Shen L, Weber CR, Raleigh DR, Yu D, Turner JR. Tight junction pore and leak pathways: a dynamic duo. Annu Rev Physiol. 2011;73:283–309.
28. Close H, Mason JM, Wilson D, Hungin AP. Hormone replacement therapy is associated with gastro-oesophageal reflux disease: a retrospective cohort study. BMC Gastroenterol. 2012;12:56.
29. Khan A, Kim A, Sanossian C, Francois F. Impact of obesity treatment on gastroesophageal reflux disease. World J Gastroenterol. 2016;22(4):1627–38.
30. Nahata M, Saegusa Y, Harada Y, Tsuchiya N, Hattori T, Takeda H. Changes in ghrelin-related factors in gastroesophageal reflux disease in rats. Gastroenterol Res Pract. 2013;2013:504816.
31. Rubenstein JH, Morgenstern H, McConell D, Scheiman JM, Schoenfeld P, Appelman H, et al. Associations of diabetes mellitus, insulin, leptin, and ghrelin with gastroesophageal reflux and Barrett's esophagus. Gastroenterology. 2013;145:1237–44.e1–5.
32. Abdelkader NA, Montasser IF, Bioumy EE, Saad WE. Impact of anthropometric measures and serum leptin on severity of gastroesophageal reflux disease. Dis Esophagus. 2015;28:691–8.
33. Kato M, Watabe K, Hamasaki T, Umeda M, Furubayashi A, Kinoshita K, et al. Association of low serum adiponectin levels with erosive esophagitis in men: an analysis of 2405 subjects undergoing physical check-ups. J Gastroenterol. 2011;46:1361–7.
34. American Gastroenterological Association. GERD care pathway. Gastroenterology. 2016;150(4):1026–30.
35. ASGE Standards of Practice Committee, Muthusamy VR, Lightdale JR, Acosta RD, Chandrasekhara V, Chathadi KV, et al. The role of endoscopy in the management of GERD. Gastrointest Endosc. 2015;81(6):1305–10.
36. Moayyedi P, Talley FMB, Vakil N. Can the clinical history distinguish between organic and functional dyspepsia? JAMA. 2006;295:1566–76.
37. Numans ME, Lau J, de Wit NJ, Bonis PA. Short-term treatment with proton pump inhibitors as a test for gastroesophageal reflux disease: a meta-analysis of diagnostic test characteristics. Ann Intern Med. 2004;140:518–27.
38. Kahrilas PJ, Shaheen NJ, Vaezi MF, Hiltz SW, Black E, Modlin IM, et al. American Gastroenterological Association Medical Position Statement on the management of gastroesophageal reflux disease. Gastroenterology. 2008;35:1383–91; 1391.e1–5.
39. Sonnenberg A, Delcò F, El-Serag HB. Empirical therapy versus diagnostic tests in gastroesophageal reflux disease: a medical decision analysis. Dig Dis Sci. 1998;43(5):1001–8.
40. Ates F, Vaezi MF. New approaches to management of PPI-refractory gastroesophageal reflux disease. Curr Treat Options Gastroenterol. 2014;12(1):18–33.
41. Johnsson F, Joelsson B, Gudmundsson K, Greiff L. Symptoms and endoscopic findings in the diagnosis of gastroesophageal reflux disease. Scand J Gastroenterol. 1987;22(6):714–8.
42. Patti MG, Diener U, Tamburini A, Molena D, Way LW. Role of esophageal function tests in diagnosis of gastroesophageal reflux disease. Dig Dis Sci. 2001;46(3):597–602.
43. Ravi K, Katzka DA. Esophageal impedance monitoring: clinical pearls and pitfalls. Am J Gastroenterol. 2016;111:1245–56.
44. Vaezi MF. Diagnosing gastroesophageal reflux disease with endoscopic-guided mucosal impedance. Gastroenterol Hepatol (N Y). 2016;12(4):266–8.
45. Saritas Yuksel E, Higginbotham T, Slaughter JC, Mabary J, Kavitt RT, Garrett CG, et al. Use of direct, endoscopicguided measurements of mucosal impedance in diagnosis of gastroesophageal reflux disease. Clin Gastroenterol Hepatol. 2012;10(10):1110–6.
46. Ates F, Yuksel ES, Higginbotham T, Slaughter JC, Mabary J, Kavitt RT, et al. Mucosal impedance discriminates GERD from non-GERD conditions. Gastroenterology. 2015;148(2):334–43.
47. Stefanidis D, Hope WW, Kohn GP, Reardon PR, Richardson WS, Fanelli RD. Guidelines for surgical treatment of gastroesophageal reflux disease. Surg Endosc. 2010;24:2647–69.
48. Moore M, Afaneh C, Benhuri D, Antonacci C, Abelson J, Zarnegar R. Gastroesophageal reflux disease: a review of surgical decision making. World J Gastrointest Surg. 2016;8(1):77–83.
49. Brethauer S. ASMBS position statement on preoperative supervised weight loss requirements. Surg Obes Relat Dis. 2011;7(3):257–60.

50. Kim JJ, Rogers AM, Ballem N, Schirmer B. American Society for Metabolic and Bariatric Surgery Clinical Issues Committee SMBS updated position statement on insurance mandated preoperative weight loss requirements. Surg Obes Relat Dis. 2016;12(5):955–9.
51. Sauerland S, Angrisani L, Belachew M, Chevallier JM, Favretti F, Finer N, et al. Obesity surgery: evidence-based guidelines of the European Association for Endoscopic Surgery (EAES). Surg Endosc. 2005;19:200–21.
52. Anderson MA, Gan SI, Fanelli RD, Baron TH, Banerjee S, Cash BD, et al. Role of endoscopy in the bariatric surgery patient. Gastrointest Endosc. 2008;68:1–10.
53. De Palma GD, Forestieri P. Role of endoscopy in the bariatric surgery of patients. World J Gastroenterol. 2014;20(24):7777–84.
54. Sharaf RN, Weinshel EH, Bini EJ, Rosenberg J, Sherman A, Ren CJ. Endoscopy plays an important preoperative role in bariatric surgery. Obes Surg. 2004;14:1367–72.
55. Kuper MA, Kratt T, Kramer KM, Zdichavsky M, Schneider JH, Glatzle J, et al. Effort, safety, and findings of routine preoperative endoscopic evaluation of morbidly obese patients undergoing bariatric surgery. Surg Endosc. 2010;24(8):1996–2001.
56. Azagury D, Dumonceau JM, Morel P, Chassot G, Huber O. Preoperative work-up in asymptomatic patients undergoing rouxen-Y gastric bypass: is endoscopymandatory? Obes Surg. 2006;16:1304–11.
57. Mong C, Van Dam J, Morton J, Gerson L, Curet M, Banerjee S. Preoperative endoscopic screening for laparoscopic roux-en-Y gastric bypass has a low yield for anatomic findings. Obes Surg. 2008;18:1067–73.
58. Zanotti D, Elkalaawy M, Hashemi M, Jenkinson A, Adamo M. Current status of preoperative oesophago-gastro-duodenoscopy (OGD) in bariatric NHS units – a BOMSS survey. Obes Surg. 2016;26:2257–62.
59. Bennett S, Gostimir M, Shorr R, Mallick R, Mamazza J, Neville A. The role of routine preoperative upper endoscopy in bariatric surgery: a systematic review and meta-analysis. Surg Obes Relat Dis. 2016;12(5):1116–25.
60. DuPree CE, Blair K, Steele SR, Martin MJ. Laparoscopic sleeve gastrectomy in patients with preexisting gastroesophageal reflux disease: a national analysis. JAMA Surg. 2014;149:328–34.
61. Chiu S, Birch DW, Shi X, et al. Effect of sleeve gastrectomy on gastroesophageal reflux disease: a systematic review. Surg Obes Relat Dis. 2011;7:510–5.
62. Padwal R, Klarenbach S, Wiebe N, Birch D, Karmali S, Manns B, et al. Bariatric surgery: a systemic review and network meta-analysis of randomized trials. Obes Rev. 2011;12:602–21.
63. Hutter MM, Schirmer BD, Jones DB, Ko CY, Cohen ME, Merkow RP, et al. First report from the American College of Surgeons bariatric center network: laparoscopic sleeve gastrectomy has morbidity and effectiveness positioned between the band and bypass. Ann Surg. 2011;254:410–20.
64. Zhang N, Maffei A, Cerabona T, Pahuja A, Omena J, Kaul A. Reduction in obesity-related comorbidities: is gastric bypass better than sleeve gastrectomy? SurgEndosc. 2013;27:1273–80.
65. Vakil N, Talley N, van Zanten SV, Flook N, Persson T, Bjorck E, et al. Cost of detecting malignant lesions by endoscopy in 2741 primary care dyspeptic patients without alarm symptoms. Clin Gastroenterol Hepatol. 2009;7(7):756–61.
66. Madhok BM, Carr WR, McCormack C, Boyle M, Jennings N, Schroeder N, et al. Preoperative endoscopy may reduce the need for revisional surgery for gastro-oesophageal reflux disease following laparoscopic sleeve gastrectomy. Clin Obes. 2016;6(4):268–72.
67. Gómez V, Bhalla R, Heckman MG, Florit PT, Diehl NN, Rawal B, et al. Routine screening endoscopy before bariatric surgery: is it necessary? Bariatric Surg Pract Patient Care. 2014;9(4):143–9.
68. Che F, Nguyen B, Cohen A, Nguyen NT. Prevalence of hiatal hernia in the morbidly obese. Surg Obes Relat Dis. 2013;9(6):920–4.
69. Sharaf RN, Weinshel EH, Bini EJ, Rosenberg J, Ren CJ. Radiologic assessment of the upper gastrointestinal tract: does it play an important preoperative role in bariatric surgery? Obes Surg. 2004;14:313–7.
70. Rosenthal RJ, Diaz AA, Arvidsson D, et al. International sleeve gastrectomy expert panel consensus statement: best practice guidelines based on experience of >12,000 cases. Surg Obes Relat Dis. 2012;8:8–19.
71. Boeckxstaens GE. Review article: the pathophysiology of gastroesophageal reflux disease. Aliment Pharmacol Ther. 2007;15(26):149–60.
72. Nelson LG, Gonzalez R, Haines K, Gallagher SF, Murr MM. Amelioration of gastroesophageal reflux symptoms following Roux – en –Y gastric bypass for clinically significant obesity. Am Surg. 2005;71:950–3.
73. Angrisani L, Santonicola A, Iovino P, et al. Bariatric surgery worldwide 2013. Obes Surg. 2015;25:1822–32.
74. Santonicola A, Angrisani L, et al. The effect of laparoscopic sleeve gastrectomy with or without hiatal hernia repair on gastroesophageal reflux disease in obese patients. Surg Obes Relat Dis. 2014;10:250–6.
75. Iannelli A, Sans A, Martini F. Hiatal hernia, GERD and Sleeve gastrectomy: a complex interplay. Obes Surg. 2016;26(10):2485–7.
76. Lyon A, et al. Gastroesophageal reflux in laparoscopic sleeve gastrectomy: hiatal findings and their management influence outcomes. Surg Obes Releat Dis. 2015;11:530–7.
77. Mahawar, et al. Simultaneous sleeve gastrectomy and hiatus hernia repair: a systematic review. Obes Surg. 2015;25:159–66.
78. Gibson SC, et al. Laparoscopic sleeve gastrectomy: review of 500 cases in single surgeon Australian. ANZ J Surg. 2013;85:673–7.
79. Chaudhry UI, Marr BM, Osayi SN, Mikami DJ, Needleman BJ, Melvin WS, Perry KA. Laparoscopic

Roux-en-Y gastric bypass for treatment of symptomatic paraesophageal hernia in the morbidly obese: medium-term results. Surg Obes Relat Dis. 2014;10(6):1063–7. https://doi.org/10.1016/j.soard.2014.02.004. Epub 2014 Feb 10
80. Pham DV, Protyniak B, Binenbaum SJ, Squillaro A, Borao FJ. Simultaneous laparoscopic paraesophageal hernia repair and sleeve gastrectomy in the morbidly obese. Surg Obes Relat Dis. 2014;10(2):257–61. https://doi.org/10.1016/j.soard.2013.08.003. Epub 2013 Aug 23.
81. Pescarus R, Reavis KM, Swanstorm LL. Gastroesophageal reflux disease in the bariatric population: when is a laparoscoic sleeve gastrectomy the right choice? Surg Obes Relat Dis: Off J Am Soc Bariatric Surg. 2014;10(5):1012.
82. Rebecchi F, Allaix ME, Giaccone C, Ugliono E, Scozzari G, Morino M. Gastroesophageal reflux disease and laparoscopic sleeve gastrectomy: a physiophathologic evaluation. Ann Surg. 2014;260(5):909–14; discussion 914 – 905.
83. Bonavina L, De Meester T, Fockens P, et al. Laparoscopic sphincter augmentation device eliminates reflux symptoms and normalizes esophageal acid exposure: one – and 2 year results of a feasibility trial. Ann Surg. 2010;252(5):857–62.
84. Asti E, Bonitta G, Lovece A, Lazzari V, Bonavina L. Longitudinal comparison of quality of life in patients undergoing laparoscopic Toupet fundoplication versus magnetic sphincter augmentation: Observational cohort study with propensity score analysis. Medicine (Baltimore). 2016;95(30):e4366.
85. Desart K, Rossidis G, Michel M, Lux T, Ben-David K. Gastroesophageal reflux management with the LINX® system for gastroesophageal reflux disease following laparoscopic sleeve gastrectomy. J Gastrointest Surg. 2015;19(10):1782–6. https://doi.org/10.1007/s11605-015-2887-z. Epub 2015 Jul 11.
86. Hawasli A. Laparoscpic management of reflux after roux en Y gastric bypass using the Linx system and repair of hiatal hernia: a case report. Surg Obes Relat Dis. 2016;12:e51–4.
87. Juan A, Largacha M. Lower esophageal magnetic sphincter augmentation for persistent reflux after roux en y gastric bypass. Obes Surg. 2016;26:464–6.
88. Csendes A, Burdiles P, Rojas J, et al. Pathological gastroesophageal reflux in patients with severe , morbid and hyper obesity. Rev Med Chil. 2001;129:1038–43.
89. Varela JE, Hinojosa MW, Nguyen NT. Laparoscopic fundoplication compared with laparoscopic gastric bypass in morbidly obese patients with gastroesophageal reflux disese. Surg Obes Relat Dis. 2009;5:139–43.
90. Kemdrich ML, Houghton SG. Gastreesophageal reflux disease in obese patients: the role of obesity in management. Dis Esophagus. 2006;19:57–63.
91. Gomez Escudero O, Herrera Hernandez MF, Valdovinos Diaz MA. Obesity and gastreesophageal reflux disease. Rev Invest Clin. 2002;54:320–7.
92. Friedenberg FK, Xanthopolous M, Foster GD, et al. The associatioin between gastroesophageal reflux disese and obesity. AM J Gaasstroenterol. 2008;103:2111–22.
93. Csendes A, Burgos AM, Smok G, Henriquez A, et al. Effect of gastric bypass on Barrett's esophagus and intestinal metaplasia of cardia in patietns with morbid obesity. J Gastrointest Surg. 2006;10:259.
94. Pereira N, Csendes A, Smok G, et al. Effect of gastric bypass on Barrett's esophagus in patients with morbid obesity. Rev Chil Cir. 2012;64:155–60.
95. Gagner M. Is sleeve gastrectomy always an absolute contraindication in patients with Barrett's? Obes Surg. 2016;26:715–7.
96. Rebecchi F, Allaix ME, Giaccone C, Uglino E, Scozzari G, Morino M. Gastreesophageal reflux disease and laparoscopic sleeve gastrectomy: a physiolophathologic evaluation. Ann Surg. 2014;260:909–14.

Obesity and Cancer

40

Samer A. Naffouje and George I. Salti

Introduction

The prevalence of obesity has been steadily increasing worldwide, coercing the World Health Organization (WHO) to consider obesity a global epidemic in 1997 [1]. Strikingly, two-thirds of adults in the United States are considered overweight or obese [2], with an alarming rapid expansion in the morbid obesity group, faster than the overall increase in the obesity prevalence [3, 4].

Obesity, as a modifiable behavioral risk factor, was proven to be one of the most common leading causes of death in the United States, second only to tobacco [5], with an estimated 300,000 deaths per year from morbidities directly related to obesity [6]. It was found that even the moderate rise of the body mass index (BMI) above 24.9 into the realm of "overweight" is associated with 20–40% increase in the risk of death [7].

Mediated by various dysregulations in lipid metabolism, obesity constitutes a strong risk factor for the development of cardiovascular disease which carries out the highest mortality rate among obese people [8–10].

Cancer has been rising as the second most common killer in the obese population, with 84,000 new cancer diagnoses per year, or 6% of all cancers, in the United States that are attributed to obesity [11]. Inversely, obesity and overweight contribute to 15–20% of cancer-related mortality [12, 13].

This interrelationship between cancer and obesity poses a significant challenge to healthcare systems presently and a greater challenge in the future. In 2008, medical costs spent on obesity-related morbidities approached $147 billion [14]. By 2030, when half of the population is projected to be obese in the United States [15] and the United Kingdom [16], medical costs associated with treatment of this preventable disease are estimated to increase by $48–66 billion/year in the United States and by £1.9–2 billion/year in the United Kingdom [15, 16].

Based on current evidence, a strong uniform correlation has been reported to exist between adiposity and several surgical malignancies of various histogenesis: endometrial cancer, postmenopausal breast cancer, renal cancer, pancreatic cancer, colorectal cancer, and esophageal/gastric cardia cancer. A less significant correlation has been established with hepatocellular carcinoma, gallbladder cancer, malignant melanoma, thyroid cancer, cervical cancer, and ovarian cancer. Moreover, obesity is considered a risk factor for more aggressive

S. A. Naffouje (✉)
Department of General Surgery, University of Illinois Hospital and Health Sciences System, Chicago, IL, USA
e-mail: snaffouj@uic.edu

G. I. Salti
Department of Surgery, Division of Surgical Oncology, University of Illinois at Chicago, Chicago, IL, USA
e-mail: geosalti@uic.edu

R. Lutfi et al. (eds.), *Global Bariatric Surgery*, https://doi.org/10.1007/978-3-319-93545-4_40

phenotypes of prostate cancer and less likely a causative factor in this case.

Biologic and Pathologic Mechanisms of Tumorigenesis in Obesity

The correlation between obesity and certain malignancies has long been noted via observational studies of various designs, most prominently of which are the reports of the International Agency for Research into Cancer (IARC) [17] and the World Cancer Research Fund (WCRF) [18].

Renehan et al. further consolidated the correlation between obesity and the broad spectrum of cancers reported above in a systematic review and meta-analysis [19]. This landmark report demonstrates an interesting sex-specific correlation and a consistent distribution across various demographic and geographic populations.

However, the matter of paramount importance remains to bridge these epidemiologic findings to a biologic elucidation. Insulin resistance and the resultant hyperinsulinemia, as sequelae of obesity, promote tumorigenesis by reducing the levels of insulin-like growth factor-binding proteins (IGF-BP) which, in turn, increase levels of the free (or unbound) insulin-like growth factor-I (IGF-I) [20, 21]. This dysregulation in the growth factors' network leads to changes in the cellular microenvironment that, in sum, promote cancer development and growth [22]. Recent meta-analyses confirmed the correlation between elevated levels of IGF-I and colorectal, prostate, and breast cancer [23, 24].

The current evidence strongly points to the insulin and the downstream insulin-dependent growth factors to be a likely candidate system for cancer progression. The hypothesis stems from the molecular outcome of the insulin receptor (IR) activation by the growth factors and ligands. The phosphorylation of the IRs by supraphysiologic levels of circulating IGF-I produces a mitogenic and antiapoptotic activity mediated by the extrinsic-regulated kinase (ERK) and phosphatidylinositol-3 (PI-3) [22]. Moreover, this system is involved in promoting cancer invasion and metastasis. Excessive activation of the IR kinase by high levels of circulating IGF-I) was found to cause a loss of integrity of the epithelial lining, thus facilitating cancer cell migration [25].

Another biological aspect linking obesity to cancer development is the sex hormone pathway. Obesity is a well-recognized risk factor for the development of postmenopausal breast cancer via the excessive conversion of androgens to estradiol by the adipose tissue [26]. Two prominent studies by the Endogenous Hormones and Breast Cancer Collaborative Group (EHBCCG) [27] and the European Prospective Investigation into Cancer and Nutrition (EPIC) [28] demonstrated a clear twofold risk of developing postmenopausal breast cancer with increasing level of circulating converted androgens, which, in turn, is correlated with increased BMI. On the other hand, the risk of endometrial cancer in obese patients was biologically proven to be more complex. Not only the elevated levels of circulating estradiol contribute to uncontrolled endothelial proliferation [29], but also IGF-I) was shown to be locally increased in the endometrial tissue due to the unopposed estrogenic shift in the estrogen-progesterone balance that normally controls the endometrial growth cycle [30]. In another field of interest, biologic studies have recently demonstrated that the fatty tissue, contrary to the common belief, is not an inert tissue. It constitutes a large source of many polypeptide hormones that play critical roles in the endocrine and metabolic equilibrium [31]. The most renowned adipokine of this family is the satiety hormone, leptin. The role of leptin in metabolism was established by the Jackson Laboratory after identification of the homozygous leptin-deficient mice *(ob^{-}/ob^{-})* that do not reach satiety and rapidly develop morbid obesity with hyperinsulinemia [32, 33]. The secretion of leptin is proportional to the body fat [34] and is biologically proven to induce mitogenesis in hematopoietic progenitor cells, epithelial cells, and vascular endothelial cells [35–37]. Another ample adipokine is adiponectin whose level, in contrary to leptin, inversely correlates with the amount of body fat [38]. Moreover, in contrast with leptin, adiponectin is considered an antiproliferative and antiapoptotic agent via blockade of

ERK-1 and ERK-2 pathways and stimulation of p53 expression [39]. It also possesses an antiangiogenic effect via induction of apoptosis in the vascular endothelium [40].

On the clinical level, low circulating levels of adiponectin correlated with increased risks of endometrial cancer [41, 42], pre- and postmenopausal breast cancer [43, 44], colorectal cancer in men [45], and advanced phenotypes of prostate cancer [46].

Lastly, many novel hypotheses are developing in an attempt to provide a well-rounded understanding of the relation between obesity and cancer, which cannot be realistically attributed to a single system failure or deviation. The migrating stromal cells [47] and the obesity-related adipose tissue hypoxia [48, 49] are prime examples of the novel theories that address the role of obesity in tumor neoangiogenesis and proliferation.

The trend of the current body of research suggests that more evidence is yet to be delivered in this regard for us to obtain a full scope of how obesity contributes to the neoplastic development and progression and, most importantly, of how we can use that knowledge in cancer screening and prevention.

Obesity and Risk of Esophageal Cancer

Esophageal cancer is the eighth most common malignancy worldwide with an estimated 450,000 new cases per year [50]. Esophageal cancer is considered a dismal diagnosis with a case fatality ratio of ~83% [51], mostly due to the delayed symptoms that do not occur until at least 60% of the circumference is involved, at which point the disease would have reached an advanced stage [52]. The American Cancer Society estimates 17,000 new cases to occur in the United States in 2016 with a male preference of 6:1 and a projected 15,500 mortalities [53]. An alarming incline in the incidence of esophageal cancer has been documented in the past few decades, with a noted fivefold increase in some countries [54]. Along with this incline in incidence, a shift in the histology of esophageal cancer started to emerge. Squamous cell carcinoma, previously the most common histology in the West, has been regressing by ~3.6% per year in the past years [55], in the face of the rise of adenocarcinoma which now constitutes slightly more than 50% of the cases [56]. Regarding the location, the incidence of distal and junctional esophageal cancer increased from 4 to 23 per million in the past three decades, indicating a true extrinsic interference in the etiology and histology of this disease.

The correlation between obesity and the increasing incidence of esophageal adenocarcinoma was first reported in the mid-1990s [57, 58], followed by numerous large population-based studies from different parts of the globe confirming the solid correlation between the increasing BMI as a marker of obesity and esophageal adenocarcinoma [59, 60]. Thereafter, many prospective studies were conducted to further assess the impact of obesity on the development of esophageal adenocarcinoma [61–71], which uniformly reported a relative risk of 2.54–5.32 for the development of esophageal cancer in obese patients compared to their normal peers. One study reported a relative risk as high as 11.3 (95% CI, 3.5–36.4; $P < 0.001$) for lower esophageal cancer when the reference cohort was constituted of patients with BMI<22 [70]. Based on this epidemiologic evidence, it is safe to conclude that obesity might have an independent carcinogenic role in the occurrence of esophageal adenocarcinoma. The research effort concerning the underlying mechanism is emerging on multiple axes [72], including, but not limited to, polymorphism in genetic coding of the IGF proteins as potential marker of esophageal adenocarcinoma, where the 1013G>A variant in obesity predisposes the patient to a higher risk of developing this malignancy [73, 74]. Also, the male preference strongly suggests a role for sex hormones in the tumorigenesis of this malignancy [75–77].

Obesity and Risk of Breast Cancer

Breast cancer remains, by far, the most common invasive malignancy in females comprising 23% of invasive and 16% of all cancers in females second only to noninvasive non-melanoma skin cancers [78, 79]. This malignancy expresses an interesting behavioral paradox in terms of its relation to obesity. Premenopausal breast cancers, which tend to be estrogen receptor (ER) and progesterone receptor (PR) negative, are not typically associated with obesity. In fact, obesity may have a protective effect in this patient group (reviewed elsewhere by Rose and Vona-Davis [80]). Nevertheless, several studies challenged this statement by reporting a positive correlation between obesity and the incidence of triple negative breast cancers [81–84], which was confirmed in a meta-analysis to be restricted to premenopausal women [85].

On the other hand, postmenopausal breast cancers are predominantly ER^{+}/PR^{+}. Therefore, the contribution of obesity to the development and progression of this cancer becomes more prominent via the converted estrogens in the abundant adipose tissue [86]. This hormonal causative theory in postmenopausal women is further confirmed by the clinical sequelae it casts on the treatment plan; obese women demonstrate lower rates of response to aromatase inhibitors due to the excess of body fat and its large capacity of estradiol synthesis [87, 88]. Hyperinsulinemia, as part of the metabolic syndrome, was also shown to place this subset of patients at a significantly higher risk of breast cancer. High circulating insulin levels in fasting nondiabetic postmenopausal women predispose the patients to at least twice the risk of developing breast cancer than the comparative control population [89, 90]. Additionally, obesity is accompanied by a diet-induced chronic inflammation in the mammary adipose tissue. The capacious release of inflammatory markers and proteins, such as TNF-α, MMP-9, VEGF, MCP-1, and leptin, by the infiltrating macrophages and stromal adipocytes is conducive to tumorigenesis by enhancing cellular proliferation, migration, invasion, and angiogenesis [91–95].

In conclusion, the current evidence highlights a palpable impact of obesity in the development of breast cancer. Simple obesity indices, such as waist-hip ratio, upper body obesity, and BMI, have repeatedly shown a positive correlation with breast cancer [96, 97], which may be interrupted by hormone replacement therapy [97], further emphasizing the impact of the adipose tissue on the hormonal balance in females.

Obesity and Risk of Colorectal Cancer

Current knowledge of colorectal cancer estimates that 5%, or 1 in 20 Americans, will be diagnosed with this disease during their lifetime [98]. Both the incidence and the mortality of colorectal cancer have been on a steady decline since the 1980s. This remarkable change in the natural course of the disease is mostly attributed to the detection and early removal of the precancerous lesions by standardizing the screening methods [99]. Therefore, the efforts are being directed to the tertiary prevention of colorectal cancer, most importantly by understanding the modifiable risk factors of this malignancy.

Adiposity, as a fundamental part of the metabolic syndrome, is reported to be involved in every step of the epithelial progression into a neoplasm by inducing the mutations in the APC, KRAS, MSI, DCC/DPC4, and p53 genes [100]. Hence, many epidemiologic studies queried about the associated risk of obesity for the development of colorectal adenomas [101–104]. All studies showed a small but significant association between obesity and colorectal adenomas across demographic, geographic, and racial variables. More specifically, greater waist circumference was reported to inflict a significantly increased risk of developing colorectal adenomas (OR = 1.32) [105].

In regard to colorectal adenocarcinoma, all large meta-analyses concluded that obesity is a significant modifiable risk factor with an RR = 1.09–1.95 and 1.12–1.15 in men and women, respectively [106–110]. A topic of prime interest in colorectal cancer is the impact of obesity on the surgical outcome, given that colectomy is considered a major intervention performed by both general and colorectal surgeons.

Numerous studies were conducted in this effort; observational studies [111–130], reviews

[131], and a meta-analysis [132], all of which were in accord that obesity increases the risk of conversion rates in laparoscopic surgeries and thus operating times and is associated with increased postoperative complications. Also, some reports indicated that the quality of the oncologic resection is hindered by the excess adiposity, with fewer lymph nodes retrieved in obese patients [111, 133].

In summary, an integrated relation exists between obesity and colorectal cancer from the early stages of development of epithelial adenomas to the incidence of colorectal adenocarcinoma and finally to influencing the surgical outcome in terms of resection quality and complication rates. Decreasing the prevalence of obesity may be a key part in the tertiary prevention of colorectal cancer in the future.

Obesity and Risk of Hepatocellular Carcinoma

Although not very common in the United States, liver cancer, or hepatocellular carcinoma (HCC), is considered the third most common killer among cancers worldwide [51], with a projected 5-year survival of only 10% of all comers at the time of diagnosis [134].

Unlike colorectal cancer, the incidence of HCC in the United States underwent an alarming threefold increase between 1975 and 2006 [135]. About half of this expansion was attributed to the increase in hepatitis C infections. However, the other common causes of hepatitis, such as hepatitis B virus and alcoholic liver disease, did not demonstrate a surge that matches or explains the inclining graph of HCC incidence [136, 137]. These facts urged the thought of other risk factors that could contribute to this significant rise in HCC occurrence. Indeed, many epidemiologic studies and analyses determined that overweight and obesity are independent risk factors for the development of HCC [138–146]. A meta-analysis by Larsson and Wolk asserted these findings with a calculated relative risk of HCC of 1.17 and 1.89 in the overweight and obese American population, respectively [147].

Aside from the pro-cancerous molecular mechanisms that were previously discussed, 90% of obese patients develop the nonalcoholic fatty liver disease (NAFLD), 30% of whom progress into nonalcoholic steatohepatitis (NASH) [148], a predisposing condition for HCC.

Like other obesity-related malignancies, the presented evidence suggests a possible role for the elimination of obesity in the prevention of HCC.

Obesity and Risk of Gallbladder and Extrahepatic Biliary Cancer

Gallbladder cancer (GBC) and the extrahepatic biliary cancer (EBC) are a group of malignancy commonly referred to as the biliary tract cancers. GBC is the most common biliary tract cancer and the sixth most common malignancy of the gastrointestinal tract [149, 150]. It typically carries a poor prognosis with an expected 5-year survival of ~30% [151]. Unlike EBC which affects more men than women, GBC has a slight preference toward females [152, 153]. Biliary tract cancers are somewhat uncommon in the United States, compared to other ethnic groups such as the American Indians and Chilean Mapuches [154], and other geographic locations such in certain areas in South America where GBC is considered the most common killer cancer in females [155].

To date, the relation between obesity and biliary tract cancers has not been clearly established. Many studies of various designs reported on this topic; cohort [63, 141, 144, 156–161] and case-control studies [152, 162–168] reported conflicting conclusion about the risk of biliary tract cancer in obese patients. Even meta-analyses were not in accord about the influence of obesity on biliary cancer incidence; one meta-analyses by Park et al. [169] concluded that obesity may contribute to benign biliary tract diseases rather than malignancies and another by Li et al. [170] whose pooled analysis demonstrated a significant risk of both overweight and obesity for the development of GBC (RR 1.17 and 1.62, respectively) and EBC (RR 1.26 and 1.48, respectively). Of note, the latter meta-analysis is more recent and inclusive of a broader range of observational studies for both GBC and EBC.

The mechanism in which obesity may contribute to the progression biliary tract cancers remains understudied and unclear. In lack of strong epidemiologic and clinical indicators that obesity functions as an independent risk factor for either GBC or EBC, the biologic evidence remains vague and hard to interpret. The deviation in incidence toward either of the genders in these cancers may suggest a role for sexual hormones, but this remains an observational extrapolation.

In conclusion, the current evidence is not considered sufficient to establish a definite association between obesity and biliary tract malignancies, despite a strong trend toward increased risk of occurrence in obese patients.

Obesity and Risk of Pancreatic Cancer

Pancreatic cancer is considered a disease of the developed world with ~70% of the new cases originating from the Western countries yearly [50]. Pancreatic malignancies of all histological types are the fourth most common cause of cancer death in the United States [171]. This disease carries a fearful reputation which stems from its substantial fatality rate with projected 1-year and 5-year survival of 25% and 5%, respectively [172]. With the best surgical treatment, 5-year survival following the diagnosis of pancreatic cancer might improve to 18–24% [173].

Like smoking, the correlation between obesity as an independent risk factor and pancreatic cancer, particularly pancreatic duct adenocarcinoma (PDAC), has been firmly instituted through large population-based epidemiologic and observational studies [29, 145, 174–176]. Obesity has been shown to increase the risk of PDAC occurrence by 10% and then 14% for each 5 kg/m^2 incremental increase above the normal BMI [177, 178]. Remarkably, obesity, as a continuous variable, is conducive of an earlier age of onset and decreased survival in a linear and dose-dependent fashion [179].

In a specific relevance to PDAC, fat-rich diet and adiposity played a critical causative role in the development of PDAC in mouse models [180–182]. This was explained by the diet-induced inflammatory state in the pancreatic tissue mediated by cyclooxygenase-2 (COX2), which leads to an increased activation of the KRAS proto-oncogene and, in consequence, increased growth and neoplasia in the ductal endothelium [183].

In the scenario of PDAC, obesity is an inveterate risk factor. Any parameter of obesity including the BMI, central obesity, waist circumference, and waist-to-hip ratio is shown to reflect an increased association with PDAC and its mortality [184–188].

Given the poor prognosis of pancreatic cancer, weight reduction is unlikely to have an impact on survival in obese patients following the diagnosis. However, weight loss carries a promise of tertiary prevention from PDAC given the strong association between obesity and this malignancy.

Bariatric Surgery and Cancer

The World Health Organization (WHO) recognized obesity as a worldwide epidemic with more than 30 million cases diagnosed per year [189], contributing by a large margin to increased healthcare-related mortality and cost, urging many international organization to initiate a call for action [190, 191].

The previously presented evidence clearly demonstrates a solid correlation between obesity and several cancers of different histogenesis, most of which fall within the scope of interest of general and/or minimally invasive surgeons. Henceforth, this raises the question of the influence of bariatric surgery on the incidence of these cancers.

All three types of bariatric or metabolic surgeries, malabsorptive, restrictive, and the combination of both, were studied in regard to their impact on cancer incidence. The overwhelming majority of registry-based data analysis, population-based studies, systematic reviews, and randomized trials corresponded in reporting reduced cancer incidence rates with successful weight loss following bariatric surgery [7, 192–202]. A meta-analysis by Casagrande et al. [203] corroborated the protective influence of bariatric surgery in morbidly obese patients, with an odds ratio of 0.12–0.88 in the reviewed controlled studies. Moreover, this meta-analysis tallied a cancer incidence density rate of 1.06 cases per 1000 persons-years following bariatric surgery versus the average incidence density rate of 5.5 per 1000 persons-years in the obese populations that have not received a metabolic intervention [203].

On the other hand, few studies disagreed with the reported benefit of bariatric surgery. Instead, they reported an increased risk of certain malignancies after bariatric surgeries, such as colorectal carcinoma [204], and attributed this phenomenon to the colonic mucosal changes following malabsorptive surgeries.

In general, the current evidence demonstrates that weight reduction, regardless of the method, results in decreased rates of cancer incidence [202]. However, parallel experiences with weight loss showed that weight loss by pharmacological means inflicts adverse outcomes on cardiovascular surgeries and increases mortality [205, 206], suggesting that bariatric surgeries might represent a safer method of weight loss in this specific group of patients. Such data are not available for the oncologic patient population where further investigation is warranted.

Nevertheless, estimating the risk reduction of cancer in the bariatric surgery population has its own inherent shortcomings; metabolic surgery is considered more frequently for young or middle-aged obese patients [207], whereas cancer is considered by large an elderly disease [149], suggesting a lead-time bias in this analysis.

Also, candidates for bariatric surgery generally undergo an extensive workup prior to their planned intervention which increases the odds of early cancer detection in this population preoperatively. Finally, the current body of literature does not dissect through the types of bariatric surgeries and their specific impact on cancer incidence creating a twofold limitation; it remains unknown whether a certain type of obesity surgeries is superior to the others in cancer prevention, which could potentially affect the procedure's choice in high-risk patients. In addition, detecting a difference between the types of bariatric surgery in their anticancer effect might help understand the mechanism through which weight reduction exerts its cancer-protective effect.

In conclusion, bariatric surgery is associated with a regression in cancer incidence of many origins. The positive correlation between obesity and cancer, along with the evidence of cancer reduction following weight loss, fulfills the pillars of the Bradford Hill criteria for the causative association between obesity and cancer [208, 209].

References

1. Caballero B. The global epidemic of obesity: an overview. Epidemiol Rev. 2007;29:1–5.
2. Flegal KM, Carroll MD, Ogden CL, Johnson CL. Prevalence and trends in obesity among US adults, 1999–2000. JAMA. 2002;288(14):1723–7.
3. Howard NJ, Taylor AW, Gill TK, Chittleborough CR. Severe obesity: investigating the socio-demographics within the extremes of body mass index. Obes Res Clin Pract. 2008;2(1):I–II.
4. Sturm R. Increases in morbid obesity in the USA: 2000–2005. Public Health. 2007;121(7):492–6.
5. Mokdad AH, Marks JS, Stroup DF, Gerberding JL. Actual causes of death in the United States, 2000. JAMA. 2004;291(10):1238–45.
6. Flegal KM, Williamson DF, Pamuk ER, Rosenberg HM. Estimating deaths attributable to obesity in the United States. Am J Public Health. 2004;94(9):1486–9.
7. Adams KF, Schatzkin A, Harris TB, Kipnis V, Mouw T, Ballard-Barbash R, et al. Overweight, obesity, and mortality in a large prospective cohort of persons 50 to 71 years old. N Engl J Med. 2006;355(8):763–78.
8. Berrington de Gonzalez A, Hartge P, Cerhan JR, Flint AJ, Hannan L, MacInnis RJ, et al. Body-mass index and mortality among 146 million white adults. N Engl J Med. 2010;363(23):2211–9.
9. de Koning L, Merchant AT, Pogue J, Anand SS. Waist circumference and waist-to-hip ratio as predictors of cardiovascular events: meta-regression analysis of prospective studies. Eur Heart J. 2007;28(7):850–6.
10. Whitlock G, Lewington S, Sherliker P, Clarke R, Emberson J, Halsey J, et al. Body-mass index and cause-specific mortality in 900 000 adults: collaborative analyses of 57 prospective studies. Lancet. 2009;373(9669):1083–96.
11. Polednak AP. Estimating the number of U.S. incident cancers attributable to obesity and the impact on temporal trends in incidence rates for obesity-related cancers. Cancer Detect Prev. 2008;32(3):190–9.

12. National Institute of Health NCI. Obesity and cancer risk. National Cancer Institute; 2012. Available from: http://www.cancer.gov/about-cancer/causes-prevention/risk/obesity/obesity-fact-sheet.
13. Society AC. Cancer facts & figures 2012. 2012. Available from: http://www.cancer.org/research/cancerfactsstatistics/cancerfactsfigures2012/.
14. Finkelstein EA, Trogdon JG, Cohen JW, Dietz W. Annual medical spending attributable to obesity: payer-and service-specific estimates. Health Aff (Millwood). 2009;28(5):w822–31.
15. Finkelstein EA, Khavjou OA, Thompson H, Trogdon JG, Pan L, Sherry B, et al. Obesity and severe obesity forecasts through 2030. Am J Prev Med. 2012;42(6):563–70.
16. Wang YC, McPherson K, Marsh T, Gortmaker SL, Brown M. Health and economic burden of the projected obesity trends in the USA and the UK. Lancet. 2011;378(9793):815–25.
17. Vainio H, Bianchini F, editors. Weight control and physical activity. Lyon: IARC Press/International Agency for Research in Cancer; 2002.
18. Food, nutrition, physical activity, and the prevention of cancer: a global perspective. Washington, DC: World Cancer Research Fund; 2007.
19. Renehan AG, Tyson M, Egger M, Heller RF, Zwahlen M. Body-mass index and incidence of cancer: a systematic review and meta-analysis of prospective observational studies. Lancet. 2008;371(9612):569–78.
20. McKeown-Eyssen G. Epidemiology of colorectal cancer revisited: are serum triglycerides and/or plasma glucose associated with risk? Cancer Epidemiol Biomark Prev. 1994;3(8):687–95.
21. Giovannucci E. Insulin and colon cancer. Cancer Causes Control. 1995;6(2):164–79.
22. Roberts DL, Dive C, Renehan AG. Biological mechanisms linking obesity and cancer risk: new perspectives. Annu Rev Med. 2010;61:301–16.
23. Renehan AG, Zwahlen M, Minder C, O'Dwyer ST, Shalet SM, Egger M. Insulin-like growth factor (IGF)-I, IGF binding protein-3, and cancer risk: systematic review and meta-regression analysis. Lancet. 2004;363(9418):1346–53.
24. Renehan AG, Harvie M, Howell A. Insulin-like growth factor (IGF)-I, IGF binding protein-3, and breast cancer risk: eight years on. Endocr Relat Cancer. 2006;13(2):273–8.
25. Chan BT, Lee AV. Insulin receptor substrates (IRSs) and breast tumorigenesis. J Mammary Gland Biol Neoplasia. 2008;13(4):415–22.
26. Renehan AG. Hormones, growth factors, and tumor growth. Oxford: Oxford University Press; 2007.
27. Key TJ, Appleby PN, Reeves GK, Roddam A, Dorgan JF, Longcope C, et al. Body mass index, serum sex hormones, and breast cancer risk in postmenopausal women. J Natl Cancer Inst. 2003;95(16):1218–26.
28. Kaaks R, Rinaldi S, Key TJ, Berrino F, Peeters PH, Biessy C, et al. Postmenopausal serum androgens, oestrogens and breast cancer risk: the European prospective investigation into cancer and nutrition. Endocr Relat Cancer. 2005;12(4):1071–82.
29. Calle EE, Kaaks R. Overweight, obesity and cancer: epidemiological evidence and proposed mechanisms. Nat Rev Cancer. 2004;4(8):579–91.
30. Kaaks R, Lukanova A, Kurzer MS. Obesity, endogenous hormones, and endometrial cancer risk: a synthetic review. Cancer Epidemiol Biomark Prev. 2002;11(12):1531–43.
31. Fischer-Posovszky P, Wabitsch M, Hochberg Z. Endocrinology of adipose tissue – an update. Horm Metab Res. 2007;39(5):314–21.
32. Friedman JM, Leibel RL, Bahary N. Molecular mapping of obesity genes. Mamm Genome. 1991;1(3):130–44.
33. Zhang Y, Proenca R, Maffei M, Barone M, Leopold L, Friedman JM. Positional cloning of the mouse obese gene and its human homologue. Nature. 1994;372(6505):425–32.
34. Schaffler A, Scholmerich J, Buechler C. Mechanisms of disease: adipokines and breast cancer – endocrine and paracrine mechanisms that connect adiposity and breast cancer. Nat Clin Pract Endocrinol Metab. 2007;3(4):345–54.
35. Vona-Davis L, Rose DP. Adipokines as endocrine, paracrine, and autocrine factors in breast cancer risk and progression. Endocr Relat Cancer. 2007;14(2):189–206.
36. Bray GA. The underlying basis for obesity: relationship to cancer. J Nutr. 2002;132(11 Suppl):3451S–5S.
37. Rose DP, Komninou D, Stephenson GD. Obesity, adipocytokines, and insulin resistance in breast cancer. Obes Rev. 2004;5(3):153–65.
38. Fasshauer M, Klein J, Neumann S, Eszlinger M, Paschke R. Hormonal regulation of adiponectin gene expression in 3T3-L1 adipocytes. Biochem Biophys Res Commun. 2002;290(3):1084–9.
39. Dieudonne MN, Bussiere M, Dos Santos E, Leneveu MC, Giudicelli Y, Pecquery R. Adiponectin mediates antiproliferative and apoptotic responses in human MCF7 breast cancer cells. Biochem Biophys Res Commun. 2006;345(1):271–9.
40. Brakenhielm E, Veitonmaki N, Cao R, Kihara S, Matsuzawa Y, Zhivotovsky B, et al. Adiponectin-induced antiangiogenesis and antitumor activity involve caspase-mediated endothelial cell apoptosis. Proc Natl Acad Sci U S A. 2004;101(8):2476–81.
41. Petridou E, Mantzoros C, Dessypris N, Koukoulomatis P, Addy C, Voulgaris Z, et al. Plasma adiponectin concentrations in relation to endometrial cancer: a case-control study in Greece. J Clin Endocrinol Metab. 2003;88(3):993–7.
42. Dal Maso L, Augustin LS, Karalis A, Talamini R, Franceschi S, Trichopoulos D, et al. Circulating adiponectin and endometrial cancer risk. J Clin Endocrinol Metab. 2004;89(3):1160–3.
43. Miyoshi Y, Funahashi T, Kihara S, Taguchi T, Tamaki Y, Matsuzawa Y, et al. Association of serum adiponectin levels with breast cancer risk. Clin Cancer Res. 2003;9(15):5699–704.

44. Mantzoros C, Petridou E, Dessypris N, Chavelas C, Dalamaga M, Alexe DM, et al. Adiponectin and breast cancer risk. J Clin Endocrinol Metab. 2004;89(3):1102–7.
45. Wei EK, Giovannucci E, Fuchs CS, Willett WC, Mantzoros CS. Low plasma adiponectin levels and risk of colorectal cancer in men: a prospective study. J Natl Cancer Inst. 2005;97(22):1688–94.
46. Goktas S, Yilmaz MI, Caglar K, Sonmez A, Kilic S, Bedir S. Prostate cancer and adiponectin. Urology. 2005;65(6):1168–72.
47. Zhang Y, Daquinag A, Traktuev DO, Amaya-Manzanares F, Simmons PJ, March KL, et al. White adipose tissue cells are recruited by experimental tumors and promote cancer progression in mouse models. Cancer Res. 2009;69(12):5259–66.
48. Bedogni B, Welford SM, Cassarino DS, Nickoloff BJ, Giaccia AJ, Powell MB. The hypoxic microenvironment of the skin contributes to Akt-mediated melanocyte transformation. Cancer Cell. 2005;8(6):443–54.
49. Bedogni B, Welford SM, Kwan AC, Ranger-Moore J, Saboda K, Powell MB. Inhibition of phosphatidylinositol-3-kinase and mitogen-activated protein kinase kinase 1/2 prevents melanoma development and promotes melanoma regression in the transgenic TPRas mouse model. Mol Cancer Ther. 2006;5(12):3071–7.
50. World Cancer Report 2014. World Health Organization; 2014.
51. Parkin DM, Bray F, Ferlay J, Pisani P. Global cancer statistics, 2002. CA Cancer J Clin. 2005;55(2):74–108.
52. Mayer RJ. Harrison's principles of internal medicine. 18th ed. New York: McGraw-Hill Medical Publishing Division; 2008.
53. American Cancer Society. Cancer facts & figures 2016. Available at http://www.cancer.org/acs/groups/content/@research/documents/document/acspc-047079.pdf. Accessed 8 Aug.
54. Pohl H, Welch HG. The role of overdiagnosis and reclassification in the marked increase of esophageal adenocarcinoma incidence. J Natl Cancer Inst. 2005;97(2):142–6.
55. Siegel R, Naishadham D, Jemal A. Cancer statistics, 2012. CA Cancer J Clin. 2012;62(1):10–29.
56. Raman R, Deorah S, McDowell BD, Abu Hejleh T, Lynch CF, Gupta A. Changing incidence of esophageal cancer among white women: analysis of SEER data (1992–2010). Contemp Oncol (Pozn). 2015;19(4):338–40.
57. Brown LM, Swanson CA, Gridley G, Swanson GM, Schoenberg JB, Greenberg RS, et al. Adenocarcinoma of the esophagus: role of obesity and diet. J Natl Cancer Inst. 1995;87(2):104–9.
58. Vaughan TL, Davis S, Kristal A, Thomas DB. Obesity, alcohol, and tobacco as risk factors for cancers of the esophagus and gastric cardia: adenocarcinoma versus squamous cell carcinoma. Cancer Epidemiol Biomark Prev. 1995;4(2):85–92.
59. Whiteman DC, Sadeghi S, Pandeya N, Smithers BM, Gotley DC, Bain CJ, et al. Combined effects of obesity, acid reflux and smoking on the risk of adenocarcinomas of the oesophagus. Gut. 2008;57(2):173–80.
60. Chow WH, Blot WJ, Vaughan TL, Risch HA, Gammon MD, Stanford JL, et al. Body mass index and risk of adenocarcinomas of the esophagus and gastric cardia. J Natl Cancer Inst. 1998;90(2):150–5.
61. Abnet CC, Freedman ND, Hollenbeck AR, Fraumeni JF Jr, Leitzmann M, Schatzkin A. A prospective study of BMI and risk of oesophageal and gastric adenocarcinoma. Eur J Cancer. 2008;44(3):465–71.
62. Reeves GK, Pirie K, Beral V, Green J, Spencer E, Bull D, et al. Cancer incidence and mortality in relation to body mass index in the Million Women Study: cohort study. BMJ. 2007;335(7630):1134.
63. Samanic C, Chow WH, Gridley G, Jarvholm B, Fraumeni JF Jr. Relation of body mass index to cancer risk in 362,552 Swedish men. Cancer Causes Control. 2006;17(7):901–9.
64. Merry AH, Schouten LJ, Goldbohm RA, van den Brandt PA. Body mass index, height and risk of adenocarcinoma of the oesophagus and gastric cardia: a prospective cohort study. Gut. 2007;56(11):1503–11.
65. MacInnis RJ, English DR, Hopper JL, Giles GG. Body size and composition and the risk of gastric and oesophageal adenocarcinoma. Int J Cancer. 2006;118(10):2628–31.
66. Engeland A, Tretli S, Bjorge T. Height and body mass index in relation to esophageal cancer; 23-year follow-up of two million Norwegian men and women. Cancer Causes Control. 2004;15(8):837–43.
67. Lagergren J, Bergstrom R, Nyren O. Association between body mass and adenocarcinoma of the esophagus and gastric cardia. Ann Intern Med. 1999;130(11):883–90.
68. Veugelers PJ, Porter GA, Guernsey DL, Casson AG. Obesity and lifestyle risk factors for gastroesophageal reflux disease, Barrett esophagus and esophageal adenocarcinoma. Dis Esophagus. 2006;19(5):321–8.
69. Figueroa JD, Terry MB, Gammon MD, Vaughan TL, Risch HA, Zhang FF, et al. Cigarette smoking, body mass index, gastro-esophageal reflux disease, and non-steroidal anti-inflammatory drug use and risk of subtypes of esophageal and gastric cancers by P53 overexpression. Cancer Causes Control. 2009;20(3):361–8.
70. Ryan AM, Rowley SP, Fitzgerald AP, Ravi N, Reynolds JV. Adenocarcinoma of the oesophagus and gastric cardia: male preponderance in association with obesity. Eur J Cancer. 2006;42(8):1151–8.
71. Corley DA, Kubo A, Zhao W. Abdominal obesity and the risk of esophageal and gastric cardia carcinomas. Cancer Epidemiol Biomark Prev. 2008;17(2):352–8.
72. Chen Q, Zhuang H, Liu Y. The association between obesity factor and esophageal cancer. J Gastrointest Oncol. 2012;3(3):226–31.
73. McElholm AR, McKnight AJ, Patterson CC, Johnston BT, Hardie LJ, Murray LJ, et al. A

population-based study of IGF axis polymorphisms and the esophageal inflammation, metaplasia, adenocarcinoma sequence. Gastroenterology. 2010;139(1):204–12 e3.
74. MacDonald K, Porter GA, Guernsey DL, Zhao R, Casson AG. A polymorphic variant of the insulin-like growth factor type I receptor gene modifies risk of obesity for esophageal adenocarcinoma. Cancer Epidemiol. 2009;33(1):37–40.
75. Armstrong RW, Borman B. Trends in incidence rates of adenocarcinoma of the oesophagus and gastric cardia in New Zealand, 1978–1992. Int J Epidemiol. 1996;25(5):941–7.
76. Lepage C, Rachet B, Jooste V, Faivre J, Coleman MP. Continuing rapid increase in esophageal adenocarcinoma in England and Wales. Am J Gastroenterol. 2008;103(11):2694–9.
77. Brown LM, Devesa SS, Chow WH. Incidence of adenocarcinoma of the esophagus among white Americans by sex, stage, and age. J Natl Cancer Inst. 2008;100(16):1184–7.
78. World Cancer Report. International Agency for Research on Cancer; 2008.
79. Breast cancer: prevention and control. World Health Organization.
80. Rose DP, Vona-Davis L. Biochemical and molecular mechanisms for the association between obesity, chronic inflammation, and breast cancer. Biofactors. 2014;40(1):1–12.
81. Millikan RC, Newman B, Tse CK, Moorman PG, Conway K, Dressler LG, et al. Epidemiology of basal-like breast cancer. Breast Cancer Res Treat. 2008;109(1):123–39.
82. Vona-Davis L, Rose DP, Hazard H, Howard-McNatt M, Adkins F, Partin J, et al. Triple-negative breast cancer and obesity in a rural Appalachian population. Cancer Epidemiol Biomark Prev. 2008;17(12):3319–24.
83. Trivers KF, Lund MJ, Porter PL, Liff JM, Flagg EW, Coates RJ, et al. The epidemiology of triple-negative breast cancer, including race. Cancer Causes Control. 2009;20(7):1071–82.
84. Yang XR, Chang-Claude J, Goode EL, Couch FJ, Nevanlinna H, Milne RL, et al. Associations of breast cancer risk factors with tumor subtypes: a pooled analysis from the Breast Cancer Association Consortium studies. J Natl Cancer Inst. 2011;103(3):250–63.
85. Pierobon M, Frankenfeld CL. Obesity as a risk factor for triple-negative breast cancers: a systematic review and meta-analysis. Breast Cancer Res Treat. 2013;137(1):307–14.
86. Rose DP, Gracheck PJ, Vona-Davis L. The interactions of obesity, inflammation and insulin resistance in breast cancer. Cancers (Basel). 2015;7(4):2147–68.
87. Sestak I, Distler W, Forbes JF, Dowsett M, Howell A, Cuzick J. Effect of body mass index on recurrences in tamoxifen and anastrozole treated women: an exploratory analysis from the ATAC trial. J Clin Oncol. 2010;28(21):3411–5.
88. Pfeiler G, Stoger H, Dubsky P, Mlineritsch B, Singer C, Balic M, et al. Efficacy of tamoxifen +/− aminoglutethimide in normal weight and overweight postmenopausal patients with hormone receptor-positive breast cancer: an analysis of 1509 patients of the ABCSG-06 trial. Br J Cancer. 2013;108(7):1408–14.
89. Kabat GC, Kim M, Caan BJ, Chlebowski RT, Gunter MJ, Ho GY, et al. Repeated measures of serum glucose and insulin in relation to postmenopausal breast cancer. Int J Cancer. 2009;125(11):2704–10.
90. Gunter MJ, Hoover DR, Yu H, Wassertheil-Smoller S, Rohan TE, Manson JE, et al. Insulin, insulin-like growth factor-I, and risk of breast cancer in postmenopausal women. J Natl Cancer Inst. 2009;101(1):48–60.
91. Kim S, Choi JH, Kim JB, Nam SJ, Yang JH, Kim JH, et al. Berberine suppresses TNF-alpha-induced MMP-9 and cell invasion through inhibition of AP-1 activity in MDA-MB-231 human breast cancer cells. Molecules. 2008;13(12):2975–85.
92. Eichbaum C, Meyer AS, Wang N, Bischofs E, Steinborn A, Bruckner T, et al. Breast cancer cell-derived cytokines, macrophages and cell adhesion: implications for metastasis. Anticancer Res. 2011;31(10):3219–27.
93. Murdoch C, Muthana M, Coffelt SB, Lewis CE. The role of myeloid cells in the promotion of tumour angiogenesis. Nat Rev Cancer. 2008;8(8):618–31.
94. Keeley EC, Mehrad B, Strieter RM. Chemokines as mediators of tumor angiogenesis and neovascularization. Exp Cell Res. 2011;317(5):685–90.
95. Engeli S, Feldpausch M, Gorzelniak K, Hartwig F, Heintze U, Janke J, et al. Association between adiponectin and mediators of inflammation in obese women. Diabetes. 2003;52(4):942–7.
96. Huang Z, Willett WC, Colditz GA, Hunter DJ, Manson JE, Rosner B, et al. Waist circumference, waist: hip ratio, and risk of breast cancer in the Nurses' Health Study. Am J Epidemiol. 1999;150(12):1316–24.
97. Connolly BS, Barnett C, Vogt KN, Li T, Stone J, Boyd NF. A meta-analysis of published literature on waist-to-hip ratio and risk of breast cancer. Nutr Cancer. 2002;44(2):127–38.
98. National Cancer Institute. DevCan: probability of developing or dying of cancer software statistical research and applications branch. National Cancer Institute.
99. Edwards BK, Ward E, Kohler BA, Eheman C, Zauber AG, Anderson RN, et al. Annual report to the nation on the status of cancer, 1975–2006, featuring colorectal cancer trends and impact of interventions (risk factors, screening, and treatment) to reduce future rates. Cancer. 2010;116(3):544–73.
100. Bardou M, Barkun AN, Martel M. Obesity and colorectal cancer. Gut. 2013;62(6):933–47.
101. Ben Q, An W, Jiang Y, Zhan X, Du Y, Cai QC, et al. Body mass index increases risk for colorectal adenomas based on meta-analysis. Gastroenterology. 2012;142(4):762–72.

102. Hong S, Cai Q, Chen D, Zhu W, Huang W, Li Z. Abdominal obesity and the risk of colorectal adenoma: a meta-analysis of observational studies. Eur J Cancer Prev. 2012;21(6):523–31.
103. Lee YJ, Myung SK, Cho B, Park BJ, Park JH, Ju W, et al. Adiposity and the risk of colorectal adenomatous polyps: a meta-analysis. Cancer Causes Control. 2011;22(7):1021–35.
104. Okabayashi K, Ashrafian H, Hasegawa H, Yoo JH, Patel VM, Harling L, et al. Body mass index category as a risk factor for colorectal adenomas: a systematic review and meta-analysis. Am J Gastroenterol. 2012;107(8):1175–85; quiz 86
105. Kim BC, Shin A, Hong CW, Sohn DK, Han KS, Ryu KH, et al. Association of colorectal adenoma with components of metabolic syndrome. Cancer Causes Control. 2012;23(5):727–35.
106. Guh DP, Zhang W, Bansback N, Amarsi Z, Birmingham CL, Anis AH. The incidence of co-morbidities related to obesity and overweight: a systematic review and meta-analysis. BMC Public Health. 2009;9:88.
107. Harriss DJ, Atkinson G, George K, Cable NT, Reilly T, Haboubi N, et al. Lifestyle factors and colorectal cancer risk (1): systematic review and meta-analysis of associations with body mass index. Color Dis. 2009;11(6):547–63.
108. Dai Z, Xu YC, Niu L. Obesity and colorectal cancer risk: a meta-analysis of cohort studies. World J Gastroenterol. 2007;13(31):4199–206.
109. Moghaddam AA, Woodward M, Huxley R. Obesity and risk of colorectal cancer: a meta-analysis of 31 studies with 70,000 events. Cancer Epidemiol Biomark Prev. 2007;16(12):2533–47.
110. Larsson SC, Wolk A. Obesity and colon and rectal cancer risk: a meta-analysis of prospective studies. Am J Clin Nutr. 2007;86(3):556–65.
111. Akiyoshi T, Ueno M, Fukunaga Y, Nagayama S, Fujimoto Y, Konishi T, et al. Effect of body mass index on short-term outcomes of patients undergoing laparoscopic resection for colorectal cancer: a single institution experience in Japan. Surg Laparosc Endosc Percutan Tech. 2011;21(6):409–14.
112. Ballian N, Yamane B, Leverson G, Harms B, Heise CP, Foley EF, et al. Body mass index does not affect postoperative morbidity and oncologic outcomes of total mesorectal excision for rectal adenocarcinoma. Ann Surg Oncol. 2010;17(6):1606–13.
113. Bege T, Lelong B, Francon D, Turrini O, Guiramand J, Delpero JR. Impact of obesity on short-term results of laparoscopic rectal cancer resection. Surg Endosc. 2009;23(7):1460–4.
114. Blee TH, Belzer GE, Lambert PJ. Obesity: is there an increase in perioperative complications in those undergoing elective colon and rectal resection for carcinoma? Am Surg. 2002;68(2):163–6.
115. Blumberg D. Laparoscopic colectomy performed using a completely intracorporeal technique is associated with similar outcome in obese and thin patients. Surg Laparosc Endosc Percutan Tech. 2009;19(1):57–61.
116. Chern H, Chou J, Donkor C, Shia J, Guillem JG, Nash GM, et al. Effects of obesity in rectal cancer surgery. J Am Coll Surg. 2010;211(1):55–60.
117. Damadi AA, Julien L, Arrangoiz R, Raiji M, Weise D, Saxe AW. Does obesity influence lymph node harvest among patients undergoing colectomy for colon cancer? Am Surg. 2008;74(11):1073–7.
118. Healy LA, Ryan AM, Sutton E, Younger K, Mehigan B, Stephens R, et al. Impact of obesity on surgical and oncological outcomes in the management of colorectal cancer. Int J Color Dis. 2010;25(11):1293–9.
119. Ishii Y, Hasegawa H, Nishibori H, Watanabe M, Kitajima M. Impact of visceral obesity on surgical outcome after laparoscopic surgery for rectal cancer. Br J Surg. 2005;92(10):1261–2.
120. Kang J, Baek SE, Kim T, Hur H, Min BS, Lim JS, et al. Impact of fat obesity on laparoscopic total mesorectal excision: more reliable indicator than body mass index. Int J Color Dis. 2012;27(4):497–505.
121. Karahasanoglu T, Hamzaoglu I, Baca B, Aytac E, Kirbiyik E. Impact of increased body mass index on laparoscopic surgery for rectal cancer. Eur Surg Res. 2011;46(2):87–93.
122. Linebarger JH, Mathiason MA, Kallies KJ, Shapiro SB. Does obesity impact lymph node retrieval in colon cancer surgery? Am J Surg. 2010;200(4):478–82.
123. Merkow RP, Bilimoria KY, McCarter MD, Bentrem DJ. Effect of body mass index on short-term outcomes after colectomy for cancer. J Am Coll Surg. 2009;208(1):53–61.
124. Nitori N, Hasegawa H, Ishii Y, Endo T, Kitagawa Y. Impact of visceral obesity on short-term outcome after laparoscopic surgery for colorectal cancer: a single Japanese center study. Surg Laparosc Endosc Percutan Tech. 2009;19(4):324–7.
125. Park JS, Choi GS, Jang YS, Jun SH, Kang H. Influence of obesity on the serum carcinoembryonic antigen value in patients with colorectal cancer. Cancer Epidemiol Biomark Prev. 2010;19(10):2461–8.
126. Poulsen M, Ovesen H. Is laparoscopic colorectal cancer surgery in obese patients associated with an increased risk? Short-term results from a single center study of 425 patients. J Gastrointest Surg. 2012;16(8):1554–8.
127. Sakamoto K, Niwa S, Tanaka M, Goto M, Sengoku H, Tomiki Y. Influence of obesity on the short-term outcome of laparoscopic colectomy for colorectal cancer. J Minim Access Surg. 2007;3(3):98–103.
128. Singh A, Muthukumarasamy G, Pawa N, Riaz AA, Hendricks JB, Motson RW. Laparoscopic colorectal cancer surgery in obese patients. Color Dis. 2011;13(8):878–83.
129. Tsujinaka S, Konishi F, Kawamura YJ, Saito M, Tajima N, Tanaka O, et al. Visceral obesity predicts surgical outcomes after laparoscopic colectomy for sigmoid colon cancer. Dis Colon Rectum. 2008;51(12):1757–65; discussion 65–7.
130. Yamamoto N, Fujii S, Sato T, Oshima T, Rino Y, Kunisaki C, et al. Impact of body mass index and

visceral adiposity on outcomes in colorectal cancer. Asia Pac J Clin Oncol. 2012;8(4):337–45.
131. Makino T, Shukla PJ, Rubino F, Milsom JW. The impact of obesity on perioperative outcomes after laparoscopic colorectal resection. Ann Surg. 2012;255(2):228–36.
132. Zhou Y, Wu L, Li X, Wu X, Li B. Outcome of laparoscopic colorectal surgery in obese and non-obese patients: a meta-analysis. Surg Endosc. 2012;26(3):783–9.
133. Park JW, Lim SW, Choi HS, Jeong SY, Oh JH, Lim SB. The impact of obesity on outcomes of laparoscopic surgery for colorectal cancer in Asians. Surg Endosc. 2010;24(7):1679–85.
134. Coleman MP, Gatta G, Verdecchia A, Esteve J, Sant M, Storm H, et al. EUROCARE-3 summary: cancer survival in Europe at the end of the 20th century. Ann Oncol. 2003;14(Suppl 5):v128–49.
135. Horner MJRL, Krapcho M, Neyman N, Aminou R, Howlader N, Altekruse SF, Feuer EJ, Huang L, Mariotto A, Miller BA, Lewis DR, Eisner MP, Stinchcomb DG, Edwards BK. SEER cancer statistics review, 1975–2006. Bethesda: National Cancer Institute; 2008.
136. El-Serag HB, Mason AC. Risk factors for the rising rates of primary liver cancer in the United States. Arch Intern Med. 2000;160(21):3227–30.
137. Hassan MM, Frome A, Patt YZ, El-Serag HB. Rising prevalence of hepatitis C virus infection among patients recently diagnosed with hepatocellular carcinoma in the United States. J Clin Gastroenterol. 2002;35(3):266–9.
138. Moller H, Mellemgaard A, Lindvig K, Olsen JH. Obesity and cancer risk: a Danish record-linkage study. Eur J Cancer. 1994;30A(3):344–50.
139. Wolk A, Gridley G, Svensson M, Nyren O, McLaughlin JK, Fraumeni JF, et al. A prospective study of obesity and cancer risk (Sweden). Cancer Causes Control. 2001;12(1):13–21.
140. Nair S, Mason A, Eason J, Loss G, Perrillo RP. Is obesity an independent risk factor for hepatocellular carcinoma in cirrhosis? Hepatology. 2002;36(1):150–5.
141. Calle EE, Rodriguez C, Walker-Thurmond K, Thun MJ. Overweight, obesity, and mortality from cancer in a prospectively studied cohort of US adults. N Engl J Med. 2003;348(17):1625–38.
142. Samanic C, Gridley G, Chow WH, Lubin J, Hoover RN, Fraumeni JF Jr. Obesity and cancer risk among white and black United States veterans. Cancer Causes Control. 2004;15(1):35–43.
143. Batty GD, Shipley MJ, Jarrett RJ, Breeze E, Marmot MG, Smith GD. Obesity and overweight in relation to organ-specific cancer mortality in London (UK): findings from the original Whitehall study. Int J Obes. 2005;29(10):1267–74.
144. Oh SW, Yoon YS, Shin SA. Effects of excess weight on cancer incidences depending on cancer sites and histologic findings among men: Korea National Health Insurance Corporation Study. J Clin Oncol. 2005;23(21):4742–54.
145. Rapp K, Schroeder J, Klenk J, Stoehr S, Ulmer H, Concin H, et al. Obesity and incidence of cancer: a large cohort study of over 145,000 adults in Austria. Br J Cancer. 2005;93(9):1062–7.
146. N'Kontchou G, Paries J, Htar MT, Ganne-Carrie N, Costentin L, Grando-Lemaire V, et al. Risk factors for hepatocellular carcinoma in patients with alcoholic or viral C cirrhosis. Clin Gastroenterol Hepatol. 2006;4(8):1062–8.
147. Larsson SC, Wolk A. Overweight, obesity and risk of liver cancer: a meta-analysis of cohort studies. Br J Cancer. 2007;97(7):1005–8.
148. Neuschwander-Tetri BA, Caldwell SH. Nonalcoholic steatohepatitis: summary of an AASLD Single Topic Conference. Hepatology. 2003;37(5):1202–19.
149. Jemal A, Bray F, Center MM, Ferlay J, Ward E, Forman D. Global cancer statistics. CA Cancer J Clin. 2011;61(2):69–90.
150. Levy AD, Murakata LA, Rohrmann CA Jr. Gallbladder carcinoma: radiologic-pathologic correlation. Radiographics. 2001;21(2):295–314; questionnaire, 549–55.
151. Lazcano-Ponce EC, Miquel JF, Munoz N, Herrero R, Ferrecio C, Wistuba II, et al. Epidemiology and molecular pathology of gallbladder cancer. CA Cancer J Clin. 2001;51(6):349–64.
152. Zatonski WA, Lowenfels AB, Boyle P, Maisonneuve P, Bueno de Mesquita HB, Ghadirian P, et al. Epidemiologic aspects of gallbladder cancer: a case-control study of the SEARCH Program of the International Agency for Research on Cancer. J Natl Cancer Inst. 1997;89(15):1132–8.
153. Hsing AW, Gao YT, Han TQ, Rashid A, Sakoda LC, Wang BS, et al. Gallstones and the risk of biliary tract cancer: a population-based study in China. Br J Cancer. 2007;97(11):1577–82.
154. Zatonski W, La Vecchia C, Levi F, Negri E, Lucchini F. Descriptive epidemiology of gall-bladder cancer in Europe. J Cancer Res Clin Oncol. 1993;119(3):165–71.
155. de Aretxabala X, Riedeman P, Burgos L, Roa I, Araya JC, Echeverria X, et al. Gallbladder cancer. Case-control study. Rev Med Chil. 1995;123(5):581–6.
156. Kuriyama S, Tsubono Y, Hozawa A, Shimazu T, Suzuki Y, Koizumi Y, et al. Obesity and risk of cancer in Japan. Int J Cancer. 2005;113(1):148–57.
157. Engeland A, Tretli S, Austad G, Bjorge T. Height and body mass index in relation to colorectal and gallbladder cancer in two million Norwegian men and women. Cancer Causes Control. 2005;16(8):987–96.
158. Ishiguro S, Inoue M, Kurahashi N, Iwasaki M, Sasazuki S, Tsugane S. Risk factors of biliary tract cancer in a large-scale population-based cohort study in Japan (JPHC study); with special focus on cholelithiasis, body mass index, and their effect modification. Cancer Causes Control. 2008;19(1):33–41.
159. Jee SH, Yun JE, Park EJ, Cho ER, Park IS, Sull JW, et al. Body mass index and cancer risk in Korean men and women. Int J Cancer. 2008;123(8):1892–6.

160. Song YM, Sung J, Ha M. Obesity and risk of cancer in postmenopausal Korean women. J Clin Oncol. 2008;26(20):3395–402.
161. Borena W, Edlinger M, Bjorge T, Haggstrom C, Lindkvist B, Nagel G, et al. A prospective study on metabolic risk factors and gallbladder cancer in the metabolic syndrome and cancer (Me-Can) collaborative study. PLoS One. 2014;9(2):e89368.
162. Grainge MJ, West J, Solaymani-Dodaran M, Aithal GP, Card TR. The antecedents of biliary cancer: a primary care case-control study in the United Kingdom. Br J Cancer. 2009;100(1):178–80.
163. Hsing AW, Sakoda LC, Rashid A, Chen J, Shen MC, Han TQ, et al. Body size and the risk of biliary tract cancer: a population-based study in China. Br J Cancer. 2008;99(5):811–5.
164. Machova L, Cizek L, Horakova D, Koutna J, Lorenc J, Janoutova G, et al. Association between obesity and cancer incidence in the population of the District Sumperk, Czech Republic. Onkologie. 2007;30(11):538–42.
165. Nakadaira H, Lang I, Szentirmay Z, Hitre E, Kaster M, Yamamoto M. A case-control study of gallbladder cancer in Hungary. Asian Pac J Cancer Prev. 2009;10(5):833–6.
166. Serra I, Yamamoto M, Calvo A, Cavada G, Baez S, Endoh K, et al. Association of chili pepper consumption, low socioeconomic status and longstanding gallstones with gallbladder cancer in a Chilean population. Int J Cancer. 2002;102(4):407–11.
167. Strom BL, Soloway RD, Rios-Dalenz JL, Rodriguez-Martinez HA, West SL, Kinman JL, et al. Risk factors for gallbladder cancer. An international collaborative case-control study. Cancer. 1995;76(10):1747–56.
168. Zhang XH, Gao YT, Rashid A, Deng J, Liu EJ, Wu K, et al. Tea consumption and risk of biliary tract cancers and gallstone disease: a population-based case-control study in Shanghai, China. Zhonghua Zhong Liu Za Zhi. 2005;27(11):667–71.
169. Park M, Song DY, Je Y, Lee JE. Body mass index and biliary tract disease: a systematic review and meta-analysis of prospective studies. Prev Med. 2014;65:13–22.
170. Li L, Gan Y, Li W, Wu C, Lu Z. Overweight, obesity and the risk of gallbladder and extrahepatic bile duct cancers: a meta-analysis of observational studies. Obesity (Silver Spring). 2016;24(8):1786–802.
171. Hariharan D, Saied A, Kocher HM. Analysis of mortality rates for pancreatic cancer across the world. HPB (Oxford). 2008;10(1):58–62.
172. Cancer facts & figures. American Cancer Society; 2010.
173. Health. NCINIo. Pancreatic Cancer Treatment, Health Professional Version; 2014.
174. Larsson SC, Permert J, Hakansson N, Naslund I, Bergkvist L, Wolk A. Overall obesity, abdominal adiposity, diabetes and cigarette smoking in relation to the risk of pancreatic cancer in two Swedish population-based cohorts. Br J Cancer. 2005;93(11):1310–5.
175. Li D, Morris JS, Liu J, Hassan MM, Day RS, Bondy ML, et al. Body mass index and risk, age of onset, and survival in patients with pancreatic cancer. JAMA. 2009;301(24):2553–62.
176. Rollins KE, Tewari N, Ackner A, Awwad A, Madhusudan S, Macdonald IA, et al. The impact of sarcopenia and myosteatosis on outcomes of unresectable pancreatic cancer or distal cholangiocarcinoma. Clin Nutr. 2016;35(5):1103–9.
177. Genkinger JM, Spiegelman D, Anderson KE, Bernstein L, van den Brandt PA, Calle EE, et al. A pooled analysis of 14 cohort studies of anthropometric factors and pancreatic cancer risk. Int J Cancer. 2011;129(7):1708–17.
178. Aune D, Greenwood DC, Chan DS, Vieira R, Vieira AR, Navarro Rosenblatt DA, et al. Body mass index, abdominal fatness and pancreatic cancer risk: a systematic review and non-linear dose-response meta-analysis of prospective studies. Ann Oncol. 2012;23(4):843–52.
179. Majumder K, Gupta A, Arora N, Singh PP, Singh S. Premorbid obesity and mortality in patients with pancreatic cancer: a systematic review and meta-analysis. Clin Gastroenterol Hepatol. 2016;14(3):355–68e; quiz e32.
180. Dawson DW, Hertzer K, Moro A, Donald G, Chang HH, Go VL, et al. High-fat, high-calorie diet promotes early pancreatic neoplasia in the conditional KrasG12D mouse model. Cancer Prev Res (Phila). 2013;6(10):1064–73.
181. Khasawneh J, Schulz MD, Walch A, Rozman J, Hrabe de Angelis M, Klingenspor M, et al. Inflammation and mitochondrial fatty acid beta-oxidation link obesity to early tumor promotion. Proc Natl Acad Sci U S A. 2009;106(9):3354–9.
182. Lashinger LM, Harrison LM, Rasmussen AJ, Logsdon CD, Fischer SM, McArthur MJ, et al. Dietary energy balance modulation of Kras- and Ink4a/Arf+/−-driven pancreatic cancer: the role of insulin-like growth factor-I. Cancer Prev Res (Phila). 2013;6(10):1046–55.
183. Philip B, Roland CL, Daniluk J, Liu Y, Chatterjee D, Gomez SB, et al. A high-fat diet activates oncogenic Kras and COX2 to induce development of pancreatic ductal adenocarcinoma in mice. Gastroenterology. 2013;145(6):1449–58.
184. Bethea TN, Kitahara CM, Sonderman J, Patel AV, Harvey C, Knutsen SF, et al. A pooled analysis of body mass index and pancreatic cancer mortality in African Americans. Cancer Epidemiol Biomark Prev. 2014;23(10):2119–25.
185. Genkinger JM, Kitahara CM, Bernstein L, Berrington de Gonzalez A, Brotzman M, Elena JW, et al. Central adiposity, obesity during early adulthood, and pancreatic cancer mortality in a pooled analysis of cohort studies. Ann Oncol. 2015;26(11):2257–66.
186. Pecorelli N, Carrara G, De Cobelli F, Cristel G, Damascelli A, Balzano G, et al. Effect of sarcopenia and visceral obesity on mortality and pancreatic fis-

tula following pancreatic cancer surgery. Br J Surg. 2016;103(4):434–42.
187. Stolzenberg-Solomon RZ, Schairer C, Moore S, Hollenbeck A, Silverman DT. Lifetime adiposity and risk of pancreatic cancer in the NIH-AARP Diet and Health Study cohort. Am J Clin Nutr. 2013;98(4):1057–65.
188. Tan BH, Birdsell LA, Martin L, Baracos VE, Fearon KC. Sarcopenia in an overweight or obese patient is an adverse prognostic factor in pancreatic cancer. Clin Cancer Res. 2009;15(22):6973–9.
189. Organization WH. Obesity and overweight fact. Sheet N311. Geneva; 2006.
190. Declaration IUACUWC. 2008.
191. Disease. GAftPoOaRC; 2008.
192. Christou NV, Lieberman M, Sampalis F, Sampalis JS. Bariatric surgery reduces cancer risk in morbidly obese patients. Surg Obes Relat Dis. 2008;4(6):691–5.
193. McCawley GM, Ferriss JS, Geffel D, Northup CJ, Modesitt SC. Cancer in obese women: potential protective impact of bariatric surgery. J Am Coll Surg. 2009;208(6):1093–8.
194. Clough A, Layani L, Shah A, Wheatley L, Taylor C. Laparoscopic gastric banding in over 60s. Obes Surg. 2011;21(1):10–7.
195. Forsell P, Hellers G. The Swedish Adjustable Gastric Banding (SAGB) for morbid obesity: 9 year experience and a 4-year follow-up of patients operated with a new adjustable band. Obes Surg. 1997;7(4):345–51.
196. Gagne DJ, Papasavas PK, Maalouf M, Urbandt JE, Caushaj PF. Obesity surgery and malignancy: our experience after 1500 cases. Surg Obes Relat Dis. 2009;5(2):160–4.
197. Gusenoff JA, Koltz PF, O'Malley WJ, Messing S, Chen R, Langstein HN. Breast cancer and bariatric surgery: temporal relationships of diagnosis, treatment, and reconstruction. Plast Reconstr Surg. 2009;124(4):1025–32.
198. Ostlund MP, Lu Y, Lagergren J. Risk of obesity-related cancer after obesity surgery in a population-based cohort study. Ann Surg. 2010;252(6):972–6.
199. Srikanth MS, Fox SR, Oh KH, Ward K, Sun H, Keskey T, et al. Renal cell carcinoma following bariatric surgery. Obes Surg. 2005;15(8):1165–70.
200. Steffen R, Potoczna N, Bieri N, Horber FF. Successful multi-intervention treatment of severe obesity: a 7-year prospective study with 96% follow-up. Obes Surg. 2009;19(1):3–12.
201. Sugerman HJ, Sugerman EL, Wolfe L, Kellum JM Jr, Schweitzer MA, DeMaria EJ. Risks and benefits of gastric bypass in morbidly obese patients with severe venous stasis disease. Ann Surg. 2001;234(1):41–6.
202. Birks S, Peeters A, Backholer K, O'Brien P, Brown W. A systematic review of the impact of weight loss on cancer incidence and mortality. Obes Rev. 2012;13(10):868–91.
203. Casagrande DS, Rosa DD, Umpierre D, Sarmento RA, Rodrigues CG, Schaan BD. Incidence of cancer following bariatric surgery: systematic review and meta-analysis. Obes Surg. 2014;24(9):1499–509.
204. Derogar M, Hull MA, Kant P, Ostlund M, Lu Y, Lagergren J. Increased risk of colorectal cancer after obesity surgery. Ann Surg. 2013;258(6):983–8.
205. James WP, Caterson ID, Coutinho W, Finer N, Van Gaal LF, Maggioni AP, et al. Effect of sibutramine on cardiovascular outcomes in overweight and obese subjects. N Engl J Med. 2010;363(10):905–17.
206. Franco M, Bilal U, Ordunez P, Benet M, Morejon A, Caballero B, et al. Population-wide weight loss and regain in relation to diabetes burden and cardiovascular mortality in Cuba 1980–2010: repeated cross sectional surveys and ecological comparison of secular trends. BMJ. 2013;346:f1515.
207. DeMaria EJ, Pate V, Warthen M, Winegar DA. Baseline data from American Society for Metabolic and Bariatric Surgery-designated Bariatric Surgery Centers of excellence using the bariatric outcomes longitudinal database. Surg Obes Relat Dis. 2010;6(4):347–55.
208. Renehan AG. Bariatric surgery, weight reduction, and cancer prevention. Lancet Oncol. 2009;10(7):640–1.
209. Ashrafian H, Ahmed K, Rowland SP, Patel VM, Gooderham NJ, Holmes E, et al. Metabolic surgery and cancer: protective effects of bariatric procedures. Cancer. 2011;117(9):1788–99.

41 Bariatric Surgery and Cancer

Yaniv Fenig and Ronald Matteotti

Background

The Centers for Disease Control and Prevention (CDC) has recently reported the prevalence of obesity, defined as a BMI ≥ 30, within the adult population in the USA to be 36.5% [1]. These numbers have been steadily growing since the 1960s. Obesity is higher in females than in males, middle-aged and older than younger adults, white, black, and Hispanic than Asian adults.

This is alarming because obesity is related to a 100% increase in all-cause mortality, and especially of cardiovascular causes, when compared to persons with a BMI of 20–25 [2]. The average life expectancy of individuals with obesity is 5–20 years shorter than nonobese individuals, depending on gender, race, and age [6]. Obesity is associated with the following morbidities: hypertension [3], type 2 diabetes mellitus [4], coronary heart disease [5], stroke [6], gallstone disease [7], osteoarthritis [8], and obstructive sleep apnea [9].

Y. Fenig
Monmouth Medical Center, Long Branch, NJ, USA

R. Matteotti (✉)
The HOPE Tower at Jersey Shore University Medical Center, Neptune, NJ, USA

Hepatobiliary and Pancreatic Program Meridian Cancer Care, Neptune, NJ, USA

Hepatobiliary and Pancreatic Surgery JSUMC, Neptune, NJ, USA
e-mail: Ronald.matteotti@hackensackmeridian.org

The Relationship of Obesity and Cancer

Studies have found a correlation between obesity and colon cancer [10–12], which is independent of physical inactivity. This correlation is stronger in males, than in females [13], possibly due to the increased abdominal adiposity in the former. Obesity is associated with increased insulin secretion and hyperinsulinemia [14], and insulin is demonstrated to act as an important growth factor for colonic mucosal cells and colonic and colonic carcinoma cells in vitro, specifically via insulin growth factor-1 (IGF-1) [15]. Thus, insulin might mediate the risk of colon cancer associated with obesity. Of interest, obesity is also an independent risk factor of lower disease-free and overall survival in colorectal cancer, although overweight status defined as a BMI 25–29 confers improved overall survival when compared with normal BMI [16]. A large Austrian population-based study has demonstrated that weight loss is inversely associated with colon cancer in males [17].

The correlation between obesity and breast cancer is more complex. Premenopausal females who are obese have lower incidence of breast cancer than their normal weight counterparts [18]. However postmenopausal females who are obese have higher incidence of breast cancer [19]. The heightened risk of postmenopausal obese females in comparison to their normal weight counterparts is thought to be related to

R. Lutfi et al. (eds.), *Global Bariatric Surgery*, https://doi.org/10.1007/978-3-319-93545-4_41

increased estrogen produced in peripheral adipose tissue. Similarly, obesity increases the risk of endometrial cancer, and weight gain in adulthood is also associated with increased risk [20].

In addition, the American Institute for Cancer Research and World Cancer Research Fund (WCRF) reported that there is convincing evidence for a relation between obesity and esophageal, pancreatic, endometrial, and kidney cancers, with probable evidence for gallbladder cancer [21]. A large meta-analysis that included 220 studies, which included some cohorts that were omitted from the WCRF report, confirmed a strong relationship in men between BMI $\geq$ 30 and esophageal cancer, thyroid cancer, kidney cancer and colon cancer, and a weak association with malignant melanoma, non-Hodgkin's lymphoma, leukemia, and rectal cancer [22]. The study also found a strong relationship in women between obesity and endometrial cancer, gallbladder cancer, kidney cancer and esophageal cancer, and a weak association with postmenopausal breast cancer, leukemia, non-Hodgkin's lymphoma, thyroid cancer, pancreatic cancer, and colon cancer.

To evaluate the attributable risk of obesity to all types of cancer in the USA, one study looked at the prevalence of cancer using the National Health and Nutrition Examination Survey (NHANES) data and the incidence of cancer using the Surveillance Epidemiology and End Results Program (SEER) data to conclude that in 2007 33,966 (4%), new cancers among males and 50,535 (7%) new cancers among females were attributable to obesity [23]. A European study using the same methods found a slightly lower attributable risk among males (2.5%), as well as among females (4.1%) [24]. The attributable risk of obesity to cancer varies with the type of malignant disease as shown by the WCRF report [21] and summarized in Table 41.1.

The Relationship of Obesity to Cancer Mortality

In regard to the effect of obesity on all-cause and cancer-related mortality, most observational studies have actually indicated that all-cause mortality is increased with weight loss [25], surprisingly. This is explained by the nature of observational studies being unable to distinguish between intentional and unintentional weight loss, which can be a consequence of conditions leading to mortality. An important finding was the dose-response relationship found between obesity and all-cause mortality and cancer mortality among participants in population-based studies [6].

The Relationship of Weight Loss and Cancer

Evaluating the association of intentional weight loss with cancer risk is challenging considering maintaining normal weight after obesity is not an easy task, and one does not want to perform a cross-sectional study evaluating long-term outcomes such as cancer incidence. Bariatric surgery is therefore a very good model to examine such a relation. A randomized controlled trial showed sustained weight loss at 10 years with laparoscopic Roux-en-Y gastric bypass achieving 69% reduction in weight and laparoscopic adjustable gastric banding – 46% [26]. On the contrary, high-

Table 41.1 WCRF attributable risk of obesity to malignancies

Malignancy	Attributable risk in the USA (%)	Hypothesized mechanism
Endometrial	49	Hyperestrogenemia
Esophageal adenocarcinoma	35	Dysplasia from acid reflux
Pancreatic adenocarcinoma	28	Inflammation
Kidney	24	Inflammation
Gallbladder	21	Inflammation
Postmenopausal breast cancer	17	Hyperestrogenemia
Colorectal	9	Inflammation

powered studies that have evaluated the ability of nonsurgical measures at maintaining weight loss have shown inferior outcomes at 10 years, ranging from a 4 kg loss to a 2 kg gain [27].

Bariatric Surgery and Cancer Risk

A cohort retrospective trial found that patients that undergo Roux-en-Y gastric bypass procedure have a reduction in all-cause mortality of 40%, as compared to matched controls, and a reduction of 60% in cancer mortality at 7-year follow-up. No difference was found in the prevalence of cancer between the control group and larger reported national institute of health figures, to ensure that differences were not due to baseline variations between the control group and the general population [28].

Another study, using nonrandomized controlled prospective methods, with slightly longer follow-up of 10 years, and a surgical intervention mostly consisting of vertical-banded gastroplasty associated with about a 15% net weight loss at 10 years showed an over 50% reduction in cancer mortality [29]. A subsequent study on the same patient population showed a reduction in the incidence of cancer in the intervention group for females only and for all three interventions: banding, vertical-banded gastroplasty, and gastric bypass [30]. Interestingly, the hazard ratios (HR) for cancer risk reduction for all three procedures were the same despite significantly different proportions of weight loss for each procedure. Gastric bypass was found to reduce insulin by twice as much as the restrictive procedure, and yet the protective effect of reduction of hyperinsulinemia did not translate to proportional cancer protection.

The most recent meta-analysis [31] performed to date of this publication employed rigorous methodology to search and analyze the known data on the subject. One of the analyses included the two abovementioned studies [28, 29], in addition to one nonrandomized controlled trial [32] and three cohort studies [33–35], and found that after pooling all the cases together – a total of 167,674 participants – the incidence of cancer was statistically lower for the surgical group [OR = 0.65, 95% CI 0.46–0.91, I^2 =86%]. In a second analysis from the same meta-analysis [31], four randomized controlled trials (RCT) [36–39] were pooled together and did not find a statistical difference in incidence of cancer between groups that were treated with bariatric surgery versus non-surgery groups. However, the data from RCTs is limited due to insufficient follow-up time and small sample size. The authors concluded that the effects of surgical treatment on cancer are consistent across the nonrandomized controlled trials and cohort studies and imply that bariatric surgeries could reduce the risk of cancer.

References

1. Ogden CL, Carroll MD, Fryar CD, Flegal KM. Prevalence of obesity among adults and youth: United States, 2011–2014. NCHS Data Brief. 2015;219(219):1–8.
2. Troiano RP, Frongillo EA Jr, Sobal J, Levitsky DA. The relationship between body weight and mortality: a quantitative analysis of combined information from existing studies. Int J Obes Relat Metab Disord. 1996;20(1):63–75.
3. Stamler R, Stamler J, Riedlinger WF, Algera G, Roberts RH. Weight and blood pressure: findings in hypertension screening of 1 million Americans. JAMA. 1978;240(15):1607–10.
4. Medalie JH, Papier CM, Goldbourt U, Herman JB. Major factors in the development of diabetes mellitus in 10,000 men. Arch Intern Med. 1975;135(6):811–7.
5. Hubert HB, Feinleib M, McNamara PM, Castelli WP. Obesity as an independent risk factor for cardiovascular disease: a 26-year follow-up of participants in the Framingham Heart Study. Circulation. 1983;67(5):968–77.
6. Prospective Studies Collaboration. Body-mass index and cause-specific mortality in 900 000 adults: collaborative analyses of 57 prospective studies. Lancet. 2009;373(9669):1083–96.
7. Stampfer MJ, Maclure KM, Colditz GA, Manson JE, Willett WC. Risk of symptomatic gallstones in women with severe obesity. Am J Clin Nutr. 1992;55(3):652–8.
8. Hart DJ, Spector TD. The relationship of obesity, fat distribution and osteoarthritis in women in the general population: the Chingford study. J Rheumatol. 1993;20(2):331–5.
9. Loube DI, Loube AA, Mitler MM. Weight loss for obstructive sleep apnea: the optimal therapy for obese patients. J Am Diet Assoc. 1994;94(11):1291–5.

10. Chute CG, Willett WC, Colditz GA, Stampfer MJ, Baron JA, Rosner B, Speizer FE. A prospective study of body mass, height, and smoking on the risk of colorectal cancer in women. Cancer Causes Control. 1991;2(2):117–24.
11. Giovannucci E, Ascherio A, Rimm EB, Colditz GA, Stampfer MJ, Willett WC. Physical activity, obesity, and risk for colon cancer and adenoma in men. Ann Intern Med. 1995;122(5):327–34.
12. Marchand L, Wilkens LR, Mi MP. Obesity in youth and middle age and risk of colorectal cancer in men. Cancer Causes Control. 1992;3(4):349–54.
13. Lew EA, Garfinkel L. Variations in mortality by weight among 750,000 men and women. J Chronic Dis. 1979;32(8):563–76.
14. Kim MK, Reaven GM, Chen YD, Kim E, Kim SH. Hyperinsulinemia in individuals with obesity: role of insulin clearance. Obesity. 2015;23(12):2430–4.
15. Watkins LF, Lewis LR, Levine AE. Characterization of the synergistic effect of insulin and transferrin and the regulation of their receptors on a human colon carcinoma cell line. Int J Cancer. 1990;45(2):372–5.
16. Sinicrope FA, Foster NR, Sargent DJ, O'Connell MJ, Rankin C. Obesity is an independent prognostic variable in colon cancer survivors. Clin Cancer Res. 2010;16(6):1884–93.
17. Rapp K, Klenk J, Ulmer H, Concin H, Diem G, Oberaigner W, Schroeder J. Weight change and cancer risk in a cohort of more than 65 000 adults in Austria. Ann Oncol. 2008;19(4):641–8.
18. Willett WC, Browne ML, Bain C, Lipnick RJ, Stampfer MJ, Rosner B, Colditz GA, Hennekens CH, Speizer FE. Relative weight and risk of breast cancer among premenopausal women. Am J Epidemiol. 1985;122(5):731–40.
19. Huang Z, Hankinson SE, Colditz GA, Stampfer MJ, Hunter DJ, Manson JE, Hennekens CH, Rosner B, Speizer FE, Willett WC. Dual effects of weight and weight gain on breast cancer risk. JAMA. 1997;278(17):1407–11.
20. Schottenfeld D, Fraumeni Jr JF. Cancer epidemiology and prevention. Oxford University Press, New York; 2006.
21. Marmot M, Diet, cancer, and NCD prevention. Lancet Oncol. 2018. pii: S1470-2045(18)30382-6.
22. Renehan AG, Tyson M, Egger M, Heller RF, Zwahlen M. Body-mass index and incidence of cancer: a systematic review and meta-analysis of prospective observational studies. Lancet. 2008;371(9612):569–78.
23. Polednak AP. Estimating the number of US incident cancers attributable to obesity and the impact on temporal trends in incidence rates for obesity-related cancers. Cancer Detect Prev. 2008;32(3):190–9.
24. Renehan AG, Soerjomataram I, Tyson M, Egger M, Zwahlen M, Coebergh JW, Buchan I. Incident cancer burden attributable to excess body mass index in 30 European countries. Int J Cancer. 2010;126(3):692–702.
25. Higgins M, D'Agostino R, Kannel W, Cobb J. Benefits and adverse effects of weight loss: observations from the Framingham study. Ann Intern Med. 1993;119(7_Part_2):758–63.
26. Angrisani L, Cutolo PP, Formisano G, Nosso G, Vitolo G. Laparoscopic adjustable gastric banding versus Roux-en-Y gastric bypass: 10-year results of a prospective, randomized trial. Surg Obes Relat Dis. 2013;9(3):405–13.
27. Diabetes Prevention Program Research Group. 10-year follow-up of diabetes incidence and weight loss in the Diabetes Prevention Program Outcomes Study. Lancet. 2009;374(9702):1677–86.
28. Adams TD, Gress RE, Smith SC, Halverson RC, Simper SC, Rosamond WD, LaMonte MJ, Stroup AM, Hunt SC. Long-term mortality after gastric bypass surgery. N Engl J Med. 2007;357(8):753–61.
29. Sjöström L, Narbro K, Sjöström CD, Karason K, Larsson B, Wedel H, Lystig T, Sullivan M, Bouchard C, Carlsson B, Bengtsson C. Effects of bariatric surgery on mortality in Swedish obese subjects. N Engl J Med. 2007;357(8):741–52.
30. Sjöström L, Gummesson A, Sjöström CD, Narbro K, Peltonen M, Wedel H, Bengtsson C, Bouchard C, Carlsson B, Dahlgren S, Jacobson P. Effects of bariatric surgery on cancer incidence in obese patients in Sweden (Swedish Obese Subjects Study): a prospective, controlled intervention trial. Lancet Oncol. 2009;10(7):653–62.
31. Zhou X, Yu J, Li L, Gloy VL, Nordmann A, Tiboni M, Li Y, Sun X. Effects of bariatric surgery on mortality, cardiovascular events, and cancer outcomes in obese patients: systematic review and meta-analysis. Obes Surg. 2016;26(11):2590–601.
32. Hofsø D, Nordstrand N, Johnson LK, Karlsen TI, Hager H, Jenssen T, Bollerslev J, Godang K, Sandbu R, Røislien J, Hjelmesæth J. Obesity-related cardiovascular risk factors after weight loss: a clinical trial comparing gastric bypass surgery and intensive lifestyle intervention. Eur J Endocrinol. 2010;163(5):735–45.
33. Arterburn D, Bogart A, Coleman KJ, Haneuse S, Selby JV, Sherwood NE, Sidney S, Theis MK, Campos GM, McCulloch D, O'Connor PJ. Comparative effectiveness of bariatric surgery vs. nonsurgical treatment of type 2 diabetes among severely obese adults. Obes Res Clin Pract. 2013;7(4):e258–68.
34. Derogar M, Hull MA, Kant P, Östlund M, Lu Y, Lagergren J. Increased risk of colorectal cancer after obesity surgery. Ann Surg. 2013;258(6):983–8.
35. Christou NV, Lieberman M, Sampalis F, Sampalis JS. Bariatric surgery reduces cancer risk in morbidly obese patients. Surg Obes Relat Dis. 2008;4(6):691–5.
36. Ikramuddin S, Billington CJ, Lee WJ, Bantle JP, Thomas AJ, Connett JE, Leslie DB, Inabnet WB, Jeffery RW, Chong K, Chuang LM. Roux-en-Y gastric bypass for diabetes (the Diabetes Surgery Study): 2-year outcomes of a 5-year, randomised, controlled trial. Lancet Diabetes Endocrinol. 2015;3(6):413–22.
37. Schauer PR, Bhatt DL, Kirwan JP, Wolski K, Brethauer SA, Navaneethan SD, Aminian

A, Pothier CE, Kim ES, Nissen SE, Kashyap SR. Bariatric surgery versus intensive medical therapy for diabetes—3-year outcomes. N Engl J Med. 2014;370(21):2002–13.

38. Halperin F, Ding SA, Simonson DC, Panosian J, Goebel-Fabbri A, Wewalka M, Hamdy O, Abrahamson M, Clancy K, Foster K, Lautz D. Roux-en-Y gastric bypass surgery or lifestyle with intensive medical management in patients with type 2 diabetes: feasibility and 1-year results of a randomized clinical trial. JAMA Surg. 2014;149(7):716–26.
39. Koehestanie P, de Jonge C, Berends FJ, Janssen IM, Bouvy ND, Greve JW. The effect of the endoscopic duodenal-jejunal bypass liner on obesity and type 2 diabetes mellitus, a multicenter randomized controlled trial. Ann Surg. 2014;260(6):984–92.

42 Bariatric Surgery and Transplantation

Giuseppe D'Amico, Kiara Tulla, and Ivo Tzvetanov

Introduction

Obesity is defined by the World Health Organization as the presence of excessive body fat that poses health risks, and body mass index (BMI) is the most common metric used by normalizing a person's weight to his/her height. Individuals with a BMI equal or greater than 30 kg/m^2 are defined as obese, and individuals with a BMI equal or greater than 40 kg/m^2 are categorized as morbidly obese. The number of adults who are obese is increasing rapidly and currently affects 35% of adults in the United States [1]. It is estimated that more than half of the US population will be obese by 2030 [2]. Obesity is a complex disease that compromises several organs including but not limited to the liver, heart, and kidney.

Obesity is affecting patients that are concurrently in need of organ transplantation frequently. Greater than 30% of kidney transplants (KT) are performed on obese patients [3]. In the last decade, the indication for liver transplantation (LT) for nonalcoholic steatohepatitis (NASH) has risen from 1.2% to 9.7% and is currently the third most common cause of liver failure and may become the leading indication for LT by 2025 [4]. Moreover, around 30% of patients referred for pancreas transplantation are diabetic and obese [5].

Bariatric surgery (BS) has been proven to be the only effective treatment for morbid obesity, leading to a significant loss of weight and reduction in obesity-related comorbid conditions. Since currently many transplant centers consider obesity as a relative contraindication for transplantation, application of highly effective obesity treatment could potentially improve the chances for transplantation for this otherwise marginalized patient group. In this regard, BS could be considered before, after, or in some circumstances during transplantation.

Bariatric Surgery

The main concerns regarding BS in patients with different types of organ failure are the rates of complications. Application of minimally invasive technics and mostly restrictive procedures, such as sleeve gastrectomy (SG), has achieved promising results with relatively low complication rates. At the same time, changes in the alimental tract hypothetically could affect the absorption of the immunosuppressive medications after transplantation. Thankfully, this process does not seem to be affected with the application of restrictive procedures (SG) [6].

G. D'Amico · K. Tulla · I. Tzvetanov (✉)
Department of Surgery, University of Illinois at Chicago, Chicago, IL, USA
e-mail: ktulla@uic.edu; itzveta@uic.edu

R. Lutfi et al. (eds.), *Global Bariatric Surgery*, https://doi.org/10.1007/978-3-319-93545-4_42

Liver Transplantation and Bariatric Surgery

Obesity, as we know, is a complex disease that compromises several organs including the liver in the form of nonalcoholic fatty liver disease (NAFLD) that may progress from simple steatosis to nonalcoholic steatohepatitis (NASH), liver cirrhosis, and eventually hepatocellular carcinoma. As a consequence, concomitant with the epidemic of obesity, a major increase in NAFLD has been recorded in Western countries, reaching an estimated prevalence between 10% and 24% in the general population and 57.5% and 74% in obese persons [7, 8]. Moreover, the progression of NAFLD to NASH has been reported in up to 42% of cases. Hence, NASH has become the third most common indication for LT, and epidemiological projections for the next decade indicate that this trend will continue and likely this pathology will probably become the most common cause of liver failure requiring LT [9].

Nevertheless, the increase in the prevalence of obesity among candidates for LT is not without concern, because obese patients seem to have less access to LT and the survival outcomes after LT for this specific population are still controversial [10]. LaMattina et al. [11] analyzed the perioperative morbidity of 813 LT patients between 1997 and 2008 and found that obese recipients had prolonged mean operative time, increased need for transfusions, higher incidence of infections, biliary complications requiring intervention, and, more importantly, decreased patient and graft survivals. In another study of 73,538 LT recipients, the overall survival was significantly lower in BMI less than 18.5 and higher than 40, compared to a control group [12]. Death in underweight patients was due to hemorrhagic and cerebrovascular complications, while infectious complications and cancer were the most common causes of demise in severely obese group. Nair et al. [13] analyzed the UNOS database on 18,172 LT patients transplanted between 1988 and 1996 and found that in primary graft dysfunction, perioperative mortality at 1, 2, and 5 years was significantly higher in the morbidly obese group due to adverse cardiovascular events. Similar outcomes were reported in 1325 obese LT recipients [14] from the United Kingdom where they had increased morbidity due to infectious complications and longer ICU and hospital stay in comparison to normal weight patients.

However, other studies suggested that higher BMI should not be considered an absolute contraindication to LT [15, 16]. In 230 LT patients stratified into a lean group (BMI 20–26 kg/m^2) and an obese group (BMI >38 kg/m^2), no significant differences were found (except that at 3-year follow-up, the obese group had a higher risk of developing MS). Similar results were noted in a retrospective study of 25,647 LT waitlist patients. When comparing patients who were on the waitlist versus those post-transplant, stratification by BMI all had a survival advantage with LT. Similar outcomes were noted by Conzen et al. [17] in a single-center study of 785 patients. A three-year patient and graft survival was similar in all groups, while a 5-year patient survival was significantly reduced in morbidly obese vs non-obese patients.

Timing for Bariatric Surgery: Before Liver Transplantation

The rationale for performing BS prior to LT would be to optimize patients' medical condition before surgery or to bring patients' BMI within the range considered acceptable by many transplant centers. However, BS performed before LT might delay transplant surgery due to the time necessary to achieve the desired BMI or to the development of perioperative complications. Another drawback of BS before LT is that recipients undergo two separate operations and two hospitalizations associated with increased financial costs, stress, and pain. Although no randomized controlled trials have ever been conducted to test whether BS is beneficial for obese patients requiring LT, case reports and observational studies have described the feasibility of BS either pre-, during, or post-LT. Lin et al. [18] published a retrospective review of all SG performed in liver (20 patients) and kidney transplant candidates (6 patients) between 2006 and 2012. The mean excess body weight loss (EBWL) at 1, 3, and 12 months was 17%, 26%, and 50% respectively without any perioperative death. Six cases (16%) experienced postoperative complications, including superficial wound infections, staple line leak, bleeding requiring transfusion, transient encephalopathy, and renal insufficiency. One-year postoperatively, all these patients became transplantable candidates by meeting institutional BMI requirements, and the authors concluded that SG is relatively safe and effective. Similar conclusions were drawn by Takata et al. [19] who evaluated the effect of BS in end-stage liver, kidney, and lung disease in 15 patients who were considered unsuitable for transplantation. Mean EBWL at or after 9 months was 61%, 33%, and 61%, respectively. Obesity-associated comorbidities improved in all patients except for two individuals (13%) who suffered from perioperative complications; no deaths occurred after surgery. More importantly, 93% of patients became transplant candidates by meeting the institutional requirements on BMI. These authors concluded that laparoscopic RYGB and SG are safe and improve the candidacy for transplantation. With gain in experience in cadaveric LT and BS, feasibility of living donor LT is being evaluated. Taneja et al. [20] published a successful outcome of SG in a patient with BMI of 55.6 and NASH undergoing living donor LT.

Timing for Bariatric Surgery: After Liver Transplantation

The main rationale for performing BS after LT would be to prevent the recurrence of metabolic syndrome (MS) and NASH and improve survival by reducing obesity-related comorbidities. In a recent publication, Duchini et al. [21] described two patients who were successfully treated by RYGB for severe graft dysfunction due to recurrent NASH. However, BS after LT comes with surgical risk of severe adhesions, wound complications, and anastomotic dehiscence due to the use of steroids and/or m-TOR inhibitors. Despite these potential drawbacks, Lin et al. [22] published a pilot study on the safety and feasibility of SG in nine obese LT recipients with the intent of improving steroid-induced diabetes, steatohepatitis, and MS. Postoperative complications occurred in three patients (33%) who developed a mesh infection with a concurrent ventral hernia repair and bile leak requiring drainage and one patient who underwent reoperation for dysphagia. At 6 months, 55% EBWL was achieved without graft rejection, and the authors concluded that SG does not adversely affect LT function. On the other hand, some technical challenges associated with BS after LT were reported by Tichansky et al. [23] who described major adhesions with complete obliteration of the gastrohepatic space during a successful laparoscopic RYGB after LT for a patient with a BMI of 54 kg/m^2.

Timing for Bariatric Surgery: During Liver Transplantation

Combining BS and LT could theoretically minimize delays and hospital stay and reduce patients' overall pain as the same incision can be used for both operations. However, one of the biggest trade-offs is that the operation for LT will take longer and that patients might suffer from more severe complications due to the increased complexity of the procedure. Campsen et al. [24] performed a successful simultaneous LT and adjustable gastric banding (AGB) and reported that at 6 months, patients' BMI went from 42 to 34 kg/m^2 with 45% EBWL and resolution of type 2 diabetes mellitus (T2DM), hypertension, and osteoarthritis. In 2013, Heimbach et al. [25] published their experience of BS in obese patients (BMI ≥35) undergoing LT. Obese patients with a BMI ≥35 were divided into two groups. Patients who successfully completed medically supervised weight loss (MSWL) underwent LT ($n = 37$) alone. Seven patients who failed MSWL underwent simultaneous LT and SG ($n = 7$). In patients who underwent LT alone, weight regain (BMI >35) was noted in 21 of 34 patients (61%), post-transplant diabetes in 12 patients (35%), steatosis in 7 (20%), and graft losses and deaths in 3 (8%). In the group of patients who underwent simultaneous LT and SG ($n = 7$), all maintained their weight loss, one had a gastrointestinal leak from the staple line (14%), and one had excessive weight loss. Although the majority of patients who did not undergo BS achieved some weight loss with a nonsurgical approach, most regained weight within a mean follow-up of 33 months. On the other hand, patients treated with combination of SG and LT achieved effective and sustained weight loss and fewer metabolic complications over a mean follow-up of 17 months.

Kidney Transplantation and Bariatric Surgery

The prevalence of obesity in patients with chronic kidney failure and renal transplant candidates has paralleled the epidemic in the general population. The associated risks of surgical complications and long-term cardiovascular death are significant. The kidney transplant operation is without a doubt technically more difficult in the obese recipient, in particular limiting the operative exposure of the external iliac vessels and the bladder in the pre-peritoneal and retroperitoneal spaces. This is reflected in the relatively longer operative times required in obese recipients, a higher rate of surgical complications, increased surgical site infections, and greater lymphoceles [26–28]. The length of stay, as a surrogate measure of a complicated recovery, is significantly longer [26]. The overall impact of postoperative complications such as surgical site infection should not be underestimated, as it has been shown to be significantly associated with graft loss [29]. Worse graft-related outcomes have been associated with obesity. Several studies have found an increased risk of delayed graft function in patients with a BMI >35 kg/m^2 [30, 31], and other studies have shown progressive risk with increased BMI [32]. Furthermore, risk of acute rejection has been found to be increased in obese recipients [33]. Obese recipients experience exacerbations of all aspects of the metabolic syndrome: hypertension, diabetes, and dyslipidemia [34]. The risks of congestive heart failure, atrial fibrillation, and myocardial infarction increase with each BMI quartile, and worse proteinuria has also been found in obese recipients [34].

Timing for Bariatric Surgery: Before Kidney Transplantation

With a scarcity of renal donors compared to demand, it is vital that recipients are selected carefully to maximize the success rates of renal transplant programs. Patient outcomes after renal transplantation are thought to be worse in obese patients. Consequently, obese patients may be refused for transplantation and those not excluded may have a lower listing priority. To improve all outcomes and to allow obese patients to undergo renal transplantation, patients need help with weight loss and maintaining weight loss before transplantation. This approach offers the advantages of (1) reducing waitlist times on dialysis, (2) increasing the proportion of patients who successfully achieve target weight loss goals, and (3) potentially decreasing post-transplant complications, including delayed graft function, and improving graft survival. It is known that diet and exercise programs rarely lead to sustained weight loss alone.

Takata et al. [19] reported a series of end-organ failure patients, including seven with end-stage renal disease (ESRD) who underwent laparoscopic gastric bypass (LGB). All patients in this series were able to reach the BMI limit for transplantation at the University of California at San Francisco of 40 kg/m^2 within a follow-up period of 3–18 months. The mean EBWL was 61% at 9 months postsurgery. The obesity-related comorbidities (hypertension, diabetes, and obstructive sleep apnea) had improved or resolved in all patients.

Focusing on KT alone, MacLaughlin et al. [35] published a series of nine patients who underwent laparoscopic sleeve gastrectomy (LSG) and reported a BMI decrease of 8.4 kg/m^2 at 6 months, representing a 43% EBWL. Concurrently, they reported a positive effect on blood pressure, diabetes, and hyperlipidemia. Subsequently, four patients were listed for KT. A larger series of 52 patients underwent LSG for failing to achieve significant weight loss with medical therapy. The mean preoperative BMI was 43.0 ± 5.4 kg/m^2; the mean BMI at last follow-up was 36.3 ± 5.3 kg/m^2. The mean EBWL was 32.1 ± 17.6%. They reported improvements in medical comorbidities. Six patients have successfully progressed to renal transplantation following LSG [36].

Timing for Bariatric Surgery: After Kidney Transplantation

Favorable results are also noted for patient undergoing BS after KT. In 1996, Marterre et al. [37] reported on three kidney transplant patients who had bypass surgery. All cases had a good response regarding weight loss, blood pressure normalization, and recovery from diabetes. Modanlou et al. [38] presented ten kidney transplant recipients who had RYGB in whom reduction of 70.5% excess body weight was attained.

Subsequently, Modanlou et al. [38] published a review of bariatric surgery among kidney transplant candidates and recipients using the US Renal Data System (USRDS) data. In this study of exclusively open surgical procedures, median EBWL of 31–61% was achieved with a 30-day mortality of 3.5% and one transplant recipient losing their graft within 30 days. Recent data in the general population shows a lower 30-day mortality in reference to laparoscopic procedures (0.15% for laparoscopic RYGB and 0.10% for LSG) [39]. Most recently, four kidney transplant patients who had LGB and one patient who had LSG achieved 50% excess weight loss, and no complications were reported [40].

Laparoscopic techniques such as LSG are now being used more commonly. LSG has been shown to be associated with effective weight loss and significant improvement in obesity-related comorbidities in the general population. The same group had previously reported on the outcome of LSG in ten kidney transplant patients. The median pre- and postoperative BMI was 42 kg/m^2 and 29 kg/m^2, respectively, and proteinuria and creatinine improved in all patients. Additionally, only three patients required minimal alterations in tacrolimus dose postsurgery [41].

Timing for Bariatric Surgery: During Kidney Transplantation

Another reported approach is a simultaneous KT and BS. The group from the University of Illinois at Chicago presented the first case of a 35-year-old woman with a BMI of 42 kg/m^2 (96.8 kg) and ESRD, who underwent combined robot-assisted kidney transplant and SG. At 24 months after transplantation, the patient's weight, BMI, creatinine, and estimated glomerular filtration rate were 81.9 kg, 35.1 kg/m^2, 0.79 mg/dL, and 81.2 mL/min per 1.73 m^2, respectively [42]. The benefits of this approach were a single anesthesia time, a single operation, and avoiding surgical complications from sequential procedures making the transplantation technically harder. The same group regularly performs minimally invasive robotic technique for kidney transplantation for their obese recipients, and the surgical technique was published previously. As a part of prospective study, they completed four more cases of combined robotic-assisted KT and SG with similar results and without surgical complications. The surgical technique of the sleeve gastrectomy did not defer from the well-established minimally invasive approaches. This data were presented at the American Transplant Congress 2015.

Pancreas Transplantation and Bariatric Surgery

Solid organ pancreas transplantation is a durable treatment to reestablish normoglycemia in diabetic patients with labile blood glucose and attenuate end-organ damage caused by diabetes. The typical pancreas transplant (PT) recipient is a patient with type 1 diabetes mellitus (T1DM), with or without concomitant renal failure. Simultaneous pancreas-kidney transplantation (SPK) accounted for approximately 77% of pancreas transplants performed in 2014. Pancreas transplant alone (PTA) in patients with preserved renal function or pancreas after kidney transplant (PAK) accounted for approximately 13.6% and 9% of pancreas transplants in 2014, respectively. As advances in surgical technique and immunosuppression have resulted in significantly improved patient and graft survival, individuals with increasing medical complexity are being considered for pancreas transplantation [43].

Obese patients are considered "unconventional recipients" of pancreas transplantation because they are a growing subgroup of the diabetic population, especially those with type 2 diabetes mellitus (T2DM). Currently, per UNOS guidelines, patients with detectable C-peptide levels (as a surrogate for T2DM) are eligible for pancreas transplantation if they are insulin-dependent with C-peptide levels more than 2 ng/ml and BMI less than 28 kg/m^2. These BMI restrictions are supported by recent data from Bedat et al. [44] who studied the impact of pancreas transplant recipient BMI in over 21,000 patients using SRTR data. The authors showed that patients who were overweight (BMI 25–29.9 kg/m^2) and obesity (>30 kg/m^2) had higher incidence of early pancreatic graft loss and early patient death (<90 days). Independently, obesity was associated with inferior long-term pancreas allograft survival. Similar findings were shown earlier by Sampiao et al. [45] who found that obesity (BMI >30 kg/m^2) was associated with increased risk of patient death and pancreas graft loss at 3 years. Very limited data exist about the safety and outcomes of BS in association with PT candidates.

Timing for Bariatric Surgery: Before Pancreas Transplantation

One series by Porubsky et al. [46] described four patients with T1DM who underwent pancreas transplantation after BS. The mean BMI before BS was 47.5 (kg/m^2), and the mean BMI at time of PT was 31 (kg/m^2). Three patients underwent RYGB and one patient underwent AGB. The postoperative course was unremarkable for all four patients. The mean follow-up time was 14 months, and the mean BMI at last follow-up was 27.6 (kg/m^2). All patients had good C-peptide and hemoglobin A1C at last visit, showing maintained graft function. Longer-term graft function was not evaluated.

Timing for Bariatric Surgery: After Pancreas Transplantation

When evaluating the effect of BS after PT, Elli et al. [47] reported their experience on 500 consecutive patients who underwent SG, 10 of which were organ transplant recipients. Two patients out of ten underwent PT before BS. The mean BMI at time of PT was 33.5 (kg/m^2), and the mean BMI at time of SG was 39.5 5 (kg/m^2). There were no surgical complications reported. The mean EBWL at 6 and 12 months was 55% and 50.5%, respectively. All two patients maintained a good graft function at 12 months.

Conclusion

The obesity epidemic is having a significant impact on the field of transplantation, as two-thirds of the adult population in the United States is overweight. Although obese patients undergoing transplantation might experience short- and long-term outcomes inferior to patients with normal BMI, their survival with transplantation is superior to best supportive care. Therefore, their exclusion from transplantation would violate the idea of fairness and should be challenged. Since medical therapies are relatively ineffective, BS might play a more distinct role in the future of transplantation. Currently, only low-quality evidence (from level 2b to level 4) [42] has shown that BS can be done either prior, during, or after LT. However, the number of publications is small, and except for a few case series, there are no studies that have systematically compared various weight loss approaches and subsequently their effect on patient outcomes (and graft function). Similarly, there is lack of data on the best timing of BS (prior, during, or after transplantation) or which type of BS (AGB vs RYGB vs SG vs DS) should be performed.

To maximize short- and long-term outcomes of these patients undergoing transplantation, prospective studies should be designed to identify if there are benefits from weight loss treatments and, if so, what interventions should be used and when they should be instituted. In the meantime, it is pertinent that the obese patients are informed of the treatment options for obesity so they are not evaluated and offered transplantation as an option for their vast array of medical conditions.

Glossary

AGB Adjustable gastric banding
BMI Body mass index
BS Bariatric surgery
DS Duodenal switch
EBWL Excess weight-loss
ESRD End-stage renal disease
KT Kidney transplant
LGB Laparoscopic gastric bypass
LSG Laparoscopic sleeve gastrectomy
LT Liver transplant
MS Metabolic syndrome
MSWL Medically supervised weight loss
PAK Pancreas after kidney transplant
PT Pancreas transplant
PTA Pancreas transplant alone
RYGB Roux-en-Y gastric bypass
SG Sleeve gastrectomy
SPK Simultaneous pancreas kidney transplant
T1DM Type 1 diabetes mellitus
T2DM Type 2 diabetes mellitus

References

1. Ng M, Fleming T, Robinson M, et al. Global, regional, and national prevalence of overweight and obesity in children and adults during 1980–2013: a systematic analysis for the Global Burden of Disease Study 2013. Lancet. 2014;384(9945):766–81.
2. Wang Y, Beydoun MA, Liang L, Caballero B, Kumanyika SK. Will all Americans become overweight or obese? Estimating the progression and cost of the US obesity epidemic. Obesity (Silver Spring). 2008;16(10):2323–30.
3. Friedman AN, Miskulin DC, Rosenberg IH, Levey AS. Demographics and trends in overweight and obesity in patients at time of kidney transplantation. Am J Kidney Dis. 2003;41(2):480–7.
4. Charlton MR, Burns JM, Pedersen RA, Watt KD, Heimbach JK, Dierkhising RA. Frequency and outcomes of liver transplantation for nonalcoholic steatohepatitis in the United States. Gastroenterology. 2011;141(4):1249–53.
5. Redfield RR, Rickels MR, Naji A, Odorico JS. Pancreas transplantation in the modern era. Gastroenterol Clin N Am. 2016;45(1):145–66.
6. Buchwald H, Avidor Y, Braunwald E, et al. Bariatric surgery: a systematic review and meta-analysis. JAMA. 2004;292(14):1724–37.
7. Kopelman PG. Obesity as a medical problem. Nature. 2000;404(6778):635–43.
8. Yanovski SZ, Yanovski JA. Long-term drug treatment for obesity: a systematic and clinical review. JAMA. 2014;311(1):74–86.
9. Halperin F, Ding SA, Simonson DC, et al. Roux-en-Y gastric bypass surgery or lifestyle with intensive medical management in patients with type 2 diabetes: feasibility and 1-year results of a randomized clinical trial. JAMA Surg. 2014;149(7):716–26.
10. Colquitt JL, Pickett K, Loveman E, Frampton GK. Surgery for weight loss in adults. Cochrane Database Syst Rev. 2014;8:CD003641.
11. LaMattina JC, Foley DP, Fernandez LA, et al. Complications associated with liver transplantation in the obese recipient. Clin Transpl. 2012;26(6):910–8.
12. Dick AA, Spitzer AL, Seifert CF, et al. Liver transplantation at the extremes of the body mass index. Liver Transpl. 2009;15(8):968–77.
13. Nair S, Verma S, Thuluvath PJ. Obesity and its effect on survival in patients undergoing orthotopic liver transplantation in the United States. Hepatology. 2002;35(1):105–9.
14. Hakeem AR, Cockbain AJ, Raza SS, et al. Increased morbidity in overweight and obese liver transplant recipients: a single-center experience of 1325 patients from the United Kingdom. Liver Transpl. 2013;19(5):551–62.
15. Perez-Protto SE, Quintini C, Reynolds LF, et al. Comparable graft and patient survival in lean and obese liver transplant recipients. Liver Transpl. 2013;19(8):907–15.
16. Pelletier SJ, Maraschio MA, Schaubel DE, et al. Survival benefit of kidney and liver transplantation for obese patients on the waiting list. Clin Transpl. 2003;(1):77–88.
17. Conzen KD, Vachharajani N, Collins KM, et al. Morbid obesity in liver transplant recipients adversely affects long-term graft and patient survival in a single-institution analysis. HPB (Oxford). 2015;17(3):251–7.
18. Lin MY, Tavakol MM, Sarin A, et al. Laparoscopic sleeve gastrectomy is safe and efficacious for pretransplant candidates. Surg Obes Relat Dis. 2013;9(5):653–8.
19. Takata MC, Campos GM, Ciovica R, et al. Laparoscopic bariatric surgery improves candidacy in morbidly obese patients awaiting transplantation. Surg Obes Relat Dis. 2008;4(2):159–64; discussion 164–155.
20. Taneja S, Gupta S, Wadhawan M, Goyal N. Single-lobe living donor liver transplant in a morbidly obese cirrhotic patient preceded by laparoscopic sleeve gastrectomy. Case Rep Transplant. 2013;2013:279651.

21. Duchini A, Brunson ME. Roux-en-Y gastric bypass for recurrent nonalcoholic steatohepatitis in liver transplant recipients with morbid obesity. Transplantation. 2001;72(1):156–9.
22. Lin MY, Tavakol MM, Sarin A, et al. Safety and feasibility of sleeve gastrectomy in morbidly obese patients following liver transplantation. Surg Endosc. 2013;27(1):81–5.
23. Tichansky DS, Madan AK. Laparoscopic Roux-en-Y gastric bypass is safe and feasible after orthotopic liver transplantation. Obes Surg. 2005;15(10):1481–6.
24. Campsen J, Zimmerman M, Shoen J, et al. Adjustable gastric banding in a morbidly obese patient during liver transplantation. Obes Surg. 2008;18(12):1625–7.
25. Heimbach JK, Watt KD, Poterucha JJ, et al. Combined liver transplantation and gastric sleeve resection for patients with medically complicated obesity and end-stage liver disease. Am J Transplant. 2013;13(2):363–8.
26. Holley JL, Shapiro R, Lopatin WB, Tzakis AG, Hakala TR, Starzl TE. Obesity as a risk factor following cadaveric renal transplantation. Transplantation. 1990;49(2):387–9.
27. Ditonno P, Lucarelli G, Impedovo SV, et al. Obesity in kidney transplantation affects renal function but not graft and patient survival. Transplant Proc. 2011;43(1):367–72.
28. Singh D, Lawen J, Alkhudair W. Does pretransplant obesity affect the outcome in kidney transplant recipients? Transplant Proc. 2005;37(2):717–20.
29. Lynch RJ, Ranney DN, Shijie C, Lee DS, Samala N, Englesbe MJ. Obesity, surgical site infection, and outcome following renal transplantation. Ann Surg. 2009;250(6):1014–20.
30. Meier-Kriesche HU, Vaghela M, Thambuganipalle R, Friedman G, Jacobs M, Kaplan B. The effect of body mass index on long-term renal allograft survival. Transplantation. 1999;68(9):1294–7.
31. Meier-Kriesche HU, Arndorfer JA, Kaplan B. The impact of body mass index on renal transplant outcomes: a significant independent risk factor for graft failure and patient death. Transplantation. 2002;73(1):70–4.
32. Molnar MZ, Kovesdy CP, Mucsi I, et al. Higher recipient body mass index is associated with post-transplant delayed kidney graft function. Kidney Int. 2011;80(2):218–24.
33. Chang SH, Coates PT, McDonald SP. Effects of body mass index at transplant on outcomes of kidney transplantation. Transplantation. 2007;84(8):981–7.
34. Armstrong KA, Campbell SB, Hawley CM, Johnson DW, Isbel NM. Impact of obesity on renal transplant outcomes. Nephrology (Carlton). 2005;10(4):405–13.
35. MacLaughlin HL, Hall WL, Patel AG, et al. Weight loss, adipokines, and quality of life after sleeve gastrectomy in obese patients with stages 3-4 CKD: a randomized controlled pilot study. Am J Kidney Dis. 2014;64(4):660–3.
36. Freeman CM, Woodle ES, Shi J, et al. Addressing morbid obesity as a barrier to renal transplantation with laparoscopic sleeve gastrectomy. Am J Transplant. 2015;15(5):1360–8.
37. Marterre WF, Hariharan S, First MR, Alexander JW. Gastric bypass in morbidly obese kidney transplant recipients. Clin Transpl. 1996;10(5):414–9.
38. Modanlou KA, Muthyala U, Xiao H, et al. Bariatric surgery among kidney transplant candidates and recipients: analysis of the United States renal data system and literature review. Transplantation. 2009;87(8):1167–73.
39. Young MT, Gebhart A, Phelan MJ, Nguyen NT. Use and outcomes of laparoscopic sleeve gastrectomy vs laparoscopic gastric bypass: analysis of the American College of Surgeons NSQIP. J Am Coll Surg. 2015;220(5):880–5.
40. Szomstein S, Rojas R, Rosenthal RJ. Outcomes of laparoscopic bariatric surgery after renal transplant. Obes Surg. 2010;20(3):383–5.
41. Golomb I, Winkler J, Ben-Yakov A, Benitez CC, Keidar A. Laparoscopic sleeve gastrectomy as a weight reduction strategy in obese patients after kidney transplantation. Am J Transplant. 2014;14(10):2384–90.
42. Ayloo SM, D'Amico G, West-Thielke P, et al. Combined robot-assisted kidney transplantation and sleeve gastrectomy in a morbidly obese recipient. Transplantation. 2015;99:1495–8.
43. Lo DJ, Sayed BA, Turgeon NA. Pancreas transplantation in unconventional recipients. Curr Opin Organ Transplant. 2016;21(4):393–8.
44. Bédat B, Niclauss N, Jannot AS, et al. Impact of recipient body mass index on short-term and long-term survival of pancreatic grafts. Transplantation. 2015;99(1):94–9.
45. Sampaio MS, Reddy PN, Kuo HT, et al. Obesity was associated with inferior outcomes in simultaneous pancreas kidney transplant. Transplantation. 2010;89(9):1117–25.
46. Porubsky M, Powelson JA, Selzer DJ, et al. Pancreas transplantation after bariatric surgery. Clin Transpl. 2012;26(1):E1–6.
47. Elli EF, Gonzalez-Heredia R, Sanchez-Johnsen L, Patel N, Garcia-Roca R, Oberholzer J. Sleeve gastrectomy surgery in obese patients post-organ transplantation. Surg Obes Relat Dis. 2016;12(3):528–34.

Part X

Research and Innovation

Interventional Radiology, Is There a Role for the Surgeon?

43

Mariano Palermo, Pablo Acquafresca, and Mariano Gimenez

Background

Obesity is a growing problem all over the world, especially in the United States, Europe, and Australia [1]. Currently, bariatric surgery offers the only effective long-term weight loss therapy for morbidly obese patients. Increased media attention to these procedures as well as the newer option of laparoscopic treatment has led patients and surgeons to embrace this surgical option in an elevated number, particularly the option of Roux-en-Y gastric bypass (RYGBP) and sleeve gastrectomy (SG). Numerous studies have demonstrated the reduction in death and disability associated with obesity surgery [2], but these surgeries also have significant rates of complications which can be as high as 32.8% [3], such as anastomotic or staple line leaks, abdominal abscess, gastrointestinal bleeding, intestinal obstruction, anastomotic strictures, choledocholithiasis in patients with modified anatomy due to RYGB, and acute gastric dilatation, among others.

It is important for the bariatric surgeon to recognize these complications and know which of them can be solved in a minimal invasive way in order to offer to the patients the best treatment.

M. Palermo (✉)
Department of Bariatric Surgery, Centro CIEN–Diagnomed, Buenos Aires, Argentina

Department of Surgery, DAICIM Foundation, Buenos Aires, Argentina

P. Acquafresca · M. Gimenez
Department of Surgery, DAICIM Foundation, Buenos Aires, Argentina

Complications Treated by IR

One of the most common complications after bariatric surgery is leaks due to inadequate tissue healing, allowing the exit of gastrointestinal material through the staple or suture line. It can be as high as 2.4% in the sleeve gastrectomy [4], while in the RYGB, it can reach the 5.6% incidence in large series [5]. Regarding the RYGB, there are five potential sites of leaking, gastrojejunostomy, gastric pouch staple line, Roux limb staple line, jejunojejunostomy, and gastric remnant staple line, while in the sleeve gastrectomy, the leaks can occur at the stapler line of the sleeve, being more common at the proximal third of the stomach in 89% of cases [4].

Although most anastomotic leaks occur 5–7 days after surgery and are thought to be related to ischemia, 95% of anastomotic leaks that occur within 2 days of surgery probably result from technical error [6]. It is important to know this because as sooner the fistula emerges more likely to have committed a technical error during the surgery, and this will indicate that a reoperation may be needed because this kind of leaks tends to come out as a peritonitis. On the other hand, if more time have passed, it is possible that the leak appears as an abdominal abscess or collection, and if this is the case, a minimally invasive approach can be attempted by draining the abscess in a percutaneous fashion.

Given the complexity of these abscesses, it is necessary in many cases to perform the drainage under computed tomography (CT) guidance, while

R. Lutfi et al. (eds.), *Global Bariatric Surgery*, https://doi.org/10.1007/978-3-319-93545-4_43

in easier cases, like big abscesses near the abdominal wall, ultrasound guidance can be used.

Materials and Technique

The technique consists in performing a puncture of the abscess with a 16-gauge needle under image guidance, and then a 0.035″ wire with "J" tip (Fig. 43.1) is inserted through the needle until it is rolled up inside the abscess in order to secure the access. Once this is confirmed with the image guidance, a multipurpose catheter (Fig. 43.2) is placed inside the abscess (Fig. 43.3) with the Seldinger technique (Fig. 43.4).

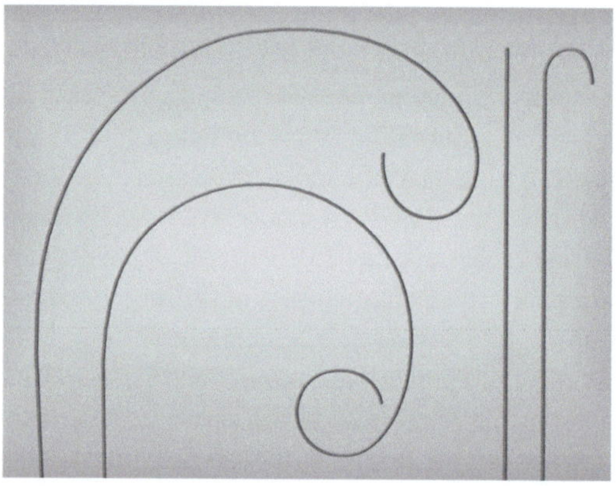

Fig. 43.1 0,035″ flexible wire with "J" tip. It is important to use a "J" tip wire in order to roll up the wire inside the abscess and not break the abscess's wall

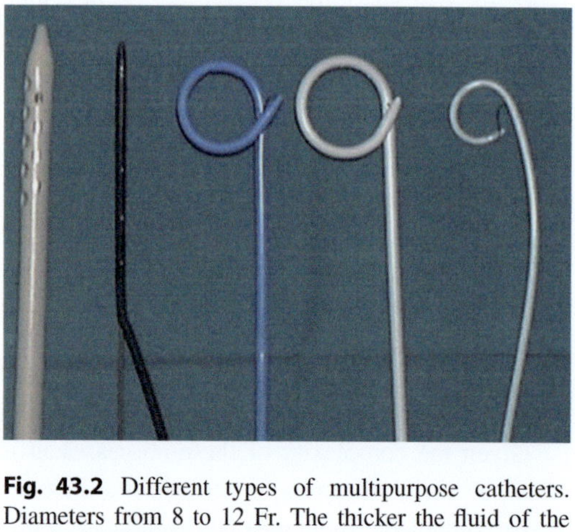

Fig. 43.2 Different types of multipurpose catheters. Diameters from 8 to 12 Fr. The thicker the fluid of the abscess, the bigger should be the diameter of the catheter. Catheters with "pig-tail" fixation must be used in order to avoid accidental dislocation

Treatment of Fistulas and Collections

The diagnosis of these abscesses sometimes can be challenging because it could be difficult to differentiate the abscess from the digestive lumen (Fig. 43.5). The absence of wall, the location, and the size of the abscess could help to differentiate it from normal structures, and in case of doubt, an upper gastrointestinal series could help to recognize the fistula (Fig. 43.6). This study must be done with water-soluble contrast in order to avoid further complications due to contrast leakage.

Once the catheter is placed, the follow-up must be done by paying attention to the patient's clinic evolution and the catheter's semiology (Fig. 43.7). If the patient persists with systemic inflammatory response syndrome (fever, increased heart rate, hypoxemia, or increased white blood cell count), a new image should be done. In case of a residual abscess or intermediate cavity along the fistula, a new drainage should be performed. On the other hand, if no abscess is present and generalized free liquid in the abdominal cavity is found, the possibility of a relaparoscopy must be considered.

It is also important to consider the drainage characteristics. If the catheter persists with a high amount of fluid and this fluid looks like gastric or intestinal fluid, a new image also must be done. In this case, a fistulography could be useful to confirm the communication between the abscess and the digestive lumen (Fig. 43.8).

Once the infection is controlled and SIRS is no more present, an adequate nutrition and a high protein level are essential to achieve the closure of the fistula. In order to accomplish this, a nasojejunal tube must be placed with the tip distal to the fistula to avoid leakage of the enteral feeding.

With this approach, 70% of the fistulas heal and no further treatment is necessary, but sometimes months should pass in order to reach the success.

In case that the fistula doesn't heal, further treatment must be performed like fully covered gastric stent placement (Figs. 43.9, 43.10, and 43.11). The goal of this procedure is to block the

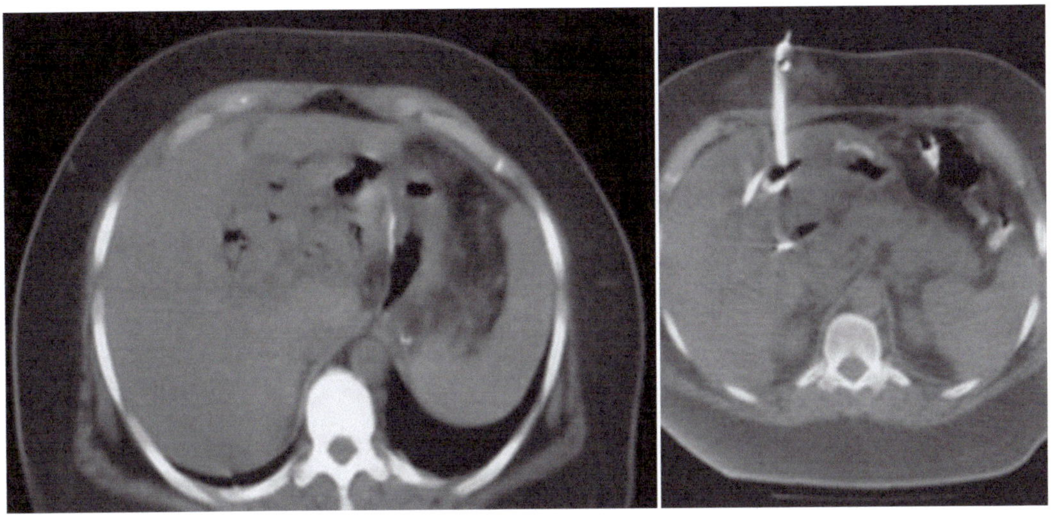

Fig. 43.3 Central abdominal abscess after sleeve gastrectomy and the multipurpose catheter placement. Notice how the catheter goes through the liver left lobe; if the patient has an adequate coagulation and platelet count, this doesn't generate further complications, but it is important not to puncture any significant vascular or biliary branch

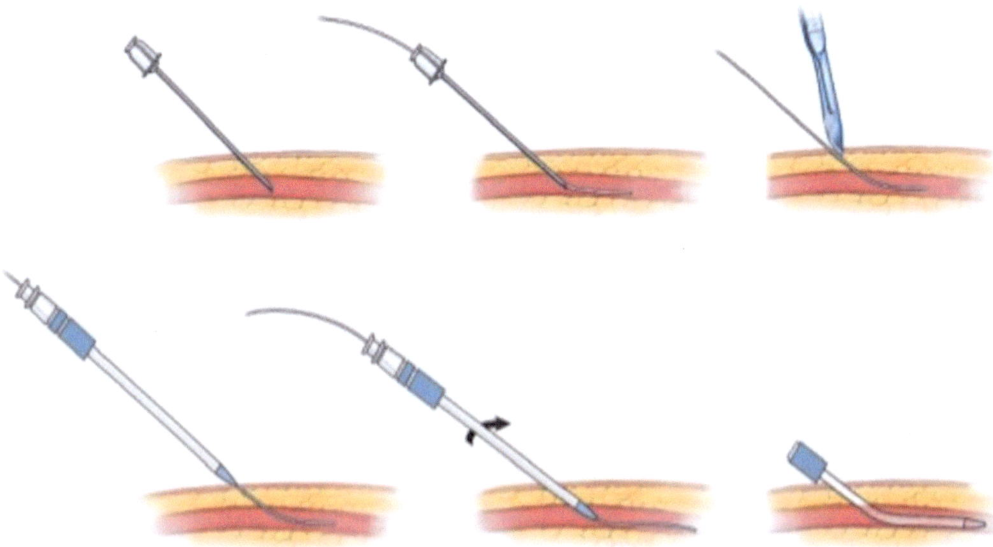

Fig. 43.4 Seldinger technique: puncture, insert of the guide wire, dilatation, and catheter placement. Same technique than a vascular access

leakage with the stent cover until the fistula heals. Although it may seem a great solution, some problems may arise like stent migration or leakage persistence due to filtration between the gastric wall and the stent cover.

Other options are also available like endoscopic clip placement (Figs. 43.12 and 43.13) or biological fibrin sealants in order to close the fistula, but further research is needed to define the success of these treatments.

Fig. 43.5 Abdominal abscess with contrast and air after sleeve gastrectomy that could be mistaken as gastric lumen. Notice the absence of thick walls and the diameter size much bigger than the usual sleeves

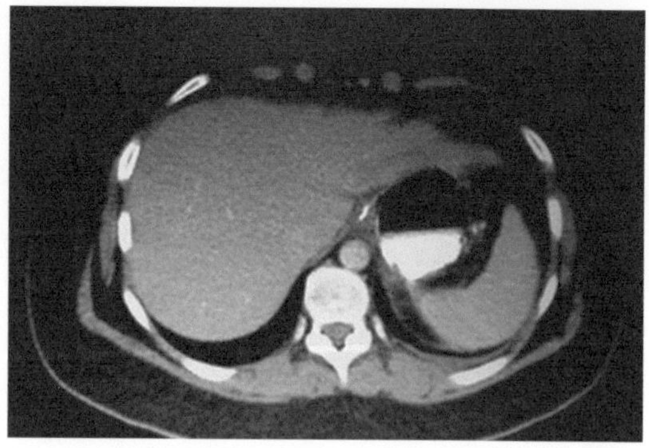

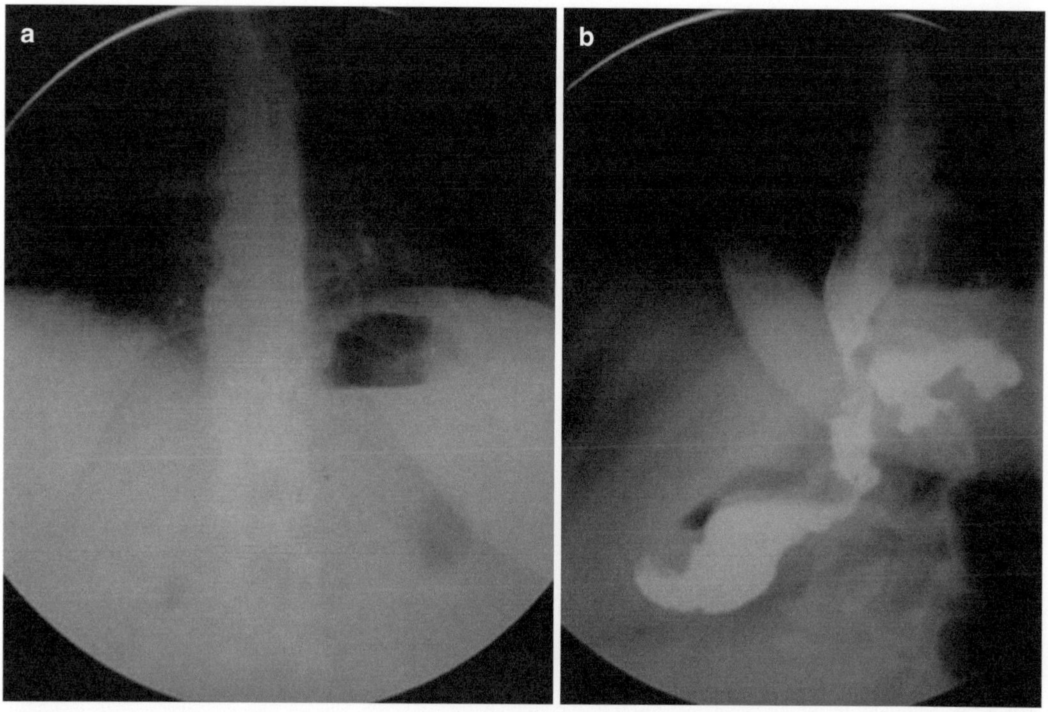

Fig. 43.6 (**a**, **b**) Upper gastrointestinal series of the same patient from Fig. 43.5 with sleeve gastrectomy where a leakage is present. Notice how the air of the abscess could be mistaken with fundus air

Fig. 43.7 Algorithm of catheter follow-up (SIRS: systemic inflammatory response syndrome)

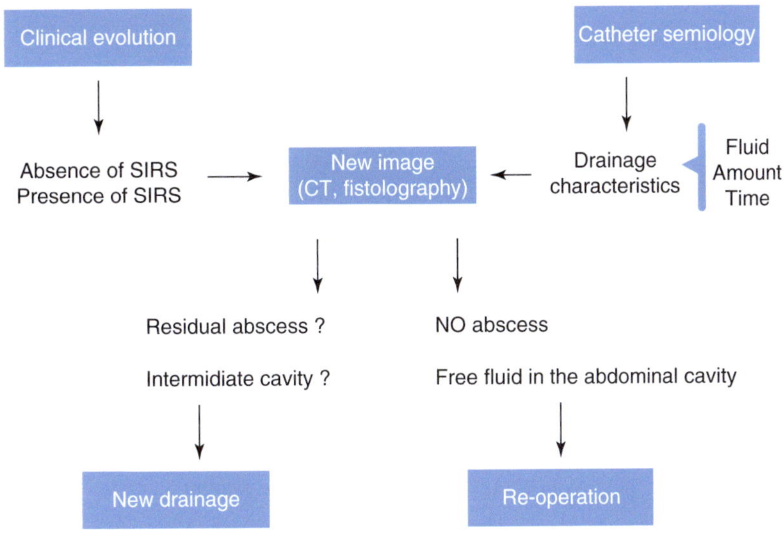

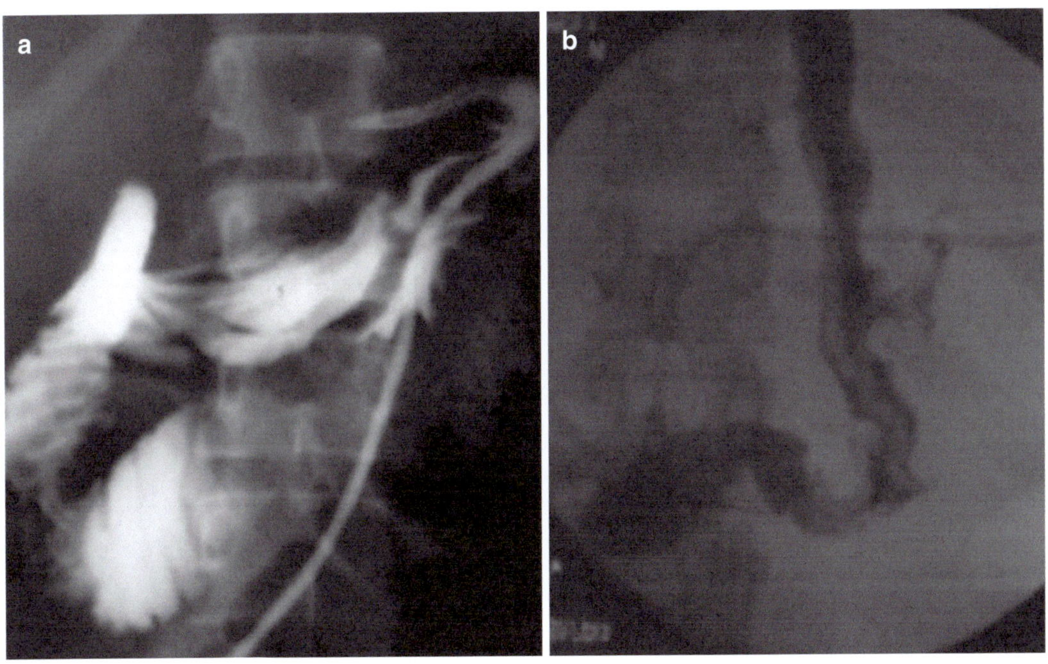

Fig. 43.8 (**a**, **b**) Fistulography of patients with sleeve gastrectomy. Contrast is instilled through the catheter and the sleeve can be seen

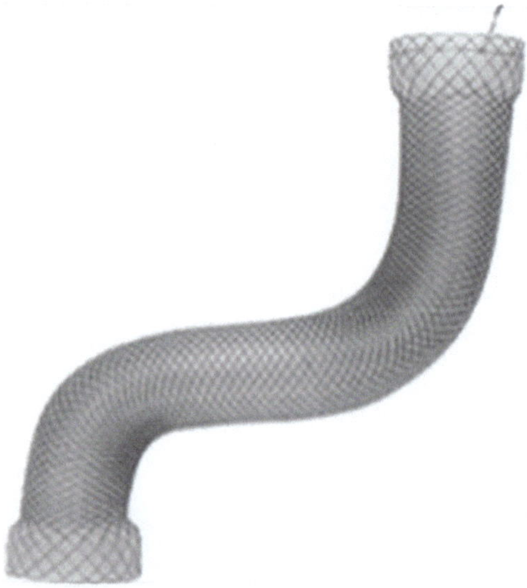

Fig. 43.9 Example of a fully covered gastric stent

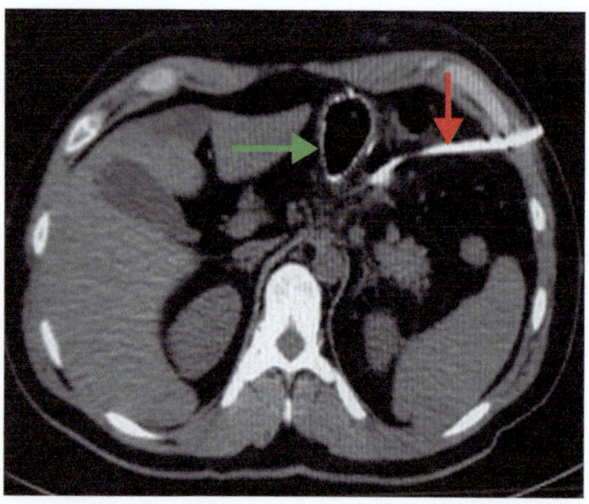

Fig. 43.10 TC scan of patient with fistula after sleeve gastrectomy. Red arrow, multipurpose catheter draining the abscess; blue arrow, gastric stent

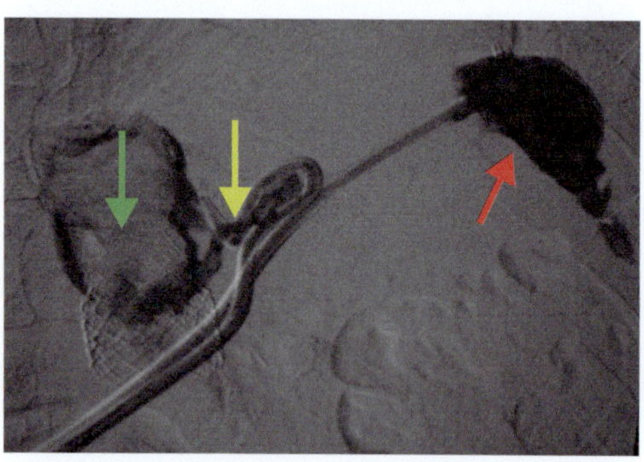

Fig. 43.11 Stent placement in a patient with sleeve gastrectomy fistula. Green arrow: gastric stent. Orange arrow: the fistula. Yellow arrow: intermediate cavity with drainage. Red arrow: abscess with drainage

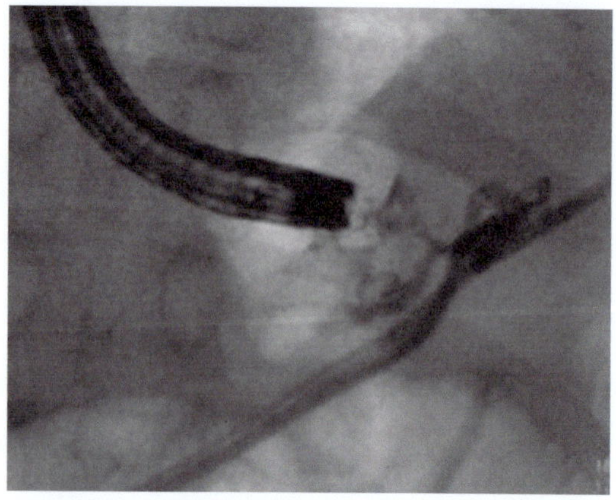

Fig. 43.12 Endoscopic clip placement under radioscopic control

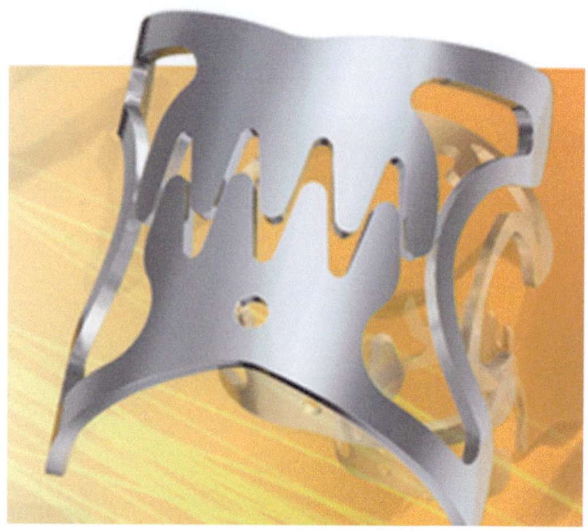

Fig. 43.13 Example of endoscopic clips

Bile Duct Stones After Bariatric Surgery

Another problem that may arise after bariatric surgery is the presence of gallstones in the common bile duct. Although it is a rare complication after RYGB (around 0.2% of the bariatric patients) [7], it represents an important challenge due to the anatomical modifications of the gastrointestinal tract (Fig. 43.14). The duodenum remains adjacent to the surgically excluded stomach. Therefore, for the endoscopist, accessing the ampulla is technically very difficult. The endoscope must pass through the mouth, esophagus, gastric pouch, and Roux limb and then return retrograde through the afferent limb to reach the ampulla. This total

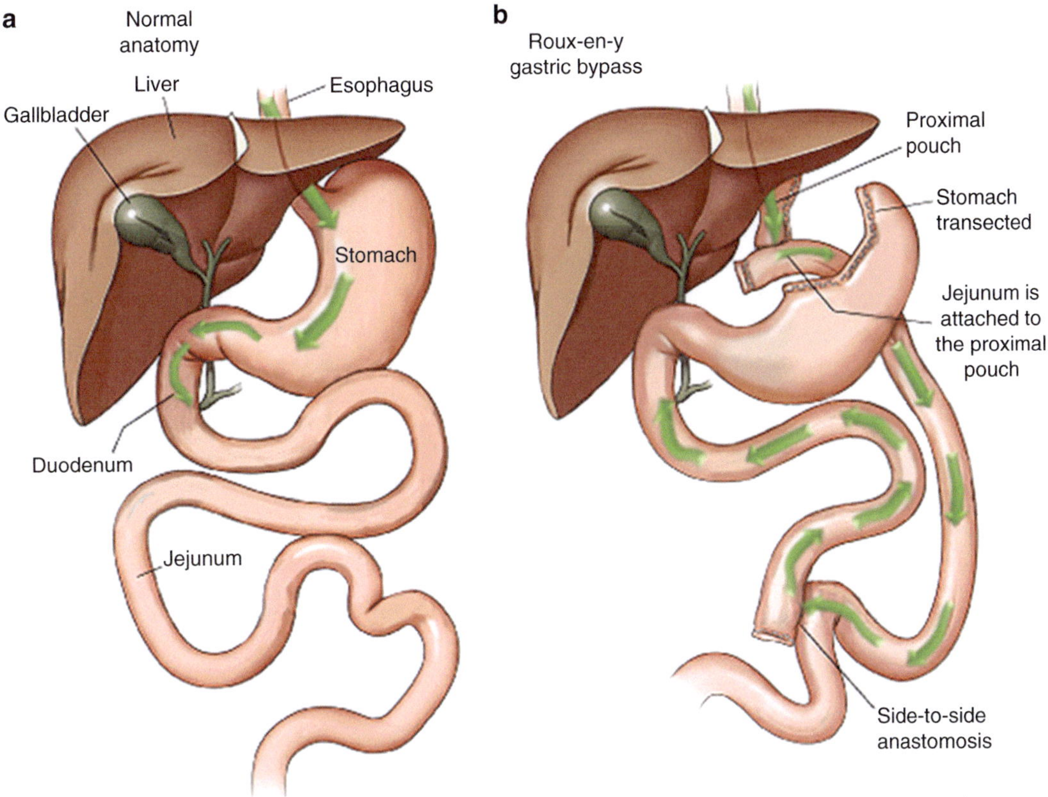

Fig. 43.14 (**a**) Green arrow showing the endoscopy path to the ampulla in normal anatomy. (**b**) Green arrow showing the endoscopy path to the ampulla in altered anatomy by gastric bypass

length may easily exceed 300 cm, making almost impossible for traditional endoscopy access to the papilla to perform an endoscopic retrograde cholangiopancreatography (ERCP).

This leads to having to pursue other methods to reach the papillae for the resolution of choledocholithiasis like laparoscopy-assisted transgastric ERCP, balloon enteroscopy-assisted ERCP, laparoscopic exploration of the common bile duct, and percutaneous biliary drainage with subsequent trans-fistula treatment, the latter being the topic of concern in this chapter.

With the percutaneous approach to treat the common bile duct gallstones, first it is necessary to perform a percutaneous biliary drainage, and later when the fistula between the biliary system and the skin is consolidated, a session to remove the stones can be performed.

The first step of the procedure consists on an ultrasound-guided puncture of the intrahepatic bile duct by using a 22G Chiba needle (Fig. 43.15), and then a percutaneous transhepatic cholangiogram should be performed to confirm the presence, location, number, and size of stones (Fig. 43.16). The choice whether to use a left-sided subxiphoid approach or a right-sided subcostal or intercostal approach must be based

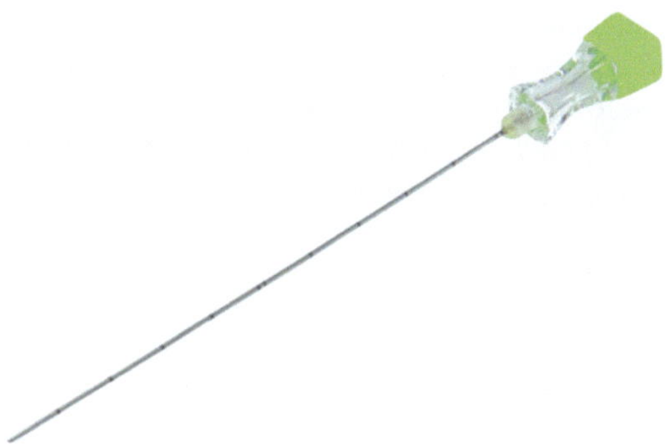

Fig. 43.15 22G Chiba needle

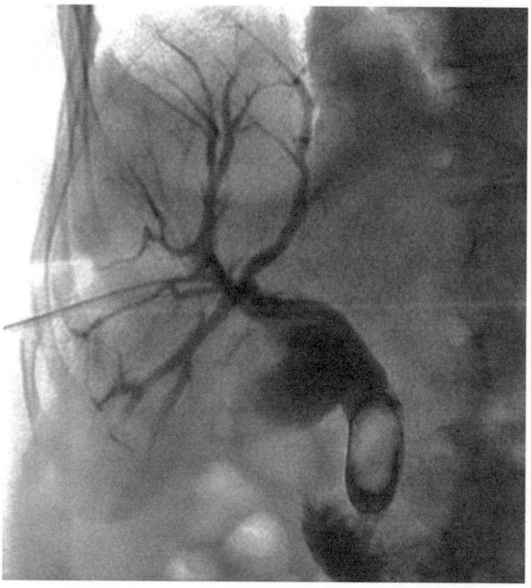

Fig. 43.16 Percutaneous transhepatic cholangiogram showing a big stone on the distal common bile duct

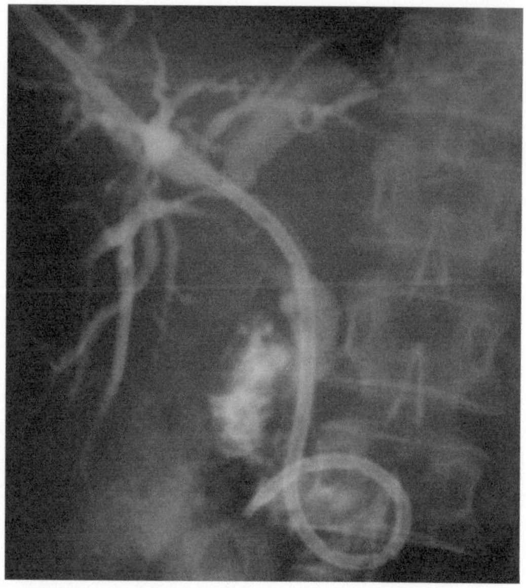

Fig. 43.17 Percutaneous biliary drainage with "pig-tail" in the duodenum

on individual and anatomic considerations, such as the position of the liver, bile duct anatomy (as seen on pre-procedural imaging), and number, position, and size of the bile duct stones.

The percutaneous transhepatic cholangiogram can be achieved in 98% of the patients with dilatation of the bile ducts and in 90% of those without dilatation [8].

Once we gain access to the biliary system with the Chiba needle, a guide wire must be introduced through the needle, and by using Seldinger technique, an 8 or 10 Fr biliary drainage must be placed (Fig. 43.17).

After 7–10 days, when the biliary system is decompressed, the symptoms of cholangitis (if were present) are relieved, and the fistula starts to consolidate, it is possible to perform the treatment of the stones. By working through the biliary-cutaneous fistula is possible to push the stones into the duodenum or extracting them through the skin's hole. In order to achieve this, a standard percutaneous transluminal angioplasty balloon catheter is advanced beyond the stones and positioned across the papilla.

Then the sphincter is dilated by an 8–12 mm balloon, depending of the size of the largest stone, until no waist could be seen in the balloon on fluoroscopy (Fig. 43.18). Once this is achieved, the balloon is deflated and the catheter withdrawn and positioned proximal to the stones. After reinflating the balloon, the stones are pushed forward through the dilated sphincter into the duodenum.

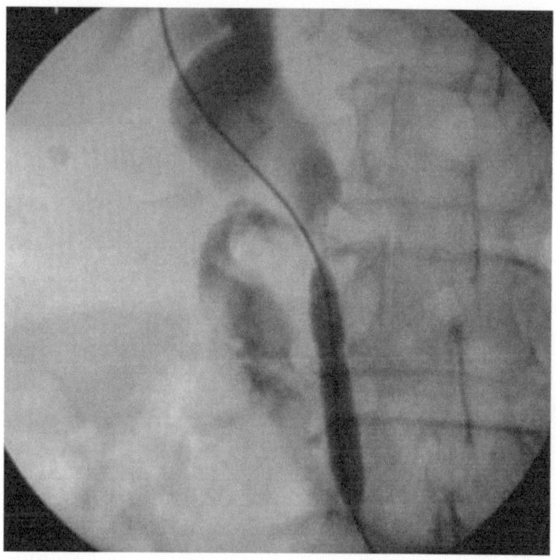

Fig. 43.18 Sphincter dilation with a 10 mm balloon. A waist can still be seen on the balloon

If the stone size exceeded 10 mm, mechanical lithotripsy with Dormia basket is recommended [9]. The stone fragments are then evacuated into

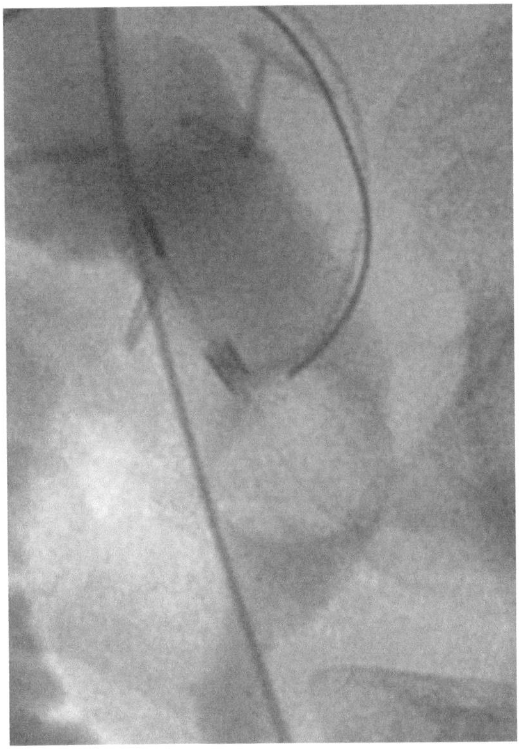

Fig. 43.19 A stone being grabbed with a Dormia basket

the duodenum by using the balloon catheter or Dormia basket (Fig. 43.19). If the stone's size is not too big, another option is to grab the stone with the Dormia basket and pull it out through the skin's hole. This maneuver could be dangerous if the stone is larger than the fistula diameter because the fistula could be damaged; thus, it is recommended to place a second (safety) wire through the papilla in order to preserve the biliary access.

When all the stones seem to have been extracted, cholangiography must be performed to confirm complete stone clearance. Then a biliary drainage is placed in the common bile duct.

After approximately 24 h later, a cholangiography must be performed to confirm common bile duct clearance, and if so, the external drainage is removed. If residual stones are found, the procedure must be repeated until all stones are removed.

The success rate reported with this approach varies between 93% and 96% and the complications between 4.7% and 6.7% [9–14]. The complications described include hemobilia, pancreatitis, cholangitis, pleural effusion due to a transpleural biliary drainage, and bile peritonitis due to fistula disruption.

In conclusion, IR strongly has a role in the treatment of complications following bariatric surgery. We think that the combination of IR, endoscopy, and laparoscopy will solve more than 90% of the complications by these approaches.

References

1. Mokdad AH, Bowman BA, Ford ES, Vinicor F, Marks JS, Koplan JP. The continuing epidemic of obesity and diabetes in the United States. JAMA. 2001;286:1195–200.
2. Buchwald H, Avidor Y, Braunwald E, et al. Bariatric surgery: a systematic review and meta-analysis. JAMA. 2004;292:1724–37.
3. Encinosa WE, Bernard DM, Du D, Steiner CA. Recent improvements in bariatric surgery outcomes. Med Care. 2009;47(5):531–5.
4. Aurora AR, Khaitan L, Saber AA. Sleeve gastrectomy and the risk of leak: a systematic analysis of 4,888 patients. Surg Endosc. 2012;26:1509–15. https://doi.org/10.1007/s00464-011-2085-3.
5. Livingston EH, Ko CY. Assessing the relative contribution of individual risk factors on surgical outcome for gastric bypass surgery: a baseline probability analysis. J Surg Res. 2002;105(1):48–52.
6. Baker RS, Foote J, Kemmeter P, Brady R, Vroegop T, Serveld M. The science of stapling and leaks. Obes Surg. 2004;14(10):1290–8.
7. Warschkow R, Tarantino I, Ukegjini K, Beutner U, Güller U, Schmied BM, Müller SA, Schultes B, Thurnheer M. Concomitant cholecystectomy during laparoscopic roux-en-Y gastric bypass in obese patients is not justified: a meta-analysis. Obes Surg. 2013;23:397–407.
8. Gimenez ME, Berkowski D, Cordoba P. Obstrucción biliar benigna. In: Gimenez M, Guimaraes M, Oleaga J, Sierre S, editors. Manual de técnicas intervencionistas guiadas por imágenes. Buenos Aires: Ediciones Journal; 2011. p. 119–38.
9. Kint JF, van den Bergh JE, van Gelder RE, Rauws EA, Gouma DJ, van Delden OM, Laméris JS. Percutaneous treatment of common bile duct stones: results and complications in 110 consecutive patients. Dig Surg. 2015;32:9–15. https://doi.org/10.1159/000370129.
10. García-García L, Lanciego C. Percutaneous treatment of biliary stones: sphincteroplasty and occlusion balloon for the clearance of bile duct calculi. AJR. 2004;182:663–70.
11. Szulman C, Giménez M, Sierre S. Antegrade papillary balloon dilation for extrahepatic bile duct stone

clearance: lessons learned from treating 300 patients. J Vasc Interv Radiol. 2011;22(3):346–53.

12. Gil S, de la Iglesia P, Verdú JF, de España F, Arenas J, Effectiveness IJ. Safety of balloon dilation of the papilla and the use of an occlusion balloon for clearance of bile duct calculi. AJR Am J Roentgenol. 2000;174(5):1455–60.
13. Aquafresca PA, Palermo M, Rogula T, Duza GE, Serra E. Complicações cirúrgicas tardias após bypass gástrico: revisão da literatura. Arq Bras Cir Dig. 2015;28(2):139–143
14. Palermo M, Gimenez M, Gagner M. Laparoscopic gastrointestinal surgery. Novel techniques, extending the limits. Agarani: AMOCA; 2015.

Accommodating Research in Busy Bariatric Practice

44

Aaron Lee Wiegmann and Alfonso Torquati

Introduction

Bariatric surgery is a field that has been shaped by the research and experimentation of the past. The modern state of bariatric surgery, most notably its ever-increasing popularity as a legitimate and safe option to the public, is a direct result of decades of clinical research in the field leading to improved outcomes and patient safety. Bariatric surgery will necessarily continue to be studied and advanced as the American population continues to suffer from the obesity epidemic. In fact, bariatric surgery research in the United States will likely see an increase in volume, funding, and scientific breakthroughs with the continued staggering prevalence of obesity and comorbid conditions over the coming decades. Currently, nearly 17% of Americans aged 2–19 are obese, and nearly 35% of adults aged 20 or higher are obese [1]. Obesity prevalence has not changed significantly since 2003–2004, but stabilization at such a high rate is quite alarming—as is the rising obesity prevalence among certain vulnerable and disadvantaged American populations, such as African-American and Mexican-American women [2]. The metabolic derangements inherent in obesity, such as diabetes, are becoming catastrophically prevalent. The CDC projects that one in three American adults could suffer from diabetes by the year 2050 [3]. This has immense implications for bariatric surgery research and funding in the future. As surgical management has been the only truly curative means of treatment for diabetes in modern medicine, bariatric surgery and its effect on the metabolic status of the obese patient will be scientifically vetted for decades to come.

A. L. Wiegmann, MD (✉) · A. Torquati, MD, MSCI, FACS
Department of Surgery, Rush University Medical Center, Chicago, IL, USA
e-mail: Aaron_L_Wiegmann@rush.edu; Alfonso_Torquati@rush.edu

Research in Bariatric Surgery Requires a Winning Team

Success in weight loss surgery research can be realized when a well-assembled research team works cohesively in a well-designed comprehensive bariatric program. Whether it is clinical, device, or basic science research, a principal investigator (PI) needs to have team members motivated and goal-oriented in a clinical environment attractive to potential patient subjects and conducive to completing the project in a timely matter. A key skill that needs to be developed by the PI is the proper delegation of tasks to research team members.

The research team is somewhat hierarchical with team members at all levels working toward publication. Clearly, a busy researching physician will likely not be able to commit all their time to a project: they have a practice to maintain. A nice way to meet this time demand is to hire a clinical research coordinator dedicated to quarterbacking ongoing projects. Having a research coordinator will also

R. Lutfi et al. (eds.), *Global Bariatric Surgery*, https://doi.org/10.1007/978-3-319-93545-4_44

lessen any increased work burden on the bariatric practice's current staff that a clinical trial could incur, thus allowing ancillary staff to focus on vital components such as maintaining subject recruitment. The physician PI's true purpose during the study is ensuring the safety of the subjects. The PI must also weigh the benefits of subject participation in the study versus any potential medical risks, monitor the subject's compliance with study parameters, oversee subject adherence to protocol, fulfill regulatory responsibilities, and ensure data quality.

A research team also has many other academic positions, all of which could contribute (in their own capacity) to the drafting and formation of the project, subject enrollment, data collection and analysis, and writing/submission of findings for peer review. Academic staff, often contributing a Ph.D. or equivalent degree in pertinent clinical knowledge, is primarily responsible for assisting the PI in achieving the goals of the ongoing research projects and could be contributing as visiting staff from another institution—possibly as co-author. Postdoctoral scholars are nonmatriculated research trainees who professionally contribute to a research project, often under the mentorship of the PI faculty member, fine-tuning their research skills in preparation for an independent academic career. Resident physicians will make substantial contributions to a project through data processing, paper writing and presenting, and surgically or medically treating patient subjects within protocol—often as co-authors during a research elective. Medical students can contribute as much as they want to; motivated students may even co-author papers but usually contribute with paper writing and data collection and analysis. All other employees of a bariatric practice become integral members of the research team by ensuring that clinical responsibilities are running smoothly.

A Comprehensive Bariatric Program Is Necessary for Research Success

Many bariatric programs in the United States boast being "comprehensive." What does this mean? The comprehensive approach to weight loss surgery was created out of three general principles: maximizing postoperative positive outcomes, ensuring appropriate patient screening for the best surgical candidates, and receiving insurance reimbursement for surgery to sustain the practice. The comprehensive bariatric practice also happens to be the ideal environment in which to conduct clinical research.

From a staff perspective, the program needs experienced, preferably well-known, surgeons specializing in bariatric surgery procedures. These surgeons are the faces of the program, and the higher the impact the surgeon has had on the field (robust web presence), the more likely primary care physicians will refer, and patient subjects will self-refer to the program. Also needed in the comprehensive program is a full complement of medical specialists (i.e., medical internists, gastroenterologists, etc.) experienced in bariatric care, for easy patient access, providing long-term medical follow-up and maintaining positive outcomes. The services of a bariatric nurse liaison are necessary to coordinate different elements of the patient's care and insurance coverage and facilitate research study recruitment. A registered dietician and nutritionist specializing in the needs of bariatric patients are necessary to work with patients preoperatively as part of the patient compliance screening process and postoperatively to ensure weight loss maintenance and adherence to dietary modifications. Clinical psychologists specializing in the mental health of bariatric patients are needed to perform psychological evaluations for preoperative screening and removal of unfit patients—something often required for insurance coverage. Clinical psychologists also provide postoperative counseling for the psychological well-being of the patient.

From a support standpoint, the comprehensive program can offer a plethora of resources to the patient. In-person educational seminars about weight loss surgery options can be offered to potential surgical subjects, and attendance often can be required to ensure proper preoperative patient education. Online videos and educational resources can also be offered to the patient on the program's website. A bariatric support group can be implemented to have both previous patients and potential surgical candidates interact and share stories. It is also important to offer certain services relevant to the treatment of certain obesity comorbidities, such as offering a sleep study lab for the diagnosis of obstructive sleep apnea (OSA) that a large cohort of obese patients will suffer from. Obviously, a comprehensive bariatric program needs to have its own clinic space for patient convenience, and privacy as surgical interventions regarding weight can often evoke feelings of embarrassment for patients. Patient support can be a very attractive element for a bariatric practice.

The importance of having a comprehensive bariatric clinic in regard to surgical research is most pertinent to the goal of this text. This can be thought of logically: in order for bariatric surgery research to be possible, bariatric surgical procedures need to be taking place. There are many moving pieces in the work-up and management of a bariatric surgical candidate, and the comprehensive clinic consolidates the entire multidisciplinary approach in one place. Thus, the comprehensive clinic is providing the PI with a steady inflow of potential study subjects that are ready for operation and enrollment into a study. It is also worth mentioning that insurance compensation for weight loss surgery is essential in keeping a busy researching practice afloat. As an example, Medicare in the United States has certain criteria that a patient must meet in order to have their weight loss surgery covered: "The beneficiary needs a body-mass index (BMI) $\geq$ 40 kg/m^2 or $\geq$ 35 kg/m^2 with at least one comorbidity related to obesity, and the beneficiary has been previously unsuccessful with medical treatment for obesity" [4]. In 2017, if a patient who has a BMI of 39.9 kg/m^2 has not seen a physician in years and has not been diagnosed with any comorbid conditions, Medicare will not cover their surgery. Therefore, they cannot be operated on, and, thus, they cannot be enrolled in a bariatric research project. But, if that same patient presents to a comprehensive clinic and endorses snoring, they can be sent to the on-site sleep study lab and potentially be diagnosed with the obesity comorbidity of obstructive sleep apnea (OSA). This would then move the patient into Medicare coverage, allowing them to receive beneficial bariatric surgery and streamlining them into potential enrollment in a research study.

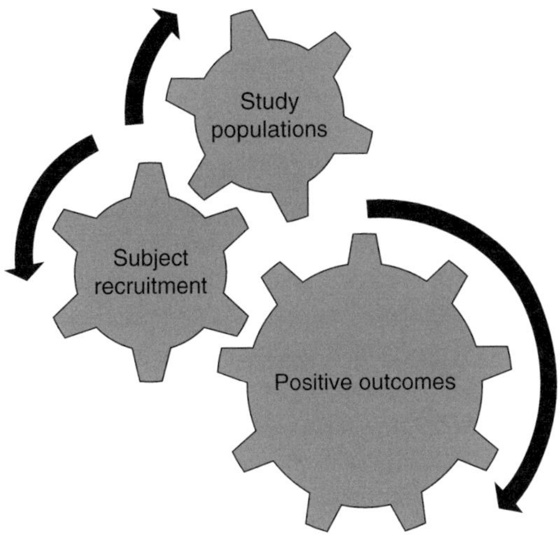

Fig. 44.1 A visual representation of the interlocking ideas of positive outcomes influencing subject recruitment and study populations for the researching bariatric PI

Another consideration regarding research in a comprehensive practice is the formation of a self-sustaining patient advertisement and recruitment cycle as increased positive outcomes from the multidisciplinary approach make it easier to recruit a meaningful patient census. Figure 44.1 shows the interlocking ideas of positive outcomes influencing patient recruitment and thus sustaining meaningful subject populations that meet inclusion and exclusion criteria. Multidisciplinary care allows the practice to advertise optimal postoperative outcomes to the public and can lead to the accreditation of the practice as a center of excellence—which can also be advertised and attract self-referrals. With a substantive patient census, study subject populations can be matured more easily. Importantly, a comprehensive clinic with good outcomes and accreditation will likely get better research funding opportunities from grants. Comprehensive practices can also incorporate research integrally into patient care with protocols and checklists for ancillary staff to use in the preoperative screening process to characterize patients based on study inclusion and exclusion criteria. Furthermore, extensive follow-up by multidisciplinary team members allows for easy collection and management of postoperative study variables.

Bariatric Surgery Research Begins with the IRB Review

In order for a PI to begin researching, they must be fluent in the clinical research process. Medical research projects involving human subjects clearly carry a more substantial ethical burden than those studies involving animals. Out of this burden, the institutional review board (IRB) was realized. The IRB is a research committee used by American medical institutions and private entities alike to grant human biomedical or behavioral research projects formal approval, monitoring, and review. It is necessary under US Food and Drug Administration (FDA) regulations in order to "assure, both in advance and by periodic review, that appropriate steps are taken to protect the rights and welfare of humans participating as subjects in the research" [5]. Specifically, the IRB examines subject recruitment, financial compensation, and a study's informed consent procedures.

IRB reviews are multifaceted and can be intra- or interinstitutional. They may also be hired by a private researching entity as a for-profit enterprise. It begins with the submission of an application to the IRB office for an initial screening and potential correspondence with the investigator regarding any necessary clarification in the submitted application. Advancing after this initial review, the application is then submitted for review by the Board where new and previously approved continuing protocols may undergo either full Board review or expedited review. Full review includes reviewing a protocol at meetings convening a majority of members of the IRB, including at least one member who has purely nonscientific interests in the review. Expedited review gives the IRB Chair, an individual Board member, or an appropriate subcommittee of the IRB the ability to review and approve research deemed as minimal risk. During this secondary review, the Board is making sure that project documentation has addressed all risks and benefits the study incurs upon potential subjects, that subject selection is done appropriately, and that consent information is adequate to allow subjects to make informed decisions. Any concerns during the IRB review are usually electronically communicated to the investigator. It is commonplace to have multiple correspondences between the Board and the investigator in order to ensure absolute study compliance.

Inherent within the IRB review process is the ability of the investigator to appeal at various levels from initial review to final approval or disapproval. Every decision the Board reaches is subject to the response of the investigator, and if the review is deemed unlikely to properly move forward by the Board, it may request an independent consultant review from a third-party entity. Studies that have been approved by the IRB may undergo further institutional/departmental review and either approval or disapproval. This more internal review, however, may not give approval to studies that have not received approval by the IRB. Any potential investigator should allot enough time, on the order of months, to the review process. This is especially important when considering submission deadlines for proposals regarding research funding. IRB approval is often required prior to any release of funding for human subjects research, and it behooves the investigator to communicate with the IRB office regarding funding submission deadlines and the IRB meeting schedule for each review interval as it pertains to sustaining study funding.

The Board has four potential determinations regarding an investigator's desire to involve human subjects in research studies:

- *"Approved as submitted"*—A letter of approval is sent to the investigator.
- *"Approved pending completion of minor modifications and/or clarifications"*—Specific requests by the Board are clarified, and an investigator's subsequent changes can undergo an expedited review. The expedited review cannot directly disapprove a response, but it can request more information from the investigator or recommend the change undergo a full Board review.
- *"Deferred"*—Protocols receiving this determination have been deemed to have substantial concerns; any changes by the investigator will automatically undergo full Board review for potential approval.

- *"Disapproved"*—Investigators maintain the right to communicate with the Board regarding the specific issues leading to disapproval; however, the IRB is resolute in its authority for granting final approval.

Evaluating the informed consent process of a study is one of the most essential tasks of the IRB. The Board must dissect how, when, and where subject consent will be obtained. Federal regulations mandate "basic" required elements of informed consent and provide additional elements of informed consent that may be included when appropriate. The IRB must conclude that informed consent is obtained from a decisional subject or a subject's legal representative, is written in language preferred by and understandable to the subject or representative, and allows for the subject or representative to sufficiently consider the subject's participation, without including language appearing to make the subject or representative waive any legal rights or exempt the investigator, sponsor, or institution from any potential negligence.

The basic elements of consent meeting the requirements of US Department of Health and Human Services 45 CFR 46.116 make sure that the IRB determines that subjects are informed of the following:

- The study involves research, the purpose of the research and the expected duration of a subject's participation, all study procedures to be followed by the subject, and any procedures that are experimental.
- Any foreseeable risks or discomforts to the subject.
- Any benefits to the subject or others.
- Appropriate alternative procedures or treatments, if any, that might be advantageous to the subject.
- The extent, if any, of which any identifying information pertaining to the subject is maintained.
- An explanation of any compensation or medical treatments available if injury occurs and what they may consist of.
- Contact information for individuals able to answer pertinent questions about the research, subject's rights, and who to contact if a research-related injury is sustained.
- Participation is voluntary and refusal to participate, or discontinuation at any time, will involve no penalty or loss of benefits to which the subject is otherwise entitled.

The US Department of Health and Human Services, per 45 CFR 46.116(b), identifies additional elements of informed consent that are required when the IRB deems them appropriate:

- A statement that any research procedures may involve risks to the subject (or embryo or fetus, if the subject becomes pregnant) that are currently unforeseeable.
- Any anticipated circumstances under which the subject's participation be terminated without the subject's consent.
- Any additional costs to the subject or their insurance provider that may result from research participation.
- Any consequences of a subject's decision to withdraw from the research study and procedures for orderly withdrawal of participation for the subject.
- A statement that any new findings of significance developed during the study that may relate to the subject's willingness to continue participation will be provided to the subject.
- The approximate number of subject participants in the study.

What Is Bariatric Surgery Research?

Weight loss surgery, as an entity, is so incredibly complex: the field involves an inseparable understanding of both surgical technique and metabolic and hormonal medicine. After gaining an understanding of the logistics behind an institutional review board, the PI can begin formulating exactly what they want to study. Because of all the moving parts in any given bariatric surgery case, there is an innumerable amount of ways that a PI could make an impact on the field through research. From the surgical perspective, novel, innovative surgical approaches and techniques can be explored and described. Also, there is an entire aspect of bariatric surgery research married to advances in technology with new device and instrument testing—think of the large-scale impact the LAP-BAND® manufacturers or laparoscopic instrument manufacturers have had on the field. Surgical outcomes, safety, perioperative medical treatment, and prophylactic protocols all have and will continue to be studied.

From a medical perspective, given the curative potential that bariatric procedures can have on different aspects of metabolic syndrome and diabetes, there has been a substantial amount of translational and basic science research undertaken to fully elucidate the consequences of the postoperative malabsorptive and restrictive physiology and endocrinology. Translational research applies findings from basic science research to enhance the health and well-being of obese patients. These medical discoveries have and will continue to open doors to future biochemical pathway targets to optimize the patient's weight loss response to bariatric surgery. Prospective clinical trials involving bariatric surgical, medical, and/or the combination of each will continue to supply data most appropriately generalized to the population at large—think of the enormous impact that the STAMPEDE trial had showing bariatric surgery contributing to superior lowering of HbA1c levels in obese diabetic patients [6].

Clinical research in weight loss surgery often involves clinical trials. These are prospective biomedical or behavioral research studies on human subjects designed to answer certain questions or make certain comparisons in bariatric surgery, usually involving new treatments, devices, and known interventions. Trials of new drugs or new devices are usually studying two aspects of these medical/surgical treatments: efficacy and safety. In clinical trials, new drugs or devices are often compared to the current "standard of care" treatment in bariatric surgery. The US National Institutes of Health (NIH) organizes clinical trials into five different types, and as it pertains to bariatric surgery, as follows [7]:

- Prevention trials look for better ways to prevent obesity in people who have never had the disease or to prevent obesity from returning postoperatively. These approaches may include medicines, vitamins, vaccines, minerals, or lifestyle changes.
- Screening trials test the best way to detect obesity and comorbid conditions.
- Diagnostic trials are conducted to find better tests or procedures for diagnosing obesity and comorbid conditions.
- Treatment trials test experimental treatments, new combinations of drugs, or new approaches to surgery for the treatment of obesity.
- Quality-of-life trials (supportive care trials) explore ways to improve comfort and the quality of life for individuals with obesity and chronic metabolic illnesses.

Useful Testing in Bariatric Surgery

Useful testing in bariatric surgery helps researchers understand the physiologic status of the preoperative patient and the physiologic outcomes of bariatric surgery. The discovery of biochemical pathways or development of useful assays will surely lead to publications in high-impact journals and competitive research funding. Useful testing research in meal stimulation in bariatric surgery has led to greater understanding of the entero-insular axis in postoperative diabetes remission, GI hormones as it pertains to food intake, postoperative changes in brain activation to food, "bariatric surgery-induced anorexia" with calorie-independent releases of glucagon-like peptide-1 (GLP-1) and peptide YY (PYY), the effect of GLP-1 on glucose metabolism postoperatively, the influence gut hormones have on weight regain after gastric bypass, etc. [8–13].

ELISA assays have been developed to elucidate the effect bariatric surgery has on gut physiology. Decreased circulating levels of leptin and increased levels of adiponectin proteins have been detected by ELISA in women after gastric bypass [14]. An assay for the anorexic hormone oxyntomodulin (OXM) showed a marked rise in OXM levels in response to glucose after Roux-en-Y gastric bypass (RYGB) compared to diet alone [15]. ELISA assays have shown that peptide YY (PYY) mediates the early weight loss observed in post-bypass patients, whereas a relative PYY deficiency during dieting may compromise weight loss attempts [16]. Assays for inflammatory markers such as sCD40L, plasminogen activator inhibitor 1, antithrombin III, and C-reactive protein showed a statistically significant decrease in these inflammatory molecules implicated in chronic obesity-related inflammation after gastric bypass surgery [17]. Clearly this work in useful testing has helped advance the understanding of the physiology relevant to bariatric surgery, and advances will continue to be made.

Diabetes remission following bariatric surgery is debatably the single greatest impact that bariatric surgeons can make on a patient's lifelong health. This curative potential has the modern scientific world reeling with excitement, and the development of useful testing to characterize a patient's preoperative and postoperative insulin sensitivity is paramount to the field, and assays will continue to be developed as researchers work toward perfecting a test to show the postoperative status of a patient's entero-insular axis. Table 44.1 shows some current tests used to objectively describe the insulin sensitivity of the bariatric patient. Useful testing for insulin sensitivity will continue to be used to evaluate adult and pediatric bariatric surgical candidates, and the development of new tests may increase. Medical societies are preparing to recommend bariatric surgery as an option for treating type 2 diabetes; thus, there may be an explosion in innovative demand, driving the development of insulin-related useful testing for bariatric patients [18].

Table 44.1 Insulin sensitivity useful testing in bariatric surgery

Insulin sensitivity test	Description
Serum glucose or glucose tolerance test (GTT)	Goal of glucose testing is to determine any impaired response to glucose
Hemoglobin A1c	Reflects blood glucose levels over 3 months
Homeostatic model assessment (HOMA)	Mathematically estimating the function of beta cells in the pancreas using measured glucose and insulin levels
Serum insulin	A common method of evaluating significant insulin resistance
Serum hs-CRP	Levels of this inflammatory marker may be elevated in insulin resistance
Insulin tolerance test (ITT)	A method for determining insulin sensitivity by IV infusion of insulin, followed by glucose and insulin measurements
Quantitative insulin sensitivity check index (QUICKI)	Mathematical calculation based on serum glucose and insulin, diagnosing insulin resistance based on where the value lies in the QUICKI

Bariatric Surgery Researchers Need Funding

With an understanding of what bariatric surgery research entails, that research in bariatric surgery is a team endeavor, is best done in a comprehensive clinic, and requires thorough institutional review, a principal investigator can understand the immense opportunities in metabolic, basic science, outcome, innovation, and epidemiology in bariatric research/useful testing and decide how they would best make an impact. At this time, the PI can focus their attention on how to fund their project.

For nearly two decades, institutions such as the National Institutes of Health (NIH) have been providing research grants to translational and clinical projects studying obesity and weight loss surgery. Previous NIH-funded obesity topics include epidemiological obesity, diabetes control and prevention, diet composition, genetics, proteomics, childhood obesity, health risk behavior, demographic disparities, disease biomarkers, bioengineering, exercise, long-term weight maintenance, development of assays, parenting and health outcomes, eating disorders, insulin resistance, computational and statistical methodologies, geographic distribution, school nutrition, human microbiome physiology, psychosocial aspects of bariatric surgery, etc. Obviously, there is a broad spectrum of research contributing to bariatric literature that is getting funded.

What is driving institutions like the NIH to fund bariatric surgery research? Apart from the obvious mission to promote the health of these high-risk patients, this funding can be thought of as an investment. They are funding research now and hoping that breakthroughs will lead to bariatric surgery alleviating the extreme healthcare cost burden of obesity and metabolic syndrome. In 2013, severe obesity cost the United States about $69BIL, which was 60% of total obesity-related costs. Eleven percent of the cost of severe obesity was covered by Medicaid, 30% by Medicare and other federal programs, 27% by private insurance companies, and 30% out of pocket. Severe obesity costs state Medicaid programs roughly $8BIL annually, and these costs will likely increase as coverage is expanded for nutritional medicine, drug therapies, and bariatric surgery [19]. The overall cost-effectiveness of bariatric surgery is a subject of debate, but recent literature is beginning to shed light on the long-term financial implications of bariatric surgery. Using a unique study design to measure healthcare expenditures from the payer perspective, Lewis et al. showed that at 3 years postoperatively, there was a significant change in the trajectory of healthcare expenditures in patients who underwent laparoscopic banding and gastric bypass. This means that there was a flattening of patient trends in total healthcare costs and prescription drug costs—which very well could result in a net savings in the long term [20]. Funding bariatric surgery research may very well lead to a lessening of the current obesity cost burden.

With these financial implications in mind, the PI can begin to look for funding opportunities. Grants for research projects in bariatric surgery are funded by the American Society for Metabolic and Bariatric Surgery (ASMBS), National Institutes of Health (NIH) obesity research fund, the Society of American Gastrointestinal and Endoscopic Surgeons (SAGES), and the National Institute of Diabetes and Digestive and Kidney Diseases (NIDDK), among others public and private funds. Obviously, there exists many other opportunities for funding within the United States and internationally from different sources and societies, but these institutions fund a substantial proportion of American bariatric surgery research. Receiving a grant from these fine entities is not only a personal and academic achievement for the PI but shows true promise in the goal of their project.

The PI must recognize the nature of their project and apply for research funding from institutions that consistently fund projects in whatever realm of bariatric surgery research that is pertinent. For instance, if the PI is undertaking a basic science project, it is best they apply for funding from a source most interested in basic science research and not apply for funding from sources interested in funding device research. Table 44.2 displays the different funding trends of the aforementioned institutions. The authors have done a review of funding and grant awards for these institutions based on their online funding data resources [21–24]. The table shows an approximate percentage of funding for the general project categories pertinent to bariatric surgery

Table 44.2 Approximate funding trends of different project types based on data available from the websites of the institutions

Funding source	Metabolic (%)	Basic science (%)	Outcome (%)	Innovation (%)	Epidemiology (%)
American Society for Metabolic and Bariatric Surgery (ASMBS) Grant Awards 2004–2013	36	50	9	0	5
National Institutes of Health (NIH) Obesity Research Funding Solicitations 2001–2015	17	23	7	12	41
Society of American Gastrointestinal and Endoscopic Surgeons (SAGES) Grant Awards 2005–2016	9	23	18	48	2
National Institute of Diabetes and Digestive and Kidney Diseases (NIDDK)-Funded Projects 2012–2015	43	25	8	8	16

research: metabolic, basic science, outcome, innovation, and epidemiology. Many of these projects span more than one of these broad categories, but they were categorized for this text based on the project's most substantive impact. Metabolic projects are those studying any of the biochemical reactions of a living cell related to energy homeostasis and the dysfunction thereof in obesity, metabolic syndrome, and diabetes. Basic science projects included any translational, fundamental, or bench research aimed at understanding the natural phenomena of obesity and its effect on the human body and mind. Outcome projects study the end results any process of the healthcare system has had on the health and well-being of patients in the bariatric surgery population. Innovation projects study a new medical or surgical method, idea, product, etc. often in terms of feasibility and efficacy. Epidemiology projects study and analyze patterns, causes, and effects of health and disease in a bariatric population of interest.

From this review, it is helpful to visualize funding trends from some of the major research funding entities in the United States over the last several years. In general, the American Society for Metabolic and Bariatric Surgery (ASMBS) has awarded the largest proportion of their grants to basic science projects, the National Institutes of Health (NIH) Obesity Research Funding Solicitations have been mostly epidemiological studies, the Society of American Gastrointestinal and Endoscopic Surgeons (SAGES) Grant Awards have been given mostly to projects in innovation, and the National Institute of Diabetes and Digestive and Kidney Diseases (NIDDK) has funded mostly metabolic projects.

This is helpful because, for instance, if a PI for a project is interested in studying a new surgical technique in a Roux-en-Y gastric bypass (RYGB), they will likely have more success in receiving funding from an entity such as the Society of American Gastrointestinal and Endoscopic Surgeons (SAGES) who has a history of funding a large percentage of innovation projects compared to others (~48% of grant awards were innovation projects). On the other hand, if the PI is leading an epidemiological investigation into an aspect of obesity, they might not have as much luck applying for a SAGES grant and should absolutely focus more on receiving funding from the NIH who clearly has a mission in better understanding obesity epidemiology based on their very robust history of funding such projects (~41% of solicited grants were epidemiological projects). Another important aspect to consider when deciding on where to apply for research funding is the amount of annual spending each of these funding entities spends on surgical or medical research relevant to bariatric surgery. The NIH estimates that in 2017 it will spend $1.04BIL on diabetes research and another $931MIL on obesity research [25]. Although a large proportion of this funding will likely go toward epidemiological and basic science projects, a surgeon PI who is studying bariatric surgical outcomes should still apply for NIH funding—if not only for the immense amount of fiscal research assets coming out of the NIH.

There are also online resources to help PIs discover what institutions and centers may be interested in their project. For example, the NIH has an online "Matchmaker tool in RePORTER" that allows the PI to use a search engine to find funding opportunities within the NIH by comparing the study abstract to abstracts that have been previously funded (projectreporter.nih.gov). This search on the NIH website can be tailored according to specific diseases, organ systems, stages of life, and keyword text search in order to find funding institutions whose mission most closely aligns with the goal of the project. It behooves the PI to be diligent and thorough in their search for funding sources, using resources such as these before applying.

Applying for Bariatric Research Funding

The funding application process is appropriately arduous given the large sums of money often going toward these projects. As previously mentioned, once the PI decides what funding entities they desire to apply to, they should thoroughly take advantage of any online resources those entities may supply regarding what they are specifically looking for in a funding application. This way, the application can be tailored to the exact specifications that the funding entity prefers. For instance, there is a robust amount of grant writing resources at www.NIH.gov, allowing applicants to fully understand the NIH application process and what makes an application competitive. General guidelines for applying include ensuring the project meets any eligibility requirements, choosing the correct type of grant program, and completing the correct type of grant application—including any specific submission requirements.

There exists a vast amount of resources to help a PI make the best decisions to ensure the best chance of getting their project funded. Many PIs are looking for the answer to the question, "How is it best to get funded?" Within the scope of this text, some broad tips and suggestions are provided regarding the best ways to get a research project funded.

- Submit research proposals studying bariatric issues that are well described and widely recognized as important.
  - Funding will come easier if the study contributes to a larger scientific question in bariatric surgery that has been studied long enough for the development of research infrastructure (i.e., specialty centers, established grants, etc.) dedicated to its understanding.
- Take into account the priorities of the funding agency.
  - Again, if the mission of the funding agency does not align with the mission of the project, successful funding is less likely.
- Make high-quality submissions with clear, attainable goals and measurable outcomes.
  - The PI should do their due diligence to ensure they are submitting what the funding agency wants to see. The more convoluted a funding application, the less likely it will make an impact on the reader. The more farfetched the goals of the project, the less believable it becomes.
- Always have a sustainability plan within the submission.
  - If the PI clearly articulates a plan for the future of the project, the funding agency can feel more comfortable investing large sums of money into the project.
- Use the past productivity and funding of group members to the research team's advantage!
  - If a team member has had consistent success in receiving funding, they are doing something right. Projects that have high-impact authors will catch the eye of the funding entity, as funding high-impact studies is in their best interest.
- Rejection is not failure.
  - Even the most decorated bariatric researchers have had countless applications for funding turn up empty. Learn from it, improve your application, and apply again!

Conclusion

Accommodating research in a busy bariatric practice is possible and fulfilling. Physician principal investigators should focus their energy on their patients and their research endeavors. They cannot afford to waste daily valuable energy on working out the logistics of being successful in research while maintaining a successful practice. With this book as a resource, a bariatric PI can begin to understand the importance of teamwork and assembling a successful practice in an ideal research environment. They can also begin to understand the research process as a whole: what type of research to undertake, how to get institutional approval for their project, and how to obtain funding for their project. With these principles in mind, a bariatric surgery PI is on the road to a successful and sustainable clinical and academic career.

References

1. Ogden CL, et al. Prevalence of childhood and adult obesity in the United States, 2011–2012. JAMA. 2014;311(8):806–14.
2. The state of obesity, better policies for a healthier America. Trust for America's Health and the Robert

Wood Johnson Foundation. 2016. http://stateofobesity.org/rates/. Accessed 20 Aug 2016.

3. Boyle JP, et al. Projection of the year 2050 burden of diabetes in the US adult population: dynamic modeling of incidence, mortality, and pre-diabetes prevalence. Popul Health Metrics. 2010;8(1):1.
4. National Coverage Determination (NCD) for bariatric surgery for treatment of co-morbid conditions related to morbid obesity (100.1). Centers for Medicare & Medicaid Services. 2017. https://www.cms.gov/medicare-coverage-database/details/ncddetails.aspx?NCDId=57&ncdver=5&bc=AgAAgAAAAQAAAA%3d%3d&. Accessed 20 Aug 2016.
5. Guidance for institutional review boards and clinical investigators, U.S. Food & Drug Administration. 01/25/2016. http://www.fda.gov/RegulatoryInformation/Guidances/ucm126420.htm Accessed 15 Aug 2016.
6. Schauer PR, et al. Bariatric surgery versus intensive medical therapy in obese patients with diabetes. N Engl J Med. 2012;366(17):1567–76.
7. clinicaltrials.gov. Accessed 18 Aug 2016.
8. Santo MA, et al. Weight regain after gastric bypass: influence of gut hormones. Obes Surg. 2016;26(5):919–25.
9. Shah M, Law JH, Micheletto F, Sathananthan M, Man CD, Cobelli C, Rizza RA, Camilleri M, Zinsmeister AR, Vella A. The contribution of endogenous glucagon-like peptide-1 to glucose metabolism after Roux-en-Y gastric bypass. Diabetes. 2013: DB_130954.
10. Evans S, et al. Gastric bypass surgery restores meal stimulation of the anorexigenic gut hormones glucagon-like peptide-1 and peptide YY independently of caloric restriction. Surg Endosc. 2012;26(4):1086–94.
11. Bruce JM, et al. Changes in brain activation to food pictures after adjustable gastric banding. Surg Obes Relat Dis. 2012;8(5):602–8.
12. Strader AD, Woods SC. Gastrointestinal hormones and food intake. Gastroenterology. 2005;128(1):175–91.
13. Patriti A, et al. The entero-insular axis and the recovery from type 2 diabetes after bariatric surgery. Obes Surg. 2004;14(6):840–8.
14. Simonyte K, et al. Weight loss after gastric bypass surgery in women is followed by a metabolically favorable decrease in 11β-hydroxysteroid dehydrogenase 1 expression in subcutaneous adipose tissue. J Clin Endocrinol Metab. 2010;95(7):3527–31.
15. Laferrere B, et al. Rise of oxyntomodulin in response to oral glucose after gastric bypass surgery in patients with type 2 diabetes. J Clin Endocrinol Metab. 2010;95(8):4072–6.
16. Chandarana K, et al. Diet and gastrointestinal bypass–induced weight loss. Diabetes. 2011;60(3):810–8.
17. Baena-Fustegueras JA, et al. Soluble CD40 ligand in morbidly obese patients: effect of body mass index on recovery to normal levels after gastric bypass surgery. JAMA Surg. 2013;148(2):151–6.
18. Mayor S. Bariatric surgery should be an option for treating type 2 diabetes, societies say. BMJ. 2016;353:i2955.
19. Wang YC, et al. Severe obesity in adults cost state Medicaid programs nearly $8 billion in 2013. Health Aff. 2015;34(11):1923–31.
20. Lewis KH, et al. Comparing medical costs and use after laparoscopic adjustable gastric banding and Roux-en-Y gastric bypass. JAMA Surg. 2015;150(8):787–94.
21. SAGES meetings/symposia/courses/workshops. Society of American Gastrointestinal and Endoscopic Surgeons. http://www.sages.org/meetings/. Accessed 22 Aug 2016.
22. Research grant awards highlights. American Society for Metabolic and Bariatric Surgery. 2014. https://asmbs.org/resources/research-grant-awards-highlights Accessed 22 Aug 2016.
23. Archive: highlights of past obesity research solicitations. NIH Obesity Research. 02/07/2017. http://obesityresearch.nih.gov/funding/archive-funding.aspx Accessed 22 Aug 2016.
24. FUNDING – project listing by category. NIH Research Portfolio Online Reporting Tools (RePORT). https://report.nih.gov/categorical_spending_project_listing.aspx. Accessed 22 Aug 2016.
25. FUNDING – estimates of funding for various research, condition, and disease categories (RCDC). NIH Research Portfolio Online Reporting Tools (RePORT). 07/03/2017. https://report.nih.gov/categorical_spending.aspx. Accessed 23 Aug 2016.

Proper Approach to New Bariatric Procedures

45

Kara J. Kallies and Shanu N. Kothari

Introduction

The field of bariatric surgery has advanced significantly from the days of Mason's original gastric bypass operation [1]. Advancement in minimally invasive surgical techniques has allowed for widespread acceptance of several bariatric procedures. Currently, the most commonly performed bariatric procedures worldwide include the laparoscopic Roux-en-Y gastric bypass (LRYGB), the laparoscopic sleeve gastrectomy (LSG), laparoscopic adjustable gastric band (LAGB), and biliopancreatic diversion with or without duodenal switch BPD/DS [2]. As our understanding of the metabolic impact of each of these operations increases, innovators are driven to develop novel and even less invasive methods to reproduce the same results as the more traditional procedures [3, 4].

While innovation and development of new surgical devices and procedures are important to advance the field of bariatric surgery, a rigorous pathway of evaluation and transparent reporting is critical to obtain approval and increase its acceptance by surgeons and patients. The challenges in obtaining acceptance include the financial burden and resources needed to conduct the appropriate clinical trials, as well as the substantial timeframe needed to gather and analyze adequate data to support the safety and effectiveness of the device or procedure.

New surgical interventions to treat obesity fall into two broad categories: devices and procedures. The development and approval process differs by category. In the United States, the Food and Drug Administration (FDA) is the federal organization which provides regulation, approval, and oversight of new medical devices. The American Society for Metabolic and Bariatric Surgery (ASMBS) is the largest professional organization dedicated to the field of bariatric surgery. The ASMBS provides critical analysis and endorsement of new bariatric devices and procedures.

Development of New Surgical Devices to Treat Obesity

Innovation of new surgical devices offers a unique opportunity to address a potential gap in therapy and benefit patients who may be suitable candidates for the device in development. Scientists and researchers developing these devices have a strong understanding of the physiology that the device is likely to impact. A "proof of concept" is established to determine initial feasibility of the device [4]. After initial feasibility and device prototypes are completed, a phase I trial may be completed. In order to market a new device, a notification and/or application is filed with the

K. J. Kallies
Department of Medical Research, Gundersen Medical Foundation, La Crosse, WI, USA
e-mail: kjkallie@gundersenhealth.org

S. N. Kothari (✉)
Department of General Surgery, Gundersen Health System, La Crosse, WI, USA
e-mail: snkothar@gundersenhealth.org

R. Lutfi et al. (eds.), *Global Bariatric Surgery*, https://doi.org/10.1007/978-3-319-93545-4_45

FDA. The FDA will then review these documents for determination of the device to be either cleared for marketing or approved for marketing [5].

- FDA Clearance: a premarket notification (PMN)/510(k) application is filed at least 90 days before marketing unless the device is exempt. A PMN is a premarketing submission to the FDA to demonstrate that the device is as safe and effective (substantially equivalent to a legally marketed device not subject to premarket approval (PMA)). In this instance, a letter must be received from the FDA which states that the device is substantially equivalent and thus "clears" the device for commercial distribution.
- FDA Approval: a PMA application to market the device is submitted and reviewed by the FDA. Unlike the PMN, a PMA is based on determination by FDA that sufficient valid scientific evidence exists to provide reasonable assurance that the device is safe and effective for its intended use(s).

Whether a PMN or a PMA application needs to be filed depends on the classification of the medical device, with PMNs used for lower risk classifications and PMA applications for higher risk classifications. FDA classification of medical devices is based on the associated risks as follows [6]:

- Class I devices are deemed to be low risk and are therefore subject to the least regulatory controls.
- Class II devices are higher risk devices than Class I and require greater regulatory controls to provide reasonable assurance of the device's safety and effectiveness.
- Class III devices are generally the highest risk devices and are therefore subject to PMA, per federal law, and these devices must be approved by the FDA before they are marketed.

Bariatric Device Case Studies: Intragastric Balloon and Vagal Blocking Therapy

Three medical devices to treat obesity were approved by the FDA in 2015: the ORBERA™ Intragastric Balloon System, the ReShape Integrated Dual Balloon System, and the EnteroMedics Maestro Rechargeable System [7]. The ORBERA™ and ReShape products are intragastric balloons, either a single or dual balloon placed within the stomach to aid in weight loss by occupying a portion of the stomach, along with lifestyle modifications. The ORBERA™ product received marketing approval in Europe in 1997. The FDA testing of the device included testing of the components, fill and force testing, leak testing, packaging, storage testing, and biocompatibility and toxicity testing. A multicenter, prospective, randomized, non-blinded comparative pivotal study was completed; 125 patients were randomized to the treatment group and 130 to the control group [8]. The safety and effectiveness were based on an analysis of 125 patients and 35 run-in patients. The serious adverse event rate was 10% (16/160, 95% CI). The mean total body weight loss at device removal was 10.2% in the balloon group vs. 3.3% in the control group. The FDA panel determined that, although limited, the overall benefits from this device outweighed the potential risks.

Similar to the ORBERA™ product, the ReShape Integrated Dual Balloon was previously approved for marketing in Europe in 2007, and the components of the device were thoroughly tested by the FDA. Two clinical studies were conducted, a feasibility study and a multicenter pivotal study (n = 187 in the balloon group and 139 in the control group) [9]. The device or procedure-related adverse event rate in the pivotal study was 7.5% (20/265, 95% CI 4.2–10.9). The mean %EWL was 25.1% in the balloon group and 11.3% in the control group ($P = 0.0041$). Both the safety and effectiveness endpoints were met, and the FDA determined that the benefit-risk model profile favored approval. Both the ORBERA™ and ReShape will complete post-approval studies.

The EnteroMedics Maestro Rechargeable System is a vagal blocking therapy (VBLOC) in which intermittent electrical blocking signals are delivered to the anterior and posterior abdominal nerve trunks of the vagus nerve to promote satiety by delaying food processing and gastric emptying. The process for approval of this device included in vivo animal studies in a porcine model and thorough testing of each of the components of the device, with subsequent modifications of early models as needed. A PMA application was filed with the FDA. Laboratory testing by the FDA included visual inspection of the device, along with testing of the kit and component packaging and shipping and temperature conditioning. Three clinical trials with human subjects (one pilot and two pivotal studies) were conducted, with a combined sample of 561 patients [10–12]. The rate of observed serious adverse events was 3.7% (6/162, 95% CI, 1.4–7.9) among the VBLOC subjects in the PMA data. Mean %EWL at 12 months was reported to be 12.1 ± 17.5 vs. 12.0 ± 20.8 and 24.4 ± 23.6 vs. 15.9 ± 17.7 in the VBLOC and sham control group respectively for the two randomized trials. The FDA review panel concluded that the device demonstrated safety, but did not demonstrate effectiveness since the primary endpoints (10% EWL difference in VBLOC and sham control groups and half of VBLOC patients would reach 20% EWL) were not met in the trials. However, since significant improvements in EWL were observed for the VBLOC vs. sham control group, the panel found that the benefits outweigh the risks. The majority of the FDA review team recommended approval for the device, with the device manufacturer agreeing to conduct two 5-year post-approval studies.

In order to be considered for approval and endorsement by the ASMBS, it is suggested that for new devices, there are at least five peer-reviewed papers of nonrandomized case series and/or randomized controlled trials with appropriate control groups [13].

Development of New Bariatric Surgical Procedures

New bariatric surgical procedures may be those consisting of a modification of an existing bariatric procedure or an entirely new procedure. The risks and benefits of the existing procedures should be carefully studied prior to development of a new procedure or surgical technique. Another challenge is when there is disagreement among experts whether a new procedure is in fact a new procedure, a major modification of an existing procedure, or a minor modification of an existing procedure. Regardless, in order for a new procedure to be considered for implementation, comparative-effectiveness studies should be planned after initial feasibility, safety, and efficacy are reported [14]. Randomized controlled trials will yield the highest level of evidence; however, if this design is not feasible, prospective, nonrandomized cohort studies may be performed to evaluate the new procedure [15].

For new procedures, the ASMBS suggests at least ten peer-reviewed publications, to include nonrandomized case series, with data reporting medium- and long-term outcomes (3–5 years) and/or randomized controlled trials [13]. The ASMBS does note that the number of trials and patients required for consideration will depend on the quality of the studies and the clinical outcomes being evaluated. Medium-term follow-up should include weight loss, comorbidity outcomes, and early and late complication rates as defined by the Standards in Outcome Reporting [16].

Bariatric Surgical Procedure Case Studies: LSG

The development of LSG as a stand-alone procedure has had a profound impact on the surgical treatment of obesity. Case volume for LSG has increased exponentially over the past 5 years [2]. The process by which the LSG has become recognized as a bariatric procedure started with a modification to an existing procedure, the biliopancreatic diversion with duodenal switch (BPD/DS). The BPD/DS has become a consistent, yet less common, procedure for select patients with class III obesity in which a staged procedure to induce initial weight loss was appropriate, thereby increasing the technical feasibility of the second stage [2, 17, 18]. The weight loss observed in many patients after the initial gastrectomy of the first stage was significant enough to negate the need for the second stage. Advantages to the LSG as a stand-alone procedure include the technical ease to perform and a similar or slightly lower risk of complications and weight loss compared to the LRYGB, often considered the "gold standard" bariatric procedure due to its favorable risk-benefit profile.

In 2007, the ASMBS endorsed LSG as a stand-alone procedure after reviewing data from 775 patients in 15 reports in the peer-reviewed literature with short-term outcomes [19]. The complication rates ranged from 0% to 24%, and the overall mortality rate was reported to be 0.39%. The mean %EWL ranged from 33% to 83%. Since the ASMBS endorsement in 2007, many subsequent studies with short- and long-term outcomes continue to be reported [20, 21]. A comparative-effectiveness study has been performed using a large, national, risk-adjusted dataset, which firmly positioned the LSG among the existing well-established bariatric procedures [21].

Challenges and Considerations in Implementation

Rigorous clinical trials are often costly. Funding required to conduct these trials may be available from industry sources, such as the device manufacturer, as well as federal and private grants. The timeline to funding dissemination is highly variable depending on the funding source. Initiation of a clinical trial can be time-intensive, particularly if it is a multi-institutional study. Study endpoints and variables must be established early and have clear definitions in order to be collected consistently by study coordinators. Consultation with a biostatistical expert is critical in order to determine the sample size needed to accurately evaluate the study endpoints with sufficient statistical power and minimal risk of error.

Ethical considerations for any initiation of a clinical trial in animal or human subjects mandate review and approval by the Institutional Animal Care and Use Committee or Institutional Review Boards at the institutions in which the trial will be carried out, as well as monitoring by the Data Safety Monitoring Boards and strict adherence to Good Clinical Practice and NIH Protection of Human Subjects standards [22, 23]. Any conflicts of interest or sponsorship by a pharmaceutical company or device manufacturer must be transparent.

After implementation of a new device or procedure, surgeons or other providers may require credentialing or privileging according to the Joint Commission standards and requirements [24]. Appropriate education and training are also necessary. A preceptorship or proctoring program may improve performance with a new procedure. Early performance should be objectively assessed using preestablished measures until any learning curve is overcome.

Pathway for Endorsement and Acceptance

The ASMBS's committees and leadership provide critical analysis and endorsement of both new bariatric devices and procedures. The Metabolic and Bariatric Surgery Accreditation and Quality Improvement Program (MBSAQIP) developed by the ASMBS and American College of Surgeons provides accreditation for bariatric surgery centers [25]. Endorsement of a new bariatric device or procedure by the ASMBS allows for the intervention to be included in the MBSAQIP program and has implications for patients and payors.

The ASMBS has developed a pathway and application process by which new bariatric procedures can be reviewed and, pending approval, endorsed by the society [13].

ASMBS Process for Approval for New Devices and Procedures

- An ASMBS member sponsor and member co-sponsor(s) in active practice may complete the application for a new procedure or removal of an approved procedure.
- The Executive Committee of the Executive Council performs an inclusive review to

ensure plausibility of new procedure and device before invoking full review. Approval by 75% of the committee is required to continue on the approval process.

- The application is assessed by the ASMBS Pathway for Approval of New Devices and Procedures Committee, which includes the chairs of Clinical Issues, Insurance, Quality Improvement and Patient Safety, Emerging Technology committees and Integrated Health president, or their designee. In the course of their review, a Clinical Issues Position Statement may be produced concurrently.
- The application is presented to the Executive Council by the ASMBS member sponsor and one co-sponsor, with pro and con advocates from the ASMBS Pathway for Approval of New Devices and Procedures Committee.
- The Executive Council will review the application and presentation by sponsors and advocates and conduct an open vote, with 75% approval required to continue.
- The ASMBS will allow a period for membership comments for the application with a summary from the ASMBS Committee Summary.
- The Executive Council will conduct a final vote, again with 75% approval required for final affirmation.
- Outcome of the ASMBS approval is sent to major insurers and MBSAQIP once application is approved.

Continuous Evaluation of Outcomes

After approval by regulatory and accrediting bodies, continuous evaluation of outcomes is critical. Reporting of device-related adverse events and mortalities to the FDA is required for the device manufacturers and importers. Device users should report these adverse events to the manufacturer or directly to the FDA if the manufacturer is unknown [26].

Patients in the early pivotal trials and those who undergo the new procedure after approval should be followed continuously, and both early and long-term outcomes should be reported. Outcomes reporting from different medical centers in different practice settings should be encouraged. The ASMBS MBSAQIP program and other large prospective datasets may offer a unique opportunity to continuously study the outcomes of a new procedure with a robust sample.

References

1. Mason EE, Ito C. Gastric bypass. Ann Surg. 1969;170(3):329–39.
2. Ponce J, DeMaria EJ, Nguyen NT, Hutter M, Sudan R, Morton JM. American Society for Metabolic and Bariatric Surgery estimation of bariatric surgery procedures in 2015 and surgeon workforce in the United States. Surg Obes Relat Dis. 2016;12(9):1637–9.
3. ASGE/ASMBS Task Force on Endoscopic Bariatric Therapy, Ginsberg GG, Chand B, CotEe GA, Dallal RM, Edmundowicz SA, Nguyen NT, Pryor A, Thompson CC. A pathway to endoscopic bariatric therapies. Gastrointest Endosc. 2011;74(5):943–53.
4. Stain SC, Pryor AD, Shadduck PP, editors. The SAGES manual ethics of surgical innovation. New York: Springer; 2016.
5. U.S. Food & Drug Administration. Device approvals, denials and clearances. Available at: https://www.fda.gov/MedicalDevices/ProductsandMedicalProcedures/DeviceApprovalsandClearances/. Last accessed 7 Apr 2017.
6. U.S. Food & Drug Administration. Device classification panels. Available at: https://www.fda.gov/MedicalDevices/DeviceRegulationandGuidance/Overview/ClassifyYourDevice/ucm051530.htm. Last accessed 7 Apr 2017.
7. U.S. FDA. Device approvals. 2015. Available at: https://www.fda.gov/MedicalDevices/ProductsandMedicalProcedures/DeviceApprovalsandClearances/Recently-ApprovedDevices/ucm430692.htm. Last accessed 1 Apr 2017.
8. Courcoulas A, Abu Dayyeh BK, Eaton L, Robinson J, Woodman G, Fusco M, Shayani V, Billy H, Pambianco D, Gostout C. Intragastric balloon as an adjunct to lifestyle intervention: a randomized controlled trial. Int J Obes. 2017;41(3):427–33.
9. Ponce J, Woodman G, Swain J, Wilson E, English W, Ikramuddin S, Bour E, Edmundowicz S, Snyder B, Soto F, Sullivan S, Holcomb R, Lehmann J, REDUCE Pivotal Trial Investigators. The REDUCE pivotal trial: a prospective, randomized controlled pivotal trial of a dual intragastric balloon for the treatment of obesity. Surg Obes Relat Dis. 2015;11(4):874–81.
10. Shikora S, Toouli J, Herrera MF, Kulseng B, Zulewski H, Brancatisano R, Kow L, Pantoja JP, Johnsen G, Brancatisano A, Tweden KS, Knudson MB, Billington CJ. Vagal blocking improves glycemic control and elevated blood pressure in obese subjects with type 2 diabetes mellitus. J Obes. 2013;2013:245683.

11. Morton JM, Shah SN, Wolfe BM, Apovian CM, Miller CJ, Tweden KS, Billington CJ, Shikora SA. Effect of vagal nerve blockade on moderate obesity with an obesity-related comorbid condition: the ReCharge study. Obes Surg. 2016;26(5):983–9.
12. Ikramuddin S, Blackstone RP, Brancatisano A, Toouli J, Shah SN, Wolfe BM, Fujioka K, Maher JW, Swain J, Que FG, Morton JM, Leslie DB, Brancatisano R, Kow L, O'Rourke RW, Deveney C, Takata M, Miller CJ, Knudson MB, Tweden KS, Shikora SA, Sarr MG, Billington CJ. Effect of reversible intermittent intra-abdominal vagal nerve blockade on morbid obesity: the ReCharge randomized clinical trial. JAMA. 2014;312(9):915–22.
13. American Society for Metabolic and Bariatric Surgery. Pathway for approval for new devices and procedures. Available at: https://asmbs.org/pathway-for-approval-for-new-devices-and-procedures. Last accessed 29 Mar 2017.
14. Stirrat GM, Farrow SC, Farndon J, Dwyer N. The challenge of evaluating surgical procedures. Ann R Coll Surg Engl. 1992;74(2):80–4.
15. Ergina PL, Cook JA, Blazeby JM, Boutron I, Clavien PA, Reeves BC, Seiler CM, Balliol Collaboration. Challenges in evaluating surgical innovation. Lancet. 2009;374(9695):1097–104.
16. Brethauer SA, Kim J, el Chaar M, Papasavas P, Eisenberg D, Rogers A, Ballem N, Kligman M, Kothari S, ASMBS Clinical Issues Committee. Standardized outcomes reporting in metabolic and bariatric surgery. Surg Obes Relat Dis. 2015;11(3):489–506.
17. Baker MT. The history and evolution of bariatric surgical procedures. Surg Clin N Am. 2011;91(6):1181–201.
18. Scopinaro N, Adami G, Marinari G, et al. Biliopancreatic diversion. World J Surg. 1998;22(9):936–46.
19. Clinical Issues Committee of American Society for Metabolic and Bariatric Surgery. Sleeve gastrectomy as a bariatric procedure. Surg Obes Relat Dis. 2007;3(6):573–6.
20. Brethauer SA, Hammel JP, Schauer PR. Systematic review of sleeve gastrectomy as staging and primary bariatric procedure. Surg Obes Relat Dis. 2009;5(4):469–75.
21. Hutter MM, Schirmer BD, Jones DB, Ko CY, Cohen ME, Merkow RP, Nguyen NT. First report from the American College of Surgeons Bariatric Surgery Center Network: laparoscopic sleeve gastrectomy has morbidity and effectiveness positioned between the band and the bypass. Ann Surg. 2011;254(3):410–20.
22. Collaborative Institutional Training Initiative (CITI) Program. Good Clinical Practice (GCP). Available at: https://about.citiprogram.org/en/series/good-clinical-practice-gcp/. Last accessed 4 Apr 2017.
23. National Institute of Health (NIH) Office of Extramural Research. Protecting human subject research participants. Available at: https://phrp.nihtraining.com/users/login.php. Last accessed 4 Apr 2017.
24. Sachdeva AK, Russell TR. Safe introduction of new procedures and emerging technologies in surgery: education, credentialing, and privileging. Surg Clin N Am. 2007;87(4):853–66.
25. Metabolic and Bariatric Surgery Accreditation and Quality Improvement Program. Available at: https://www.facs.org/quality-programs/mbsaqip. Last accessed 7 Apr 2017.
26. U.S. Food and Drug Administration. Medical Device Reporting (MDR). Available at: https://www.fda.gov/MedicalDevices/Safety/ReportaProblem/default.htm. Last accessed 1 Apr 2017.

Index

R. Lutfi et al. (eds.), *Global Bariatric Surgery*, https://doi.org/10.1007/978-3-319-93545-4

M

N

O

T

MIX
Papier aus verantwortungsvollen Quellen
Paper from responsible sources
FSC® C105338

If you have any concerns about our products,
you can contact us on
ProductSafety@springernature.com

In case Publisher is established outside the EU,
the EU authorized representative is:
Springer Nature Customer Service Center GmbH
Europaplatz 3, 69115 Heidelberg, Germany

Printed by Libri Plureos GmbH
in Hamburg, Germany